THE YOUNG ATHLETE

VOLUME XIII OF THE ENCYCLOPAEDIA OF SPORTS MEDICINE

AN IOC MEDICAL COMMISSION PUBLICATION

IN COLLABORATION WITH

THE INTERNATIONAL FEDERATION OF SPORTS MEDICINE

EDITED BY

HELGE HEBESTREIT

and

ODED BAR-OR

Blackwell
Publishing

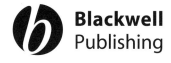

Published by Blackwell Publishing Ltd

Blackwell Publishing, Inc., 350 Main Street, Malden, Massachusetts 02148-5020, USA
Blackwell Publishing Ltd, 9600 Garsington Road, Oxford OX4 2DQ, UK
Blackwell Publishing Asia Pty Ltd, 550 Swanston Street, Carlton, Victoria 3053, Australia

First published 2008

1   2008

Library of Congress Cataloging-in-Publication Data
The young athlete / edited by Helge Hebestreit and Oded Bar-Or.
       p. ; cm. – (Encyclopaedia of sports medicine ; v. 13)
    "An IOC Medical Commission Publication in collaboration with the International Federation
of Sports Medicine."
    Includes bibliographical references and index.
    ISBN 978-1-4051-5647-9 (alk. paper)
    1. Pediatric sports medicine–Encyclopedias.   I. Hebestreit, Helge.   II. Bar-Or, Oded.
    III. IOC Medical Commission.   IV. International Federation of Sports Medicine.   V. Series.
    [DNLM: 1. Sports Medicine.   2. Adolescent.   3. Athletic Injuries.   4. Child.
    5. Physical Education and Training.   6. Sports–physiology.   QT 261 Y68 2008]
    RC1218.C45Y678 2008
    617.1′02703—dc22

                                                                                2006102161
ISBN: 978-1-4051-5647-9

A catalogue record for this title is available from the British Library

Set in 9/12pt Palatino by Graphicraft Limited, Hong Kong
Printed and bound in Singapore by Fabulous Printers Pte Ltd

Commissioning Editor: Gina Almond
Editorial Assistant: Jamie Hartmann-Boyce
Development Editors: Adam Gilbert and Victoria Pittman
Production Controller: Debbie Wyer

For further information on Blackwell Publishing, visit our website:
http://www.blackwellpublishing.com

The publisher's policy is to use permanent paper from mills that operate a sustainable forestry
policy, and which has been manufactured from pulp processed using acid-free and elementary
chlorine-free practices. Furthermore, the publisher ensures that the text paper and cover board
used have met acceptable environmental accreditation standards.

Contents

List of contributors

NEIL ARMSTRONG, PhD, DSc
Children's Health and Exercise Research Centre
University of Exeter
Exeter EX1 2LU
UK

ODED BAR-OR, MD
DECEASED
Department of Pediatrics
McMaster University
Hamilton, ON
Canada

SHONA L. BASS, PhD
Center for Physical Activity and Nutrition Research
Deakin University
Burwood
Australia 3125

RALPH BENEKE, MD, PhD
Centre for Sports and Exercise Science
Department of Biological Sciences
University of Essex
Colchester CO4 3SQ
UK

DAVID T. BERNHARDT, MD
Department of Pediatrics, Orthopedics and Rehabilitation
Division of Sports Medicine
University of Wisconsin School of Medicine and Public Health
Madison, WI 53705
USA

GASTON BEUNEN, PhD
Faculty of Kinesiology and Rehabilitation Sciences
Katholieke Universiteit Leuven
Belgium

JENNIFER A. BHALLA, MS
Curry School of Education
University of Virginia
Charlottesville, VA 22903
USA

CAMERON J.R. BLIMKIE, PhD
Department of Kinesiology
McMaster University
Hamilton, ON
Canada

SARAH CARSON, MS
Institute for the Study of Youth Sports
Michigan State University
East Lansing, MI 48824-1049
USA

MICHELINA CASSELLA, PT, BS
Department of Physical Therapy and Occupational Therapy
* Services*
Children's Hospital
Boston, MA 02115
USA

MICHAEL CHIA, PhD
Faculty of Physical Education and Sports Science
National Institute of Education
Nanyang Technological University
Singapore

ROBIN M. DALY, PhD
Center for Physical Activity and Nutrition Research
Deakin University
Burwood
Australia

RAFFY DOTAN, PhD
Department of Physical Education and Kinesiology
Faculty of Applied Health Science
Brock University
St Catharines, ON L2S 3A1
Canada

ROBERT C. EKLUND, PhD
Educational Psychology and Learning Systems
Florida State University
Tallahassee, FL 32306
USA

BAREKET FALK, PhD
Department of Physical Education and Kinesiology
Faculty of Applied Health Science
Brock University
St Catharines, ON L2S 3A1
Canada

BO FERNHALL, PhD
Kinesiology and Community Health Department
College of Applied Life Studies
University of Illinois at Urbana-Champaign
Champaign, IL 61820
USA

STEFANIE GILBERT, PhD
Department of Psychology
Howard University
Washington, DC 20059
USA

SCOTT B. GOING, PhD
Department of Nutritional Sciences
University of Arizona
Tucson, AZ 85721
USA

DANIEL GOULD, PhD
Institute for the Study of Youth Sports
Michigan State University
East Lansing, MI 48824-1049
USA

HELGE HEBESTREIT, MD
Children's Hospital
University of Würzburg
97080 Würzburg
Germany

BRADLEY R. HERRIN, BS
Department of Physiology
University of Arizona
Tucson, AZ 85721
USA

OMRI INBAR, PhD
Zinman College, Wingate Institute
Netania, 24902
Israel

KATHERINE E. ISCOE, BA
School of Kinesiology and Health
York University
Toronto, ON M3J 1P3
Canada

DAVID A. JONES, PhD
School of Sport and Exercise Sciences
The University of Birmingham
Edgbaston, Birmingham B15 2TT
UK

HAN C.G. KEMPER, MD
Emeritus Professor
VU University Medical Center
Institute for Research in Extramural Medicine
NL-1081 BT Amsterdam
The Netherlands

FELIPE LOBELO, MD
Department of Exercise Science
Arnold School of Public Health
University of South Carolina
Columbia, SC 29208
USA

TIMOTHY G. LOHMAN, PhD
Department of Physiology
Ina Gittings Building
University of Arizona
Tucson, AZ 85721
USA

PATRICIA E. LONGMUIR, MSc
PEL Consulting
Don Mills, ON M3A 1K1
Canada

ANTHONY LUKE, MD, MPH
Departments of Orthopedics and Family and Community
  Medicine
University of California, San Francisco
San Francisco, CA 94115
USA

ROBERT M. MALINA, PhD
Tarleton State University
Stephenville, TX 76402-0370
USA

LYLE J. MICHELI, MD
Division of Sports Medicine
Department of Orthopaedic Surgery
Children's Hospital and Harvard Medical School
Boston, MA 02115
USA

JASON H. NIELSON, MD
Children's Bone and Spine Surgery
Sunrise Children's Hospital
Las Vegas, NV 89109
USA

DAVID M. ORENSTEIN, MD
Antonio J. and Janet Palumbo Cystic Fibrosis Center
Children's Hospital of Pittsburgh
Pittsburgh, PA 15213
USA

RUSSELL R. PATE, PhD
Department of Exercise Science
University of South Carolina
Columbia, SC 29208
USA

ADAM M. PERSKY, PhD
Division of Pharmacotherapy and Experimental Therapeutics
School of Pharmacy
University of North Carolina at Chapel Hill
Chapel Hill, NC 27599-7360
USA

KARIN A. PFEIFFER, PhD
Institute for the Study of Youth Sports
Michigan State University
East Lansing, MI 48824
USA

MELISSA S. PRICE, MEd
Curry School of Education
University of Virginia
Charlottesville, VA 22903
USA

ERIC S. RAWSON, PhD
Department of Exercise Science and Athletics
Bloomsburg University
Bloomsburg, PA 17815
USA

KATHLEEN RICHARDS, BS, PT, PCS
Department of Physical Therapy and Occupational Therapy
  Services
Children's Hospital
Boston, MA 02115
USA

MICHAEL C. RIDDELL, PhD
Kinesiology and Health Science, York University
Toronto, ON M3J 1P3
Canada

ALAN D. ROGOL, MD, PhD
Department of Pediatrics
University of Virginia
Charlottesville, VA 22911-8441
USA

JOAN M. ROUND, PhD
School of Sport and Exercise Sciences
The University of Birmingham
Edgbaston, Birmingham B15 2TT
UK

THOMAS W. ROWLAND, MD
Department of Pediatrics
Baystate Medical Center
Springfield, MA 01199
USA

LAUREN K. SILBERSTEIN, MS
Department of Psychology
Howard University
Washington, DC 20059
USA

ERIC SMALL, MD
Department of Pediatrics, Orthopedics, and Rehabilitation
*   Medicine*
Mount Sinai School of Medicine
New York, NY 10029
USA

J. KEVIN THOMPSON, PhD
Department of Psychology
University of South Florida
Tampa, FL 33620-8200
USA

BRIAN W. TIMMONS, PhD
Children's Exercise and Nutrition Centre
Chedoke Hospital
Hamilton, ON L8N 3Z5
Canada

WILLEM VAN MECHELEN, MD,
PhD
Institute for Research in Extramural Medicine and Department
*   of Public and Occupational Health, and Research Center*
*   Body@Work TNO VUmc*
VU University Medical Center
NL-1081 BT Amsterdam
The Netherlands

EMMANUEL VAN PRAAGH, PhD,
DHC
Laboratory of Exercise Physiology
Université Blaise Pascal

BP. 104, 63172-Aubiere
France

EVERT VERHAGEN, PhD
Institute for Research in Extramural Medicine and Department
*   of Public and Occupational Health, and Research Center*
*   Body@Work TNO VUmc*
VU University Medical Center
NL-1081 BT Amsterdam
The Netherlands

DIANNE S. WARD, EdD
Department of Nutrition
University of North Carolina
Chapel Hill, NC 27599
USA

MAUREEN R. WEISS, PhD
Curry School of Education
University of Virginia
Charlottesville, VA 22904
USA

JOANNE R. WELSMAN, PhD
University of Exeter
Exeter, EX1 2LU
UK

MELVIN H. WILLIAMS, PhD
Department of Exercise Science
Old Dominion University
Norfolk, VA 23529
USA

Foreword

During the second half of the 20th century, participation in competitive sports attained high levels of popularity. In response to the rapid increase in sports participation, in particular among children and adolescents, the IOC Medical Commission added a volume in 1996 to its series, Encyclopaedia of Sports Medicine, Vol. VI entitled *The Child and Adolescent Athlete*, edited by Prof. Oded Bar-Or, MD. This volume provided medical doctors and sports scientists with comprehensive and authoritative information on such important topic areas as physical conditioning, the relationship of physical performance to growth and maturation, nutrition, prevention and treatment of injuries, and non-orthopaedic health concerns.

During the past 10 years, the large and rapid increase of scientific information has, in all of these topic areas, led to a greater need for a volume to expand upon and update the original publication.

The present publication, Vol. XIII *The Young Athlete* began under the editorial leadership of Dr. Bar-Or together with Professor Helge Hebestreit, MD. As Dr. Bar-Or passed away mid-way through its development, we owe a great debt of appreciation to Dr. Hebestreit for seeing the project through to its successful completion.

It gives me great pleasure to welcome the addition of *The Young Athlete* to The Encyclopaedia of Sports Medicine collection. Medical doctors, sports scientists, allied health personnel, team coaches and the athletes, themselves, will benefit greatly from the information that has been gathered and provided. I congratulate all of the clinicians and scientists who have contributed to this excellent publication.

Dr. Jacques Rogge
President of the International Olympic Committee

Preface

Intense involvement in competitive sports often begins during childhood. During adolescence, many athletes reach their peak performance and some may participate in World Championships and Olympic Games at a relatively young age. Thus, knowledge about specific physiologic characteristics, responsiveness to training, and possible health hazards is imperative for all individuals involved in the training, coaching, and medical care of young athletes. The current volume of the *Encyclopaedia of Sports Medicine* summarizes up-to-date information on physiologic and medical aspects relevant to the care of children and adolescents involved in exercise and competitive sports. This specific group has been addressed only in one previous volume of the Encyclopaedia, *The Child and Adolescent Athlete*, which was published 11 years ago. Since then, based on new non-invasive methodologies and long-term longitudinal studies, new information has been gathered in most areas covered in the previous volume of the Encyclopaedia, and several new interesting areas have emerged.

When the idea for this new volume of the Encyclopaedia evolved, Dr. Oded Bar-Or and I were asked to assume editorial responsibility. I felt especially honored to work with my mentor and personal friend on this prestigious project. Dr. Bar-Or's immense knowledge of the field helped tremendously in identifying important chapter topics to be covered and in recruiting the best possible authors. Unfortunately, while the project was progressing, Dr. Bar-Or fell seriously ill. Despite his illness, he kept working harder than anybody could expect or even imagine for more than a year. Only shortly before his death on December 8, 2005, did he stop his engagement with this new volume of the Encyclopaedia, which was always of great importance to him.

The Young Athlete is subdivided in seven parts. Part 1 summarizes the information on the physiologic bases of physical performance in view of growth and development. The important topic of trainability and the consequences of a high level of physical activity during childhood and adolescence for future health are covered in Part 2. Part 3 addresses the epidemiology of injuries, their prevention, treatment, and rehabilitation. Non-orthopedic health concerns including the preparticipation examination are covered in Part 4. Part 5 covers psychosocial issues relevant to young athletes, while Part 6 reviews diseases and disabilities relevant to child and adolescent athletes, from infections through bronchial asthma and diabetes mellitus to motor and mental disabilities. The methodology relevant to the assessment of young athletes is summarized in Part 7.

The available information relevant to exercise and training in youth has been reviewed and summarized by authors who are recognized as leaders in their respective fields. Although the focus of the volume is on young athletes, several chapters include valuable information also relevant to the general pediatric population. This volume summarizes a large database of information from thousands of studies and provides a valuable reference to all professionals who are interested in the effects of exercise and sports on young people. It will be especially relevant to sports physicians, pediatricians, general practitioners, physiotherapists, dietitians, coaches, students, and researchers in the exercise sciences.

I am grateful to all authors of *The Young Athlete* for their excellent contributions, to Howard Knuttgen and the IOC medical commission for their continuing support during the editorial process, and to the staff of Blackwell Publishing who made the book become reality.

Helge Hebestreit
Würzburg, Germany, 2007

Oded Bar-Or, MD
(August 28, 1937–December 8, 2005)

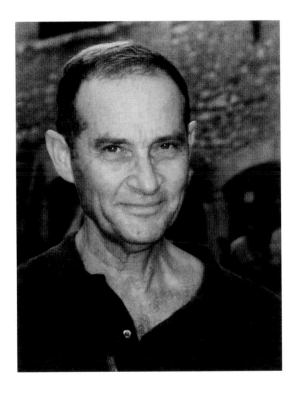

Dr. Oded Bar-Or was born in Jerusalem on August 28, 1937. He received his medical training at the Hebrew University-Hadassah Medical School in Jerusalem and qualified as a medical doctor in 1965. Thereafter, Dr. Bar-Or worked first as research assistant and then as assistant professor with Dr. E.R. Buskirk at the Human Performance Laboratory at Pennsylvania State University, USA. In 1969, he returned to Israel and became director of the Department of Research and Sports Medicine at the Wingate Institute for Physical Education and Sport. Twelve years later, Dr. Bar-Or spent a sabbatical in the Cardio-Respiratory department of McMaster University in Hamilton, Ontario, Canada. He stayed for an extra year at the behest of the then Chairman of the Department of Paediatrics, who offered him the possibility of setting up a center where he could put his theories and experience into practice.

After returning to Israel for a year, Dr. Bar-Or returned to Hamilton to head the Children's Exercise and Nutrition Center, a unique and innovative facility, which combines clinical care for children and adolescents—both athletes and individuals with chronic health conditions—with pioneering scientific work. Dr. Bar-Or was director of the center until he retired from clinical work in 2003. However, he continued to work part-time as research director of the Hamilton Health Sciences Center at Hamilton and served as part-time scientific advisor to the Alpine Children's Hospital at Davos, Switzerland.

Possibly the most outstanding characteristic of Dr. Bar-Or was his open mind to all people, questions, and problems. He maintained close contacts with many colleagues on all continents and attracted many postgraduate students and post-doctoral fellows from all over the world. Many of these returned to their home countries to establish facilities similar to the Children's Exercise and Nutrition Center.

During his career, Dr. Bar-Or produced scientific work that covered nearly all areas of research in the field of children and exercise. He published more than 180 articles in peer-reviewed journals, wrote 79 review articles and book chapters, and edited eight books on pediatric exercise physiology and medicine such as the *Encyclopaedia of Sports Medicine* Volume VI *The Child and Adolescent Athlete*. His monograph *Pediatric Sports Medicine for the Practitioner* was the key reference in the field for almost 20 years, until a second edition of *Pediatric Exercise Medicine: from Physiologic Principles to Health Care Application*, co-authored by Thomas Rowland, was published in 2004.

Dr. Bar-Or served on many scientific committees and organizations all over the world. Among his appointments, he was president of the International Council on Physical Fitness Research 1984–1992, president of the Canadian Association of Sports Sciences 1987–1988, and vice president of the American College of Sports Medicine 1992–1994.

Dr. Bar-Or's enormous impact in the field of pediatric exercise medicine has been acknowledged by numerous honors, including a Citation Award of the American College of Sports Medicine, an Honorary Award from the North American Society for Pediatric Exercise Medicine, and honorary memberships of several professional societies. He further received an honorary doctoral degree from Blaise Pascal University in Clermont-Ferrand, France, from Brock University in St. Catharine's, Ontario, Canada, and from the Józef Pilsudski Academy of Physical Education in Warsaw, Poland.

It was a tremendous loss to his family, friends, and colleagues when Oded Bar-Or died on December 8, 2005. He will be remembered through various lectures given in his memory, at scientific conferences, and through the Bar-Or Travel Award in Pediatric Exercise Medicine offered at Brock University, Canada.

Helge Hebestreit
on behalf of the contributors
to this book and all past
students and fellows of
Dr. Oded Bar-Or
Würzburg, Germany, 2007

Part 1

Growth, Maturation, and Physical Performance

Chapter 1

Growth and Biologic Maturation: Relevance to Athletic Performance

GASTON BEUNEN AND ROBERT M. MALINA

Growth refers to measurable changes in size, physique and body composition, and various systems of the body, whereas maturation refers to progress toward the mature state. Maturation is variable among bodily systems and also in timing and tempo of progress. The processes of growth and maturation are related, and both influence physical performance.

Chronologic age (CA) is the common reference in studies of growth and performance. However, there is considerable variation in growth, maturity, and performance status among individuals of the same CA, especially during the pubertal years.

Interrelationships among growth, maturation, and performance during childhood and adolescence are the focus of this chapter. It specifically considers:

1 Age-, sex-, and maturity-associated variation in physical performance;
2 Growth and maturity characteristics of young athletes;
3 The influence of training on growth and maturation; and
4 Matching of opponents for sport.

Overview of growth and performance

Somatic growth

Growth in stature is rapid in infancy and early childhood, rather steady during middle childhood, rapid during the adolescent spurt, and then slow as adult stature is attained. This pattern of growth (size-attained and rate) is generally similar for body weight and other dimensions with the exception of

subcutaneous fat and fat distribution. The growth rate of stature is highest during the first year of life then gradually declines until the onset (take-off) of the adolescent growth spurt (about 10 years in girls and 12 years in boys). With the spurt, growth rate increases, reaching a peak (peak height velocity, PHV) at about 12 years in girls and 14 years in boys, and then gradually declines and eventually ceases with the attainment of adult stature (Tanner 1962, 1978; Malina *et al.* 2004). There is evidence for a small mid-growth spurt in childhood in stature and probably in other dimensions in many, but not all, children (Malina *et al.* 2004; see Chapter 31). Daily, half-weekly, or weekly measurements of length and height indicate that growth is episodic rather than continuous over short periods (Lampl *et al.* 1992), although "mini growth spurts" superimposed on a continuous growth pattern have been suggested (Hermanussen *et al.* 1988).

Physical performance

Physical performance is commonly measured as the outcome (product) of standardized motor tasks requiring speed, agility, balance, flexibility, explosive strength, local muscular endurance, and static muscular strength.

Isometric strength increases linearly with age during childhood and the transition into adolescence in both sexes. At approximately 13 years, strength development accelerates considerably in boys (adolescent spurt), but continues to increase linearly in girls through about 15 years with less evidence for a clear adolescent spurt, although data vary among specific strength tests. Sex differences in strength are consistent, although small, through childhood and the transition into adolescence. Thereafter, the differences become increasingly larger so that at the age of 16 years and later only a few girls perform at the same level as the average boy. Among Belgian youth, for example, the median arm pull strength of 17-year-old girls falls below the corresponding third percentile for boys (Beunen et al. 1989). Strength is related to body size and muscle mass, so that sex differences might relate to a size advantage in boys. During childhood and adolescence boys tend to have greater strength per unit body size, especially in the upper body and trunk than girls, but corresponding sex differences in lower extremity strength are negligible. In fact, isometric strength in boys and girls increases during childhood and adolescence more than predicted from height alone (Asmussen & Heeboll-Nielsen 1955). The disproportionate strength increase is most apparent during male adolescence, and is greater in the upper extremities than in the trunk or lower extremities (Asmussen 1962; Carron & Bailey 1974).

Performance in a variety of standardized tests such as dashes (speed), shuttle runs (agility, speed), vertical and standing long jumps and distance throw (coordination and explosive strength), flexed arm hang and sit-ups (local muscular endurance), and beam walk and flamingo stand (balance) also improve, on average, from childhood through adolescence in boys. The performances in girls increase until the age of 13–14 years, with little subsequent improvement, although some more recent evidence suggests that the plateau for some motor tasks has shifted to a slightly older age. The growth pattern for flexibility differs. Mean scores in the sit and reach are stable or decline slightly during childhood, increase during adolescence, and reach a plateau at about 14–15 years in girls and decline from childhood through mid-adolescence and then increase in boys (Haubenstricker & Seefeldt 1986; Beunen & Simons 1990; Malina et al. 2004).

Performances of girls fall, on average, within 1 standard deviation (SD) below average performances of boys in late childhood and early adolescence, with the exception of softball throw for distance. However, after 14 years average performances of girls are consistently beyond the bounds of 1 SD below the means of boys in most tasks. In contrast, girls are more flexible than boys at virtually all ages (Beunen et al. 1989; Malina et al. 2004).

Correlations between somatic dimensions and performance in motor tasks during childhood are generally low (0 to about 0.35). Performance in tasks in which the body is projected (jumps and dashes) correlates negatively and performance in tasks in which an object is projected (throws) correlates positively with body mass. Correlations during adolescence are of the same magnitude and in the same direction as during childhood (Malina 1975; Malina et al. 2004).

Most fitness test batteries include a direct or indirect estimate of aerobic power. Absolute aerobic power ($\dot{V}O_{2max}$, $L\cdot min^{-1}$) increases from childhood through adolescence in boys, but reaches a plateau at 13–14 years of age in girls. Before the age of 10–12 years, $\dot{V}O_{2max}$ of girls reaches about 85–90% of the mean values of boys, but after the adolescent spurt average $\dot{V}O_{2max}$ in girls reaches only 70% of mean scores in boys (Krahenbuhl et al. 1985; Armstrong & Welsman 1994; Malina et al. 2004).

The dependence of aerobic power on body size during growth is indicated in the growth curve of relative aerobic power (i.e., per unit body mass, $mL\cdot kg^{-1}\cdot min^{-1}$). The values are rather stable throughout the growth period in cross-sectional samples of boys (Krahenbuhl et al. 1985), but trends in longitudinal samples suggest a decline through adolescence (Mirwald & Bailey 1986). On the other hand, relative $\dot{V}O_{2max}$ decreases systematically with age in girls (Krahenbuhl et al. 1985; Mirwald & Bailey 1986; Armstrong & Welsman 1994). Sex differences in relative $\dot{V}O_{2max}$ are generally smaller than in absolute $\dot{V}O_{2max}$, with girls reaching 80–95% of boys' values. Several authors demonstrated that expressing $\dot{V}O_{2max}$ to body mass may confound the understanding of changes in oxygen uptake with growth and maturation (see Chapter 5). Power functions, allometric equations, and multilevel modeling have been used more recently. Results are mixed because of the various techniques used, the age ranges considered, and sample bias (Armstrong & Welsman 1994). When size and mass are included in the scaling, mass exponents close to the theoretical scaling coefficient of k = 0.67 are obtained (Arsmtrong & Welsman 1994).

Adolescent spurts in performance

Most data for performance are derived from cross-sectional samples which are inadequate for quantifying the timing and tempo of the adolescent growth spurt. Individuals pass through adolescence at their own pace and consequently have their growth spurts over a wide range of CAs, the so-called time-spreading effect (Tanner 1962). Only longitudinal or mixed longitudinal data properly analysed provide adequate information about tempo and timing of spurts in a variety of characteristics.

In addition to documenting the occurrence of growth spurts per se in performance, the timing of the spurts is ordinarily viewed relative to the timing of PHV (i.e., relative to a biologic milestone) rather than to CA. This serves to reduce the time spread along the CA axis and provides more specific information about the timing and magnitude of adolescent spurts in other body dimensions than height and in performance. Note that this concept was first realized by Boas (1892).

In such analyses, individual velocities for a body dimension or performance item are aligned on the individual's PHV so that growth rates are viewed in terms of years before and after the individual's PHV, regardless of the age at which PHV occurred. A mean constant velocity curve is obtained from these individual values in which the aligned individual values are combined. When mathematical functions are used, the mean–constant curve is obtained by fitting the function to each individual, estimating the constants for each individual, and then averaging the constants to yield the curve.

Longitudinal data show well-defined adolescent spurts in strength, several motor performances, and absolute aerobic power of boys. Corresponding data for girls are less extensive and show a spurt in absolute aerobic power while data for strength are variable.

The male adolescent spurt in static strength occurs about 0.5–1.0 year after PHV and is more coincident with peak weight velocity (PWV) (Stolz & Stolz 1951; Carron & Bailey 1974; Kemper & Verschuur 1985; Beunen et al. 1988; Beunen & Malina 1988).

The strength spurt (arm pull) of Dutch girls occurs at about the same time as in boys, 0.5 years after PHV. Peak strength (arm pull) gain in boys is, on average, about 12 kg·year^{-1} compared to 6 kg·year^{-1} in girls. Among California girls, however, a composite strength score of four tests shows an inconsistent pattern; the spurt in strength preceded PHV in about 40% of the girls, coincided with PHV in 11%, and followed PHV in 49% (Faust 1977).

Half-yearly velocities for six performance tasks in Belgian boys are summarized in Fig. 1.1. On the average, peak velocities in static strength (arm pull), explosive strength (vertical jump), and muscular endurance (bent arm hang) occur after PHV. The adolescent spurt in these characteristics appears to begin about 1.5 years prior to PHV and reach a peak 0.5–1.0 year after PHV. In contrast, maximum velocities in speed tests (shuttle run and plate tapping) and flexibility (sit and reach) occur before PHV. The lower age limit in the Leuven Growth Study of Belgian boys, 12 years of age, does not permit an accurate estimate of the onset of the spurts in flexibility and speed. Results for small samples of Spanish boys ($n = 18$–27) and girls are generally consistent with those observed for Belgian boys. The data for Spanish girls ($n = 25$–35) are consistent with the trends for Belgian boys for strength and power, but the flexibility and speed tasks show peak gains after PHV which is in contrast to the findings in Belgian boys (Heras Yague & de la Fuente 1998). Data for girls are limited; however, when performance is related to age at menarche, which occurs on average after PHV, there is no tendency for motor performance to peak before, at, or after menarche (Espenschade 1940).

An overview of the timing in strength and motor performance relative to PHV, PWV, and peak strength velocity (PSV) is given in Table 1.1. Because PWV and PSV follow PHV, it is obvious that maximum velocities in running speed (shuttle run), speed of limb movement (plate tapping), and flexibility (sit and reach) also precede PWV and PSV. Maximum velocities in strength and muscular endurance follow PWV and coincide with PSV. The evidence thus indicates that during adolescence boys are first stretched (spurt in stature) and then filled-out (spurt in muscle mass, weight, and strength).

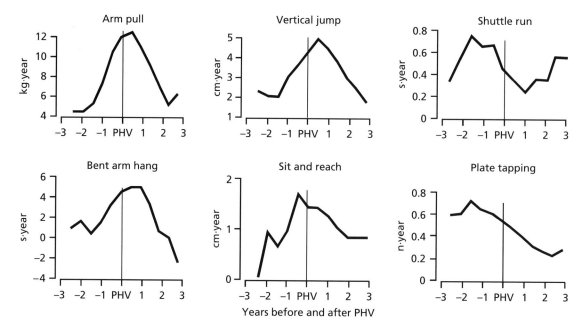

Fig. 1.1 Median velocities of several tests of strength and motor performance aligned on peak height velocity (PHV) in the Leuven Growth Study of Belgian Boys. Velocities for the performance items are plotted as years before and after PHV. Drawn from data reported by Beunen *et al.* (1988).

Table 1.1 Timing of maximum observed velocities of several motor performance items relative to adolescent spurts in stature, body weight and arm pull strength in Belgian boys (after Beunen *et al.* 1988).

Performance	Height spurt			Weight spurt			Strength spurt		
	Precedes	Coincides	Follows	Precedes	Coincides	Follows	Precedes	Coincides	Follows
Arm pull		×				×			
Vertical jump		×				×		×	
Plate tapping	×			×			×		
Shuttle run	×			×			×		
Sit & reach	×			×			×		
Bent arm hang		×				×		×	

Absolute $\dot{V}o_{2max}$ (L·min^{-1}) shows a clear adolescent spurt in both sexes in samples of Belgian and Canadian children (Mirwald & Bailey 1986; Geithner *et al.* 2004). Estimated peak velocities are greater in boys (1.01 L·min^{-1}·year^{-1} in Belgian boys and 0.41 L·min^{-1}·year^{-1} in Canadian boys) than in girls (0.59 L·min^{-1}·year^{-1} in Belgian girls and 0.28 L·min^{-1}·year^{-1} in Canadian girls). Note, however, that in the Belgian sample $\dot{V}o_{2peak}$ reached a plateau or declined after reaching a maximal value. Corresponding data for Dutch (Kemper 1985),

German, and Norwegian (Rutenfranz *et al.* 1982) adolescents, although not analyzed in the same manner, suggest a similar trend. On average, $\dot{V}o_{2max}$ begins to increase several years before PHV and continues to increase after PHV. $\dot{V}o_{2max}$ per unit body mass (mL O$_2$·kg^{-1}·min^{-1}), on the other hand, generally begins to decline 1 year before PHV and continues to decline after PHV. The decline reflects the rapid changes in stature and body mass so that, per unit body mass, oxygen uptake declines during the growth spurt. The significance of relative aerobic power as expressed per body weight or other body dimensions can be questioned because the relationships between aerobic power and several body dimensions and systemic functions during growth are complex. Relative aerobic power masks the sex-specific changes in body composition, size, and function. Changes in relative aerobic power during adolescence probably reflect changes in body composition and not changes in aerobic function, which increases at this time. Power functions, allometric equations, and multilevel modeling have been used to scale changes in aerobic function during adolescence (Armstrong & Welsman 1994; Beunen et al. 2002; see Chapter 5). Although $\dot{V}o_{2peak}$ is associated with biologic maturity status after controlling for height and weight (Armstrong & Welsman 2000), studies utilizing multilevel modeling do not provide at present additional information about changes in $\dot{V}o_{2peak}$ normalized for height and/or weight relative to the timing of the adolescent growth spurt.

Maturity-associated variation in performance

Individual differences in maturity status at a given age and in the timing of the adolescent spurt influence growth status and performance. Moreover, youth who are successful in sport tend to differ, on average, in maturity status and rate compared with the general population. It is thus important to review maturity-associated variation in performance.

Variation in maturity status influences body dimensions, composition and proportions, and also performance. The effect of variation in maturity status can operate through associated variation in body size and/or composition and through a direct influence on performance. Maturity-associated variation in somatic growth is discussed in more detail elsewhere (Malina et al. 2004). The subsequent discussion focuses on the influence of variation in matutity status on performance, summarizing first correlational analyses and then comparisons of youth of contrasting maturity status.

Correlations between skeletal age (SA) as one indicator of maturity and several indicators of motor performance, including tests of speed, flexibility, explosive strength or power, and muscular endurance, range from low to moderate in children and adolescents (Espenschade 1940; Seils 1951; Rarick & Oyster 1964; Beunen et al. 1981b, 1997a; Malina et al. 2004). Static strength is positively correlated with SA at all ages in pre-adolescent boys and girls, while muscular endurance (functional strength or dynamic strength) is negatively correlated to SA in adolescent girls 11–13 years and boys 12–13 years of age. The negative associations reflect the negative influence of body weight at this time. In boys, from 14 years onwards all gross motor abilities are positively associated with SA. The greater strength that accompanies male adolescence compensates for the higher body weight so that from 14 years positive associations are apparent between SA and muscular endurance.

More comprehensive analyses considering the interactions of CA, SA, height, and weight indicate that variation in maturity status influences performance indirectly. Among children 7–12 years of age, skeletal maturity status influenced strength and motor performance mainly through its interaction with size and body mass (Katzmarzyk et al. 1997). Among 6- to 11-year-old girls, SA by itself appeared only sporadically among the predictors of performance (Beunen et al. 1997a). Among adolescent boys, CA and SA by themselves or in combination with height and body mass accounted for a small percentage (0–17%) of the variance in speed, flexibility, explosive strength, and muscular endurance, but for static strength the explained variance was as high as 58% (Beunen et al. 1981b). The corresponding analyses of adolescent girls indicated a significant influence of the interaction between SA and body size on static strength (up to 33% of explained variance), but relatively little influence (generally, less than 10%) on motor performance (speed, flexibility, explosive strength, and muscular endurance). By inference, the results may suggest an important role for variation in neuromuscular maturation as a factor influencing performance during childhood. Skeletal maturity perhaps does not reflect neuromuscular maturation and probably exerts its influence on performance through associated variation in somatic features.

In a longitudinal analysis of boys and girls of contrasting maturity status (Jones 1949; see also Malina *et al*. 2004), early maturing boys had higher muscular strength than late maturing boys at all ages between 11 and 17 years, while early maturing girls performed only slightly better than late maturing girls only in early adolescence (i.e., 11–13 years of age). Subsequently, there were no differences in strength among girls of contrasting maturity status. Associations among various maturity indicators and measures of static or isometric strength have consistently documented a positive relationship between maturity status and strength in boys and girls (Clarke 1971; Carron & Bailey 1974; Beunen *et al*. 1981b; Bastos & Hegg 1986; Malina *et al*. 2004).

Motor performances (vertical jump, sit and reach, shuttle run, plate tapping) of early maturing boys grouped by age at PHV, are, on average, better than those of average and late maturing boys of the same age from 12 to 18 years, with the exception of the flexed arm hang (Lefevre *et al*. 1990). Controlling for body size reduces some of the differences between adolescent boys of contrasting maturity status, but the advantage for early maturing boys persists in strength and power tasks compared to speed tasks (Beunen *et al*. 1978). Among adolescent girls, on the other hand, maturity-associated variation in performance is not consistent among tasks and from age to age (Beunen *et al*. unpublished data [see Malina *et al*. 2004]; Little *et al*. 1997).

Some evidence for boys suggests the performance advantage associated with early maturation disappears at adult age (Lefevre *et al*. 1990). Performances of 30-year-old men grouped on the basis of their age at PHV do not significantly differ for static strength (arm pull), muscular endurance of the lower trunk (leg lifts), running speed (shuttle run), and flexibility (sit and reach). However, early maturers still perform better at 30 years for speed of limb movement (plate tapping), while late maturers perform better in muscular endurance of the upper body (bent arm hang) and explosive strength (vertical jump). The results also indicate that late maturing males improve significantly in performance between 18 and 30 years, more so than early or average maturing males (Lefevre *et al*. 1990).

Skeletal maturation and absolute aerobic power are significantly related. The correlations are higher (0.89) when a broad age range, 8–18 years, is considered (Hollmann & Bouchard 1970) compared to a narrower range, 8–14 years (0.55–0.68; Labitzke 1971). When $\dot{V}O_{2max}$ is expressed per kilogram body mass, correlations are not significant (Hollmann & Bouchard 1970; Labitzke 1971; Savov 1978; Shephard *et al*. 1978). Non-significant and generally lower associations are apparent between several indices of submaximal performance capacity and maturity status, except around the growth spurt in boys when correlations are higher (Hebbelinck *et al*. 1971; Kemper *et al*. 1975; Bouchard *et al*. 1976, 1978). In a national sample of Belgian girls, submaximal power output (PWC) at heart rates of 130, 150, and 170 beats·min^{-1} is significantly related to skeletal maturation. The correlations generally increase with age and reach a maximum between 11 and 13 years (Beunen 1989).

Early maturing boys have, on average, a higher absolute $\dot{V}O_{2max}$ than late maturing boys except in late adolescence. A similar trend is evident for early and late maturing girls, but the differences are smaller than in boys. On the other hand, relative $\dot{V}O_{2max}$ is higher in late maturers of both sexes (Kemper *et al*. 1986; Malina *et al*. 1997). This observation most probably reflects the higher absolute and relative fatness of early maturing girls. However, among boys, early maturers have an absolutely larger fat-free mass and relatively less fat mass than late maturers. The better relative $\dot{V}O_{2max}$, expressed per kilogram body mass, of late maturers more likely reflects the rapid growth of body mass with advancing maturation, so that oxygen uptake per unit body mass becomes progressively less. Allometric analyses indicate that early maturing boys have higher coefficients for body mass and height compared with average and late maturing boys. In girls from 11 to 14 years the increase in $\dot{V}O_{2peak}$ is not associated with increases in body mass or stature (Beunen *et al*. 1997b; Malina *et al*. 2004).

Maturity status of elite young athletes

The biologic maturity status of athletes has been studied rather extensively, especially age at menarche.

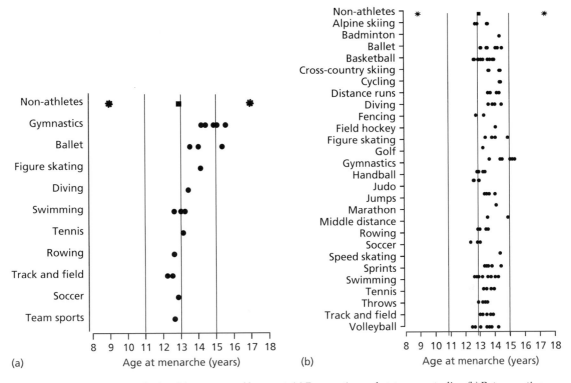

Fig. 1.2 Mean ages at menarche in athletes grouped by sport. (a) Prospective and status quo studies. (b) Retrospective studies. Assuming a mean age at menarche of 13.0 ± 1.0 years for non-athletes, about 95% of girls will attain menarche between 11.0 and 15.0 years of age. These ages are indicated by vertical lines in the figure; the range of reported ages at menarche in a large sample of university students who were non-athletes, 9.2–17.2 years of age, is also indicated with asterisks.

The subject has been reviewed by Beunen (1989), Malina (1983, 1994a, 1998a, 2002), and Malina *et al.* (2004). Studies of young athletes have a number of limitations. First, the definition of an athlete is vague and a wide variety of skill and competitive levels are represented. Second, young athletes are a highly selected group, not only with regard to skill and performance level, but also with regard to size and physique. The selection may be made by the individual, parents, coach, influential others, or some combination of these. Third, earlier maturation is intrinsically related to growth in size and both are associated with performance. Finally, athletic performance is influenced by many factors, many of which are not biologic.

Age at menarche is the maturational landmark most often studied in elite athletes (Malina 1983, 1991, 1998b, 2002). Mean ages at menarche based

on longitudinal and status quo studies of adolescent athletes, and on retrospective ages at menarche of older adolescent and young adult athletes are summarized in Fig. 1.2. Data collected by questioning adolescent athletes are limited (Fig. 1.2a). Most samples of adolescent athletes have mean or median ages at menarche within the normal range, but mean ages for samples of adolescent gymnasts, ballet dancers, figure skaters, and divers tend to be later than those of athletes in other sports. It should be noted that the samples of adolescent athletes are rather small, which suggests that more data are needed. Mean recalled ages at menarche for late adolescent and young adult athletes are more extensive (Fig. 1.2b). The majority of mean ages are above 13.0 years, but variation within and between sports is apparent. The retrospective data for gymnasts, divers, ballet dancers, and soccer players are generally consistent with the longitudinal or status quo data (Fig. 1.2a). Differences between ages at menarche in younger and older athletes in a given sport merit attention. For tennis, rowing, track and field, and swimming the longitudinal or status quo data show earlier ages at menarche than the retrospective data. Allowing for error of recall associated with the retrospective method, data suggest that late adolescent and young adult athletes in these sports tend to attain menarche later than athletes involved in the same sports during the circumpubertal years (prospective and longitudinal data). This trend is especially apparent in swimmers. Status quo and retrospective data indicate mean ages at menarche that approximate the mean of the general population; however, retrospective data for university level swimmers indicate later mean ages at menarche, 14.3 and 14.4 years. This trend reflects, in part, more opportunities for adolescent girls in swimming, most probably because of improved or additional swim programs at university level (Title IX legislation). A related factor is differential success of later maturing girls in the sport at more advanced competitive levels (Malina *et al.* 2004).

Data for other maturity indicators in female athletes are less extensive (Beunen 1989; Malina *et al.* 2004). Local level age group athletes and non-athletes do not differ in the distributions of stages 2–4 of breast and pubic hair development (Plowman *et al.* 1991). Gymnasts are not as advanced in both breast and pubic hair development compared with swimmers or control subjects of the same age, who do not differ from each other (Bernink *et al.* 1983; Peltenburg *et al.* 1984). Among 113 gymnasts competing at the 1987 World Championships at Rotterdam, the SA–CA difference was –1.9 years, indicating late maturation (Claessens *et al.* 1991). These observations are consistent with earlier reports documenting slower maturation in female gymnasts (Novotny & Taftlova 1971; Beunen *et al.* 1981a). In a small sample of ballet dancers ($n = 15$) followed from 12 to 15 years, breast development occured at later ages, while pubic hair developed at expected ages (Warren 1980). In contrast, among 30 girls training in rowing and light athletics in Polish sport schools (about 8–12 hours·week^{-1}) and followed

longitudinally from 11 to 14 years, breast and pubic hair development, age at menarche (prospectively obtained), and estimated growth velocities did not differ from reference data for the general population (Malina *et al.* 1990).

With few exceptions, male athletes of different competitive levels in various sports are characterized by average or advanced biologic maturity status. Whatever the biologic maturity indicator used or the competitive level considered, the evidence points in the same direction (Beunen 1989; Malina 1998a, 2002; Malina *et al.* 2004). Boys average and advanced in maturity status tend to be overrepresented among young athletes. The most marked advancement in maturity status occurs in adolescence, which is probably a result of the size, physique, fat-free mass, and performance (strength, power, speed) advantages of the early maturers. This advantage is reduced as boys approach late adolescence or early adulthood, when late maturers catch up or even tend to outperform the early maturers (see above). In a select national sample of Belgian male track athletes, all 15- to 16-year-olds except one had an SA in advance of CA. Among 17- to 18-year-old athletes, about two-thirds had an SA equal to or in advance of that expected for CA, while one-third had an SA that was less than their CA (Malina *et al.* 1986). The statures of 16-year-old athletes advanced in SA, of 17- to 18-year-old athletes who had already attained skeletal maturity, and of 17- to 18-year-old athletes who had reached skeletal maturity did not differ, although athletes 16–18 years old advanced in skeletal maturity were heavier. Although the data are cross-sectional, the trend suggests catch-up in stature of those late in skeletal maturation, but persistent differences in body weight.

Training and the growth and maturation of young athletes

Training refers to systematic, specialized practice for a specific sport or sport discipline for most of the year or to specific short-term experimental programs. Physical activity is not the same as regular training. The measurement, quantification, and specification of training programs by sport need further attention. Training programs are ordinarily specific (e.g., endurance running, strength training, sport skill training) and vary in intensity and duration.

Many of the changes attributed to regular training, although not all, are in the same direction as those that accompany normal growth and maturation. It is difficult to partition training effects from those of normal growth and maturation in the currently available data. Many studies of young athletes tend to focus on training per se and overlook other factors that are capable of influencing growth and maturation. An obvious factor is selection; young athletes in many sports are rigorously selected for specific morphologic and maturational features. Allowing for these caveats, a discussion of training, growth, and maturation follows.

Growth in stature

Longitudinal data for young athletes that span childhood and adolescence are extremely limited. Data for active and inactive boys followed from late childhood through adolescence indicate no differences in stature, while corresponding data for boys active in several sports indicate statures consistent with average to advanced maturity status (Beunen *et al.* 1992; Malina 1994a,b; Malina & Bielicki 1996). Longitudinal data for girls are less extensive. Girls regularly active in a variety of team and individual sports (track, rowing, swimming, basketball, volleyball) present a pattern of growth that is characteristic of average maturing individuals (Malina 1994a,b; Malina & Bielicki 1996). Young female athletes in a variety of sports tend to have less weight-for-height than non-athletes, suggesting a linear and lean build. There is, of course, variation by event and/or position within a sport. This is especially evident in track and field. Mean heights of adolescent female distance runners and sprinters 10–18 years of age tend to be at or above reference medians; mean weights of distance runners are consistently below the reference medians, while those of sprinters are generally quite close to the medians. Distance runners thus have less weight-for-height. Data for jumpers and throwers indicate greater heights in jumpers than throwers, and greater weights in throwers than jumpers. The heights of jumpers and throwers often exceed the 90th percentiles; in contrast, mean weights of the throwers are close to or above the 90th percentiles, while those of the jumpers are at or above the reference medians (Malina 2004).

Available short- and long-term longitudinal data indicate mean statures that maintain their position relative to the reference values over time, which suggests that they are not apparently influenced by the regular training for sport. Short-term longitudinal studies of male and female athletes in a variety of sports (volleyball, diving, distance running, track, basketball, rowing, cycling, ice hockey) indicate growth rates within the range expected for non-athletes (Malina 1994a,b). Intensive training for distance running has received considerable scrutiny, but longitudinal data indicate growth rates in male and female runners similar to those for reference values for non-athletes (Eisenmann & Malina 2002; Malina 2004).

In the context of these short- and long-term longitudinal observations, and allowing for selective criteria in some sports, regular participation in sport and training for sport has no apparent effect on attained stature and rate of growth in stature. Nevertheless, it is consistently suggested that regular gymnastics training "blunts" growth velocities in female gymnasts with the inference that the adolescent growth spurt is also "blunted" (Theintz *et al.* 1993; Daly *et al.* 2005). These conclusions are based on samples of female gymnasts followed over short periods (2.0–3.7 years) that do not cover the age span needed to capture the adolescent growth spurt in individual girls (see below).

The adolescent growth spurt

Age at PHV is not apparently affected by regular physical activity and training for sport. The observations for male athletes are consistent with the data for SA (i.e., ages at PHV tend to occur early or close to the average in male athletes). Available data for female athletes indicate ages at PHV that approximate the average (Malina *et al.* 2004). Longitudinal data for females in ballet, figure skating, and diving, sports in which later maturing girls commonly excel during adolescence, are insufficient to estimate ages at PHV. Samples of ballet dancers show shorter statures during early adolescence, but late adolescent statures that do not differ from non-dancers (i.e., later attainment of adult stature) (Malina 1994a). This is a growth pattern characteristic of late maturers (Malina *et al.* 2004).

Data for gymnasts of both sexes indicate later ages at PHV (Malina 1999; Thomis *et al.* 2005). The parameters of the adolescent spurt in male and female gymnasts are similar to those for short, but healthy, late maturing children with short parents (Malina 1999). Nevertheless, it has been suggested that the adolescent growth spurt in female gymnasts is "blunted" or absent (Theintz *et al.* 1993; Daly *et al.* 2005). Note that the inference of growth "blunting" is not discussed for male gymnasts who, relative to reference data for males, are as short as and later maturing as female gymnasts (Malina 1994a, 1999). As noted, the duration of the studies of female gymnasts was not sufficient to accommodate the entire duration of the growth spurt which leads to biased estimates of PHV and age at PHV (Zemel & Johnston 1994). Individually fitted growth curves for 13 female gymnasts followed, on average, from 8.7 to 15.5 years, indicate a later age at PHV compared to a reference for the general population (Thomis *et al.* 2005). Estimated peak velocities of growth in height, leg length, and sitting height are only slightly less than in non-athletes and well within the range of normal variability (Malina *et al.* 2004).

Skeletal maturation

Skeletal age does not differ between active and inactive boys followed longitudinally from 13 to 18 years (Beunen *et al.* 1992). In boys active in sport, SA and CA show similar gains prior to the adolescent spurt, but SA progresses faster than CA during the growth spurt and puberty in boys, reflecting their advanced maturity status. In a corresponding sample of girls active in sport, SA and CA progress at the same pace from late childhood through the growth spurt and puberty (Malina & Bielicki 1996). Although young athletes in several sports, including gymnasts of both sexes, differ in skeletal maturity status, short-term longitudinal observations indicate similar gains in both SA and

CA (Malina 1994a, 1998a). The data thus imply no effect of training for sport on skeletal maturation of the hand and wrist.

Sexual maturation

The pubertal progress of boys and girls active in sport is similar to the progress observed in boys or girls not active in sport. The effect of training for sport on the sexual maturation of boys has not generally been considered. This may not be surprising because early and average maturation are characteristic of the majority of young male athletes. Wrestling is the primary sport among males that has an emphasis on weight regulation. The emphasis on weight control, however, is short term, and longitudinal observations over a season indicate no significant effects on maturation and hormonal profiles (Roemmich & Sinning 1997a,b).

Later mean ages at menarche in young gymnasts, figure skaters, and ballet dancers, and in late adolescent and adult athletes in many sports are often attributed to regular training for the respective sports (Malina 1983, 1991, 1998b, 2002). Although some data are prospective, the majority are status quo and retrospective, which does not permit establishment of causality. Many biologic and environmental factors are related to the timing of menarche (e.g., genotype, diet, family size, family composition and interactions, stress) (Clapp & Little 1995; Ellis 2004; Malina *et al.* 2004). Given the complexity of factors, it is essential that they be considered before inferring causality for training before and/or during puberty as a factor influencing the timing of menarche in presumably healthy adolescent athletes (Loucks *et al.* 1992; Clapp & Little 1995). The conclusion of a comprehensive evaluation of exercise and female reproductive health merits attention in this regard: "it has yet to be shown that exercise delays menarche in anyone" (Loucks *et al.* 1992, p. S288).

The available evidence thus suggests that regular training for and participation in sport do not affect growth in stature, the timing and magnitude of PHV, and skeletal and sexual maturation in young athletes. In contrast to the commonly used indicators of growth and maturation, systematic training has potentially beneficial effects on body composition and specific tissues—skeletal (bone), skeletal muscle and adipose—but discussion of these is beyond the scope of this chapter (Malina *et al*. 2004). Functional effects of systematic training also have implications for performance. Resistance and aerobic training leads to improvements in muscular strength and maximal aerobic power, respectively, in youth of both sexes, while improvements in sport-related skills associated with sport-specific training have not been systematically evaluated although are often taken for granted (Malina *et al*. 2004).

Matching opponents in youth sports

Youth sport programs are ordinarily structured into chronologic age categories. Given the wide range of variation in body size, body composition, biologic maturation, physical performance, skill, psychosocial characteristics, personality, and behaviour among children of the same age and especially in the transition from childhood to adolescence, attempts to equalize competition are often discussed and occasionally attempted. Nevertheless, size, maturity, strength, performance, and skill mismatches are rather common in spite of attempts to equate participants for competition. The potential competitive inequity and perhaps risk for injury associated with such mismatches are especially evident in contact and collision sports (for a classification of contact and collision sports see American Academy of Pediatrics 1988). Matching participants by size and biologic maturity has often been proposed as a means for reducing differences in size, strength, motor performance, and skill (e.g., Gallagher 1969; Seefeldt 1981; Caine & Broekhoff 1987).

Matching criteria

Children and adolescents are ordinarily grouped for sport by CA and sex. As noted, interindividual variation in body dimensions, biologic maturity, body composition, physical performance, and skill is considerable within a single chronologic year (e.g., 10.0–10.99 years).

The limitation of CA for grouping youth was already recognized by Crampton (1908) and Rotch (1909). Although Crampton did not specifically refer to sport (his focus was child labor), he advocated the use of "physiological age" based on the development of pubic hair; Rotch, on the other hand, advocated "anatomical age" based on X-rays of the carpals and indicated the potential utility of this approach for sport.

Sports vary with season of the year and this implies differential cut-off dates to define age for a given season. Participants born after the cut-off date are grouped in a younger age category than those born before the cut-off date. Moreover, coaches tend to select participants who are born in the months immediately after the cut-off date.

Although matching participants by size and/or biologic maturation is often proposed, matching by size or biologic maturity status independent of CA is misleading; CA, size, and biologic maturity status are highly interrelated. Matching by body mass is common in some sports (e.g., American football, weight lifting, judo, and wrestling). Weight categories are often quite broad so that mismatches are still possible. Moreover, some American youth football programs place weight limits on primary ball carriers (offensive players). The rationale for limiting body weight of ball carriers is that a markedly heavier athlete will not be able to run into a lighter athlete playing on defense. However, the weight limitation on ball carriers does not apply for any defensive position (i.e., a heavier player could run into a lighter player while making a tackle).

The most commonly used indicators of biologic maturity are secondary sex characteristics (see Chapter 31; Malina *et al*. 2004). An important issue is the invasiveness of the assessment of sexual maturity, although self-assessments are available. The question remains which indicators should be used (pubic hair, genital development in boys; pubic hair, breast development, or age at menarche in girls)? Although these indicators are correlated there is considerable variation in the tempo of the transition from one stage to the next stage and in the sequence of the stages and indicators (Malina *et al*. 2004). This variation presents a practical problem. If secondary sex characteristics are used to group participants, how are changes in status that occur during a season taken into consideration? It is likely that some participants will change in status quite quickly over a season whereas others will remain in the same stage leading again to potential mismatches.

SA is the best single indicator of biologic maturity because it spans childhood and adolescence (Tanner 1962; Malina *et al.* 2004). However, it requires an X-ray of the hand and wrist with, although minimal, exposure to radiation. It is certainly not to be recommended for use on a large scale in youth sports. An alternative could be to use percentage of adult height as a criterion, which implies the prediction of mature height, or the prediction of maturity-offset from age at PHV (see Chapter 31). Similar variability in tempo of biologic maturation in SA, percentage of mature height and maturity offset can be expected as for secondary sex characteristics, which presents a practical problem for the matching process.

While matching based on secondary sex characteristics, SA, or other valid indicators of biologic maturity may be a practical tool for equitable matching in youth sports, it may not necessarily be accurate or valid for matching opponents on behavior and psychologic factors. A younger physically mature athlete may be matched with older athletes, who are biologically similar but psychologically more mature and tactically more proficient as a result of longer experience. Potential psychologic effects associated with moving up (e.g., increased competitive stress, behavioral insecurity) or moving down (e.g., drop-out, lower self-esteem) associated with maturity matching also need to be considered (Hergenroeder 1998; Kontos & Malina 2003).

The prudent implementation of matching using a combination of physical size and maturity, as well as psychologic, behavioral, and other factors, needs to be more systematically evaluated. In spite of being logistically difficult to implement, a matching system, if implemented properly, may be beneficial to equalizing competition, to maintaining interest in participation, and to reducing potential for injury (Kontos & Malina 2003).

In the context of national or international competition in early entry sports (e.g., gymnastics, diving, tennis, and figure skating) the issue of CA and biologic age limits needs careful evaluation. Should biologic age limits be imposed (e.g., skeletal age of 15 years)? Such changes may be desirable for the sake of the health and well-being of the children involved.

Challenges for future research

Longitudinal or mixed longitudinal studies of growth and performance (strength, motor, aerobic, anaerobic) on sufficiently large samples of female adolescents are needed. Mixed longitudinal studies are recommended because information can be collected over a shorter period, but such studies need to be carefully planned to include cohorts that are followed over a short period but are selected so that they overlap in time (Goldstein 1979). Control for test or learning effects needs to be built into the study design (van't Hof *et al.* 1976).

The impact of intensive training on saltatory growth (Lampl *et al.* 1992) and/or mini-growth spurts (Hermanussen *et al.* 1988) needs evaluation.

Muscular strength and endurance and aerobic power show well-defined adolescent spurts in boys. Can performance be enhanced by training during the spurts? This question implies that knowledge about somatic growth and maturation be incorporated into experimental studies of various training programs.

There is need for prospective longitudinal studies of youth training for different sports from the prepubertal years through puberty. Such studies should include a variety of somatic, maturity, and performance characteristics together with specific information about training programs, nutrition, and hormonal secretions.

For issues that require invasive methods, animal models that closely replicate the human situation may permit experimental control of intervening variables.

The genetic determination of physical performance capacities and genotype–environment interactions (training, physical activity, nutrition) needs study in children and youth.

In the context of national or international competitions in early entry sports (e.g., gymnastics, diving, tennis, and figure skating), the issue of age limits—chronologic and/or biologic—needs consideration. Should biologic age limits be imposed? Such changes may be desirable for the sake of the health and well-being of young athletes.

References

American Academy of Pediatrics, Committee on Sports Medicine (1988) Recommendations for participation in competitive sports. *Pediatrics* **81**, 737–739.

Armstrong, N. & Welsman, J.R. (1994) Assessment and interpretation of aerobic fitness in children and adolescents. *Exercise and Sport Sciences Reviews* **22**, 435–476.

Armstrong, N. & Welsman, J.R. (2000) Aerobic fitness. In: *Paediatric Exercise Science and Medicine* (Armstrong, N. & van Mechelen W., eds.) University Press, Oxford: 173–182.

Asmussen, E. (1962) Muscular performance. In: *Muscle as a Tissue* (Rodahl, K. & Horvath, S.M., eds.) McGraw Hill, New York: 161–175.

Asmussen, E. & Heebøll-Nielsen, K. (1955) A dimensional analysis of performance and growth in boys. *Journal of Applied Physiology* **7**, 593–603.

Bastos, F.V. & Hegg, R.V. (1986) The relationship of chronological age, body build, and sexual maturation to handgrip strength in schoolboys ages 10 through 17 years. In: *Perspectives in Kinanthropometry* (Day, J.A.P., ed.) Human Kinetics, Champaign, IL: 45–49.

Bernink, M.J.E., Erich, W.B.M., Peltenburg, A.L., Zonderland, M.L. & Huisveld, I.A. (1983) Height, body composition, biological maturation and training in relation to socio-economic status in girl gymnasts, swimmers, and controls. *Growth* **47**, 1–12.

Beunen, G. (1989) Biological age in pediatric exercise research. In: *A dvances in Pediatric Sport Sciences* Volume 3: *Biological Issues* (Bar-Or, O., ed.) Human Kinetics, Champaign, IL: 1–39.

Beunen, G., Baxter-Jones, A., Mirwald, R.L., *et al.* (2002) Intraindividual allometric development of aerobic power in 8- to 16-year-old boys. *Medicine and Science in Sports and Exercise* **33**, 503–510.

Beunen, G., Claessens, A. & Van Esser, M. (1981a) Somatic and motor characteristics of female gymnasts. *Medicine and Sport* **15**, 176–185.

Beunen, G., Colla, R., Simons, J., *et al.* (1989) Sexual dimorphism in somatic and motor characteristics. In: *Children and Exercise XIII* (Oseid, S. & Carlsen, K.-H., eds.) Human Kinetics, Champaign, IL: 83–90.

Beunen, G. & Malina, R.M. (1988) Growth and physical performance relative to the timing of the adolescent spurt. *Exercise and Sport Science Reviews* **16**, 503–540.

Beunen, G.P., Malina, R.M., Lefevre, J., *et al.* (1997a) Skeletal maturation, somatic growth and physical fitness of girls 6–16 years of age. *International Journal of Sports Medicine* **18**, 413–419.

Beunen, G.P., Malina, R.M., Renson, R., Simons, J., Ostyn, M. & Lefevre, J. (1992) Physical activity and growth, maturation and performance: a longitudinal study. *Medicine and Science in Sports and Exercise* **24**, 576–585.

Beunen, G.P., Malina, R.M., Van't Hof, M.A., *et al.* (1988) *Adolescent Growth and Motor Performance: A Longitudinal Study of Belgian Boys.* Human Kinetics, Champaign, IL.

Beunen, G., Ostyn, M., Renson, R., Simons, J. & Van Gerven, D. (1978) Motor performance as related to chronological age and maturation. In: *Physical Fitness Assessment: Principles, Practice and Application* (Shephard, R.J. & Lavallée, L., eds.) C.C. Thomas, Springfield, IL: 229–236.

Beunen, G., Ostyn, M., Simons, J., Renson, R. & Van Gerven, D. (1981b) Chronological and biological age as related to physical fitness in boys 12 to 19 years. *Annals of Human Biology* **8**, 321–331.

Beunen, G.P., Rogers, D.M., Woynarowska, B. & Malina, R.M. (1997b) Longitudinal study of ontogenetic allometry of oxygen uptake in boys and girls grouped by maturity status. *Annals of Human Biology* **24**, 33–43.

Beunen, G.P. & Simons, J. (1990) Physical growth, maturation and performance. In: *Growth and Fitness of Flemish Girls: The Leuven Growth Study* (Simons, J., Beunen, G.P., Renson, R., Claesens, A.L.M., Vanreusel, B. & Lefevre, J.A.V., eds.) Human Kinetics, Champaign, IL: 69–118.

Boas, F. (1892) The growth of children. *Science* 19–20, 256–257, 281–282, 351–352.

Bouchard, C., Leblanc, C., Malina, R.M. & Hollmann, W. (1978) Skeletal age and submaximal capacity in boys. *Annals of Human Biology* **5**, 75–78.

Bouchard, C., Malina, R.M., Hollmann, W. & Leblanc, C. (1976) Relationship between skeletal maturity and submaximal working capacity in boys 8 to 18 years. *Medicine and Science in Sports* **8**, 186–190.

Carron, A.V. & Bailey, D.A. (1974) Strength development in boys from 10 through 16 years. *Monographs of the Society for Research in Child Development* **39** (Serial No. 157).

Caine, D.J. & Broekhoff, J. (1987) Maturity assessment: A viable preventive measure against physical and psychological insult to the young athlete? *The Physician and Sports Medicine* **15**, 67–80.

Claessens, A.L., Veer, F.M., Stijnen, V., *et al.* (1991) Anthropometric characteristics of outstanding male and female gymnasts. *Journal of Sports Sciences* **9**, 53–74.

Clapp, J.F. & Little, K.D. (1995) The interaction between regular exercise and selected aspects of women's health. *American Journal of Obstetrics and Gynecology* **173**, 2–9.

Clarke, H.H. (1971) *Physical and Motor Tests in the Medford Boys' Growth Study.* Prentice-Hall, Englewood Cliffs, NJ.

Crampton, C.W. (1908) Physiological age: A fundamental principle. *American Physical Education Review* **13**, 141–154.

Daly, R.M., Caine, D., Bass, S.L., Pieter, W. & Broekhoff, J. (2005) Growth of highly versus moderately trained competitive female artistic gymnasts. *Medicine and Science in Sports and Exercise* **37**, 1053–1060.

Eisenmann, J.C. & Malina, R.M. (2002) Growth status and estimated growth rate of young distance runners. *International Journal of Sports Medicine* **23**, 168–173.

Ellis, B.J. (2004) Timing of pubertal maturation in girls: An integrated life history approach. *Psychological Bulletin* **130**, 920–958.

Espenschade, A. (1940) Motor performance in adolescence, including the study of relationships with measures of physical growth and maturity. *Monographs of the Society for Research in Child Development* **5** (Serial No. 24).

Faust, M.S. (1977) Somatic development of adolescent girls. *Monograph of the Society for Research in Child Development* **42** (Serial No. 169).

Gallagher, J.R. (1969) Problems in matching competitors: Adolescents, athletics and competitive sports. *Clinical Pediatrics* **8**, 434–436.

Geithner, C.A., Thomis, M.A., Vanden Eynde, B., *et al.* (2004) Growth in peak aerobic power during adolescence. *Medicine and Science in Sport and Exercise* **36**, 1616–1624.

Goldstein, H. (1979) *The Design and Analysis of Longitudinal Studies.* Academic Press, London.

Haubenstricker, J.L. & Seefeldt, V.D. (1986) Acquisition of motor skills during childhood. In: *Physical Activity and Well-being* (Seefeldt V., ed.) AAHPERD, Reston, VA: 41–102.

Hebbelinck, M., Borms, J. & Clarys, J. (1971) La variabilité de l'âge squelettique et les corrélations avec la capacité de travail chez des garçons de 5me année primaire. *Kinanthropologie* **3**, 125–135.

Heras Yague, P. & de la Fuente, J.M. (1998) Changes in height and motor performance relative to peak height velocity: A mixed longitudinal study of Spanish boys and girls. *American Journal of Human Biology* **10**, 647–660.

Hergenroeder, A.C. (1998) Prevention of sports injuries. *Pediatrics* **101**, 1057–1063.

Hemanussen, M., Geiger-Benoit, K., Burmeister, J. & Sippel, W.G. (1988) Periodical changes of short term growth velocity ("mini growth spurts") in human growth. *Annals of Human Biology* **15**, 103–109.

Hollmann, W. & Bouchard, C. (1970) Untersuchungen über die Beziehungen zwischen chronologischem und biologischem Alter zu spiroergometrischen Messgrössen, Herzvolumen, anthropometrischen Daten und Skelettmuskelkraft bei 8–18 jährigen Jungen. *Zeitschrift für Kreislaufforschung* **59**, 160–176.

Jones, H.E. (1949) *Motor Performance and Growth: A Developmental Study of Static Dynamometric Strength.* University of California Press, Berkeley, CA.

Katzmarzyk, P.T., Malina, R.M. & Beunen, G.P. (1997) The contribution of biological maturation to the strength and motor fitness of children. *Annals of Human Biology* **24**, 493–505.

Kemper, H.C.G. (ed.) (1985) *Growth, Health and Fitness of Teenagers.* Karger, Basel.

Kemper, H.C.G. & Verschuur, R. (1985) Motor performance fitness tests. In: *Growth, Health and Fitness of Teenagers* (Kemper, H.C.G., ed.) Karger, Basel: 96–106.

Kemper, H.C.G., Verschuur, R., Ras, K.G.A., Snel, J., Splinter, P.G., & Tavecchio, L.W.C. (1975) Biological age and habitual physical activity in relation to physical fitness in 12- and 13-year-old schoolboys. *Zeitschrift für Kinderheilkunde* **119**, 169–179.

Kemper, H.C.G., Verschuur, R. & Ritmeester, J.W. (1986) Maximal aerobic power in early and late maturing teenagers. In: *Children and Exercise XII* (Rutenfranz, J., Mocellin, R. & Klimt, F., eds.) Human Kinetics, Champaign, IL: 220–221.

Kontos, A.P. & Malina, R.M. (2003) Youth sports in the 21st centery: Overview and directions. In: *Youth Sports: Perspectives for a New Century* Malina, R.M. & Clark, M.A., eds.) Coaches Choice, Monterey, CA: 240–253.

Krahenbuhl, G.S., Skinner, J.S. & Kohrt, W.M. (1985) Developmental aspects of maximal aerobic power in children. *Exercise and Sports Science Reviews* **13**, 503–538.

Labitzke, H. (1971) Über Beziehungen zwischen biologischen Alter (Ossifikationsalter) und der Körperlänge, den Körpergewicht und der Körperoberfläche sowie der maximalen Sauerstoffaufnahme. *Medizin und Sport* **11**, 82–86.

Lampl, M., Veldhuis, J.D. & Johnson, M.L. (1992) Saltation and stasis: A model of human growth. *Science* **258**, 801–803.

Lefevre, J., Beunen, G., Steens, G., Claessens, A. & Renson, R. (1990) Motor performance during adolescence and age thirty as related to age at peak height velocity. *Annals of Human Biology* **17**, 423–434.

Little, N.G., Day, J.A.P. & Steinke, L. (1997) Relationship of physical performance to maturation in perimenarcheal girls. *American Journal of Human Biology* **9**, 163–171.

Loucks, A.B., Vaitukaitis, J., Cameron, J.L., *et al.* (1992) The reproductive system and exercise in women. *Medicine and Science in Sports and Exercise* **24** (Suppl 6), S288–S289.

Malina, R.M. (1975) Anthropometric correlates of strength and motor performance. *Exercise and Sport Sciences Reviews* **3**, 249–274.

Malina, R.M. (1983) Menarche in athletes: a synthesis and hypothesis. *Annals of Human Biology* **10**, 1–24.

Malina, R.M. (1991) Darwinian fitness, physical fitness and physical activity. In: *Applications of Biological Anthropology to Human Affairs* (Mascie-Taylor, C.G.N. & Lasker, G.W., eds.) Cambridge University Press, Cambridge: 143–184.

Malina, R.M. (1994a) Physical growth and biological maturation of young athletes. *Exercise and Sport Sciences Reviews* **22**, 389–433.

Malina, R.M. (1994b) Physical activity and training: effects on stature and the adolescent growth spurt. *Medicine and Science in Sports and Exercise* **26**, 759–766.

Malina, R.M. (1998a) Growth and maturation of young athletes: Is training for sport a factor? In: *Sport and Children* (Chang, K.M. & Micheli, L., eds.) Williams & Wilkins, Hong Kong: 133–161.

Malina, R.M. (1998b) Physical activity, sport, social status and Darwinian fitness. In: *Human Biology and Social Inequality* (Strickland, S.S. & Shetty, P.S., eds.) Cambridge University Press, Cambridge: 165–192.

Malina, R.M. (1999) Growth and maturation of elite female gymnasts: Is training a factor. In: *Human Growth in Context* (Johnston, F.E., Zemel, B. & Eveleth, P.B., eds.) Smith-Gordon, London: 291–301.

Malina, R.M. (2002) The young athlete: Biological growth and maturation in a biocultural context. In: *Children and Youth in Sport: A Biopsychosocial Perspective*, 2nd edn. (Smoll, F.L. & Smith, R.E., eds.) Brown and Benchmark, Dubuque, IA: 261–292.

Malina, R.M. (2004) *Growth and maturation of child and adolescent track and field athletes: Final report.* The International Athletic Foundation, Monaco.

Malina, R.M., Beunen, G., Wellens, R. & Claessens, A. (1986) Skeletal maturity and body size of teenage Belgian track and field athletes. *Annals of Human Biology* **13**, 331–339.

Malina, R.M. & Bielicki, T. (1996) Retrospective longitudinal growth study of boys and girls active in sport. *Acta Paediatrica* **85**, 570–576.

Malina, R.M., Bouchard, C. & Bar-Or, O. (2004) *Growth, Maturation and Physical Activity*, 2nd edn. Human Kinetics, Champaign, IL.

Malina, R.M., Eveld, D.J. & Woynarowska, B. (1990) Growth and sexual maturation of active Polish children 11–14 years of age. *Hermes (Leuven)* **21**, 341–353.

Malina R.M., Beunen, G., Lefevre, J. & Woynarowska, B. (1997) Maturity-associated variation in peak oxygen uptake in active adolescent boys and girls. *Annals of Human Biology* **24**, 19–31.

Mirwald, R.L. & Bailey, D.A. (1986) *Maximal Aerobic Power: A Longitudinal Analysis*. Sports Dynamics, London, Ontario.

Novotny, V.V. & Taftlova, R. (1971) Biological age and sport fitness of young gymnast women. In: *Anthropological Congress Dedicated to Ales Hrdlicka* (Novotny, V.V., ed.) Academia, Prague: 123–130.

Peltenburg, A.L., Erich, W.B.M., Berninck, M.J.E., Zonderland, M.L. & Huisveld, I.A. (1984) Biological maturation, body composition, and growth of female gymnasts and control group of schoolgirls and girls swimmers aged 8 to 14 years: a cross-sectional survey of 1064 girls. *International Journal of Sports Medicine* **5**, 36–42.

Plowman, S.A., Liu, N.Y. & Wells, C.L. (1991) Body composition and sexual maturation in premenarcheal athletes and non-athletes. *Medicine and Science in Sports and Exercise* **23**, 23–29.

Rarick, G.L. & Oyster, N. (1964) Physical maturity, muscular strength, and motor performance of young school-age boys. *Research Quarterly* **35**, 523–531.

Roemmich, J.N. & Sinning, W.E. (1997a) Weight loss and wrestling training: Effects on nutrition, growth, maturation, body composition, and strength. *Journal of Applied Physiology* **82**, 1751–1759.

Roemmich, J.N. & Sinning, W.E. (1997b) Weight loss and wrestling training: Effects on growth-related hormones.

Journal of Applied Physiology **82**, 1760–1764.

Rotch, T.M. (1909) A study of the development of the bones in early childhood by the Roentgen method, with the view of establishing a developmental index for the grading of and the protection of early life. *Transactions of the Association of American Physicians* **24**, 603–624.

Rutenfranz, J., Andersen, K., Seliger, V., *et al*. (1982) Maximal aerobic power affected by maturation and body growth during childhood and adolescence. *European Journal of Pediatrics* **139**, 106–112.

Savov, S.G. (1978) Physical fitness and skeletal maturity in girls and boys 11 years of age. In: *Physical Fitness Assessment: Practice and Application* (Shephard, R.J. & Lavallée, H., eds.) C.C. Thomas, Springfield, IL: 222–228.

Seefeldt, V. (1981) Equating children for sports competition: Some common problems and suggested solutions. *Motor Development: Theory into Practice* **3**, 13–22.

Seils, L.R.G. (1951) The relationship between measurements of physical growth and gross motor performance of primary-grade school children. *Research Quarterly* **22**, 244–260.

Shephard, R.J., Lavallée, H., Rajic, K.M., Jéquier, J.C., Brisson, G., & Beaucage, C. (1978) Radiographic age in the interpretation of physiological and

anthropological data. In: *Pediatric Work Physiology* (Borms, J. & Hebbelinck, M., eds.) Karger, Basel: 124–133.

Stolz, H.R. & Stolz, L.M. (1951) *Somatic Development of Adolescent Boys*. Macmillan, New York.

Tanner, J.M. (1962) *Growth at Adolescence*, 2nd edn. Blackwell, Oxford.

Tanner, J.M. (1978) *Foetus into Man: Physical Growth from Conception to Maturity*. Open Books, London.

Theintz, G.E., Howald, H., Weiss, U. & Sizonenko, P.C. (1993) Evidence for a reduction of growth potential in adolescent female gymnasts. *Journal of Pediatrics* **122**, 306–313.

Thomis, M., Claessens, A.L., Lefevre, J., Philippaerts, R., Beunen, G.P. & Malina, R.M. (2005) Adolescent growth spurts in female gymnasts. *Journal of Pediatrics* **146**, 239–244.

Van't Hof, M.A., Roede, M.J. & Kowalski, C.J. (1976) Estimation of growth velocities from individual longitudinal data. *Growth* **40**, 217–240.

Warren, M.P. (1980) The effects of exercise on pubertal progression and reproductive function in girls. *Journal of Clinical Endocrinology and Metabolism* **51**, 1150–1156.

Zemel, B.S. & Johnston, F.E. (1994) Application of the Preece–Baines growth model to cross-sectional data: Problems of validity and interpretation. *American Journal of Human Biology* **6**, 563–570.

Chapter 2

Muscle Development During Childhood and Adolescence

DAVID A. JONES AND JOAN M. ROUND

When it comes to skeletal muscle, size really does matter for the adult athlete. Quality is also important, the power athlete needs large, fast muscles while the endurance athlete must have relatively small, slow, and highly oxidative muscles. Skeletal muscle is very adaptable, responding to different training regimens but the muscle characteristics of the elite performers are the result of prolonged training and the raw material that was laid down in the embryo, during childhood and adolescence. We will therefore trace the development of muscle from its earliest appearance through to the young adult.

Embryonic origins

Skeletal muscle is derived from myogenic cells in the embryonic mesoderm. At about 6 weeks' gestation these mesodermal stem cells migrate to appropriate sites and begin to differentiate to form myoblasts which proliferate and eventually fuse to form multinucleate primary myotubes attached at each end to the developing tendons and skeleton. Within the developing myotubes a central chain of nuclei forms surrounded by basophilic cytoplasm rich in polyribosomes. The transition from myoblasts to myotubes is initiated by the expression of a group of muscle transcription factors, products of the *myf* genes. Myoblast proliferation in tissue culture is strongly stimulated by insulin-like growth factor 1 (IGF1) and their fusion to form myotubes can be induced by reducing the IGF1 concentration in the medium but whether this mechanism applies *in vivo* is not clear.

Mid-way along the primary myotubes further myoblasts aggregate and fuse to form secondary myotubes. At first the primary and secondary myotubes share a common basement membrane but eventually the secondary myotubes develop a separate membrane, make contact with the tendon, and become independent of the primaries. The proportions of primary and secondary myotubes may vary between muscles and between individuals. The soleus, a "slow" muscle, contains a predominance of fibers derived from primary myotubes, while in faster muscles the majority of fibers originate from secondary myotubes.

In the human fetus the transition from myoblasts to primary myotubes takes place at around 7–9 weeks' gestation and by the end of this period the primordia of most muscle groups are well defined. At this time the synthesis of the contractile proteins, actin and myosin, begins and the first signs of cross-striation are visible within the myotubes (Fig. 2.1).

From 11 weeks onwards there is a proliferation of myofibrils leading to an increase in diameter of the myotubes, which also grow in length. At 16–17 weeks a further population of myotubes becomes apparent, known as the tertiary myotubes adhering to the secondary myotubes and enclosed within the same basement membrane but by 18–23 weeks the tertiary myotubes have become independent. At around this time the nuclei of the more mature myotubes move to the periphery and this marks the appearance of fibers that have the characteristic structure of adult muscle fibers, although being much smaller in size.

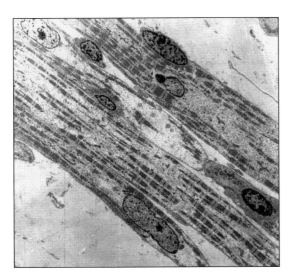

Fig. 2.1 Myoblasts fusing to form myotubes and starting to synthesize contractile proteins arranged in the characteristic sarcomeres of skeletal muscle.

Satellite cells

Muscle fibers constitute a syncitium, each fiber being multinucleate and in this respect they differ from every other tissue in the body. Although the majority of myoblasts fuse to form myotubes, about 10% of myoblasts remain as undifferentiated muscle stem, or satellite, cells that will provide the nuclear material for future growth and repair. The satellite cells lie between the plasma membrane and the basement membrane of muscle fibers and each consists of a large nucleus with a thin layer of cytoplasm. Nuclei within the muscle fibers are post-mitotic and do not divide. Consequently, the only source of new nuclear material for growth is the satellite cells. It is not clear, however, whether this pool of cells is sufficient for all future requirements or if the pool can be replenished, or expanded, by multipotent stem cells from sources outside the muscle.

Developing fibers express a number of different myosin heavy chains, these include an embryonic form and an intermediate fast type 2c form which is also seen in regenerating adult muscle. The primary myotubes can be identified throughout embryonic development as they alone express adult slow myosin from about 9 weeks' gestation (Draeger *et al.* 1987). In response to the contractile activity imposed by the motor nerve following innervation by axons growing out from the spinal cord, the fibers begin to differentiate so that, eventually, fetal myosins are no longer expressed and about half the fibers express slow myosin and half fast myosin. This process, which is apparent by about 32 weeks' gestation, is probably not fully completed in human muscle until a few months after birth.

Connections between nerve and muscle

In the human embryo, as early as 10–11 weeks' gestation, axons from motoneurons grow out of the spinal cord and invade the fetal muscle. At first a number of axons form synapses with each embryonic fiber but as the muscle matures all but one of the synapses are lost. The loss of multiple innervation appears to be brought about by the contractile activity of the developing fiber which, paradoxically, is the result of stimulation by the same attached nerve endings (Vrbová *et al.* 1995). The first contacts between nerve and muscle occur between axons and the primary myotubes, leading, at first, to multiple innervation as described above. Later, as the multiple innervation is lost, the secondary myotubes become innervated by the axons that have been rejected by the primary myotubes. This sequence of innervation may have consequences for the later development of different fiber types because many of the fibers derived from primary myotubes are constrained to become slow type 1 fibers with, apparently, little opportunity for change. The fibers derived from secondary myotubes, however, have the ability to change the expression of a wide range of contractile and other proteins depending on the pattern of activity imposed on the muscle.

The athletic potential of an individual is determined to a large extent by the size and contractile characteristics of their muscles. Although training over many years will modify the size, speed, and fatiguability of their muscles, some individuals, usually with a mesomorphic body shape, are naturally heavily muscled while others are of a relatively slight build. Top class sprinters are heavily muscled all over their body, not just in the major propulsive muscles in the lower body and limbs, and their muscles have a predominance of fast type 2 fibers. Endurance athletes, on the other hand, tend to be ectomorphic, with a smaller skeleton and musculature that has a predominance of slow type 1 fibers. It is unproven, but nevertheless tempting to speculate, that the difference between these two extremes may originate in the numbers of secondary and tertiary myotubes. Where there is an excess of the secondary and tertiary myotubes these can develop into large, fast muscles. Individuals with minimal secondary and tertiary myotube development will have a predominance of slower fibers because the primary myotubes seem predestined to remain slow. It is possible therefore that the potential for elite athletic performance is laid down in the embryo in the 6–7-week period when the secondary and tertiary myotubes are developing.

Muscle fiber growth

In the rat, muscle fiber numbers have been shown to remain constant during life while the mean fiber cross-sectional area increases nearly 10-fold from the newborn to adult animal (Rowe & Goldspink 1969). There are considerable practical and ethical problems involved in making measurements of fiber size and number in children and adults although it is clear that there are major changes in muscle fiber size during development (Fig. 2.2). The cross-sectional area of fibers in a biopsy from the quadriceps muscle in a normal man range from means of 3500 to 7500 μm^2 and in normal women from 2000 to 5000 μm^2 (Round et al. 1982). The average cross-sectional area of the quadriceps muscle, measured at mid femur, is approximately 60 cm^2 in women and 80 cm^2 in men (Chapman et al. 1984), roughly in proportion to the muscle fiber cross-sectional areas, which suggests that the number of fibers is similar between the sexes. There are very limited data of this type on children but the indications are that the ratio of muscle cross-sectional area to that of the fibers is the same as found for adults, suggesting that the number of fibers remains constant during development, as is the case in rats.

Muscle growth requires the deposition of new proteins and this can occur in two ways. The first is

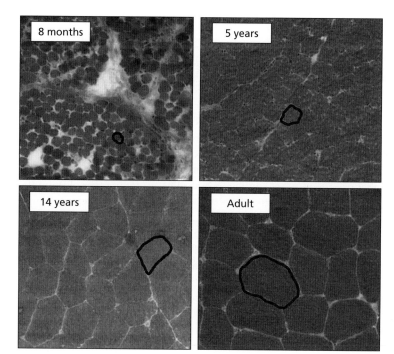

Fig. 2.2 Growth of muscle fiber cross-sectional area. Biopsies from an 8-month-old baby, a 5-year-old child, a 14-year-old boy, and a large 23-year-old man. Transverse sections of quadriceps muscle samples, stained with trichrome. An individual fiber has been outlined in each section to emphasize the change in fiber size with growth and maturation.

an increase in the amount of protein synthesized per unit of DNA, either by increasing transcription or translation. A decrease in the rate of protein breakdown would also have the same effect. The second major mechanism for growth is by nuclear division and it is established that it is the satellite cell nuclei that divide (Mauro 1961). In postnatal life the dividing satellite cells are incorporated into existing fibers, rather than forming new fibers, thereby increasing the nuclear material available within the fiber to support protein synthesis. The notion is that a muscle fiber nucleus can support a certain maximum volume of cytoplasm (nuclear domain) and in order to increase in volume the fiber must acquire more nuclei. Clearly, both mechanisms are possible. Cheek (1985) suggested that during the course of human development there is a 14–20-fold increase in the DNA content of skeletal muscle and a twofold increase in the DNA unit size (i.e., growth being predominantly caused by an increase in nuclear number). Short-term fluctuations in size and strength, such as with dietary manipulation or as the result of prolonged bed rest or immobilization, may be the result of a change in the protein synthesis per unit DNA. Long-term increases in muscle size, such as seen during growth, certainly require nuclear proliferation. The precise details of which phase of growth depends on nuclear proliferation and which on expanding the nuclear domain remain to be elucidated.

Relationship between muscle size and strength

In an idealized parallel fiber muscle, the isometric force generated is proportional to its cross-sectional area; however, muscle fibers work within a mechanical system of tendons and bones which modifies the forces exerted on the external world.

Angle of muscle fiber insertion

Very few muscles have fibers that simply run from end to end; in most cases fibers insert obliquely into their tendons at angles of around 10–20° and consequently the force transmitted by the tendon is somewhat less than that generated by the muscle fibers (Alexander & Vernon 1975). It is possible that during development the angle of pennation may change, thus changing the force produced in relation to the anatomic cross-section of muscle, but there is no information available on this point.

Lever ratios

Muscle strength is measured indirectly through the lever system of the skeleton. Consequently, the force measured at the ankle or wrist is the force of the muscle multiplied by the mechanical advantage (or disadvantage) of the lever system. For knee extension, the force measured at the ankle is the force generated by the quadriceps in the patella tendon multiplied by the ratio of the size of the patella tuberocity and the length of the tibia. The ratio is about 1 : 10 so that a force of 500 N measured at the ankle represents a force of about 5000 N in the patella tendon. Because the patella tuberocity is relatively small, a change in relative location of a few millimeters could have a major effect on the ratio and consequently the force measured at the ankle (Jones & Round 2000). During childhood and adolescence there is continual remodeling of the bones and we do not know if the relative dimensions remain constant or change during development.

Measurement of force, practical considerations

Much of the information about muscle development comes from measurements of force because repeated biopsies are unsuitable for children and until the recent developments of magnetic resonance imaging (MRI) and ultrasound, X-ray and computed tomography (CT) scanning were likewise of limited application. Strength can be assessed in many ways. There is sometimes a conflict between the interests of athletic coaches and sports scientists. The former need a measure that is "relevant" to their sport while the physiologist is concerned to make measurements that reflect the structure and contractile properties of individual muscle groups. The difficulty is that "relevant" measurements usually involve complex muscle groups where performance will depend not only on the size and strength of individual muscles, but also on their coordinated activation. As an example, in most people the individual muscles in left and right arms are much the same size and can generate similar forces, yet if asked to perform some task such as hitting or throwing they will do far better with their dominant side. Even a simple test such as pushing or pulling requires the coordinated action of stabilizing muscles all over the body for optimal performance. For these reasons the measurement of isometric force of major muscle groups such as the knee extensors (quadriceps), the forearm flexors (mainly biceps), or plantar flexors (calf muscles) represents the best option for physiologic assessment. It is generally most convenient to measure force with the appropriate joint at 90° because it is usually easiest to stabilize the limb in this position and problems of compensating for the weight of the limb do not arise. However, it should be remembered that a joint angle of 90° may not set the muscle at its optimal length. The optimal angle depends on both muscle fiber and tendon length so it is possible that the angle, and thus the force recorded, will change during development.

It is often suggested that dynamic shortening contractions are a more "natural" movement and should be measured. The force generated during a dynamic contraction, however, is difficult to measure and the commercial equipment available is not portable or particularly accurate. If dynamic measurements are made it should be remembered that the force recorded will depend on the speed of the muscle as well as its size, and that speed is influenced both by the intrinsic fiber type composition and the overall length of the muscle.

There are two further complications to be aware of when making measurements of strength. The first is that a voluntary effort may not fully activate the muscle. This can be checked by superimposing electrical stimulation on the voluntary effort and in healthy adults this reveals that most people can produce 90–95% full activation (Rutherford *et al.* 1986). There is generally a reluctance to use electrical stimulation with children but our experience is that over the age of about 6–7 years children can activate their muscles in a similar way to adults. However, below that age children seem to find it difficult to isolate the movement required.

The other complicating factor is that with every contraction of an agonist there may also be co-contraction of the antagonist muscles which will reduce the force that is measured (Kellis & Baltzopoulos 1999). Estimates of antagonist activity during knee extension in adults vary widely and may well depend on the joint angle, but generally amount to about 10% of the measured force. Thus, taking the shortfall in voluntary activation and the action of the antagonist muscles, the measured force of the quadriceps may be 15–20% less than the force the muscle is truly capable of. Provided this proportion remains constant it will not affect the conclusion of any survey but the difficulty is that we do not know if this is the case for children.

Growth studies and the measurement of strength

There have been a number of longitudinal studies charting the development of strength during adolescence and a few that include younger children. Tanner (1962) provides a comprehensive review of the earlier work. The most frequently quoted early work relating to strength is that of Jones (1949) on the adolescent group in the University of California Child Welfare Study. The static strength of hand grip, arm pull, and arm thrust were measured using an isometric dynamometer. The most striking feature of the results is the clear separation in strength between boys and girls that occurs at the time of puberty (Fig. 2.3).

Stoltz & Stoltz (1951) reported data on Californian boys during adolescence (part of the Fells Growth Study) and Faust (1977) complemented the Stoltzs' work with her study of a group of Californian girls with similar findings to those of Carron & Bailey (1974) on boys from the Saskatchewan Growth Study. All of these studies emphasize the fact that, in sharp contrast to girls, there is a major increase in strength of boys during puberty. More recently, Beunen *et al.* (1988) have measured static, dynamic, and explosive strength in Belgian boys as part of the Leuven Growth Study, and motor performance and similar tests have been used by Kemper & Verschuur (1985a,b) with Dutch children in the Amsterdam Growth Study. Round *et al.* (1999) reported the

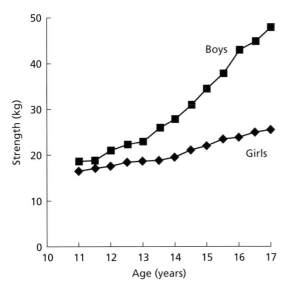

Fig. 2.3 Changes in arm strength with age. Data for "arm pull" taken from the mixed longitudinal study of Jones (1949). Note that strength is reported in kilogram force, equivalent to 9.81 N.

isometric strength of quadriceps and biceps in a longitudinal study of British children from north London (Fig. 2.4).

It is generally agreed that during childhood there is a steady increase in strength with little difference seen between boys and girls until puberty when both sexes show a significant increase in the velocity of

strength gain. At this time boys increase to a greater final strength than girls and show a disproportionate increase in the upper limb musculature which reaches a final strength that is nearly double that of young women.

The only suggestion of a sex difference in strength before puberty involves muscular actions of the arms. Jones (1949) reported greater handgrip strength and others have commented on the superiority of over arm throwing in boys (reviewed by Malina 1998). After puberty it is clear that boys' strength increases but Jones (1949) remarked that girls seem to decrease in strength after menarche. This suggestion was supported by Faust (1977) but she cautioned that dynamometer strength testing might be unreliable as a measure of strength in teenage girls and that the decrease she found was most likely a result of the teenage girls not trying so hard. Our own experience of post-menarchial girls is that they showed no loss of strength (Round et al. 1999); this may be because we were using isometric strength testing in which the components of skill and coordination are minimized.

Early reports on the timing of the adolescent spurt in strength suggested that it occurred around the time of the peak of height velocity (Jones 1949; Tanner 1962) but more recent reports place it about 1 year after peak height velocity and roughly coincident with that of weight velocity (Beunen et al. 1988).

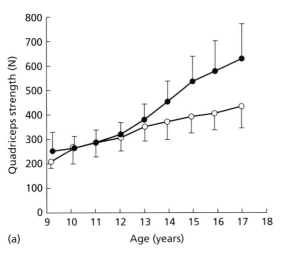

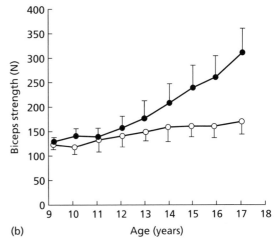

Fig. 2.4 Changes in strength with age. Mixed longitudinal study in which the isometric strength of the quadriceps (a) and elbow flexors (biceps, b) was measured in boys (filled symbols) and girls (open symbols). Data from Round et al. (1999).

The old adage that boys may outgrow their strength at some period during puberty was questioned by Tanner in the 1960s and finds no support from modern studies. Neither in the Leuven study (Beunen *et al.* 1988) nor the north London study (Round *et al.* 1999) was there any time during puberty where strength failed to increase.

Stimuli for muscle growth during development

Growth and maintenance of all tissues is dependent on the presence of an extracellular environment containing the appropriate mixture of amino acids, carbohydrates, and growth factors and it is evident that muscle is the same as all other tissues in this respect. Thyroid and growth hormones are obviously required for normal growth and in their absence the main consequence is a general retardation of growth affecting all tissues. However, in the case of growth hormone deficiency in children there is a change in body composition such that more adipose tissue is laid down at the expense of muscle (Rutherford *et al.* 1990). What is not clear for muscle, or any tissue, is what drives growth in the early years when, for instance, growth hormone levels are relatively low, or what causes growth to stop when the adult size has been reached.

As the young body grows we might expect the muscles attached to the long bones to increase in proportion to the linear dimensions and, if this were the case, the cross-sectional area of the muscle (which is the main determinant of isomeric strength) would then be proportional to the square of the linear dimensions (Jones *et al.* 2004). It is evident, however, that in this situation, strength would lag behind body weight because weight is proportional to the third power of the linear dimensions. The observation is that for the quadriceps, strength is very nearly proportional to body weight during childhood growth so the stimulus for muscle growth must be more than the lengthening of the long bones and the muscle is probably responding to the load imposed upon it (Parker *et al.* 1990). Interestingly, for the biceps, a muscle that is not weight bearing, strength increases roughly as the square of the linear dimensions, at least in girls and also for boys up to the age of puberty.

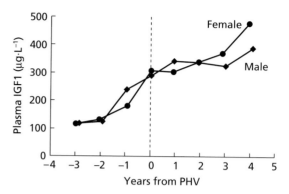

Fig. 2.5 Circulating insulin-like growth factor 1 (IGF1) levels and the changes with puberty. Mean values for plasma IGF1 measured in a mixed longitudinal study of boys and girls going through puberty. Data have been aligned to the time of peak height velocity (PHV; vertical dotted line). Unpublished data from the study of Round *et al.* (1999).

At puberty there is a general rapid increase in body size, including the skeletal musculature, which is associated with increased secretion of growth hormone and circulating IGF1 (Fig. 2.5). For girls, there is an increase in quadriceps strength which is commensurate with the increase in weight, while biceps strength increases minimally. For boys, however, puberty is a time of considerable increase in strength with the increases in both quadriceps and biceps strength far outstripping what would be expected from the change in body size (Fig. 2.4; Round *et al.* 1999).

It is widely believed that testosterone causes muscle hypertrophy although there is relatively little evidence about the effects of physiologic levels, as opposed to the supra-physiologic levels that are abused in many sports. However, the association between the increase in muscle strength (especially of the biceps) in boys and increasing circulating testosterone is very strong (Fig. 2.6; Round *et al.* 1999). Testosterone leads to muscle fiber hypertrophy which is associated with an increase in the number of myonuclei per fiber (and thus, presumably, maintaining a constant nuclear domain) and an increase in satellite cell number (Sinha-Hikim *et al.* 2002, 2003). It is not clear, however, whether testosterone causes proliferation of existing satellite cells or the differentiation of mesenchymal stem cells into a myogenic line.

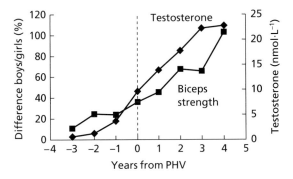

Fig. 2.6 Increases in biceps strength and circulating testosterone in boys. Biceps strength of boys, expressed as a percentage of the strength of girls, compared with the rise in circulating testosterone levels. Data have been aligned to the time of peak height velocity (PHV; vertical dotted line). Data from the study of Round *et al.* (1999).

On average, 17-year-old boys are 50% stronger than girls in the quadriceps but have biceps strength that is almost double that of the girls (Fig. 2.4). This preferential development of the upper limb musculature has been noted in a number of studies. Carron & Bailey (1974) found that measures of upper body strength in boys increased 3.9-fold between the ages of 10 and 16 years while for lower body strength the increase was 2.5-fold. Tanner *et al.* (1981) estimated that peak growth velocity of arm muscles in boys was about twice that in girls while there were no sex differences in the calf. Kemper and Verschuur (1985a), in a longitudinal study measuring muscle volumes, showed that sex differences became apparent at puberty, with a suggestion of greater differences between boys and girls in the upper body musculature.

It would appear therefore that muscles of the upper limb girdle are particularly sensitive to testosterone and it is interesting to speculate on the evolutionary significance of the differences in upper body strength between the sexes. In terms of hunting and gathering, there would seem to be little point in women not having the same strength in the upper body as men, and this leads to the conclusion that it may be a secondary sexual characteristic analogous to the shoulder girdle development seen in many mammalian species, including other primates and cattle. An unscientific survey of female staff and students suggests that excessive

muscular development in men is not particularly attractive to the opposite sex and consequently the upper body development seems more likely to have served in the past as a way of asserting dominance over other males rather than attracting mates.

Muscle growth, strength, and performance

The development of motor performance has been reviewed by Malina & Bouchard (1991) and Malina (1998) and it is important to consider the role that development of muscle strength has in this vital process. Even the simplest task such as jumping or running depends on the interplay of strength and coordination with the complex biomechanics of the musculoskeletal system. For running and explosive tasks such as jumping, the strength to body weight ratio would seem to be a critical factor, yet it is interesting to note that while running speed and jumping performance improve steadily throughout childhood, and often dramatically in teenage boys, the ratio of isometric strength to body weight remains remarkably constant or decreases somewhat until puberty (Jones & Round 2000). One aspect of muscle function that may explain this observation is the influence of changing muscle length. Isometric strength is not dependent on muscle length but the velocity of shortening is directly proportional to the number of sarcomeres in series and this will increase approximately in parallel with height. A faster muscle means that larger forces can be generated at high speeds, generating more power so the muscle will be able to impart a greater impulse to the ground during jumping or move a longer limb at the same angular velocity to impart a greater momentum to the hand or foot when throwing or kicking.

One of the consequences of the greater upper limb girdle development in the male is that performance in throwing events is very much better than that of female competitors. In most track events the differential between men and women is of the order of 10%, which may be explained (albeit with some difficulty) by the differences in strength and length of male and female muscles. For the throwing events, however, the difference is so marked that women throw lighter javelins, hammers, and shots and still do not achieve the same distances as men. World class men throw an 800-g javelin about 90 m while women throw 600 g but achieve only about 70 m. Although it is tempting for a muscle physiologist to ascribe all these differences to the preferential muscle development of the male upper limb girdle, it is notable that, of all performance indicators, over arm throwing is superior in boys and is seen long before the time when sex hormones play their part in promoting upper limb girdle development (Malina 1998). Although prepubertal boys throw better than girls, they are not noticeably stronger in the arms compared with girls at this stage (Fig. 2.4). It is possible therefore that boys acquire the skill of over arm throwing very early in development and that it is one of the social or behavioural markers of maleness.

Muscle development is clearly central to normal growth and development and the growing child provides fascinating information about the factors that regulate muscle growth. When trying to account for changes in performance with increasing maturity, again muscle strength has a central part to play but the relationships are complex and muscle strength has to be seen in the context of many other changes, in development of the skeletal lever system, of skill acquisition, and probably also social attitudes towards certain types of activity and exercise.

References

Alexander, R.McN. & Vernon, A. (1975) The dimensions of the knee and ankle muscles and the forces they exert. *Journal of Human Movement Studies* 1, 115–123.

Beunen, G.P., Malina, R.M., Van't Hof, M.A., *et al.* (1988) *Adolescent Growth and Performance. A Longitudinal Study of Belgian Boys.* Human Kinetics, Champaign, IL.

Carron, A.V. & Bailey, D.A. (1974) Strength development in boys from 10 through 16 years. *Monographs of the Society for Research in Child Development* 39, 1–37.

Chapman, S.J., Grindrod, S.R. & Jones, D.A. (1984) Cross-sectional area and force production of the quadriceps muscle. *Journal of Physiology* 353, 53P.

Cheek, D.B. (1985) The control of cell mass and replication. The DNA unit: a personal 20-year study. *Early Human Development* 12, 211–239.

Draeger, A., Weeds, A.G. & Fitzsimmons, R.B. (1987) Primary, secondary and tertiary myotubes in developing muscle: a new approach to the analysis of human myogenesis. *Journal of the Neurological Sciences* 81, 19–43.

Faust, M.S. (1977) Somatic development of adolescent girls. *Monographs of the Society for Research in Child Development* 42, 1–90.

Jones, D.A. & Round, J.M. (2000) Strength and muscle growth. In: *Paediatric Exercise Science and Medicine* (Armstrong, A. & van Mechelen, W., eds.) Oxford University Press, Oxford: 133–142.

Jones, D.A., Round, J.M. & de Haan, A. (2004) *Skeletal Muscle from Molecules to Movement.* Churchill Livingstone, Edinburgh.

Jones, H.E. (1949) *Motor performance and growth. A Developmental Study of Static Dynamometric Strength.* University of California Press, Berkeley, CA: 34–52.

Kellis, E. & Baltzopoulos, V. (1999) The effects of the antagonist muscle force on intersegmental loading during isokinetic efforts of the knee extensors. *Journal of Biomechanics* 32, 19–25.

Kemper, H.C.G. & Verschuur, R. (1985a) Body build and composition. *Medicine & Sport Science* 20, 88–95.

Kemper, H.C.G. & Verschuur, R. (1985b) Motor performance fitness tests. *Medicine & Sport Science* 20, 96–106.

Malina, R.M. (1998) Motor development and performance. In: *The Cambridge Encyclopaedia of Human Growth and Development* (Ulijaszek, S.J., Johnston, F.E. & Preece, M.A., eds.) Cambridge University Press, Cambridge: 247–250.

Malina, R.M. & Bouchard, C. (1991) *Growth, Maturation and Physical Activity.* Human Kinetics, Champaign, IL.

Mauro, A. (1961) Satellite cell of skeletal muscle fibres. *Journal of Biophysics, Biocemistry and Cytology* 9, 493–494.

Parker, D.F., Round, J.M., Sacco, P. & Jones, D.A. (1990) A cross sectional survey of upper and lower limb strength in boys and girls during childhood and adolescence. *Annals of Human Biology* 17, 199–211.

Round, J.M., Jones, D.A. & Edwards, R.H.T. (1982) A flexible microprocessor system for the measurement of cell size. *Journal of Clinical Pathology* 35, 620–624.

Round, J.M., Jones, D.A., Honour, J.W. & Nevill, A.M. (1999) Hormonal factors in the development of differences in strength between boys and girls during adolescence: a longitudinal study. *Annals of Human Biology* 26, 49–62.

Rowe, R.W.D. & Goldspink, G. (1969) Muscle fibre growth in five different muscles in both sexes of mice: I, normal mice. *Journal of Anatomy* 104, 519–530.

Rutherford, O.M., Jones, D.A. & Newham, D.J. (1986) Clinical and experimental application of the twitch superimposition technique for the study of human muscle activation. *Journal of Neurology, Neurosurgery and Psychiatry* 49, 1288–1291.

Rutherford, O.M., Jones, D.A., Round, J.M. & Preece, M.A. (1990) Changes in skeletal muscle after discontinuation of growth hormone treatment in young adults with hypopituitarism. *Acta Peadiatrica Scandinavia* (Suppl) 356, 61–63.

Sinha-Hikim, I., Artaza, J., Woodhouse, L. *et al.* (2002) Testosterone-induced increase in muscle size in healthy young men is associated with muscle fiber hypertrophy. *American Journal of Physiology, Endocrinology and Metabolism* 283, E154–164.

Sinha-Hikim, I., Roth, S.M., Lee, M.I. & Bhasin, S. (2003) Testosterone-induced muscle hypertrophy is associated with an increase in satellite cell number in healthy, young men. *American Journal of Physiology, Endocrinology and Metabolism* 285, E197–205.

Stoltz, H.R. & Stoltz, L.M. (1951) *Somatic development of adolescent boys.* Macmillan, New York.

Tanner, J.M. (1962) *Growth at Adolescence.* Blackwell, Oxford.

Tanner, J.M., Hughes, P.C. & Whitehouse, R.H. (1981) Radiographically determined widths of bone muscle and fat in the upper arm and calf from age 3–18 years. *Annals of Human Biology* 8, 495–517.

Vrbová, G., Gordon, T. & Jones, R. (1995) *Nerve-muscle interactions.* Chapman & Hall, London.

Chapter 3

Development of Maximal Anaerobic Performance: An Old Issue Revisited

OMRI INBAR AND MICHAEL CHIA

During unsupervised play and exercise, young people derive energy from the interplay of aerobic and anaerobic metabolisms. Although there is increasing recognition of the importance of maximal anaerobic exercise, research and documentation of the capability of young people to perform maximal anaerobic exercise lag behind that for maximal aerobic exercise. The reasons for this imbalance in research attention include:

1 The absence of a "gold standard" measure of anaerobic fitness comparable to that of maximal oxygen uptake for aerobic fitness;

2 The opinion that anaerobic fitness is less important than aerobic fitness because the association between aerobic fitness and health is more apparent and accepted while the links between anaerobic fitness and health remain contentious;

3 The importance of aerobic fitness to sports is more established than that documented for anaerobic fitness;

4 The relative difficulty in measuring anaerobic fitness compared to aerobic fitness;

5 Maximal anaerobic exercise is considered as more strenuous than maximal aerobic exercise for young and elderly people; and

6 While aerobic fitness is more encompassing of a person's overall fitness, anaerobic fitness is more localized to the muscle or group of muscles.

There are many merits in studying the maximal anaerobic exercise of young people: (i) many team sports require young people to perform maximal anaerobic exercise, interspersed with varying recovery periods; (ii) there is greater relevance and resemblance of anaerobic than aerobic tasks to daily activities, exercise, and play patterns of young people; (iii) tests of maximal anaerobic exercise usually last less than a minute compared to tests of maximal aerobic exercise, which take 10–20 times longer to complete; and (iv) the motivation and attention span of young people can be better harnessed and ensured during the shorter anaerobic fitness tests.

Knowledge about how maximal anaerobic power changes with age also provides useful information about the maturational stages of the anatomic, biochemical, physiologic, and neurologic systems and functions that are inherently linked to the performance of maximal anaerobic exercise. Sport scientists should pay equal attention to the anaerobic and aerobic fitness of young people because the combined knowledge base provides a composite picture of the exercising young person.

Maximal anaerobic exercise nomenclature

A plethora of terms is used to describe maximal anaerobic exercise in the pediatric exercise literature. Jargon such as alactacid, lactacid, anaerobic power, anaerobic capacity, anaerobic work capacity, instantaneous power, peak power, mean power, and short-term power are commonly and often indiscriminately used to describe non-identical aspects of maximal anaerobic exercise in textbooks of exercise physiology and in sports science journals.

Short-term or short duration "all-out exercise" is different from "maximal intensity exercise"; the latter is often used to describe the terminal stages of exercise in a maximal oxygen uptake test. This is because the mechanical power elicited during an all-out anaerobic-type cycling (or running) task is 2–4 times that elicited during a maximal oxygen uptake cycle test in young people (Bar-Or 1987). To differentiate between the two distinct types of exercise, the terms "maximal anaerobic exercise" and "maximal aerobic exercise" are recommended. Maximal anaerobic exercise refers to exercise that requires an all-out exertion, where the predominant, although not exclusive, energy for the accomplishment of the exercise comes from anaerobic or non-oxidative metabolism.

Anaerobic fitness can be explained as the capability of a person to perform maximal anaerobic exercise. In essence, the competence to generate the highest mechanical power (peak power, PP) over a few seconds (an indicator of maximal anaerobic power) and to sustain the high power output over a short period of time (usually less than 60 s) (mean power, MP, an indicator of maximal anaerobic endurance or maximal muscular endurance) can be considered as prime indicators of anaerobic fitness (Inbar et al. 1996; Chia 2000). In describing the maximal anaerobic exercise competence of young people, it is important to state explicitly the indicator(s) of choice (i.e., PP or MP), because although PP and MP are related, they are not identical (Inbar et al. 1996).

Longitudinal and cross-sectional studies

Data on the evolution of exercise fitness are more reliable when the results are derived from longitudinal studies that encompass the prepubescent, pubescent and post-pubescent periods (Kemper 1986; Armstrong et al. 2000). However, as longitudinal approaches are a heavy burden on resources and logistics, cross-sectional studies are more common. Furthermore, cross-sectional studies tend to focus on male subject cohorts (Inbar & Bar-Or 1986; Falgairette et al. 1991; Mercier et al. 1992) and even though there are some data on girls (Inbar 1985, 1996; Dore et al. 2001; Chia 2001), more are necessary to consolidate and expand the knowledge base.

Performance data on the anaerobic fitness of young people are derived mainly from results of the Margaria stair-running test (Margaria et al. 1966; di Prampero & Ceretelli 1969; Kuroski 1977), and the Wingate Anaerobic Test (WAnT) (Ben-Ari & Inbar 1978; Inbar 1985; Blimkie et al. 1986; Inbar & Bar-Or 1986; Falk & Bar-Or 1993; Armstrong & Welsman 1997; Chia 1998). Other performance data on the anaerobic fitness of young people are based on smaller subject populations using force–velocity cycle tests (Sargeant & Dolan 1987; Mercier et al. 1992; Santos et al. 2003), an inertia-corrected force–velocity test (Dore et al. 1997), a combination of force–velocity and WAnT (Van Praagh et al. 1990; Falgairette et al. 1991), a motorized treadmill test (Paterson et al. 1986), a non-motorized treadmill test (Fargreas et al. 1993; Falk et al. 1996; Sutton et al. 2000), an isokinetic cycling test (Sargeant & Dolan 1987; Williams & Keen 2001), and the Quebec-10-s maximal cycle and maximal knee extension and flexion performances lasting 10, 30, and 90 s (Saavedra et al. 1991; Calvert et al. 1993). These data, which are derived from different laboratories employing dissimilar test apparatus and protocols and using different subject cohorts, cannot be directly compared and the different results often obfuscate research in the area.

Anaerobic fitness in relation to chronologic age

Figure 3.1 summarizes anaerobic muscle power and muscle endurance of the lower limbs and the upper limbs derived from the WAnT in male ($n = 306$) and female ($n = 70$) subjects plotted over age (Inbar 1985; Inbar et al. 1996). WAnT performance expressed in absolute power units is positively related to age in both female and male subjects and the relationship between power and age is stronger for the lower limbs than for the upper limbs. However, even when the WAnT power is normalized for body mass, the power produced by a 9-year-old boy is still only 70–80% of that generated by a young male adult.

In Fig. 3.1, apex values for WAnT power for the lower limbs are achieved at the end and middle of the third decade for male and female subjects, respectively. The highest WAnT power for the upper limbs is correspondingly achieved in the beginning of the third decade in male subjects. Data on the WAnT power of the upper limbs in female subjects are sparse and more data beyond the age of 14 years are required.

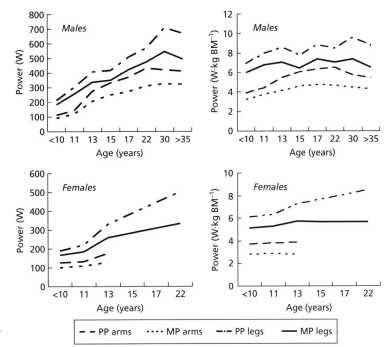

Fig. 3.1 Maximal anaerobic performance and chronologic age. Cross-sectional data for absolute (W) and relative (W·kg^{-1}) PP and MP outputs. Data are based on 306 male subjects and 70 female subjects who performed the Wingate Anaerobic Test (WAnT) by the upper and lower limbs. Based on data from Inbar 1985. MP, mean power; PP, peak power.

In the female subject sample examined by Inbar (1985), it is not possible to determine the age at which peak anaerobic performance occurred, because there was still a definite rise in absolute PP and MP up to age 25 years for the lower limbs and up to age 14 years for the upper limbs.

The typical 5-s PP values normalized for body mass (BM) of young male subjects (age 10–12 years) are 80.0% (6.90 ± 1.15 vs. 8.63 ± 0.78 W·kg BM^{-1}) while 30-s MP of young male subjects are 81.3% (5.95 ± 0.46 vs. 7.32 ± 0.34 W·kg BM^{-1}) of that of male adults (25–35 years) for WAnT power generated by the lower limbs. In young females (age 10–12 years), the equivalent 5-s PP are 72.3% (6.10 ± 1.33 vs. 8.43 ± 1.07 W·kg BM^{-1}) and the 30-s MP are 91.6% (5.21 ± 1.08 vs. 5.69 ± 0.59 W·kg BM^{-1}) of that of adult female subjects (18–25 years). Throughout the age span described, the WAnT power generated by the upper limbs is 60–70% that of WAnT power generated by the lower limbs. Although the increase in absolute anaerobic power (W) is about threefold from 9 to 30 years, the increase of the BM-independent anaerobic fitness (W·kg^{-1}) within the same age range is still 1.3–1.5 times that of age 8–9 years (Fig. 3.2).

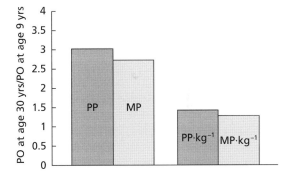

Fig. 3.2 Improvement in absolute and relative (to body mass) anaerobic fitness from 9 to 30 years in male subjects. Based on data from Inbar & Bar-O 1986. PO, power output; PP, peak power; MP, mean power.

The majority of research dealing with the issue of growth and development of anaerobic fitness in young people involves subject samples ranging in age from 8 years through to 15–16 years (Bedu *et al.* 1991; Falgairette *et al.* 1991; Naughton *et al.* 1992). Very few studies have included broader age ranges in their comparisons of maximal anaerobic performance (Inbar 1985; Inbar & Bar-Or 1986). Nonetheless, ample data suggest that the indicators of mechanical power (i.e., PP and MP) as well as various anaerobic field performances (i.e., 100 m sprint, high jump and long jump) increase with calendar age, even with BM accounted for, long after sexual maturation is achieved (Fig. 3.1). It is interesting to note that in male subjects between the ages of 16 years (assuming full sexual maturation) and 30 years (when male apex values of maximal power for the lower limbs are attained), absolute maximal anaerobic performance and values relative to BM continue to increase with age by 55% and 45%, respectively. More recent studies support the above observations, demonstrating similar changes in indicators of anaerobic fitness using cycle ergometry in absolute and relative terms during the periods of childhood, adolescence, and early adulthood (Hebestreit *et al.* 1993; Armstrong *et al.* 2001; Doré *et al.* 2001; Williams & Keen 2001; Santos *et al.* 2003).

Data in Fig. 3.1 suggest that the anaerobic fitness of female subjects is markedly lower than that of male subjects, even when BM or muscle mass is accounted for. For example, PP·kg BM^{-1} generated by the lower limbs in female subjects is 40% lower than in male subjects; MP·kg BM^{-1} generated by the lower limbs is 15% lower in female subjects than in male subjects. For power generated by the upper limbs, PP·kg BM^{-1} and MP·kg BM^{-1} in female subjects are 5–8% and 10–15% lower than in male subjects, respectively.

As shown above, at least in male subjects, anaerobic fitness continues to increase after the attainment of sexual maturation and peak physical growth into early adulthood, irrespective whether a correction for BM has been made or not. These results of laboratory tests of anaerobic fitness are also buttressed by exercise performances in track and field events under competitive situations (Fig. 3.3). Factors other

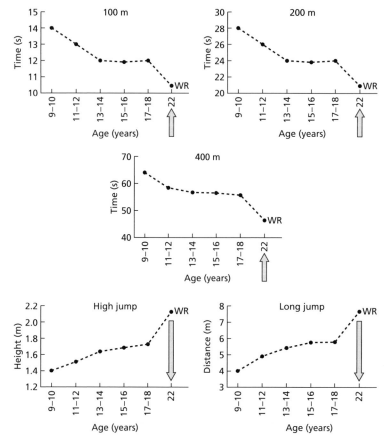

Fig. 3.3 Maximal anaerobic field performances as a function of age. Data from Van Praagh & Franca (1998).

than muscle mass and/or sexual maturation (such as neural activation, intramuscular coordination) are suggested to have additional and significant roles in the development of this essential component of the human fitness.

To summarize, children and adolescents attain lower PP and MP than adults during maximal anaerobic exercise, whether the performance is expressed in absolute terms (Margaria *et al.* 1966; Di Prampero & Cerretelli 1969; Davies *et al.* 1972; Kurowski 1977; Inbar *et al.* 1996; Armstrong & Welsman 1997), per unit BM (Inbar & Bar-Or 1986; Falgairette *et al.* 1991; Bar-Or 1995; Inbar *et al.* 1996; Armstrong & Welsman 1997), per unit fat-free mass (FFM) (Blimkie *et al.* 1988; Dore *et al.* 2000), per unit lean limb volume (LLV) (Blimkie *et al.* 1988; Saavedra *et al.* 1991), or even per unit lower limb muscle mass (LLMM) (Chia 2001). More recently, such data have also been scaled to various dimensions of body size using the analysis of covariance (ANCOVA) (Dore *et al.* 2000), and allometric modeling (Chia 1998; Welsman & Armstrong 2000; Santos *et al.* 2003).

When comparing subjects of different body size, the simple division of power by a body size descriptor using simple ratio standards does not always produce a body size-independent variable, and alternative scaling techniques such as allometric modeling may be more appropriate as they can better accommodate the characteristics of the data sets (Winter *et al.* 1991; Armstrong & Welsman 1994; Nevill & Holder 1995; Welsman *et al.* 1996). Despite a greater recognition of the pitfalls of using the simple ratio standards to normalize maximal anaerobic exercise data in young people, its use remains rife (see Chapter 5).

It is yet not entirely clear why children have a deficient maximal anaerobic performance when compared to adolescents and adults because much of the available data are equivocal and incomplete. Both quantitative and qualitative factors are proposed to help explain child–adult and male–female differences in anaerobic fitness.

Anatomic factors

The capability of a muscle to generate force depends on its cross-sectional area, while the shortening velocity during muscle contraction depends on its length, among other factors. As mechanical power is the product of force and velocity, power depends on the volume or mass of the muscle (each of which is a function of the product of cross-sectional area and length). Martin and Malina (1998) reported that the rate of increase in muscle volume during childhood and adolescence is similar to the rate of increase in peak and mean anaerobic power, when the power indicators are normalized for body mass.

Peak muscle mass in male subjects is attained at about 30 years of age, while female subjects attain peak muscle mass just before age 20 years. After 7 years of age, male subjects have greater absolute and relative muscle volume (kg muscle mass·kg BM^{-1}). Female subjects have about 50% muscle size of the upper limb and about 70% of the muscle size of the lower limb of male subjects after adolescence. The increase in muscle fiber size is about 3.5 times in female subjects and 4.5 times in male subjects between the periods of early childhood and adolescence (Van Praagh & Dore 2000).

The patterns of muscle mass development are suggested to account for a significant variance in age- and sex-related differences in power development during childhood and adolescence. However, these previous insights are based on studies using subject samples with a relatively narrow age range and the use of simple ratio standards in accounting for differences in body size. In describing the evolution of anaerobic fitness of young people and adults, future studies should encompass subject cohorts that represent the whole pediatric range (8–21 years) and possibly into early adulthood (22–35 years) because changes in anaerobic fitness continues beyond the attainment of adulthood, defined by chronologic age (i.e., 21 years). Researchers should also use the appropriate statistical approach to analyze the data when describing anaerobic fitness that is independent of body size.

Some muscle biopsy data suggest a greater percentage distribution of fast twitch muscle fibers in adults than in children but these data are not very convincing because they are based mainly on male participants, involve very small sample sizes, and involve participants who are trained and untrained (Saltin 1977). It is plausible that there could be differences in muscle fiber type distribution in the male and female adults and in children and adolescents. The appreciable age and sex differences in the fatigue index (FI) obtained during WAnT, at all ages and for both the upper and lower limbs (Inbar *et al.* 1996), and the close association between power decay (FI) during the WAnT and muscle fiber distribution (Bar-Or *et al.* 1980; Inbar *et al.* 1981) allude to such a possibility.

Neurologic factors

Sprint running, sprint cycling, or skipping at maximal speed require coordination among muscle groups. It is well documented that neuromuscular performance undergoes strong developmental alterations, because neuromuscular components are fully developed after puberty (Bosco & Komi 1980; Blimkie 2001). One of the major changes that occurs throughout childhood is the myelination of the nerve fibers. Full myelination is completed in adolescence, and so until then coordination and reactions will be limited and will not be equivalent to those documented in adults. Indeed, skills that require short bursts of high-intensity activities develop gradually during childhood (Martin & Malina 1998).

Some evidence suggests that muscle recruitment and the angle of muscle pennation improve with age; adults are able to recruit more motor units when performing maximal exercise tasks compared to children (Fournier *et al.* 1982; Blimkie & Sale 1998).

In addition, the coordination of synergistic and antagonistic muscles also develops with age. It is not until all the stabilizing muscle groups are developed and become correctly coordinated with the prime movers, that the optimal exercise form can be achieved when performing various types of maximal anaerobic exercise tasks. Also, adult male subjects have a greater capacity to utilize stored elastic energy of muscle, known to be produced during activities such as running, cycling, or jumping, than prepubertal male subjects (Moritani *et al.* 1989).

Although apparently no attempt has been made to correlate maximal anaerobic performance with neuromuscular coordination, some data suggest that such a relationship exists and that it is not inconceivable that changes in neural factors can influence young people's capability to perform maximal anaerobic exercise.

Hormonal and sexual maturation factors

During a short span of 3–4 years that encompass puberty, the pediatric subject undergoes tremendous hormonal (as well as metabolic, emotional, and behavioral) changes, which affect responses to acute exercise. Studies in rats suggest that lactate production is related to the level of circulating testosterone (Krotkiewski *et al.* 1980). Extrapolating the results of animal studies to humans, it is suggested, but not confirmed, that the ability of young boys to produce lactate (Eriksson *et al.* 1971) or to generate peak anaerobic power (Ferretti *et al.* 1994) depends on circulating levels of testosterone and other hormonal changes during puberty, such as increases in growth hormone and insulin-like growth factors. The relative lower anaerobic performance of mature female subjects, when compared to male subjects, and the smaller age-related difference in generated maximal anaerobic power among females lend support to such a hypothesis. However, there is insufficient evidence to allow researchers to state categorically that the difference between the rate of glycolysis in boys and men is explained by differences in male hormone concentrations.

The data presented in Fig. 3.4 demonstrate the uncertainty of hormonal influence on anaerobic fitness, by implying a linear increase in mass-independent anaerobic performance with increased chronologic age before, during, and after sexual maturity (Falk & Bar-Or 1993). Such a linear increase in maximal anaerobic power suggests that sexual maturation, with all the possible accompanying hormonal and other physiologic changes, does not exert any "unusual" or independent influence on the development of the anaerobic fitness with age. That is, there is no "maximal anaerobic performance spurt" at peak height velocity (PHV).

Data presented in a previous volume of this Encyclopedia (Inbar 1996) further reinforce the above assertion by demonstrating that the largest relative change in muscle endurance (MP) of the upper and lower limbs seems to occur before late or even

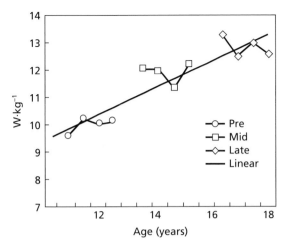

Fig. 3.4 Body mass-independent peak anaerobic power as a function of developmental stage. Data from Falk & Bar-O 1993.

mid-puberty and prior to the occurrence of PHV in both sexes.

Nindl *et al.* (1995) reported significantly greater ANCOVA-adjusted upper and lower limb WAnT PP and MP, adjusted for BM, FFM, or muscle cross-section area (CSA), in 20 adolescent male (age 16.5 ± 0.9 years) than in 20 female (age 16.1 ± 1.0 years) subjects. These gender-related dissimilarities are evident despite similar sexual maturity status as assessed using Tanner indices. These findings also refute the importance of sexual maturity as a dominant explanatory factor for the competence to perform maximal anaerobic exercise.

In a series of studies that examined the changes in WAnT PP and MP in 10- to 12-year-old children and adolescents (Armstrong *et al.* 1997, 2001) and in a force–velocity test (FVT)-derived optimized peak power (PP_{opt}) in 12- to 14-year-old adolescents (Santos *et al.* 2003), using multilevel modeling, no significant sex or maturity effect is observed either for PP or MP, or for PP_{opt}. These data also disprove the assertion that sexual maturation accounts for a significant change in young people's competence to perform maximal anaerobic exercise.

It is important to distinguish between the effects of body size (mass or stature) and the level of sexual maturation (hormonal and system development) on young people's competence in maximal anaerobic

exercise tasks. Although increases in body size and the onset of sexual maturation are both age-related, they may have co-dependent as well as independent impact on the competence of young people to perform maximal anaerobic exercise. Therefore, research that attempts to prove that sexual maturity and its associated hormonal effects are a prime factor for the development of maximal anaerobic performance, within subjects of a narrow age span (e.g., 9–15 years), may be missing important information.

Biochemical factors

The markedly lower anaerobic performance of children reflects, among other aspects, their lower capability for anaerobic energy turnover. Several findings support this notion. Table 3.1 summarizes the characteristics of biochemical substrates within the muscle that are utilized for muscle contraction. The main age-related difference between children and adults is in the glycolytic capability. The resting concentration of glycogen, and especially the rate of its anaerobic utilization, is lower in the child, who is therefore at a relative functional disadvantage compared to the adult when performing strenuous activities that last 5–60 s.

One method of estimating glycogen utilization during anaerobic metabolism is by measuring maximal lactate concentration in the muscle. For ethical reasons, this method has rarely been used on children. Figure 3.5 summarizes the few data on maximal muscle lactate concentration as a function of age in male subjects. There is an increase in maximal muscle lactate concentration after maximal

Table 3.1 Qualitative differences in child–adult substrate availability and utilization. Based on data from Eriksson *et al.* 1971, 1974; Haralambi 1982; Berg *et al.* 1986.

Substrate	Concentration in muscles* ($mmol \cdot kg^{-1}$)	Compared with adults	Utilization rate during exercise
ATP	3–5	Same	Same
PCr	12–22	Lower	Same or less
Glycogen	50–60	Lower	Much less

ATP, adenosine triphosphate; PCr, phosphocreatine.
* Values reflect wet weight of muscle.

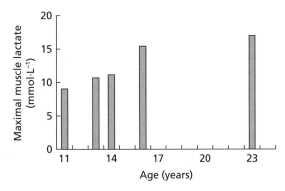

Fig. 3.5 Maximal muscle lactate levels as a function of age. After Eriksson *et al.* 1974.

anaerobic exercise in the second decade of life and this continues into early adulthood.

Despite its methodologic shortcomings, data on maximal blood lactate concentration support the notion that lactate production is limited in children compared to adolescents or adults (Robinson 1938; Astrand 1952; Blimkie *et al.* 1978; Matejkova *et al.* 1980; Williams & Armstrong 1991; Hebestreit *et al.* 1996; Ratel *et al.* 2002). There is, however, some evidence to show that the lower maximal blood lactate concentration in children may be the result of faster lactate removal and not necessarily because of lower lactate production (Beneke *et al.* 2005).

The rate of glycolysis is limited by the activity of enzymes such as phosphorylase, pyruvate dehydrogenase, and phosphofructokinase. The latter enzyme has been found to be less active in the muscle cells of 11- to 13-year-old boys (Eriksson *et al.* 1973, 1974) or 16- to 17-year-old boys (Fournier *et al.* 1982) than in young adults.

Recent data of Kuno *et al.* (1995), using phosphorus 31 nuclear magnetic resonance spectroscopy (^{31}P-NRS) support the earlier findings of muscle biopsy studies, where children and adolescents are reported to be less able than adults to regenerate adenosine triphosphate (ATP) via glycolysis during high-intensity exercise. Additionally, in the cited study, the activity of the enzyme phosphofructokinase, a major regulator of glycolysis, is reported to be lower in children and adolescents than in adults.

An additional indicator of anaerobic capability is the degree of acidosis at which a muscle can still contract. On the basis of ^{31}P-(RS), Zanconato *et al.* (1993) showed that during intense contraction of the calf muscles, children do not attain the low muscle pH levels that adults do. Kuno *et al.* (1995) also reported less acidosis in the thigh muscles of adolescents compared to adults, following maximal anaerobic exercise. These findings are also buttressed by the results of other studies showing less acidosis in children compared to adults after intense exercise (Gaisl & Buchberger 1977; Von Ditter *et al.* 1977; Kinderman *et al.* 1979; Matejkova *et al.* 1980; Ratel *et al.* 2002).

Based on the evidence, it is speculated that the metabolic pathways involved in maximal anaerobic exercise and the tolerance of acidosis are not fully mature until after the adolescent growth spurt and perhaps into early adulthood. These maturational changes are, however, more pronounced in male subjects than in female subjects.

Genetic factors

The exercise performances of young people is a function of environmental, genetic, and interactive genetic–environmental influences. Thus, anaerobic characteristics depend, at least to a certain extent, on a person's genotype. However, data on the genetic influence on maximal anaerobic exercise in young people are scarce, with previous estimates of genetic contribution ranging from virtually 0 to 100% of the performance variance (Komi & Karlsson 1979). Malina and Bouchard (1991) reported that, based on the results of a maximal 10-s cycle sprint using siblings and twins, the genetic effects account for about 50% of the maximal anaerobic performance variance. However, a heritability estimate of 97% was reported for the maximal anaerobic power of the arms in 17 pairs of male twins aged between 11 and 17 years (Malina & Bouchard 1991). In a separate study, the heritability index (HI) (number to express the extent of heredity of a certain property) was reported (Calvo *et al.* 2002), using the computation method of Rodas *et al.* (1998) on a series of exercise tests of 32 male monozygotic and dizygotic twins (age 21.3 ± 2.1 years) with similar backgrounds.

Their results revealed significant ($P < 0.05$) HI for 5-s PP (HI = 0.74) and 30-s MP (HI = 0.84) in the WAnT and for maximal post-exercise blood lactate concentration (HI = 0.82). However, the HI for FI was not significant (HI = 0.43; $P > 0.05$). The HI for the accumulated oxygen deficit (AO_2D) test was also not significant (HI = 0.22; $P > 0.05$). It is noteworthy that the genetic effect on performance using different maximal anaerobic exercise tests in the same subjects varied and therefore results must not be extrapolated to tests with dissimilar characteristics. Other studies also show that genetic factors accounted for up to 65% and up to 82% for maximal anaerobic concentric and eccentric exercises, respectively (Thomis *et al.* 1997, 1998a,b). It was recently suggested that the genetic effect is more likely to account for about 50% of the variance in maximal anaerobic exercise phenotype (Van Praagh & Dore 2000).

Furthermore, heredity also affects FFM (Bouchard *et al.* 1988), muscle size (Hewitt 1957), proportion of muscle fiber types (Simoneau & Bouchard 1995), the ratio between glycolytic and oxidative muscle enzymes (Bouchard *et al.* 1986), and the trainability of high-intensity muscle performance (Simoneau *et al.* 1986), all of which could, conceivably, affect the individual's anaerobic performance capability.

Conclusions

The assessment of short-term power output in young people is important considering that daily tasks in children and adolescents involve both aerobic and anaerobic function, albeit fewer data are available for the latter. Researchers have to grapple with methodologic and ethical constraints when dealing with young people and this has limited somewhat the proliferation of the knowledge base on the maximal anaerobic exercise competence of children and adolescents.

The competence to perform maximal anaerobic exercise improves with age and appears to culminate in mid-adulthood in male subjects and in late adolescence in female subjects. The timing and tempo of anaerobic fitness development is distinctly different in male and female subjects.

Both quantitative and qualitative factors account for the development of maximal anaerobic exercise capability of young people. Quantitative factors include increases in muscle mass, muscle CSA, and muscle fiber diameter, while qualitative factors include genetics, muscle metabolism, and neural and hormonal influences. Increases in muscle mass and CSA (hence muscle size) in male and female subjects between childhood and early adulthood are suggested to explain the age- and sex-related increases and differences in young people's maximal anaerobic functionality, but not entirely.

Genetics appear to exert a moderate-to-strong influence on young people's maximal anaerobic performance, especially on PP and MP in the WAnT. The HI for short-term power generation measured in the WAnT range from 0.74 to 0.82. Longer tests such as the AO_2D test have no significant HI, which suggests a greater plasticity to environmental influences such as experience, training, and motivation. Some data suggest a greater preponderance of type 2 muscle fibers in adolescence and adulthood than in childhood and therefore help explain the increase of maximal anaerobic capability from childhood through adolescence and into adulthood. Caution is advised, however, in the interpretation of muscle biopsy studies because of methodologic limitations and limited sample size, and also the plasticity of some fiber types to non-genetic factors. Differences in the muscle metabolism between young people and adults in their responses to maximal anaerobic exercise show a reduced reliance on anaerobic metabolism and perhaps a different regulation of pH concentration in young people compared to adults. Improvements in neural adaptations with age (complete myelination of nerve fibers, improved muscle coordination during multijoint exercise, improved capability to recruit motor units, or the ability to activate muscles more fully) can also help to explain age-related improvements in maximal anaerobic exercise in young people. However, the suggested postulations to account for the maximal anaerobic exercise of young people await further research attention, a more secure data base, and further confirmation in male and female subjects within the pediatric age span.

It is noteworthy that some 20 years ago Inbar and Bar-Or (1986), in their review article on this same topic, had already postulated that "Anaerobic performance, irrespective of sex, is closely related to body mass and probably more so to lean tissue mass, of the growing individual. However, during growth *and even after full physical development*, many modifications occur at the cellular, biochemical, and physiological levels that sustain the developmental changes in maximal anaerobic performance beyond those obtained by physical growth alone."

It is surprising that not much has come forth in terms of new knowledge of maximal anaerobic performance and its development, although there have been some refinements in methodology as well as in statistical approaches used in data analysis.

Future research directions worthy of consideration include: (i) affirming the relevance of documenting short term power output for sports, exercise performance or physical health; (ii) embarking on longitudinal studies and using appropriate statistical techniques to model short-term power data from childhood into mid-adulthood; and (iii) using non-invasive technologies such as magnetic resonance imaging (MRI) and magnetic resonance spectroscopy (MRS), on their own or in combination with other emerging technologies, to examine mechanisms that may influence the maximal anaerobic performance of male and female children and adolescents.

References

Armstrong, N. & Welsman, J.R. (1994) Assessment and interpretation of aerobic fitness in children and adolescents. *Exercise and Sport Sciences Reviews* **22**, 435–476.

Armstrong, N. & Welsman, J.R. (1997) *Young People and Physical Activity*. Oxford University Press, Oxford: 79–96.

Armstrong, N., Welsman, J.R. & Chia, Y.H.M. (2001) Short term power output in relation to growth and maturation. *British Journal of Sports Medicine* **35**, 118–124.

Armstrong, N., Welsman, J.R. & Kirby, B.J. (1997) Performance on the Wingate anaerobic test and maturation. *Pediatric Exercise Science* **9**, 253–261.

Armstrong, N., Welsman, J.R., Williams, C.A. & Kirby, B.J. (2000) Longitudinal changes in young people's short-term power output. *Medicine and Science in Sports and Exercise* **32**, 1140–1145.

Astrand, P.O. (1952) *Experimental Studies of Physical Working Capacity in Relation to Sex and Age*. Copenhagen: Munksgaard.

Bar-Or, O. (1987) The Wingate anaerobic test. An update on methodology, reliability and validity. *Sports Medicine* **4**, 381–394.

Bar-Or, O. (1995) The young athlete: some physiological considerations. *Journal of Sports Sciences* 13 Spec. no S31–S33.

Bar-Or, O., Dotan, R., Inbar, O., Rotstein, A., Karlsson, J. & Tesch, P. (1980) Anaerobic capacity and muscle fiber type distribution in non-athletes and in athletes. *International Journal of Sports Medicine* **1**, 82–85.

Bedu, M., Fellmann, N., Spielvogel, H., Falgairette, G., Van Praagh, E. & Coudert, J. (1991) Force–velocity and 30-s Wingate tests in boys at high and low altitude. *Journal of Applied Physiology* **70**, 1031–1037.

Ben-Ari, E. & Inbar, O. (1978) Leg and arm anaerobic capacity of 30 to 40-year-old men and women. In: *Biomechanics of Sports and Kin: Anthropometry*. Proceedings of the 5th International symposium on kinanthropometry and ergometry. (Landry F. & Organ W.A.R., eds.) Pelican: Quebec, 427–433.

Beneke, R., Hütler, M., Jung, M. & Leithäuser, R.M. (2005) Modeling the blood lactate kinetics at maximal short-term exercise conditions in children, adolescents and adults. *Journal of Applied Physiology* **99**, 499–504.

Berg, A., Kim, S.S. & Keul, J. (1986) Skeletal muscle enzyme activities in healthy young subjects. *International Journal of Sports Medicine* **7**, 236–239.

Blimkie, C. (2001) Age- and sex-associated variation in strength during childhood: anthropometric, morphologic, neurologic, biomechanical, endocrinologic, genetic, and physical activity correlates. In: *Perspectives in Exercise Science and Sports Medicine, Youth, Exercise, and Sport* (Gisolfi, C. & Lamb, D., eds.) Cooper Publishing Group, MI: 99–163.

Blimkie, C.J.R., Cunningham, D.A. & Leung, F.Y. (1978) Urinary catecholamine excretion during competition in 11- to 23-year-old hockey players. *Medicine and Science in Sports and Exercise* **10**, 188–193.

Blimkie, C.J.R., Roche, P. & Bar-Or, O. (1986) The anaerobic-to-aerobic power ratio in adolescent boys and girls. In: *Children and Exercise XIII* (Rutenfranz, J., Mocellin, R. & Klimt, F. eds.) Human Kinetics, Champaign, IL: 31–37.

Blimkie, C.J.R., Roche, P., Hay, J.T. & Bar-Or, O. (1988) Anaerobic power of arms in teenage boys and girls: relationship to lean tissue. *European Journal of Applied Physiology* **57**, 677–683.

Blimkie, C.J.R. & Sale, D.G. (1998) Strength development and trainability during childhood. In: *Pediatric Anaerobic Performance* (Van Praagh, E., ed.) Human Kinetics, Champaign, IL: 193–224.

Bosco, C. & Komi, P. (1980) Influence of aging on the mechanical behavior of leg extensor muscles. *European Journal of Applied Physiology* **45**, 209–219.

Bouchard, C., Perusse, L., Leblanc, C., Tremblay, A. & Theriault, G. (1988) Inheritance of the amount and distribution of human body fat. *International Journal of Obesity* **12**, 205–215.

Bouchard, C., Simoneau, A.-L., Lortie, G., Boulay, M.R., Marcotte, M. & Thibault, M.C. (1986) Genetic effects in human skeletal muscle fiber type distribution and enzyme activities. *Canadian Journal of Physiology and Pharmacology* **64**, 1245–1251.

Calvert, R.E., Bar-Or, O., McGillis, L.A. & Suei, K. (1993) Total work during an isokinetic and Wingate endurance tests in circumpubertal males. *Pediatric Exercise Sciences* **5**, 60–71.

Calvo, M., Rodas, G., Vallejo, M., *et al.* (2002) Heritability of explosive power and anaerobic capacity in humans.

European Journal of Applied Physiology **86**, 218–225.

Chia, Y.H.M. (1998) Anaerobic fitness of young people. PhD thesis. Exeter University, UK.

Chia, Y.H.M. (2000) Assessing young people's exercise using anaerobic performance tests. *European Journal of Physical Education* **5**, 231–258.

Chia, Y.H.M. (2001) Power recovery in the Wingate Anaerobic Test in girls and women following prior sprints of a short duration. *Biology of Sport* **18**, 45–53.

Davies, C.T.M., Barnes, C. & Godfrey, S. (1972) Body composition and maximal exercise performance in children. *Human Biology* **44**, 195–214.

Di Prampero, P.E. & Cerretelli, P. (1969) Maximal muscular power (aerobic and anaerobic) in African natives. *Ergonomics* **12**, 51–59.

Dore, E., Bedu, M., Franca, N.M. & Van Praagh, E. (2001) Anaerobic cycling performance characteristics in prepubescent, adolescent and young adult females. *European Journal of Applied Physiology* **84**, 476–481.

Dore, E., Diallo, O., Franca, N.M., Bedu, M. & Van Praagh, E. (2000) Dimensional changes cannot account for all differences in short-term cycling power during growth. *International Journal of Sports Medicine* **21**, 360–365.

Dore, E., Franca, N.M., Bedu, M. & Van Praagh, E. (1997) The effect of flywheel inertia on short-term cycling power output in children (abstract). *Medicine and Science in Sports and Exercise* **29** Supplement, p. 170.

Eriksson, B.O., Gollnick, P.D. & Saltin, B. (1973) Muscle metabolism and enzyme activities after training in boys 11–13 years old. *Acta Physiologica Scandinavica* **87**, 485–497.

Eriksson, B.O., Gollnick, P.D. & Saltin, B. (1974) The effect of physical training on muscle enzyme activities and fiber composition in 11-year-old boys. *Acta Paediatrica Belgica (Suppl)* **28**, 245–252.

Eriksson, B.O., Karlsson, J. & Saltin, B. (1971) Muscle metabolites during exercise in pubertal boys. *Acta Paediatrica Scandinavica (Supplement)* **217**, 154–157.

Falgairette, G., Bedu, M., Fellmann, N., Van Praagh, E. & Coudert, J. (1991) Bioenergetic profile in 144 boys aged from 6 to 15 years with special reference to sexual maturation. *European Journal of Applied Physiology* **62**, 151–156.

Falk, B. & Bar-Or, O. (1993) Longitudinal changes in peak aerobic and anaerobic mechanical power of circum-pubertal boys. *Pediatric Exercise Science* **5**, 318–331.

Falk, B., Weinstein, Y., Dotan, R., Abramson, D.A., Mann-Segal, D. & Hoffman, J.R. (1996) A treadmill test of sprint running. *Scandinavian Journal of Medical Sciences and Sports* **6**, 259–264.

Fargeas, M., Van Praagh, E., Leger, L., Fellman, N. & Coudert, J. (1993) Comparison of cycling and running power outputs in trained children. *Pediatric Exercise Science* **5**, 415 (abstract).

Ferretti, G., Narici, M.V., Binzoni, T., et al. (1994) Determinants of peak muscle power: effects of age and physical conditioning. *European Journal of Applied and Occupational Physiology* **68**, 111–115.

Fournier, M., Ricci, J., Taylor, A.W., Ferguson, R.J., Montpetit, R.R. & Chaitman, B.R. (1982) Skeletal muscle adaptation in adolescent boys: sprint and endurance training and detraining. *Medicine and Science in Sports and Exercise* **14**, 453–456.

Gaisl, G. & Buchberger, J. (1977) The significance of stress acidosis in judging the physical working capacity of boys aged 11 to 15. In: *Frontiers of Activity and Child Health* (Lavallee, H. & Shephard, R.J., eds.) Pelican, Quebec: 161–168.

Haralambie, G. (1982) Enzyme activities in skeletal muscle of 13–15 year old adolescents. *Bulletin Européen de Physiopathologie Respiratoire* **18**, 65–74.

Hebestreit, H., Meyer, F., Htay, H., Heigenhäi, G.J. & Bar-Or, O. (1996) Plasma metabolites, volume and electrolytes following 30-s high-intensity exercise in boys and men. *European Journal of Applied and Occupational Physiology* **72**, 563–569.

Hebestreit, H., Minura, K-I. & Bar-Or, O. (1994). Recovery of muscle power after high intensity short-term exercise: comparing boys to men. *Journal of Applied Physiology* **74**, 2875–2880.

Hewitt, D. (1957) Some familial correlations in height, weight and skeletal maturity. *Annals of Human Genetics* **22**, 26–35.

Inbar, O. (1985) *The Wingate Anaerobic Test: its performance, characteristics, applications, and norms*. Wingate Book Publications [Hebrew].

Inbar, O. (1996) Development of anaerobic power and local muscular endurance. *Encyclopedia of Sports Medicine: The Child and the Adolescent Athlete*. Blackwell Science, Oxford: 42–53.

Inbar, O. & Bar-Or, O. (1986) Anaerobic characteristics in male children and adolescents. *Medicine and Science in Sports and Exercise* **18**, 264–266.

Inbar, O., Bar-Or, O. & Skinner, J. (1996) *The Wingate Anaerobic Test*. Human Kinetics Publication, Champaign IL.

Inbar, O., Kaiser, P. & Tesch, P. (1981) Relationships between leg muscle fiber type distribution and leg exercise performance. *International Journal of Sports Medicine* **3**, 154–159.

Kemper, H.C. (1986) Longitudinal studies on the development of health and fitness and the interaction with physical activity of teenagers. *Pediatrician* **13**, 52–59.

Kindermann, W., Keul, J. & Lehmann, M. (1979) Prolonged exercise in adolescents, metabolic and cardiovascular changes. *Fortschritte der Medizin* **97**, 659–665.

Komi, P.V., Karlsson, J. (1979) Physical performance, skeletal muscle enzyme activities and fiber types in monozygous and dizygous twins of both sexes. *Acta Physiologica Scandinavica* **462**, 1–28.

Krotkiewski, M., Kral, J.G. & Karlsson, J. (1980) Effects of castration and testosterone substitution on body composition and muscle metabolism in rats. *Acta Physiologica Scandinavica* **109**, 233–237.

Kuno, S., Takahashi, H., Fujimoto, K., et al. (1995) Muscle metabolism during exercise using phosphorus-31 nuclear magnetic resonance spectroscopy in adolescents. *European Journal of Applied Physiology* **70**, 301–304.

Kurowski, T.T. (1977) Anaerobic power of children ages 9 through 15 years. MSc thesis. Florida State University.

Malina, R. & Bouchard, C. (1991) *Growth, Maturation and Physical Activity*. Human Kinetics, Champaign, IL.

Margaria, R., Aghemo, P. & Rovelli, E. (1966) Measurement of muscular power (anaerobic) in man. *Journal of Applied Physiology* **21**, 1662–1674.

Martin, J.C. & Malina, R.M. (1998) Developmental variations in anaerobic performance associated with age and sex. In: *Pediatric Anaerobic Performance* (Van Praagh, E., ed.) Human Kinetics, Champaign, IL: 45–64.

Matejkova, J., Koprivova, Z. & Placheta, Z. (1980) Changes in acid–base balance after maximal exercise. In: *Youth and Physical Activity* (Placheta, Z. & Brno, J.E., eds.) Purkyne University: 191–199.

Mercier, B., Mercier, J., Granier, P., Le Gallais, D. & Prefaut, C. (1992) Maximal anaerobic power: relationship to anthropometric characteristics during growth. *International Journal of Sports Medicine* **13**, 21–26.

Moritani, T., Oddsson, L., Thorstensson, A. & Astrand, P.O. (1989) Neural and biomechanical differences between men and young boys during a variety of motor tasks. *Acta Physiologica Scandinavica* **137**, 347–355.

Naughton, G., Carlson, J. & Fairweather, I. (1992) Determining the variability of performance on Wingate anaerobic tests in children aged 6–12 years. *International Journal of Sports Medicine* **13**, 512–517.

Nevill, A.M. & Holder, R.L. (1995) Scaling, normalizing and per ratio-standards: an allometric modeling approach. *Journal of Applied Physiology* **79**, 1027–1031.

Nindl, B.C., Mahar, M.T., Harman, E.A. & Patton, J.F. (1995) Lower and upper body anaerobic performance in male and female adolescent athletes. *Medicine and Science in Sports and Exercise* **27**, 235–241.

Paterson, D.H., Cunningham, D.A. & Bumstead, L.A. (1986) Recovery O_2 and blood lactic acid: longitudinal analysis in boys aged 11 to 15 years. *European Journal of Applied Physiology* **55**, 93–99.

Ratel, S., Duche, P., Hennegrave, A., Van Praagh, E. & Bedu, M. (2002) Acid–base balance during repeated cycling sprints in boys and men. *Journal of Applied Physiology* **92**, 479–485.

Robinson, S. (1938) Experimental studies of physical fitness in relation to age. *Arbeitsphysiologie* **10**, 251–323.

Rodas, G., Calvo, M., Estruch, A., *et al.* (1998) Heritability of running economy: a study made on twin brothers. *European Journal of Applied and Occupational Physiology* **77**, 511–516.

Saavedra, C., Lagasse, C.P., Bouchard, C. & Simoneau, J.-A. (1991) Maximal anaerobic performance of the knee extensor muscles during growth. *Medicine and Science in Sports and Exercise* **23**, 1083–1089.

Saltin, B., Henriksson, J., Nygaard, E., Andersen, P. & Janson, E. (1977) Fiber types and metabolic potentials of skeletal muscles in sedentary men and endurance runners. *Annals of New York Academy of Sciences* **301**, 3–39.

Santos, A.M.C., Armstrong, N., De Ste Croix, M.B.A., Sharp, P. & Welsman, J. (2003) Optimal peak power in relation to age, body size, gender and thigh muscle volume. *Pediatric Exercise Science* **15**, 406–418.

Sargeant, A.J. & Dolan, P. (1987) Effect of prior exercise on maximal short-term power output in humans. *Journal of Applied Physiology* **63**, 1475–1480.

Simoneau, J.-A. & Bouchard, C. (1995) Genetic determinism of fiber type proportion in human skeletal muscle. *Federation of American Societies for Experimental Biology* **9**, 1091–1095.

Simoneau, J.-A., Lortie, G., Boulay, M.R., Marcotte, M., Thibault, M.-C. & Bouchard, C. (1986) Inheritance of human skeletal muscle and anaerobic capacity adaptation to high-intensity intermittent training. *International Journal of Sports Medicine* **7**, 167–171.

Sutton, N.C., Childs, D., Bar-Or, O., *et al.* (2000) A non-motorized treadmill test to assess children's short-term power output. *Pediatric Exercise Sciences* **12**, 91–100.

Thomis, M.A., Van Leemputte, M., Maes, H.H., *et al.* (1997) Multivariate genetic analysis of maximal isometric muscle force at different elbow angles. *Journal of Applied Physiology* **82**, 959–967.

Thomis, M.A., Beunen, G.P., Maes, H.H., *et al.* (1998) Strength training: importance of genetic factors. *Medicine and Science in Sports and Exercise* **30**, 724–731.

Thomis, M.A., Beunen, G.P., Van Leemputte, M., *et al.* (1998) Inheritance of static and dynamic arm strength and some of its determinants. *Acta Physiologica Scandinavica* **163**, 59–71.

Van Praagh, E. & Dore, E. (2000) Development of anaerobic function during childhood and adolescence. *Pediatric Exercise Sciences* **12**, 150–173.

Van Praagh, E., Fellmann, N., Bedu, M., *et al.* (1990) Gender difference in the relationship of anaerobic power output to body composition in children. *Pediatric Exercise Sciences* **2**, 336–348.

Van Praagh, E. & Franca, N.M. (1998) Measuring maximal short-term power output during growth. In: *Pediatric Anerobic Performance* (Van Praagh, E., ed.). Human Kinetics, Champaign, IL: 155–189.

Von Ditter, H., Nowacki, P., Simai, E. & Wmkier, U. (1977) Das Verhaltan des Saurebasen-haushalts nach erschopfender Belastung bei untrainierten und trainerten Jungen und Vergleich zu Leistungssportlern. *Sportarzt Sport Medicine* **28**, 45–48.

Welsman, J.R. & Armstrong, N. (2000) Scaling performance for differences in body size. In: *Paediatric Exercise and Sports Medicine* (N. Armstrong & W.V. Mechlen, eds.) Oxford University Press: 7–23.

Welsman, J.R., Armstrong, N., Nevill, A.M., Winter, E.M. & Kirby, B.J. (1996) Scaling peak VO_2 for differences in body size. *Medicine and Sciences in Sports and Exercise* **28**, 259–265.

Williams, C.A. & Keen, P. (2001) Isokinetic measurement of maximal muscle power during leg cycling: a comparison of adolescent boys and adult men. *Pediatric Exercise Sciences* **13**, 154–166.

Williams, J.R. & Armstrong, N. (1991) The influence of age and sexual maturation on children's blood lactate responses to exercise. *Pediatric Exercise Sciences* **3**, 111–120.

Winter, E.M., Brooks, F.B.C. & Hamley, E.J. (1991) Maximal exercise performance and lean leg volume in men and women. *Journal of Sports Sciences* **9**, 3–13.

Zanconato, S., Buchthal, S., Barstow, T.J. & Cooper, D.M. (1993) ^{31}P magnetic resonance spectroscopy of leg muscle metabolism during exercise in children and adults. *Journal of Applied Physiology* **74**, 2214–2218.

Chapter 4

Cardiorespiratory Responses During Endurance Exercise: Maturation and Growth

THOMAS W. ROWLAND

Heart and lung function are essential for satisfying the metabolic, thermoregulatory, and hormonal demands of sustained exercise and have long been recognized as critical in defining athletic performance. Not unexpectedly, a considerable body of research has focused on identifying the unique anatomic and physiologic characteristics of adult distance cyclists, runners, and swimmers. The extent to that these features are evident in child and adolescent endurance athletes has been less thoroughly investigated. However, there are particular reasons for understanding cardiopulmonary characteristics and responses to exercise in growing young athletes.

1 Endurance performance normally improves during the pediatric years. The extent that improvements in cardiopulmonary functional reserve from sports training might alter this performance curve, or define its ultimate limits, needs to be delineated. Particularly poorly understood is the relative importance of genetically endowed talent versus training effects on cardiopulmonary function in the development of endurance fitness in this age group. In addition, the timing of expression of endurance fitness aptitude as the child ages is pertinent to those interested in early talent identification.

2 Training studies have suggested that the ability to improve aerobic fitness (i.e., increase maximal oxygen uptake) is dampened in the prepubertal years. It is not clear if limitations in cardiopulmonary function can explain this "ceiling" of response.

3 While proper training regimens for optimizing cardiopulmonary function and performance have been developed in adult athletes, it is not altogether clear if these regimens can be appropriately transferred to younger athletes. Indeed, given information

suggesting maturation-related differences in training responses, it might be suspected that training programs in young athletes should be approached differently.

4 It is important that physicians caring for children know whether the clinical features of ventricular enlargement and/or hypertrophy ("athlete's heart") can be expected in highly trained young endurance athletes. If not, such findings in this age group would be approached with much greater levels of concern.

5 Whether limitations should be placed on volume of training or distance of competitions in child athletes is problematic. Safety of training regimens needs to be established to allow coaches greater confidence in managing young competitors. This is important not only from a cardiopulmonary standpoint but involves nutritional, musculoskeletal, and psychologic aspects as well.

This chapter focuses on a number of these issues, particularly the cardiac and ventilatory responses to exercise in young endurance athletes, how these differ from non-training children as well as adult athletes, and whether the findings of "athlete's heart" are observed in the pediatric age group. Chapter 19 examines potential cardiac risks associated with intense endurance training in children and adolescents.

Cardiovascular responses to acute exercise

The usual model for examining cardiovascular responses to exercise in youth has involved measurement of variables during a bout of progressive upright cycle exercise. Techniques for assessing

39

cardiac output, particularly Doppler ultrasound, generally require the stability offered by this approach but leave the possibility that responses might differ using other testing modalities. This creates a problem when testing athletes, for only competitive cyclists will be performing exercise specific to their sport.

Non-trained youth

It is useful when evaluating cardiac responses to exercise to examine empirically observed patterns and then consider mechanisms based on what is "known" from these findings. That is, any proposed mechanisms for cardiovascular responses to exercise must be consistent with empirically derived testing data. What follows is a set of observations of cardiovascular responses to acute exercise in healthy, non-trained children. From these, comparisons with athletes can be made and proposed mechanisms considered.

Alterations in cardiac stroke volume do not contribute to circulatory responses during acute progressive exercise. Stroke volume rises by 30–40% in the initial stages of a progressive cycle test and then plateaus, or remains stable, at intensities above 50% $\dot{V}o_{2max}$. This pattern has been consistently recorded in children by numerous techniques (for references see Rowland 2005a). However, when exercise is performed supine, no such initial increase is typically seen. Values of stroke volume usually remain stable throughout progressive exercise and are similar to those observed during the plateau phase of upright exercise (Rowland *et al.* 2003) (Fig. 4.1).

These observations imply that the initial rise in stroke volume during upright exercise represents a mobilization of blood which was displaced by gravity into the lower extremities when assuming the upright position. In the adult this can amount to 500–1000 mL, a volume that returns to the heart with contraction of the skeletal muscles of the leg with onset of exercise. This concept is supported by measurements of stroke volume supine before beginning upright exercise (Fig. 4.2). Values that fall when assuming the sitting position are regained at the onset of exercise. The early rise in stroke volume in the upright posture therefore appears to be simply a "refilling" phenomenon and not part of

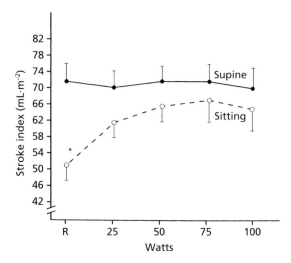

Fig. 4.1 Stroke index responses to progressive exercise with subjects supine and sitting in boys aged 10–15 years. From Rowland *et al.* 2003.

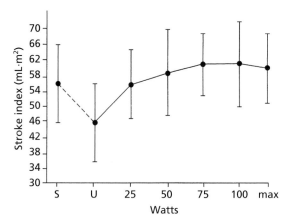

Fig. 4.2 Average values for stroke index while supine (S), assuming the sitting position (U), and during progressive upright cycle exercise to exhaustion in 12-year-old boys. From Rowland 2001.

the intrinsic mechanisms that determine circulatory responses to the demands of exercise.

Left ventricular diastolic size and filling volume do not increase with exercise. Echocardiographic measurements indicate, in fact, that left ventricular end-diastolic size actually slowly declines as cycling intensity increases (Rowland & Whatley-Blum 2000a; Nottin *et al.* 2002a). (The exception to this is a small rise in volume at the onset of upright exercise which is consistent with augmented mobilization of blood from the dependent legs noted above.) This indicates that ventricular pre-load does not substantially change as cardiac output rises.

Cardiac contractility increases with greater work intensity. While left ventricular diastolic size is stable or slowly declines, end-systolic volume progressively falls. Consequently, ventricular shortening fraction (or ejection fraction), reflecting the extent of myocardial contraction, is heightened as work intensifies. Nottin *et al.* (2002a) reported an increase in average left ventricular shortening fraction from 37% at rest to 47% at maximal exercise in boys. These findings mimic those of Rowland and Blum (2000a) who found a mean rise from 31% before exercise to 47% at exhaustion.

Systemic vascular resistance declines rapidly, mirroring increases in ventricular shortening fraction. During progressive exercise, mean arterial pressure rises only slightly (about 20 mmHg), while cardiac output increase about 4 times above resting levels. This indicates that peripheral vascular resistance falls dramatically as work increases, a reflection of arteriolar dilatation in exercising muscle. In the boys studied by Rowland *et al.* (2003), resistance values at maximal exercise fell to less than half of those at rest.

These empiric observations are consistent with the following mechanistic scenario. The rise in circulatory flow with exercise is facilitated by peripheral arteriolar dilatation, which is effected by local factors sensing metabolic demands of muscular work. Following the Poiseuille law, $Q = P/R$, cardiac output (Q) increases as resistance (R) falls, the heart output maintaining P, systemic pressure. In a sense, then, the rise in blood circulation with exercise mimics that of the effects of a low-resistance peripheral arteriovenous fistula. The pumping action of the contracting skeletal muscle contributes to this peripheral control of circulation, but its dynamics remain uncertain (Rowland 2001).

The observation that diastolic filling volume of the ventricles remains constant while systemic venous return increases fourfold can only be explained by a rise in heart rate that matches blood volume returning from the periphery (the Bainbridge reflex). The increase in heart rate in effect "defends" left ventricular size, preventing an increase in left ventricular diastolic volume which would augment wall stress (Laplace law).

The left ventricle contracts more vigorously and completely as work increases, but stroke volume does not change. This apparent paradox can be solved by recognizing that the greater contractility serves to eject the same amount of blood (i.e., stroke volume) in a shorter systolic time as heart rate increases. That is, the effect of improved contractility is to *maintain* rather than increase stroke volume. If the myocardium fails in this task, as observed in patients with congestive heart failure, stroke volume falls during exercise (Rowland *et al.* 1999b).

This scenario, which is based on contemporary studies of children mainly using Doppler ultrasound, is consistent with traditional concepts of control of circulation from animal and adult human studies over the past 100 years (Rowland 2005b). Moreover, studies involving direct comparisons of adults and children have revealed no maturational qualitative differences in these patterns of circulatory adaptations (Rowland *et al.* 1997, 1999a; Nottin *et al.* 2002a). Once variables are adjusted for body size, current data suggest no maturational influences on cardiovascular responses to exercise in healthy subjects.

Responses in young endurance athletes

The circulatory responses to an acute bout of upright cycle exercise in young athletes have been examined in five echocardiographic studies reported to date (Unnithan *et al.* 1997; Rowland *et al.* 1998, 2000b, 2002; Nottin *et al.* 2002b). With the exception of one involving distance runners (Rowland *et al.* 1998), all describe findings in young male adolescent cyclists. Each but one (that in runners) reveals patterns of cardiovascular dynamics in this testing model that are identical to those described above in non-athletes. The distinguishing feature of young athletes in these studies—as witnessed in adult athletes—is the magnitude of cardiac variables, specifically stroke volume and left ventricular filling dimensions. These observations imply that the factors controlling and limiting circulatory responses to acute exercise are no different in child and adolescent athletes than non-athletes.

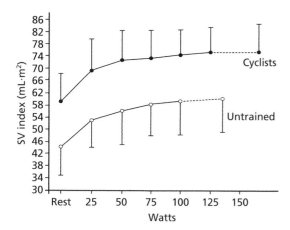

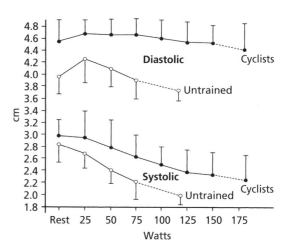

Fig. 4.3 Stroke index responses to progressive cycle exercise in well-trained male cyclists (age 12–15 years) and non-athletic boys. From Rowland *et al*. 2002.

Fig. 4.4 Changes in left ventricular end-diastolic and systolic dimensions during progressive cycle exercise in young male cyclists and non-athletic boys. From Rowland *et al*. 2002.

The two most comprehensive studies (Nottin *et al*. 2002b; Rowland *et al*. 2002) can be discussed together, as both revealed identical findings. At rest, highly trained cyclists (ages 10–15 years) demonstrated significantly greater stroke index and left ventricular end-diastolic and end-systolic dimensions (adjusted for body size) when compared with non-athletes. The pattern of initial rise and plateau of stroke volume with increasing work intensity was the same in both groups, the curve in the athletes simply shifted up and parallel to that of the non-trained boys (Fig. 4.3). Compared to the non-athletes, values of stroke index at maximal exercise were 13% higher in the cyclists described by Nottin *et al*. (2002b) and 25% greater in those reported by Rowland *et al*. (2002). These data suggest that the factors responsible for the larger stroke index in the athletes at maximal exercise are the same as those that define stroke volume differences from non-athletes at rest.

Left ventricular shortening fraction at rest was not significantly different in the athletes and non-athletes. Although values were always greater in the athletes, the patterns of change in left ventricular diastolic and systolic size with increasing work intensity in the cyclists mimicked those seen in non-athletes, with a gradual fall in the former and a more precipitous decline in the latter (Fig. 4.4). Subsequently, shortening fraction increased equally

in both groups (Fig. 4.5). That is, there was no indication of differences in cardiac contractility before or during exercise in the cyclists and non-athletes.

These studies indicated that maximal stroke volume was the factor that accounted for the higher maximal cardiac output and $\dot{V}o_{2max}$ in the cyclists, as heart rate and arterial venous oxygen difference at peak exercise were no different than those in

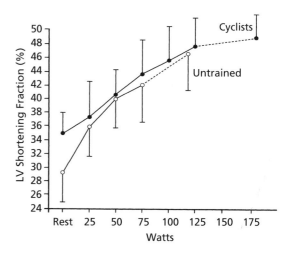

Fig. 4.5 Left ventricular shortening fraction changes during progressive upright cycle exercise in young male cyclists and untrained boys. From Rowland *et al*. 2002.

non-athletes. Maximal stroke volume was a reflection of resting stroke volume, which, in turn, was a manifestation of factors affecting left ventricular filling volume, or pre-load. It can be concluded that determinants such as greater plasma volume, vagal-induced bradycardia, inherent larger cardiac dimensions, and chronic volume overload from training which affect resting ventricular preload are, at least in part, responsible for the differences in cardiovascular fitness observed in young cyclists and non-athletes.

These findings and conclusions in young athletes are consistent with those traditionally described in adult endurance athletes. In a comparison study, Rowland & Roti (2004) reported cardiac adaptations to acute exercise in eight highly trained adult male cyclists (mean age 30.5 years). Patterns of response of stroke volume, shortening fraction, and left ventricular systolic and diastolic dimensions were identical to those seen in the studies in young cyclists. Compared to child cyclists studied in the same laboratory (Rowland et al. 2000b), values of maximal stroke index and cardiac index were greater in adult cyclists (15.38 ± 2.40 vs. 13.94 ± 1.37 L·min^{-1}·m^{-2} for cardiac index, 85 ± 13 vs. 76 ± 6 mL·m^{-2} for stroke index). Maximal arterial venous oxygen difference was 18.3 ± 3.0 mL·100 mL^{-1} in men and 13.1 ± 0.8 mL·100 mL^{-1} in boys, the difference presumably reflecting higher hemoglobin levels in the former.

Some studies in adult athletes (Gledhill et al. 1994) have indicated a rise in stroke volume throughout the course of progressive exercise, without plateau (this was also observed among the young runners by Rowland et al. 1998). This would imply that factors occurring during exercise (myocardial contractility, diastolic function) contribute to differences in maximal stroke volume and cardiac output in athletes. The explanation for these different findings of stroke volume patterns in athletes is unclear.

The above observations provided only limited insights into physiologic differences responsible for the augmented cardiovascular fitness of young athletes. There is no information regarding those peripheral factors that appear to be most crucial to facilitate (and also presumably limit) these circulatory responses. Whether child athletes are, in fact,

characterized by greater plasma volume, enhanced muscle capillarization, enhanced vasodilatory properties, and superior muscle pump function as described in adult endurance athletes (Ingjer 1978; Hopper et al. 1988; Cameron & Dart 1994) remains to be revealed. Such information awaits the development of non-invasive measurement techniques that are ethically acceptable in immature subjects.

Based on current research data, however, it appears that the primary distinguishing factor of young athletes that defines their superior cardiovascular fitness is a generalized expansion of the circulatory system. Advantages in size and volume rather than alterations in function appear to differentiate these athletes from non-athletic youth. In this regard, most data suggest that, at least qualitatively, the patterns of response to exercise and the factors defining superior cardiovascular fitness are similar in children and adults. Whether quantitative differences between the two age groups reflect factors such as length and intensity of training or instead indicate a "ceiling" of cardiovascular responses to training in immature subjects is uncertain.

"Athlete's heart"

Highly trained adult endurance athletes typically exhibit a set of clinical findings known collectively as "athlete's heart." This includes left ventricular enlargement, sinus bradycardia, and electrocardiographic features such as left ventricular hypertrophy, varying degrees of atrioventricular block, and ST-T wave changes. Although these findings may mimic those of heart disease (particularly cardiomyopathies), it is generally agreed that "athlete's heart" reflects salutary responses to long-term endurance training (Rost & Hollman 1983).

It is important for health care providers of children and adolescents to know whether these findings of "athlete's heart" are expected to be observed in young competitors as well. If they are, these characteristics should not be confused with cardiac abnormalities, a conclusion that would lead to unnecessary restriction from sports play. On the other hand, if "athlete's heart" is not typically seen in this age group, detecting these features in the young competitor should be viewed with more concern.

"Athlete's heart" in adults

Adult endurance athletes typically demonstrate mild left ventricular chamber enlargement, with a diastolic diameter of 54–56 mm (compared to 40–52 mm in non-athletes). This enlargement is accompanied by a mild degree of eccentric wall hypertrophy, which minimized wall tension. The hearts of athletes who train in resistance sports (weight lifting, wrestling), on the other hand, more often demonstrate more impressive concentric wall hypertrophy without chamber dilatation.

The electrocardiogram in the highly trained runner, swimmer, or cyclist characteristically reveals sinus bradycardia, with heart rate commonly <60 beats·min^{-1}. An adult endurance athlete has a resting heart rate that is, on average, about 11 beats·min^{-1} lower than that of the non-athlete. Voltage criteria for left ventricular hypertrophy are commonly seen, and a variety of other electrocardiographic findings have been described, including atrioventricular block, wandering atrial pacemaker, right ventricular conduction delay, and T-wave inversion.

The etiology for the development of "athlete's heart" is not entirely clear. Certainly, autonomic responses to training, particularly increased vagal tone, have a role. The general expansion of the circulatory system is manifest by increased ventricular size. While some have implicated intrinsic cardiac responses for this left ventricular enlargement (i.e., a response to recurrent volume overload of training), it is likely that non-cardiac factors such as augmented plasma volume and increased diastolic filling from bradycardia are more important (Perrault & Turcotte 1993).

Equally uncertain are the relative contributions of genetic endowment and training effects to the findings of "athlete's heart." Detraining studies have usually indicated some regression of these features, but values of left ventricular dimension stills remain greater than those typically seen in non-athletes (Fagard 1997). It is reasonable to suggest that both training and genetic factors influence cardiovascular features in endurance athletes.

Is "athlete's heart" observed in children and adolescents?

Assessment of findings of "athlete's heart" in young endurance athletes have largely involved male runners, swimmers, and cyclists. Overall, these studies indicate that young competitors demonstrate some but not all of the features seen in adult athletes.

RESTING BRADYCARDIA

Table 4.1 outlines 11 studies that have compared pre-exercise (resting but not basal) heart rate in trained male prepubertal endurance athletes (generally, ages 10–13 years) with those of non-athletes. In all but two of these reports, heart rates were substantially lower in the athletes. If one averages the values in these studies, mean resting heart rate in

Table 4.1 Pre-exercise resting heart rates (beats·min^{-1}, mean and standard deviation) in studies of prepubertal male endurance athletes compared to non-trained children.

Study	Age (years)	Gender	Sport	Athletes	Non-athletes
Sundberg & Elovainio (1982)	12–14	M	Runners	96 (9)	83 (14)
Rowland et al. (1994)	11–13	M	Runners	71 (6)	73 (8)
Rowland et al. (1998)	11–13	M	Runners	67 (10)	90 (14)
Obert et al. (1998)	10–11	M, F	Swimmers	69 (7)	83 (14)
Rowland et al. (1987)	8–13	M	Swimmers	65 (7)	74 (8)
Triposkiadis et al. (2002)	9–13	M, F	Swimmers	62 (9)	79 (11)
Rowland et al. (2000b)	10–13	M	Cyclists	71 (12)	85 (15)
Rowland et al. (2002)	12–15	M	Cyclists	73 (10)	90 (14)
Nottin et al. (2002b)	9–13	M	Cyclists	75 (6)	78 (11)
Nottin et al. (2004)	11–14	M	Cyclists	56 (7)	70 (11)

Table 4.2 Mean value for echocardiographic resting left ventricular end-diastolic dimension (mm) in studies of prepubertal endurance athletes compared to non-athletes.

Study	n	Age	Sex	Athletes	Non-athletes	Size adjustment
Swimmers						
Obert *et al.* (1998)	9	10–11	M, F	41.6	39.0*	BSA$^{0.33}$
Rowland *et al.* (1987)	11	8–13	M	39.5	36.2*	BSA$^{0.33}$
Ozer *et al.* (1994)	82	7–14	M, F	46.2	40.4*	
Lengyel & Gyarfas (1979)	9	14	M, F	30.3	27.9*	BSA
Medved *et al.* (1986)	72	8–14	M	45.2	40.5*	
Triposkiadis *et al.* (2002)	25	9–13	M, F	32.3	29.5*	BSA
Runners						
Gutin *et al.* (1988)	8	8–11	M	34.3	34.3	BSA
Shepherd *et al.* (1988)	13	5–12	M	41.0	41.0	
Rowland *et al.* (1994)	10	11–13	M	33.2	33.5	BSA
Telford *et al.* (1988)	48	11–12	M	46.6	45.9	
	37	11–12	F	45.7	45.9	
Cyclists						
Rowland *et al.* (2000b)	7	10–13	M	38.1	36.4	BSA$^{0.5}$
Rowland *et al.* (2002)	8	12–15	M	41.0	36.4*	BSA$^{0.5}$
Nottin *et al.* (2002b)	10	9–13	M	40.0	37.0*	BSA$^{0.5}$
Nottin *et al.* (2004)	12	11–14	M	38.6	36.0*	BSA$^{-0.5}$

BSA, body surface area.
* $P < 0.05$ compared to athletes.

the athletes is 11 beats·min^{-1} lower than in the non-athletes (70 vs. 81). The magnitude of this difference is comparable to that observed between adult endurance athletes and non-athletes.

ELECTROCARDIOGRAPHIC CHANGES

Studies that have examined electrocardiograms in child endurance athletes have found no differences other than lower heart rate from those obtained in non-athletic youth (Rowland *et al.* 1987, 1994, 1998; Nudel *et al.* 1989). Specifically, the athletes did not demonstrate right or left ventricular hypertrophy, conduction delays, arrhythmias, or repolarization abnormalities.

LEFT VENTRICULAR ENLARGEMENT

Table 4.2 outlines studies of resting left ventricular end-diastolic dimension in prepubertal endurance athletes compared with non-athletes as determined by echocardiography. Reports in young highly trained

swimmers and cyclists are consistent with data in adult endurance athletes: left ventricular size is consistently greater in the young athletes (by about 9%) but with values still within the normal range. It is an interesting but puzzling observation that a similar expression of "athlete's heart" has not been observed in distance runners.

Fewer studies have been performed in older, post-pubescent adolescent endurance athletes. Petridis *et al.* (2004) found a mean left ventricular end-diastolic dimension of 51.8 ± 2.5 mm in a group of 15- to 16-year-old male endurance athletes compared to 46.1 ± 4.3 mm in non-athletes with similar body surface area. Makan *et al.* (2005) assessed echocardiographic findings in 664 males and 236 females aged 14–18 years who were athletes training intensely in a wide variety of endurance and non-endurance sports. Compared with non-training adolescents, the athletes demonstrated a greater ventricular diastolic dimension (50.8 ± 3.7 vs. 47.9 ± 3.5 mm, a 6% difference). Similar findings were reported by Larsen *et al.* (2000) who found an 11% greater ventricular diastolic diameter in 17 members of the Danish national cycling team (ages 19–20 years) compared with non-athletes.

CONCLUSIONS

This information indicates that highly trained pre-pubertal endurance athletes can be expected to manifest some but not all of the features of "athlete's heart." Resting bradycardia and small increases in left ventricular size—albeit still within normal limits—are characteristic of at least swimmers and cyclists. Moreover, the magnitude of these variations from non-athletes is similar to that observed in post-pubertal athletes. Limited data suggest, however, that electrocardiographic findings of "athlete's heart" are not typically observed in young endurance athletes.

Ventilatory responses to acute exercise

Differences in ventilatory responses to exercise between athletes and non-athletes should not necessarily be expected to mimic those of circulatory adaptations. Besides adjusting for demands of gas exchange, respiratory patterns during exercise are dictated by the carbon dioxide released from buffering of lactic acid as well as compensation for metabolic acidosis. Thus, the responses seen in V_E with acute exercise reflect not only demands of increased metabolic rate, but also challenges to maintaining acid–base balance.

Moreover, although critical for aerobic fitness, the respiratory system is not pushed to its functional limits during an acute bout of maximal progressive exercise. In defining limits of endurance exercise, the contributions of respiratory muscle fatigue, terminal hypoxemia, and energy "steal" of ventilatory work are less than minor in highly trained adult endurance athletes (Wetter & Dempsey 2000). However, ventilatory factors have not generally been considered to define limitations of endurance exercise.

Descriptive studies

In contrast to circulatory findings, no increased dimensions of the lungs and airways are witnessed in adult athletes, and in most studies these competitors do not demonstrate any characteristic findings in resting lung function or airway dynamics (Wetter & Dempsey 2000). The same appears to be true in child and adolescent endurance athletes (Vaccaro & Clarke 1978; Vaccaro & Poffenbarger 1982). There have, however, been exceptions. Andrew et al. (1972), for example, found greater values of vital capacity and forced expiratory volumes in 8- to 18-year-old swimmers compared to non-athletes.

At maximal exercise, young endurance athletes demonstrate higher levels of size-relative minute ventilation than non-athletic children, consistent with their superior $\dot{V}O_{2max}$. Unnithan (1993) found mean peak $\dot{V}_E$ values (in $L \cdot kg^{-1} \cdot min^{-1}$) of 1.92 in a group of trained child runners (mean age 11.3 ± 0.9 years) and 1.63 in non-runners. Respective $\dot{V}O_{2max}$ for the two groups was 60.5 and 51.1 $mL \cdot kg^{-1} \cdot min^{-1}$. Similarly, in the 11- to 13-year-old runners studied by Rowland and Green (1990), $\dot{V}_{Emax}$ per kg was 16% greater than that of non-athletes (2.05 vs. 1.75 $L \cdot kg^{-1} \cdot min^{-1}$). The greater minute ventilation in the athletes reflected their larger tidal volume at peak exercise (mean 35 vs. 28 $mL \cdot kg^{-1}$) as maximal breathing rates were similar to the non-trained children.

These characteristics are similar to those observed in adult endurance athletes. The extent that other ventilatory features, such as resistance to respiratory muscle fatigue and alterations in pulmonary diffusion capacity, contribute to ventilatory responses to exercise in trained athletes has not been clarified in adult athletes and remains unstudied in younger competitors (Wetter & Dempsey 2000).

At submaximal exercise, both child and adult endurance athletes demonstrate a lower minute ventilation at a given work rate than non-athletes. This difference typically is not evident at low work levels but becomes more pronounced as intensity rises, becoming most prominent near the anaerobic threshold. Rowland & Green (1990) demonstrated this finding during treadmill running in trained versus untrained children. Group differences in minute ventilation rose with increasing treadmill speed, and at 9.6 $km \cdot hr^{-1}$ (6 mph), $\dot{V}_E$ was 17% higher in the non-athletes, a magnitude typically seen in studies of adult athletes. This dampened ventilatory response at submaximal exercise in athletes could reflect lower blood lactate levels, increased fat utilization (with less carbon dioxide production), or diminished central command (Wetters & Dempsey 2000).

Maturational influences

It can be inferred from the above descriptive information that ventilatory responses to acute exercise are different in child athletes and non-athletes in the same way that these patterns vary between trained and untrained adults. Moreover, these data imply no obvious maturational influences on these adaptations. However, there are recognized differences in ventilatory responses to exercise in populations of non-athletic children compared with adults (for review see Rowland 2005a), and these maturational features may be manifest in athletes as well.

Children have a lower glycolytic capacity than adults and hence generate less lactic acid during exercise. Consequently, the ventilatory anaerobic threshold (VAT, or exercise intensity at which $\dot{V}_E$ begins to rise disproportionally to $\dot{V}O_2$ because of CO_2 produced by lactate buffering) is higher relative to $\dot{V}O_{2max}$ in children. Highly aerobically fit athletes are also expected to demonstrate a higher VAT than non-athletes. Reported relative values during treadmill running in endurance trained children are typically 70–80% $\dot{V}O_{2max}$ (Wolfe et al. 1986; Faria et al. 1989; Nudel et al. 1989), compared with approximately 60% in untrained youth. In untrained adult subjects, VAT is usually about 10% lower than that seen in children. No direct comparisons of VAT in child and adult athletes have been performed. Values of 75% $\dot{V}O_{2max}$ are typically observed in adult distance runners (Withers et al. 1981).

Children breath more frequently (f_R) than adults to achieve a given minute ventilation. The explanation for this higher ratio of breathing rate to tidal volume, even when adjusted for body size, is not immediately obvious. The same phenomenon is observed in child athletes. The runners and non-athletes studied by Rowland & Green (1990) had similar f_R/V_T per kg while running at 9.6 km·hr^{-1} (6 mph), but values were almost twice that seen in adults.

Prepubertal subjects hyperventilate during exercise compared to adults. That is, they demonstrate a greater V_E for any given metabolic rate (the ventilatory equivalent for oxygen, or $V_E/\dot{V}O_2$). Whether this reflects maturational differences in ventilatory neural drive, airway dimensional factors, or even testing artefact (higher equipment dead space) is unclear.

Little information is available in child athletes. Rowland and Green (1990) found that $\dot{V}_E/\dot{V}O_2$ at a treadmill speed of 9.6 km·hr^{-1} was 27.6 ± 3.5 in non-athletic children and 25.1 ± 2.2 in child runners, a difference that was not statistically significant.

Challenges for future research

It is evident from the foregoing discussion that considerable gaps exist in our understanding of cardiopulmonary responses to exercise in young athletes. Virtually nothing is known, for example, of the characteristics of the peripheral mechanisms that facilitate and control circulatory adaptations to exercise. Do young athletes have enhanced skeletal muscle pump function, enhanced arteriolar dilatation, and improved muscle capillarization compared to non-athletes? If so, are there qualitative or quantitative differences in these characteristics from adult endurance athletes?

All studies in child athletes to date have described cardiovascular responses in the same testing model–progressive cycle exercise to exhaustion. Because not even competitive cycling mimics this pattern of exercise, there is a need to better define cardiovascular adaptations to various forms of exercise in the manner they are performed in sports training and competition.

Virtually all studies of cardiopulmonary features of young athletes have involved males. There is a need to understand if gender differences exist in these characteristics.

Do anatomic and physiologic features of young athletes reflect inherent or training-acquired traits? If training itself is influential, which mechanism triggers the development of these features? We know little regarding the extent that physiologic (and performance) improvements that can be gained from training of prepubertal endurance athletes. Until this is understood, appropriate training regimens in this group can only be surmised.

References

Andrew, G.M., Becklake, M.R., Guleria, J.S. & Bates, D.V. (1972) Heart and lung functions in swimmers and non-athletes during growth. *Journal of Applied Physiology* **32**, 245–251.

Cameron, J.D. & Dart, A.M. (1994) Exercise training increases total systemic arterial compliance in humans. *American Journal of Physiology* **266**, H693–H701.

Fagard, R.H. (1997) Impact of different sports and training on cardiac structure and function. *Cardiology Clinics* **15**, 397–412.

Faria, I.E., Faria, E.W., Roberts, S. & Yoshimura, D. (1989) Comparison of physical and physiological characteristics in elite young and mature cyclists. *Research Quarterly for Exercise and Sport* **60**, 388–395.

Gledhill, N., Cox, D. & Jamnik, R. (1994) Endurance athletes' stroke volume does not plateau: major advantage is diastolic function. *Medicine and Science in Sports and Exercise* **26**, 1116–1121.

Gutin, B., Mayers, N., Levy, J.A. & Herman, M.V. (1988) Physiologic and echocardiographic studies of age-group runners. In: *Competitive Sports for Children and Youth* (Brown, E.W. & Branta, C.F., eds.) Human Kinetics, Champaign, IL: 117–128.

Hopper, M.K., Coggan, A.R. & Coyle, E.F. (1988) Exercise stroke volume is relative to plasma volume expansion. *Journal of Applied Physiology* **64**, 404–408.

Ingjer, F. (1978) Maximal aerobic power related to the capillary supply of the quadriceps femoris muscle in man. *Acta Physiolica Scandinavia* **104**, 238–240.

Larsen, S.E., Hansen, H.S., Froberg, K. & Nielsen, J.R. (2000) Left ventricular structure and function in young elite cyclists. *Pediatric Exercise Science* **12**, 382–387.

Lengyel, M. & Gyarfas, I. (1979) The importance of echocardiography in the assessment of left ventricular hypertrophy in trained and untrained schoolchildren. *Acta Cardiologica* **34**, 63–69.

Makan, J., Sharma, S., Whyte, G., Jackson, P.G. & McKenna, W.J. (2005) Physiological upper limits of ventricular cavity size in highly-trained adolescent athletes. *Heart* **91**, 495–499.

Medved, R., Fabecic-Sabadi, V. & Medved, V. (1986) Relationship between echocardiographic values and body dimensions in child swimmers. *Journal of Sports Cardiology* **2**, 28–31.

Nottin, S., Agnes, V., Stecken, F., *et al.* (2002a) Central and peripheral cardiovascular adaptations during maximal cycle exercise in boys and men. *Medicine and Science in Sports and Exercise* **33**, 456–463.

Nottin, S., N'Guyen, L-D., Terbah, M. & Obert, P. (2004) Left ventricular function in endurance-trained children by tissue Doppler imaging. *Medicine and Science in Sports and Exercise* **36**, 1507–1513.

Nottin, S., Vinet, A., Stecken, F., *et al.* (2002b) Central and peripheral cardiovascular adaptations to exercise in endurance-trained children. *Acta Physiologica Scandinavia* **175**, 85–92.

Nudel, D.B., Hassett, I., Gurain, A., Diamant, S., Weinhouse, E. & Gootman, N. (1989) Young long distance runners: physiologic characteristics. *Clinical Pediatrics* **28**, 500–505.

Obert, P., Stecken, F., Courteix, D., Lecoq, A.-M. & Guenon, P. (1998) Effect of long-term intensive endurance training on left ventricular structure and diastolic function in prepubertal children. *International Journal of Sports Medicine* **19**, 149–154.

Ozer, S., Cil, E., Baltaci, G., Ergun, N. & Ozme, S. (1994) Left ventricular structure and function by echocardiography in childhood swimmers. *Japanese Heart Journal* **35**, 295–300.

Perrault, H.M. & Turcotte, R.A. (1993) Do athletes have "the athlete's heart?" *Progress in Pediatric Cardiology* **2**, 40–50.

Petridis, L., Kneffel, Z., Kispeter, Z., Horvath, P., Sido, Z. & Pavlik, G. (2004) Echocardiographic characteristics in adolescent junior male athletes of different sport events. *Acta Physiologica Hungaria* **91**, 99–109.

Rost, R. & Hollman, W. (1983) Athlete's heart: a review of its historical assessment and new aspects. *International Journal of Sports Medicine* **4**, 147–165.

Rowland, T.W. (2001) The circulatory response to exercise: role of the peripheral pump. *International Journal of Sports Medicine* **22**, 558–565.

Rowland, T.W. (2005a) *Children's Exercise Physiology.* Human Kinetics, Champaign, IL.

Rowland, T.W. (2005b) Circulatory responses to exercise. Are we misreading Fick? *Chest* **127**, 1023–1030.

Rowland, T.W. & Whatley-Blum, J.W. (2000a) Cardiac dynamics during upright exercise in boys. *American Journal of Human Biology* **12**, 749–757.

Rowland, T.W., Delaney, B.C. & Siconolfi, S.F. (1987) "Athlete's heart" in prepubertal children. *Pediatrics* **79**, 800–804.

Rowland, T.W., Garrison, A. & DeIulio, A. (2003) Circulatory responses to progressive exercise: insights from positional differences. *International Journal of Sports Medicine* **24**, 512–517.

Rowland, T., Goff, D., Popowski, B., DeLuca, P. & Ferrone, L. (1998) Cardiac responses to exercise in child distance runners. *International Journal of Sports Medicine* **19**, 385–390.

Rowland, T.W. & Green, G.M. (1990) The influence of biological maturation and aerobic fitness on ventilatory responses to treadmill exercise. In: Dotson, C.O. & Humphrey, J.H., eds.) *Exercise Physiology. Current Selected Research.* AMS Press, New York: 51–59.

Rowland, T.W., Miller, K., Vanderburgh, P., Goff, D., Martel, L. & Ferrone, L. (1999a) Cardiovascular fitness in premenarcheal girls and young women. *International Journal of Sports Medicine* **20**, 117–121.

Rowland, T.W., Popowski, B. & Ferrone, L. (1997) Cardiac responses to maximal upright cycle exercise in healthy boys and men. *Medicine and Science in Sports and Exercise* **29**, 1146–1151.

Rowland, T.W., Potts, J., Potts, T., Son-Hing, J., Harbison, G. & Sandor, G. (1999b) Cardiovascular responses to exercise in children and adolescents with myocardial dysfunction. *American Heart Journal* **137**, 126–133.

Rowland, T.W. & Roti, M.W. (2004) Cardiac responses to progressive upright exercise in adult male cyclists. *Journal of Sports Medicine and Physical Fitness* **44**, 179–185.

Rowland, T.W., Unnithan, V., Fernhall, B., Baynard, T. & Lange, C. (2002) Left ventricular response to dynamic exercise in young cyclists. *Medicine and Science in Sports and Exercise* **34**, 637–642.

Rowland, T.W., Unnithan, V.B., MacFarlane, N.G., Gibson, N.G. & Paton, J.Y. (1994) Clinical manifestations of the "athlete's heart" in prepubertal male runners. *International Journal of Sports Medicine* **15**, 515–519.

Rowland, T.W., Wehnert, M. & Miller, K. (2000b) Cardiac responses to exercise in competitive child cyclists. *Medicine and Science in Sports and Exercise* **32**, 747–752.

Shepherd, T.A., Eisenman, P.A., Ruttenburg, H.D., Adams, T.G. & Johnson, S.C. (1988) Cardiac dimensions of highly trained prepubescent boys [abstract]. *Medicine and Science in Sports and Exercise* **20** (Supplement), S53.

Sundberg, S. & Elovainio, R. (1982) Cardiorespiratory function in competitive runners aged 12–16 years compared with normal boys. *Acta Paediatrica Scandinavia* **91**, 987–992.

Telford, R.D., McDonald, I.G., Ellis, L.B., Chennells, H.M.D., Sandstrom, E.R. & Fuller, P.J. (1988) Echocardiographic dimensions in trained and untrained 12-year old boys and girls. *Journal of Sports Science* **6**, 49–57.

Triposkiadis, F., Ghiokas, S., Skoularigis, I., Kotsakis, A., Giannakoulis, I. & Thanopoulos, V.

(2002) Cardiac adaptations to intensive training in prepubertal swimmers. *European Journal of Clinical Investigation* **32**, 16–23.

Unnithan, V.B. (1993) Factors affecting submaximal running economy in children. Doctoral thesis. University of Glasgow, Scotland.

Unnithan, V.B., Rowland, T.W., Cable, N.T. & Raine, N. (1997) Cardiac responses to exercise in elite male junior cyclists. In: *Children and Exercise XIX* (Armstrong, N., Kirby, B. & Welsman, J., eds.) E & FN Spon, London: 501–506.

Vaccaro, P. & Clarke, D.H. (1978) Cardiorespiratory alterations in 9 to 11 year old children following a season of competitive swimming. *Medicine and Science in Sports* **10**, 204–207.

Vaccaro, P. & Poffenbarger, A. (1982) Resting and exercise respiratory function in young female runners. *Journal of Sports Medicine* **22**, 102–107.

Wetter, T.J. & Dempsey, J.A. (2000) Pulmonary system and endurance exercise. In: *Endurance in Sport* (Shephard, R.J. & Astrand, P-O., eds.) Blackwell Science, Oxford: 52–67.

Withers, R.T., Sherman, W.M., Miller, J.M. & Costill, D.L. (1981) Specificity of the anaerobic threshold in endurance trained cyclists and runners. *European Journal of Applied Physiology* **47**, 93–104.

Wolfe, R.R., Washington, R., Daberkow, E., Murphy, J.R. & Brammel, H.E. (1986) Anaerobic threshold as a predictor of athletic performance in prepubertal female runners. *American Journal of Diseases of Children* **140**, 922–924.

Chapter 5

Scaling for Size: Relevance to Understanding the Effects of Growth on Performance

JOANNE R. WELSMAN AND NEIL ARMSTRONG

Examination of any graph of children's physiologic performance (such as peak oxygen uptake (peak $\dot{V}o_2$, short term power, or peak torque) expressed in absolute terms plotted against body mass will reveal a strong positive relationship. The data presented in Fig. 5.1 exemplify this relationship with the Pearson correlation between body mass and peak $\dot{V}o_2$ in 11- to 14-year-old girls and boys of r = 0.87 and 0.86, respectively. Even within a narrow chronologic age range, body mass varies widely between individuals and the effect is accentuated during the pubertal years as a result of individual differences in maturational status. For example, in our longitudinal study of 10- to 17-year-olds the magnitude of the difference in body mass between the lightest and heaviest boy was 37.8 kg at 10–11 years, 54.8 kg at 12–13 years, and

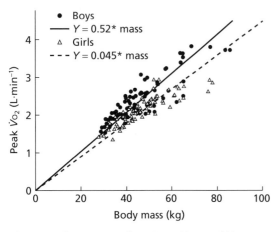

Fig. 5.1 Peak oxygen uptake in 11- to 14-year-old boys and girls. The line is showing the simple linear relationship assumed by conventional ratio scaling ($Y = aX$).

51.8 kg at the final test at 16–17 years (unpublished data). Therefore, if we wish to elucidate age and maturational effects upon physiologic performance we need appropriate methods for controlling or removing the effects of body size. This process is often referred to as scaling.

The aim of any scaling technique is to remove the effects of the body size variable (usually body mass but it can be stature, lean body mass, leg volume) such that the computed scaled variable (e.g., peak $\dot{V}o_2$ in mL·min^{-1}·kg^{-b}) retains no significant correlation with the performance variable. The importance of selecting an appropriate scaling technique cannot be overemphasized; applying a scaling technique that does not remove size effects can lead to erroneous interpretation of the physiologic data. Therefore, this chapter both critically reviews the techniques available and demonstrates simple techniques for evaluating whether or not a scaling method has achieved this objective using examples both from the literature and from unpublished data collected in the Children's Health and Exercise Research Centre, Exeter, UK.

Traditional approaches to scaling cross-sectional data

Conventional ratio scaling

Since the pioneering laboratory studies of young people's physiologic performance by Robinson (1938) and Astrand (1952), interindividual size differences have been traditionally controlled for by simply dividing the absolute value of the measure by body mass. Thus, a simple "per body mass ratio" is constructed (e.g., mL·kg^{-1}·min^{-1} for oxygen uptake, W·kg^{-1} for mechanical power, and Nm·kg^{-1} for maximal torque). Although this approach has long been criticised on both theoretical and practical grounds (Tanner 1949, 1964; Astrand & Rodahl 1986), and alternative approaches embraced in other disciplines (Schmidt-Nielsen 1984), within pediatric exercise science the use of simple ratio scaling still appears to dominate despite increasing documentation of its limitations when applied to pediatric exercise data (Armstrong et al. 1995; Welsman et al. 1996; Armstrong & Welsman 2001). That is not to say, however, that ratio scaling should never be used. There are instances where it remains appropriate, notably in the interpretation of running performance (Nevill et al. 1992, 2004a); however, only where this is statistically verified.

Ratio scaling implies the following statistical relationship between the performance measure (Y) and the body size variable (X):

$$Y = aX + \varepsilon$$

a relationship that describes a straight line passing from the origin (zero) through the intersection of the mean values of the Y and X variables. The additive error term (ε) suggests that error variance is consistent throughout the numerical range of the data. In Fig. 5.1 this relationship has been superimposed upon the data. It is immediately clear that the assumption of constant error does not hold for this data set. Instead, the distance between the data point and the regression line (called the error or residual) is greater at higher levels of body mass and peak $\dot{V}O_2$. Thus, the data display non-uniform error or "heteroscedasticity" suggesting that the simple linear model will be unable to provide a good statistical fit to the data. This "fanning" of error is very typical of size-related physiologic measures and is observed in both adults and young people.

Several authors have emphasized the importance of evaluating that ratio adjustments are performing as intended (i.e., are truly removing the influence of body size) (Tanner 1949; Albrecht et al. 1993). The following summarize the methods these authors suggest which are easily computed to check the validity of a ratio adjustment. Tanner (1949) demonstrated how a ratio standard was only appropriate where the following relationship could be demonstrated between the dependent (X) and independent (Y) variables:

$$V_X/V_Y = r_{XY}$$

where V is the coefficient of variation and r is the Pearson product moment correlation coefficient. For the girls' data summarized in Fig. 5.1 the values for this relationship are as follows: $V_X/V_Y = 1.31$ and $r = 0.86$. Clearly, this data set does not comply with this criterion suggesting that the application of a per body mass ratio would be inappropriate.

The three criteria suggested by Albrecht et al. (1993) are based upon statistical, graphical, and algebraic evaluation of the data. To satisfy the statistical criterion, the Pearson product moment correlation coefficient between the mass-adjusted value and body mass should not be significantly different from zero. If this criterion is applied to the data set presented in Fig. 5.1, significant ($P < 0.01$) negative coefficients of $r = -0.472$ and -0.622 are obtained for boys and girls, respectively (Fig. 5.2).

The graphical criterion examines in more detail the exact nature of the relationship between the adjusted variable and body size. If the influence of body size has been removed effectively from the criterion variable, the relationship between the mass-adjusted variable and body mass should result in a horizontal line when plotted against each other.

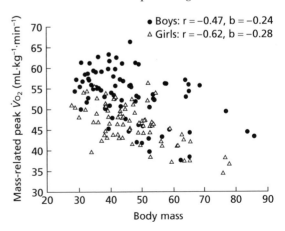

Fig. 5.2 Mass-adjusted peak oxygen uptake in 11- to 14-year-olds illustrating residual significant ($P < 0.05$) negative relationship and negative slope coefficient.

In other words, the slope of the least-squares regression line should not be significantly different from zero. It is evident from the data presented in Fig. 5.2 that mass-related peak $\dot{V}O_2$ remains size-dependent with significant ($P < 0.01$) negative regression slope coefficients of b = −0.24 and −0.28 for boys and girls, respectively.

The algebraic criterion states that the expected value of adjusted Y is algebraically equal to a constant (e.g., b). It is important to emphasize that these three criteria are equivalent when assessing a linear relationship between two variables (i.e., a correlation coefficient of zero implies a horizontal regression line whose equation is equal to a constant) (Albrecht *et al.* 1993).

The problems of using ratio scaling where not justified are illustrated in more detail below, but to summarize this model will overestimate fitness in light individuals and penalize heavy people. This effect is particularly critical in comparisons of overweight or obese children with normal weight counterparts. For example, in unpublished data collected in our laboratory we identified a 13.6% difference between the mass-related peak $\dot{V}O_2$ of overweight (>120% mass for stature for age) vs. lean 11-year-old children. This difference was reduced to 5.2% when comparisons were based upon allometrically adjusted values.

Further inaccuracies in interpretation can arise where ratio-adjusted scores are used in subsequent correlational or regression analyses. To exemplify this, Bloxham *et al.* (2005) examined the influence of scaling technique upon the interpretation of relationships between peak $\dot{V}O_2$ and short-term power in 12-year-olds. Their findings demonstrated that in all comparisons the magnitude of the relationship decreased substantially when allometric scaling was used to adjust for body mass compared to ratio scaled values. In one comparison a significant relationship (between Wingate anaerobic test mean power and cycle peak $\dot{V}O_2$) became non-significant once appropriately adjusted.

Alternative approaches for cross-sectional data

If we accept that the simple linear model implied by the per body mass ratio often fails to provide a size-free variable, what alternative scaling techniques are available and what evidence is there that these represent a better solution for scaling young people's physiologic data?

Linear regression scaling

Several authors (Williams *et al.* 1992; Eston *et al.* 1993; Welsman *et al.* 1996) have applied a scaling technique based upon standard linear regression, the equation for which is:

$$Y = a + bX + \varepsilon$$

where Y is the dependent variable, X the independent (body size) variable, a represents the intercept of the regression line on the y axis, b describes the slope of the line and ε is an additive error term. Using this technique, regression lines are constructed for each group (or groups) in a comparative study and the slopes and intercepts of these individual regression lines compared using a standard statistical technique, analysis of covariance. The data presented in Fig. 5.3 are unpublished data drawn from our database and replicate the findings of Williams *et al.* (1992). They represent the peak $\dot{V}O_2$ values of 13-year-old boys divided into two groups by maturity status (prepubertal vs. post-pubertal). Based upon a traditional per body mass ratio, the interpretation of these data would be that there was no significant difference ($P > 0.05$) in peak $\dot{V}O_2$ between

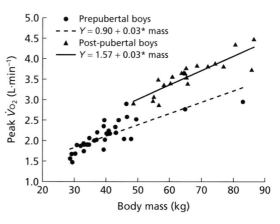

Fig. 5.3 The linear regression relationship between peak oxygen uptake and body mass in prepubertal and post-pubertal boys.

the two groups, with values of 54 ml·kg^{-1}·min^{-1} compared to 55 ml·kg^{-1}·min^{-1} for the prepubertal and post-pubertal groups, respectively.

However, the results of the analysis of covariance suggest otherwise. The data for each maturity group have been fitted separately with least-squares linear regression lines. The regression slopes identified were 0.028 and 0.035 for prepubertal and post-pubertal groups, respectively. Analysis of covariance demonstrated that these were not significantly different ($P > 0.05$) (i.e., examination of interaction effect of maturity group by body mass yielded a non-significant result) and a common slope of b = 0.030 was identified.

Statistical verification of common slope is an important underlying assumption of analysis of variance and if this is violated the analysis should not be pursued. Subsequent comparison of the elevations (intercept values) of the group regression lines yielded significantly different values of 1.57 and 0.90, respectively, confirming the higher peak $\dot{V}o_2$ of the post-pubertal group.

Using this technique, "adjusted means" or "regression standards" can be computed by adding the value of each individual subject's residual from the least-squares regression line to the group mean value. Although these are reported in absolute terms, the adjusted values have had the influence of body mass covaried out. Therefore, for this data set the observed mean absolute peak $\dot{V}o_2$ values were 2.12 and 3.57 L·min^{-1} for prepubertal and post-pubertal groups, respectively. Once adjusted for body mass the absolute values change to 2.51 and 3.18 L·min^{-1}, confirming that once adjusted for body mass, post-pubertal boys score higher for peak $\dot{V}o_2$ than prepubertal boys of the same age.

Although in this example linear regression scaling was able to distinguish an important group difference in peak $\dot{V}o_2$ that was masked by the conventional per body mass ratio, there are well-documented limitations with linear regression scaling, recently reviewed by Nevill et al. (2005), which caution against its routine use. Specifically, the assumption that the relationship between the Y and X variable is linear with constant error variance is clearly violated in this heteroscedastic data set (Fig. 5.3). Furthermore, the biologically implausible intercept parameter "a," suggesting a physiologic response exists for a body size of zero, has been highlighted by several authors (Welsman et al. 1996; Nevill et al. 2005).

Allometric (log-linear) scaling and power function ratios

From the discussion so far some of the requirements of a statistical model for scaling pediatric exercise data are becoming clearer: in contrast to simple ratio and linear regression scaling techniques, the model must be able to accommodate heteroscedastic data (i.e., a multiplicative rather than additive error term is required). Second, in order to provide biologically plausible results the technique should regress through zero.

The simple allometric model:

$$Y = aX^b \cdot \varepsilon$$

fulfills both of these requirements. This equation describes the curvilinear relationship depicted in Fig. 5.4(a) where it has been applied to the relationship between peak $\dot{V}o_2$ and body mass in 13-year-old girls. The exponent "b" describes the curvature of the line. Where, as in this example, the Y variable (e.g., peak $\dot{V}o_2$) increases at a slower rate to the X variable (e.g., body mass), b is less than 1.0. In cases where the opposite is true and Y increases faster than X, the b exponent is greater than 1.0 and the line curves upwards. Where a directly proportional relationship exists, the relationship is linear with a slope equal to 1.0 (i.e., the data conform to the simple ratio relationship described earlier).

The curvilinear allometric relationship can be transformed into a linear one simply by taking the natural logarithms ($\log_e$) of the Y and X data. This linearizes the relationship to:

$$\log_e Y = \log_e a + b \log_e X + \log_e \varepsilon$$

and simple linear regression can be used to solve for the values of a and b. This is illustrated in Fig. 5.4(b). Thus, intergroup comparisons are facilitated as analysis of covariance can be applied to compare the slope and intercept terms for different groups as described for linear regression modeling above. This analysis can also be extended to include other concurrent covariates (e.g., stature or thigh muscle volume) (Nevill 1994; Welsman et al. 1996).

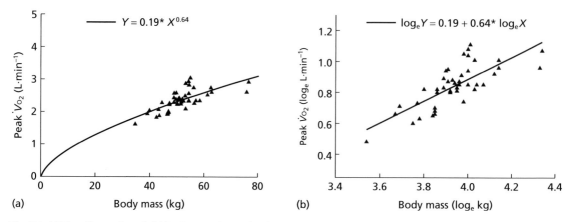

Fig. 5.4 (a) The allometric and (b) log linear relationship between peak oxygen uptake and body mass in 13-year-old girls.

Identification of the value of the b exponent also enables the calculation of power function ratios (Welsman *et al.* 1996; Nevill *et al.* 2005). Here, the absolute value of the performance variable is divided by body mass raised to the power "b". For example, in Fig. 5.4, the b exponent of the allometric relationship (slope of the log linear regression) in the girls was 0.64. Therefore to remove the effects of body mass in this sample, peak $\dot{V}O_2$ in mL·min^{-1} should be divided by mass$^{0.64}$ to yield the power function ratio mL·kg$^{-0.64}$·min^{-1}.

Theoretical vs. sample-specific exponents

A question that has long challenged proponents of allometric scaling and continues to be strongly debated relates to the "true" value of the exponent that describes the relationship between body mass and metabolic rate, both at rest and at peak $\dot{V}O_2$. Within the pediatric literature some authors have recommended using allometric mass exponents of either 0.67 (Rogers *et al.* 1995) or 0.75 (Svedenhag 1995) to express young people's peak $\dot{V}O_2$ and these recommendations have been taken up in recent studies (Eisenmann *et al.* 2001; Dencker *et al.* 2006).

These values of 0.67 and 0.75 have derivations which are comprehensively reviewed elsewhere (Astrand & Rodahl 1986) but, to summarize briefly, the value 0.67 is most simply explained with reference

to two cubes—one small and one large. The two cubes can be described as geometrically similar or "isometric," as corresponding linear dimensions are related in the same proportion and corresponding surface areas are related in the same proportion squared. The volumes of the cubes are related in the same proportion to the third power. These relationships can be summarized as:

Surface area $\propto$ length^2
Volume $\propto$ length^3
Surface area $\propto$ volume$^{2/3}$

Extrapolating this theory to human physiology, assuming that individuals are isometric, all linear measures such as stature and breadths have the dimension L, all measurements of area including body surface area and muscle cross-sectional area have the dimension L^2 and body mass and volume (e.g., heart and lung volumes) have the dimension L^3. In physiologic systems time has the dimension L. Therefore, as peak $\dot{V}O_2$ is a volume per unit time it should be proportional to L^3·L^{-1} = L^2. This relates to stature^2 or its analog in isometric bodies, mass$^{2/3}$ (i.e., mass$^{0.67}$).

The alternative value of 0.75 derives from empirical observations that in many homeotherm species metabolic rate increases proportional to mass$^{0.75}$ (analogous to stature$^{2.25}$) and does not conform to these theoretical predictions (Kleiber 1932). In the biologic sciences arguments have been put forward to both explain (McMahon 1973) and refute (Heusner 1982) the 0.75 exponent but both values continue to be explored as valid alternatives for the interpretation of performance data in children.

Identifying a universal alternative is an attractive proposition as it both simplifies data analysis and facilitates comparisons between studies. However, to establish whether or not one of the proposed exponents offers a valid alternative for generic acceptance vs. traditional ratio scaling requires consideration of both theoretical concerns and the empirical evidence.

A fundamental assumption of the mass exponent 0.67 is that individuals demonstrate geometric similarity. Although it is well documented that body proportions alter during the first decade of life (e.g., the characteristic shorter limbs and longer torso of babies and young children), it has been generally accepted that from the age of around 10 years geometric similarity can be assumed (Astrand & Rodahl 1986). Recent work has challenged this assumption, albeit in adult subjects: Studies by Nevill et al. (2004b) have demonstrated that human physiques are not geometrically similar in that body circumferences and limb girths develop at rates different to that anticipated by geometric similarity. These authors have also used this information to demonstrate that the exponent mass$^{0.75}$ derived in many studies reflects a disproportionate increase in muscle girth which, if subsequently accounted for in an allometric analysis, reduces the mass exponent to values approximating 0.67 (Nevill et al. 2004c). A similar effect has been noted in a previous study of scaling of adolescent thigh volume, where a mass exponent of 1.1 confirmed that muscle volume increases at a faster rate than body mass even in younger subjects (Nevill 1994).

With regard to the empirical evidence, Table 5.1 summarizes the range of body mass exponents reported in the literature for children encompassing the age range 6–18 years. The data are arranged by magnitude of exponent to facilitate insight into the

Table 5.1 Allometric body mass exponents for peak $\dot{V}o_2$ in children and adolescents: cross-sectional studies.

Study	Age (years)	Sex (M/F) Trained (T)	n	Mass exponent (SE)	Mode of exercise
McMiken 1976*	10–15	M (T)	14	1.07	Treadmill
Paterson et al. 1987	11–15	M	18	1.02 (0.04)	Treadmill
Cooper et al. 1984	6–18	M, F	109	1.01 (0.06)	Cycle
McMiken 1976†	12–16	F (T)	30	0.97	Cycle
Loftin et al. 2001	7–18	F	47	0.92	Treadmill
McMiken 1976‡	7–13	M	50	0.88	Treadmill
Welsman et al. 1996	10–11, 13–14, 22–23	M, F	156	0.80 (0.04)	Treadmill
Sjödin & Svedenhag 1992	11–15	M (T)	8	0.78 (0.07)	Treadmill
Chamari et al. 2005	14	M (T)	21	0.72 (0.04)	Treadmill
Nevill et al. 2004a	12	M	36	0.71 (0.09)	Cycle
Armstrong & Welsman, unpublished	13–14	M, F	105	0.69 (0.06)	Cycle
Armstrong et al. 1995	10–11	M, F	164	0.66	Treadmill
Bloxham et al. 2005	11–12	M, F	58	0.65 (0.06)	Cycle
Bloxham et al. 2005	11–12	M, F	58	0.65 (0.06)	Treadmill
Winsley et al. 2006	13–14	M, F	52	0.61	Treadmill
Fawkner & Armstrong 2004	10–11	M, F	48	0.55 (0.09)	Cycle
Rogers et al. 1995	7–9	M, F	42	0.52	Treadmill
Rowland et al. 2000	11.3–13.2	F	24	0.52 (0.02)	Cycle
Fawkner et al. 2002	11–12	M, F	30	0.44 (0.12)	Cycle

* Data from Daniels and Oldridge (1971).
† Data from Astrand et al. (1963).
‡ Data from Klissouras (1971).

factors influencing the value derived. Standard errors are included where reported in the original papers. It is immediately evident that the highest exponents have been identified where the age of the subject group varies widely. In subject groups encompassing a single chronologic age values approximate or are lower than 0.67. In the very large, single age group data sets, values are closest to 0.67, signaling sample size as having a critical influence upon the value of the mass exponent obtained—a finding echoed by other authors (Jensen *et al.* 2001).

A further factor contributing to variability in the value of the mass exponent is the extent to which the sample size is heterogeneous for body mass. It has been suggested that a wide spread of body mass within a subject group will yield a mass-exponent closer to the theoretical value than in a restricted set (Calder 1987) and this has been supported by the results of our studies (Armstrong *et al.* 1995; Welsman *et al.* 1997).

Taken together, the available evidence does not yet support the adoption of a single body mass exponent as a universal alternative to ratio scaling—at least for peak $\dot{V}O_2$. Mass exponents are clearly sample-specific and if differences between groups or relationships between performance variables are to be examined sample-specific mass exponents should be used.

Allometric scaling in longitudinal comparisons

Longitudinal studies are optimal for understanding the interactions between physical growth, chronologic age, maturation and physical performance. In such studies a wealth of information is usually collected and controversy exists as to the best way to analyze the findings.

Traditionally, the interpretation of longitudinal data has been fraught with methodologic problems —particularly where an allometric framework is desired. Extending the analysis of covariance described for cross-sectional data sets to a repeated measures ANCOVA is not a satisfactory option as varying covariates are not usually allowed (i.e., only one measure of mass can be covaried out) which is clearly unsatisfactory, particularly when

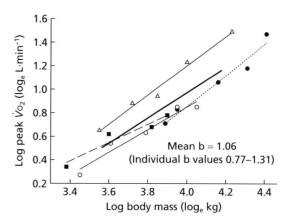

Fig. 5.5 Longitudinal changes in peak oxygen uptake and body mass in four individuals tested between the ages 10 and 17 years.

children are measured longitudinally throughout their adolescent growth spurt.

Ontogenetic allometry

One solution reported by several studies has been to apply ontogenetic allometry (Rowland *et al.* 1997; Beunen *et al.* 2002). This reflects the dimensional relationship between peak $\dot{V}O_2$ and body mass over time at the individual level. Figure 5.5 illustrates the ontogenetic relationship between peak $\dot{V}O_2$ and body mass in five individuals who participated in a longitudinal study in our laboratory spanning the age range 10–17 years. Peak $\dot{V}O_2$ was determined at approximately yearly intervals from 10 to 14 years and again at 17 years. In the small subsample illustrated individual exponents ranged from b = 0.77 to 1.31 with a mean value of b = 1.06. Other studies have reported a similarly large interindividual range in ontogenetic exponents. For example, Beunen *et al.* (2002) reported values in 8- to 16-year-old boys ranging from 0.56 to 1.18 with a mean of 0.87. Such variation in ontogenetic exponents is not surprising and exemplifies the difficulties of interpreting size-related performance during growth and maturation. Although using this scaling technique the individual relationship between mass and performance is well-described, it neither allows for quantification of the average magnitude of change in peak $\dot{V}O_2$ over the adolescent period nor enables the influence of other covariates to be examined simultaneously.

Multilevel regression modeling

Our understanding of longitudinal changes in size-related exercise performance data has been revolutionized in recent years by the availability of programs enabling multilevel modeling (Rasbash *et al.* 2000).

The data collected in longitudinal studies of growth, fitness, or performance can be seen to exist at different levels. This hierarchical structure is illustrated in Fig. 5.5. Within the multilevel structure, each individual's measurement occasions represent level 1 of the analysis. As shown in Fig. 5.5 these individual data points can be summarized by an individually computed regression line that represents the second level of the analysis.

What is clear from Fig. 5.5 is that the slope and intercept values for each individual vary reflecting each individual's rate of growth and maturation. Furthermore, it is evident that some individual's measurement occasions vary more markedly around their regression line (i.e., greater residual error) while others scarcely deviate from it. The advantage of a multilevel analysis is that it allows the mean response of the subject population to be described while simultaneously capturing the element of variation both within the individual (level 1 variation) and between individuals (level 2 variation). A two-level multilevel analysis thus comprises two components: a "fixed" part describing the average value of slope and intercept for the subject group, and a "random" part consisting of variances which summarize variability in individual slopes and intercepts from the mean values and also the extent of any covariance between slope and intercept values at different levels of the analysis if required.

Additional and higher levels of analysis may be defined as necessary; for example, in a mixed longitudinal design the responses of similar populations belonging to different cohorts may be of interest, with cohort forming a third level of analysis (Martin *et al.* 2003).

A major advantage of a multilevel approach is that complete longitudinal data sets are not required.

That is, both the number of measurement occasions per individual and the temporal spacing of these occasions may vary. For example, in Fig. 5.5 two of the subjects were only tested on four occasions. Furthermore, the age at each test occasion varied between individuals; for example, at the first test occasion from 10.4 to 11.5 years. Such variation is unavoidable in large-scale longitudinal studies but, in contrast to traditional repeated measures analyses, all available data points can be incorporated into and contribute to the final multilevel analysis.

Although multilevel analyses can be conducted using both polynomial (linear) and multiplicative (allometric) approaches it is the latter that is preferable when modeling size-related performance measures during growth and maturation for the reasons described in earlier sections. For example, Baxter-Jones *et al.* (1993) used a polynomial, additive approach to analyze peak $\dot{V}o_2$ and strength data in young athletes. Subsequently, these data were reanalyzed following logarithmic transformation to provide an allometric framework (Nevill *et al.* 1998) with a variety of statistical techniques used to evaluate model fit. This latter study demonstrated that the multiplicative, allometric approach produced a solution that was not only physiologically plausible but represented a significantly better statistical fit, requiring fewer fitted parameters than the original solution, and accommodating the heteroscedasticity evident in the raw data.

Subsequent to these reports, the number of publications applying multilevel allometric modeling to the understanding of growth and maturational influences upon health and exercise performance have burgeoned providing valuable insights into the factors influencing the development of peak $\dot{V}o_2$ (Armstrong *et al.* 1999, 2001; Beunen *et al.* 2002); submaximal $\dot{V}o_2$ (Welsman & Armstrong 2000); cardiovascular responses (Armstrong & Welsman 2002); isokinetic strength (De Ste Croix *et al.* 2002); short-term power (Armstrong *et al.* 2000b, 2001; De Ste Croix *et al.* 2001; Martin *et al.* 2003; Santos *et al.* 2003); and physical activity (Armstrong *et al.* 2000a).

To illustrate the way in which multilevel modeling has enabled insights into the development of aerobic fitness, Table 5.2 presents the results of our study (Armstrong & Welsman 2001) describing the longitudinal development of peak $\dot{V}o_2$ in healthy, untrained 11- to 17-year-olds.

The focus of this study was to elucidate the development of peak $\dot{V}o_2$ in relation to age, sex, and maturation having simultaneously controlled for the influence of selected variables related to body size and composition. Following evaluation of several model formulations, Nevill and Holder (1994) proposed the following equation as an initial model for investigation in multilevel analyses:

$$Y = mass^{k1} \cdot stature^{k2} \cdot exp\,(a_j + b_j \cdot age)\,\varepsilon_{ij}$$

In this model all parameters are fixed with the exception of the constant (intercept, a) and age parameters which are allowed to vary randomly at level 2 (between individuals) and the multiplicative error ratio (ε_{ij}) which varies randomly at level 1, describing the error variance between test occasions. With logarithmic transformation this equation is linearized to:

$$Log_e Y = Log_e mass \cdot k_1 + Log_e stature \cdot k_2 + a_j + b_j \cdot age + Log_e \varepsilon_{ij}$$

and thus can be solved using multilevel regression. From this baseline model, additional explanatory variables can be investigated, including in this example sum of two skinfolds, blood hemoglobin concentration. Sex and stage of maturity are also investigated by incorporating them into the model as "dummy" or indicator variables. For example, sex is coded "0" for boys and "1" for girls. A similar procedure is followed for maturity stage. By doing this, the baseline model reflects the average response of a prepubertal boy from which responses for girls and children of different maturity status deviate. Interaction terms may also be computed and investigated such as age by sex or maturity stage by sex.

During the multilevel modeling process, explanatory variables can be entered into and taken out of the analysis. If a variable is making a significant contribution to the dependent variable, the value of the estimate is more than twice the value of the standard error (Duncan et al. 1996). The -2*loglikelihood is a measure of the overall statistical fit of the model; the more negative the value, the better the statistical fit.

In Table 5.2 the results are interpreted thus. In model 1, both body mass and stature proved to be significant explanatory variables with exponents of 0.44 and 1.01, respectively. These values are interpreted exactly as for the b exponent in the allometric

Parameter	Model 1 Estimate (SE)	Model 2 Estimate (SE)
Fixed		
Constant	-1.2023 (0.1474)	-1.9005 (0.1400)
Log_e mass	0.4454 (0.0460)	0.8752 (0.0432)
Log_e stature	1.0082 (0.1607)	Not significant ($P > 0.05$)
Log_e skinfolds	Not entered	-0.1656 (0.0174)
Age	0.0452 (0.0101)	0.0470 (0.0094)
Sex	-0.1608 (0.0135)	-0.1372 (0.0121)
Age × Sex	-0.258 (0.0051)	-0.0214 (0.0053)
Maturity 2	0.0511 (0.0116)	0.0341 (0.0094)
Maturity 3	0.0665 (0.0135)	0.0361 (0.0102)
Maturity 4	0.0988 (0.0169)	0.0537 (0.0116)
Maturity 5	0.0770 (0.0301)	Not significant ($P > 0.05$)
Random		
Level 2 constant	0.0042 (0.0007)	0.0030 (0.0005)
Level 2 age	0.0002 (0.0001)	0.0004 (0.0001)
Level 1 constant	0.0033 (0.0004)	0.0032 (0.0004)
-2*loglikelihood	-844.2189	-870.6431

Table 5.2 Multilevel regression models for peak oxygen uptake ($n = 388$). Age centred on the group mean age of 12.9 years. Data from Armstrong and Welsman (2001).

equation described above. The positive estimate for age demonstrates that even with effects of body size accounted for, peak $\dot{V}O_2$ increases with age in 11- to 17-year-olds (supporting the findings of previous cross-sectional allometric comparisons; Welsman et al. 1996). However, this increase with age is substantially greater in boys than girls as shown by the negative coefficient for the age by sex interaction which is deducted from the age coefficient for girls only. Furthermore, the negative effect of sex reflects the overall lower peak $\dot{V}O_2$ of girls compared with boys. This analysis also showed positive, incremental increases in peak $\dot{V}O_2$ with maturation—an effect over and above that due to chronologic age.

In model 2, sum of two skinfolds was entered as an additional fixed explanatory variable yielding a significant, negative coefficient. As a result, the effect of stature was negated and the value of the mass exponent was increased to 0.88, highlighting that the value of the mass exponent is to a large extent dependent upon what additional covariates are included. The addition of a measure of body fatness also explained some of the variation due to maturity as the coefficients for stages 2–4 were reduced and that for maturity stage 5 became non-significant. Similarly, the age and sex coefficients were slightly reduced but remained significant. Therefore, overall the combined effect of the positive coefficient for mass and the negative effect for skinfold thickness indicate that lean body mass is a key factor in explaining developmental changes in peak $\dot{V}O_2$ and, in particular the divergence in male and female scores throughout the age range examined.

That model 2 provides a better fit for the data is reflected in the change in the −2*loglikelihood (sometimes referred to as the deviance statistic). Where models are "nested" (in this example where model 1 was modified by the addition of skinfold thickness), the smaller the number the better the model fit. The change in this value is interpreted relative to the change in the number of fitted parameters. Thus, in model 2, there is a deviance of −26.42 for one fewer fitted parameters (i.e., one fewer degrees of freedom as maturity stage 5 becomes non-significant) compared with model 1. This exceeds the χ^2 critical value of 3.84 for significance at $P < 0.05$.

The random parameters reflect the error associated with specified terms at both levels of the analysis (i.e., they represent the part of the model unexplained by the fixed parameter estimates). The random structure of the models presented in Table 5.2 was comparatively simple. In models 1 and 2, the random variation associated with the intercept (constant) reflects the degree of variation from the average intercept both between (level 2) and within (level 1) individuals. There was significant random variation at level 2 (between individuals) for age, allowing each child to have their own growth trajectory.

To briefly return to the earlier discussion of what factors influence the value of the mass exponent, the results of studies using multilevel modeling, both alone and in comparison with preceding cross-sectional analyses of the same data sets, provide some interesting and informative insights. For example, Armstrong et al. (1995) reported a mass exponent for peak $\dot{V}O_2$ in prepubertal children of 0.66. Data from these children were subsequently reported after 3 and 7 years follow-up, respectively (Armstrong et al. 1999; Armstrong & Welsman 2001). In the latter studies, when modeled with mass as the sole covariate in the multilevel model, values identified for the mass exponent were 0.67 and 0.73, respectively. However, as already discussed and illustrated in Table 5.2, these values altered markedly as other covariates were entered into the analysis. This raises interesting questions regarding the interpretation of longitudinal data, the relative importance of explanatory variables, and how the interpretation of a performance variable may change according to which covariates are available for incorporation into a model.

Beunen et al. (2002) used multilevel modeling to interpret growth and maturational influences upon peak $\dot{V}O_2$ in boys aged 8–16 years. In addition to body mass they identified a significant effect of physical activity and significant interactive effects of maturity age (years from peak height velocity) and physical activity upon peak $\dot{V}O_2$. However, they did not include any measure of body fatness, which has been shown to be a key covariate in the interpretation of peak $\dot{V}O_2$, nor did they separate the contributions of chronologic age vs. maturational age. In contrast, our longitudinal study (Armstrong *et al.* 1999), albeit with a smaller age range, identified no significant effect of physical activity once age, sex, maturity, body mass, and sum of skinfolds had been controlled for. Clearly, there are methodologic differences between these studies that may explain the discrepant findings but they do serve to illustrate how the interpretation of a given physiologic variable may be influenced by the availability of covariates in a multilevel analysis and also highlight the importance of careful consideration of variables of interest in the design of prospective longitudinal studies.

Conclusions

In summary, this chapter has illustrated the pitfalls of conventional ratio scaling and demonstrated simple methods for verifying that a given scaling technique is performing as intended (i.e., is creating an adjusted variable that retains no correlation with body size).

The application of simple ratio scaling without verification of its goodness of fit is likely to lead to erroneous interpretation of results particularly with reference to age, sex, and maturational effects.

The pros and cons of alternative scaling techniques have been reviewed and allometric scaling shown to be preferable from both statistical and theoretical standpoints. Using studies reporting allometric scaling of peak $\dot{V}_{O_2}$, variability in mass exponents has been highlighted and related to sample size and composition. Although theoretical alternatives to simple ratio scaling have been proposed, a review of published exponents does not yet support universal acceptance of either 0.67 or 0.75 and suggests that sample-specific mass exponents should be derived

to examine group differences or relationships among variables within a given study.

The application of allometry to longitudinal data is complex. Ontogenetic allometry describes the individual growth process but cannot be used to quantify changes in performance or fully describe group or population responses. In this respect, multilevel regression modeling offers many advantages. Using an allometric framework, underlying group trends can be modeled while concurrently investigating individual growth trajectories. This process thus enables the effects of body size and other explanatory variables upon the performance measure to be examined in a sensitive and flexible manner although the availability of covariates for inclusion will ultimately influence the interpretation of the data.

Directions for future research

The vast majority of studies to date have applied allometric scaling techniques to the interpretation of peak $\dot{V}_{O_2}$. This has enabled insights into age and maturational differences masked by traditional scaling techniques. Further insights into relationships between body size and function during growth and maturation are possible with the application of these techniques to the studies of strength, short-term power, cardiovascular function, and ventilatory responses. The description of longitudinal trends in the development of these physiologic responses is fundamental but a particular interest lies in understanding how allometric relationships evolve in individuals at different stages of maturity and how this is influenced by other factors such as intensive training.

References

Albrecht, G.H., Gelvin, B.R. & Hartman, S.E. (1993) Ratios as a size adjustment in morphometrics. *American Journal of Physical Anthropology* **91**, 441–468.

Armstrong, N., McManus, A.M., Welsman, J.R. & Kirby, B. (1995) Aerobic fitness of pre-pubescent children. *Annals of Human Biology* **22**, 427–441.

Armstrong, N. & Welsman, J.R. (2001) Peak oxygen uptake in relation to

growth and maturation in 11–17 year olds. *European Journal of Applied Physiology* **85**, 546–551.

Armstrong, N. & Welsman, J. (2002) Cardiovascular responses to submaximal treadmill running in 11 to 13 year olds. *Acta Pediatica* **91**, 125–131.

Armstrong, N., Welsman, J.R. & Chia, M.Y.H. (2001) Short term power output

in relation to growth and maturation. *British Journal of Sports Medicine* **35**, 118–124.

Armstrong, N., Welsman, J.R. & Kirby, B.J. (2000a) Longitudinal changes in 11–13 year olds' physical activity. *Acta Paediatrica* **89**, 775–780.

Armstrong, N., Welsman, J.R. & Kirby, B.J. (2000b) Longitudinal changes in young people's short term power output.

Medicine and Science in Sports and Exercise **32**, 1140–1145.

Armstrong, N., Welsman, J.R., Nevill, A.M. & Kirby, B.J. (1999) Modeling growth and maturation changes in peak oxygen uptake in 11–13-year olds. *Journal of Applied Physiology* **87**, 2230–2236.

Astrand, P.O. (1952) *Experimental Studies of Physical Working Capacity in Relation to Sex and Age*. Munksgaard, Copenhagen.

Astrand, P.-O. *et al.* (1963) Girl swimmers. *Acta Paediatrica (Supplement)* 147.

Astrand, P.O. & Rodahl, K. (1986) *Textbook of Work Physiology*. McGraw-Hill, New York.

Baxter-Jones, A., Goldstein, H. & Helms, P. (1993) The development of aerobic power in young athletes. *Journal of Applied Physiology* **75**, 1160–1167.

Beunen, G., Baxter-Jones, A.D.G., Mirwald, R.L., *et al.* (2002) Intraindividual allometric development of aerobic power in 8- to 16-year-old boys. *Medicine and Science in Sports and Exercise* **33**, 503–510.

Bloxham, S.R., Welsman, J.R. & Armstrong, N. (2005) Ergometer-specific relationships between peak oxygen uptake and peak power output in children. *Pediatric Exercise Science* **17**, 136–148.

Calder, W.A.III (1987) Scaling energetics of homeothermic vertebrates: An operational allometry. *Annual Reviews in Physiology* **49**, 107–120.

Chamari, K., Moussa-Chamari, I., Boussaïdi, L., Hachana, Y., Kaouech, F. & Wisløff, U. (2005) Appropriate interpretation of aerobic capacity: allometric scaling in adult and young soccer players. *British Journal of Sports Medicine* **39**, 97–101.

Cooper, D.M., Weiler-Ravell, D., Whipp, B.J. & Wasserman, K. (1984) Aerobic parameters of exercise as a function of body size during growth. *Journal of Applied Physiology* **56**, 628–634.

Daniels, J.T. & Oldridge, N. (1971) Oxygen consumption and growth of young boys during running training. *Medicine and Science in Sports* **3**, 161–165.

De Ste Croix, M.B.A., Armstrong, N., Chia, M.Y.H., Welsman, J.R., Parsons, G. & Sharpe, P. (2001) Changes in short term power output in 10–12 year olds. *Journal of Sports Sciences* **19**, 141–148.

De Ste Croix, M.B.A., Armstrong, N., Welsman, J.R. & Sharpe, P. (2002) Longitudinal changes in isokinetic leg strength in 10–14 year olds. *Annals of Human Biology* **29**, 50–62.

Dencker, M., Thorsson, O., Karlsson, M.K., *et al.* (2006) Daily physical activity and its relation to aerobic fitness in children aged 8–11 years. *European Journal of Applied Physiology* **96**, 587–592.

Duncan, C. Jones, K. & Moon, G. (1996) Health-related behaviour in context: A multilevel modelling approach. *Social Science in Medicine* **42**, 817–830.

Eisenmann, J.C., Pivarnik, J.M. & Malina, R.M. (2001) Scaling peak $\dot{V}o_2$ to body mass in young male and female distance runners. *Journal of Applied Physiology* **90**, 2172–2180.

Eston, R.G., Robson, S. & Winter, E. (1993) A comparison of oxygen uptake during running in children and adults. In: *Kinanthropometry*, Vol. IV (Duquet, W. & Day J., eds.) E and FN Spon, London: 236–241.

Fawkner, S.G. & Armstrong, N. (2004) Sex differences in the oxygen uptake kinetic response to heavy-intensity exercise in prepubertal children. *European Journal of Applied Physiology* **93**, 210–216.

Fawkner, S.G., Armstrong, N., Potter, C.R. & Welsman, J.R. (2002) Oxygen uptake kinetics in children and adults after the onset of moderate-intensity exercise. *Journal of Sports Sciences* **20**, 319–326.

Heusner, A.A. (1982) Energy metabolism and body size. Is the 0.75 mass exponent of Kleiber's equation a statistical artefact? *Respiration Physiology* **48**, 1–12.

Jensen, K., Johansen, L. & Secher, N.H. (2001) Influence of body mass on maximal oxygen uptake: effect of sample size. *European Journal of Applied Physiology* **84**, 201–205.

Kleiber, M. (1932) Body size and metabolism. *Hilgardia* **6**, 315–353.

Klissouras, V. (1971) Heritability or adaptive variation. *Journal of Applied Physiology* **31**, 338–344.

Loftin, M., Sothern, M., Trosclair, L., O'Hanlon, A., Miller, J. & Udall, J. (2001) Scaling VO_2 peak in obese and non-obese girls. *Obesity Research* **9**, 290–296.

McMahon, T. (1973) Size and shape in biology. Elastic criteria impose limits on biological proportions, and consequently on metabolic rates. *Science* **174**, 1201–1204.

McMiken, D.F. (1976) Maximum aerobic power and physical dimensions of children. *Annals of Human Biology* **3**, 141–147.

Martin, R.J.F., Dore, E., Twisk, J., Van Praagh, E., Hautier, C.A. & Bedu, M. Longitudinal changes in maximal short-term peak power in girls and boys during growth. *Medicine and Science in Sports and Exercise* **36**, 498–503.

Nevill, A.M. (1994) Evidence of an increasing proportion of leg muscle mass to body mass in male adolescents and its implication on performance. *Journal of Sports Science* **12**, 163–163.

Nevill, A.M., Bate, S. & Holder, R.L. (2005) Modelling physiologic and anthropometric variables known to vary with body size and other confounding variables. *Yearbook of Physical Anthropology* **48**, 141–153.

Nevill, A.M. & Holder, R.L. (1994) Modelling maximum oxygen uptake: a case-study in non-linear regression model formulation and comparison. *Applied Statistics* **43**, 653–666.

Nevill, A.M., Holder, R.L., Baxter-Jones, A., Round, J.M. & Jones, D.A. (1998) Modelling developmental changes in strength and aerobic power in children. *Journal of Applied Physiology* **84**, 963–970.

Nevill, A.M., Markovic, G., Vucetic, V. & Holder, R.L. (2004c) Can greater muscularity in larger individuals resolve the $^3/4$ power-law controversy when modelling maximum oxygen uptake? *Annals of Human Biology* **31**, 62–68.

Nevill, A., Ramsbottom, R. & Williams, C. (1992) Scaling physiological measurements for individuals of different body size. *European Journal of Applied Physiology* **65**, 110–117.

Nevill, A.M., Rowland, T., Goff, D., Martel, L. & Ferrone, L. (2004a) Scaling or normalising maximum oxygen uptake to predict 1-mile run time in boys. *European Journal of Applied Physiology* **92**, 285–288.

Nevill, A.M., Stewart, A.D., Olds, T. & Holder, R. (2004b) Are adult physiques geometrically similar? The dangers of allometric scaling using body mass power laws. *American Journal of Physical Anthropology* **124**, 177–182.

Paterson, D.H., McLellan, T.M., Stella, R.S. & Cunningham, D.A. (1987) Longitudinal study of ventilation threshold and maximal O_2 uptake in athletic boys. *Journal of Applied Physiology* **62**, 2051–2057.

Rasbash, J., Browne, W., Goldstein, H., *et al.* (2000) *A user's guide to MLwiN version 2.1*. Institute of Education, University of London.

Robinson, S. (1938) Experimental studies of physical fitness in relation to age. *Arbeitsphysiology* **10**, 251–323.

Rogers, D.M., Turlwy, K.R., Kujawa, K.I., Harper, K.M. & Wilmore, J.H. (1995) Allometric scaling factors for oxygen uptake during exercise in children. *Pediatric Exercise Science* **7**, 12–25.

Rowland, T., Miller, K., Vanderburgh, P., Goff, D., Martel, L. & Ferrone, L. (2000) Cardiovascular fitness in premenarcheal girls and young women. *International Journal of Sports Medicine* **20**, 117–121.

Rowland, T., Vanderburgh, P. & Cunningham, L. (1997) Body size and the growth of maximal aerobic power in children: A longitudinal analysis. *Pediatric Exercise Science* **9**, 262–274.

Santos, A.M.C., Armstrong, N., De Ste Croix, M.B.A., *et al.* (2003) Optimal peak power in relation to age, body size, gender and thigh muscle volume. *Pediatric Exercise Science* **15**, 405–417.

Schmidt-Nielsen, K. (1984) *Scaling: Why is Animal Size so Important?* Cambridge University Press, Cambridge.

Sjödin, B. & Svedenhag, J. (1992) Oxygen uptake during running as related to body mass in circumpubertal boys: a longitudinal study. *European Journal of Applied Physiology* **65**, 150–157.

Svedenhag, J. (1995) Maximal and submaximal oxygen uptake during running: how should body mass be accounted for? *Scandinavian Journal of Medicine and Science in Sports* **5**, 175–180.

Tanner, J.M. (1949) Fallacy of per-weight and per-surface area standards and their relation to spurious correlation. *Journal of Applied Physiology* **2**, 1–15.

Tanner, J.M. (1964) *The Physique of the Olympic Athlete*. Allen & Unwin, London.

Welsman, J.R. & Armstrong, N. (2000) Longitudinal changes in submaximal oxygen uptake in 11–13 year olds. *Journal of Sports Sciences* **18**, 183–189.

Welsman, J., Armstrong, N., Kirby, B.J., Nevill, A.M. & Winter, E. (1996) Scaling peak oxygen uptake for differences in body size. *Medicine and Science in Sports and Exercise* **28**, 259–265.

Welsman, J.R., Armstrong, N., Kirby, B.J., Winsley, R.J., Parsons, G. & Sharpe, P. (1997) Exercise performance and MRI determined muscle volume in children. *European Journal of Applied Physiology* **76**, 92–97.

Williams, J.R., Armstrong, N., Winter, E.M. & Crichton, N. (1992) Changes in peak oxygen uptake with age and sexual maturation in boys: physiological fact or statistical anomaly? In: *Children and Exercise*, Vol. XVI (Coudert, J. & Van Praagh, E., eds.) Masson, Paris: 35–37.

Winsley, R.J., Armstrong, N., Middlebroode, A.R., Ramos-Ibanez, N. & Williams, C.A. Aerobic fitness and visceral adipose tissue in children. *Acta Paediatrica* **95**, 1435–1438.

Part 2

Training: Principles, Trainability, and Consequences

Chapter 6

Muscle Strength, Endurance, and Power: Trainability During Childhood

CAMERON J.R. BLIMKIE AND ODED BAR-OR

Regrettably, there has been a paucity of new studies on the trainability of muscle strength and power in childhood since our earlier overview of this topic in Volume VI of the *Encyclopaedia of Sports Medicine: The Child and Adolescent Athlete* (Blimkie & Bar-Or 1996). The current chapter supplements the previous review and provides an update of the published literature on this topic. The main focus of the chapter is the trainability of strength, muscle endurance, and power in normal healthy children; however, a brief section is also included relating to the rationale for, and application of strength training in selected pediatric clinical populations, some of whom may also be involved in sports participation (e.g., children with a specific pediatric condition or illness such as asthma or obesity), as some of these children might benefit from this type of training.

Strength is defined as the maximal force or torque generated by a muscle or muscle group either during a single maximal voluntary effort or in response to electrical stimulation. Muscle endurance is defined as the number of repetitions of a given strength exercise at a certain intensity (usually expressed as a percentage of the 1 repetition maximum [1 RM] load). Power is defined as the rate at which mechanical work is performed during a given period of time (Sale 1991). Strength and power are inextricably linked as depicted in the well-known force–velocity–power relationship (Fig. 6.1). Muscle strength, endurance, and power are important prerequisites for activities of daily living and success in sports during childhood; however, the relative importance of these capacities may vary, depending on the nature of the activity or sport, and the health status of the child.

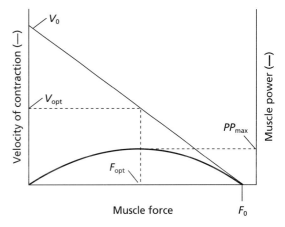

Fig. 6.1 Theoretical relationship between muscle force, velocity of muscle contraction, and muscle power. F_0, peak force during an isometric contraction at 0 velocity; V_0, peak rate of muscle contraction; PP_{max}, maximum peak power; V_{opt}, rate of contraction that elicits PP_{max}; F_{opt}, muscle force that elicits PP_{max} at V_{opt}.

There is substantial information about the factors that determine strength, endurance, and power, and the trainability of these capacities in adults (Green 1991; Komi 1992). Although not as extensively studied as in adults, there is increasing information about the developmental determinants of strength and power in children (Blimkie 1989; also see Chapters 2 and 3 in this volume). By comparison, little is known about the trainability of these capacities during childhood.

Skeletal muscle strength

There has been substantial interest during the past two decades, from both the general public and the

65

scientific community, in resistance or strength train-ing during childhood. The key areas of concern relate to the risk of injury, the effectiveness of training to increase strength especially during the prepubertal and early pubertal years, and the mech-anisms underlying training induced strength gains, and changes in strength during detraining. Many of these topics have been addressed thoroughly in recent reviews and position papers (Kraemer *et al.* 1989; Sale 1989; Weltman 1989; American Academy of Pediatrics 1990, 2001; Freedson *et al.* 1990; Webb 1990; Blimkie 1992, 1993a,b; Faigenbaum *et al.* 1996; Faigenbaum 2001; Guy & Micheli 2001; Strong *et al.* 2005). The first part of this review is restricted to the topics of the trainability of strength and muscle endurance, the mechanisms underlying training induced strength gains, and changes in strength during detraining at different developmental stages during childhood.

Muscle strength, at a given velocity will increase as a function of growth during childhood (Blimkie 1989; Froberg & Lammert 1996; see also Chapters 2 and 5). Strength or resistance training has been proven effective in increasing strength in adults (Fleck & Kraemer 1988) and the possibility also exists that it may be effective in increasing strength beyond growth-related increases during childhood. Resistance training in the context of this review implies the use of progressive resistance training methods to exert or resist force (Cahill 1988) and this term will be used interchangeably with strength training. Resistance training methods vary in terms of program design, in training mode, and in rela-tive strain or intensity of the applied resistance. Resistance training studies involving children have incorporated a variety of training methods, and these differences have confounded interpretation of resistance training studies in this population.

Effectiveness of resistance training

Until the mid-1980s, it was generally believed that resistance training would be ineffective in increas-ing strength prior to adolescence. This belief was based partly on the presumption that strength gains were not possible until circulating testosterone levels increased substantially during mid- to late puberty, and partly on results from a limited num-ber of training studies, which, despite their design limitations, were interpreted as lending support to this notion.

Several studies in this area failed to show any increase in back (Kirsten 1963) or arm and leg strength (Ainsworth 1970; Vrijens 1978; Docherty *et al.* 1987) in prepubertal children following various types of strength training programs. These studies either utilized fairly modest training loads by today's standards or were of very short duration. The largely negative results from these studies can therefore not be taken as proof of the ineffectiveness of strength training during the pre-adolescent years.

Studies that have controlled for the confounding effects of growth and motor skill acquisition on strength gain, and have incorporated moderate to high training loads, provide rather convincing evid-ence that strength training can result in substantial and significant increases in strength in either sex during pre-adolescence (Nielsen *et al.* 1980; Pfeiffer & Francis 1986; Sewall & Micheli 1986; Weltman *et al.* 1986; Sailors & Berg 1987; Hakkinen *et al.* 1989; Mersch & Stoboy 1989; Hassan 1991; Ozmun *et al.* 1991; Fukunga *et al.* 1992; DeRenne *et al.* 1996; Lillegard *et al.* 1997; Morris *et al.* 1997; Tsolakis *et al.* 2004; Feigenbaum *et al.* 2005).

The results of the longest and perhaps most inten-sive randomized controlled trial of strength training to date involving pre-adolescents (Ramsay *et al.* 1990) also support this view. In this study, emphasis was placed on providing high resistive loads to the elbow flexor and knee extensor muscle groups using dynamic resistance training (Global Gym). The training involved progressive resistance load-ing (resistance was increased as subjects became stronger), a similar frequency and intensity of train-ing as commonly used in strength training pro-grams for adults (Fleck & Kraemer 1987), and strength testing that was both training mode specific (1 RM lifts) and non-specific (isometric and isokinetic test-ing). Additionally, the effects of skill acquisition or motor learning were controlled by performing interim testing. Twenty weeks of training resulted in significant increases (Fig. 6.2) in the 1 RM bench press (35%), the 1 RM double leg press (22%), maximal voluntary isometric elbow flexion (37%) and knee

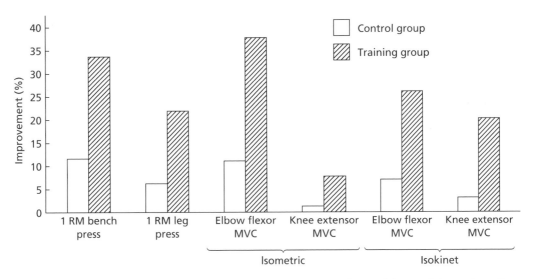

Fig. 6.2 Effects of 20 weeks of heavy resistance training on various measures of strength in pre-adolescent boys. From Ramsey *et al.* 1990.

extension (25%) strength, and maximal voluntary isokinetic elbow flexion (26%) and knee extension (21%) strength (Ramsay *et al.* 1990). More recently, a non-randomized school-based study of even longer duration reported significantly larger strength gains in prepubertal boys who performed multiple sets of twice weekly low to moderate intensity resistance training for 21 weeks, compared with controls who participated in standard physical education classes (Sadres *et al.* 2001).

Collectively, the results from these longer term studies and the other studies cited above provide fairly compelling evidence that strength training can be effective in increasing strength during the pre-adolescent period. The results of these studies have been summarily reported in meta-analyses of this topic (Falk & Tenenbaum 1996; Payne *et al.* 1997). The effectiveness of training appears, as it does also in adults, to be dependent primarily on the provision of a sufficient training intensity and volume, and to a lesser degree on training duration. Strength improvements have been reported using isometric, isotonic, and isokinetic training methods involving high-intensity loading. However, the optimal combination of training method, mode, intensity, volume, and duration of training for maximal strength gain during pre-adolescence has yet to be deter-

mined. Recent studies suggest that strength gains are realized in prepubertal children within 8 weeks of training, with as little as one set of moderate (15–20 repetitions at 60–75% of the 1 RM: 15–20 RM) or high (6–10 repetitions at 75–85% of the 1 RM: 6–10 RM) intensity strength exercises (Faigenbaum *et al.* 2005), and with as few as 2 weekly training sessions (Falk & Mor 1996; Sadres *et al.* 2001; Faigenbaum *et al.* 2005). While the data are limited, there appears to be little difference in maximal strength gains (1 RM) between moderate and high intensity training programs in prepubertal children; however, adaptations in local muscle endurance (number of repetitions at the pre-training test load) seem more specifically related to type of training, as improvement was greater with lower intensity, higher repetition training compared to higher intensity, lower repetition training (Faigenbaum *et al.* 2005). The relationships between training intensity, strength, and endurance gains in children remain to be more clearly established.

Compared to pre-adolescence, the trainability of strength for both sexes during adolescence is a less contentious issue. Significant strength gains have resulted from isometric training (Wolbers & Sills 1956; Rarick & Larsen 1958; Kirsten 1963; Fukunaga 1976; Komi *et al.* 1978; Nielsen *et al.* 1980;

DeKoning *et al.* 1984), dynamic or isotonic weight training (Gallagher & DeLorme 1949; Delorme *et al.* 1952; Kusinitz & Keeney 1958; Vrijens 1978; Westcott 1979, 1991; Gillam 1981; Munson *et al.* 1985; Pfeiffer & Francis 1986; Witzke & Snow 2000), isokinetic (McCubbin & Shasby 1985), and hydraulic resistance training (Blimkie *et al.* 1993). With dynamic or isotonic training, strength gains appear to be directly related to the frequency of training (Gillam 1981); nevertheless, as for the pre-adolescent population, the optimal combination of training mode, intensity, volume, and duration of resistance training for strength increases during adolescence has yet to be established.

Comparative trainability

Although it appears that significant improvements can be made in strength during pre-adolescence, the question remains as to the relative effectiveness of strength training at this stage of development compared to training during adolescence, and adulthood. This question can be considered both in terms of percentage or proportional strength gains (relative strength gain), as well as in terms of the absolute strength gains, compared to pre-training levels.

Results from a number of early studies in this area suggested that pre-adolescent children had either the same or lower relative trainability, but lower absolute trainability for isometric back, arm, and leg strength than adolescents and young adults (Hettinger 1958; Kirsten 1963; Vrijens 1978). However, the conclusions from these studies are questionable, given the relatively low training loads used, and the failure in some cases to clearly formulate groups on the basis of distinct maturity levels, especially during the circumpubertal years.

Results from studies that used similar training programs across developmental stages, incorporated moderate to high training intensities and volumes, and that separated groups more clearly on the basis of maturity, have consistently reported comparable, and sometimes greater relative strength trainability in pre-adolescents, compared to adolescents and adults (Westcott 1979; Nielsen *et al.* 1980; Pfeiffer & Francis 1986; Sailors & Berg 1987; Sale 1989). One of the more recent studies (Hakkinen *et al.* 1989)

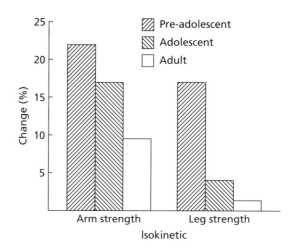

Fig. 6.3 Comparative strength changes in pre-adolescent, adolescent, and adult males in response to 9 weeks of resistance training. From Pfeiffer & Francis (1986).

likewise reported greater relative squat extension strength gains in pre-adolescent boys, compared with a group of elite junior weightlifters following 1 year of weight training. The results from this study, however, cannot be taken as support of greater relative strength trainability of pre-adolescents because there were differences in initial level of training experience, and the training programs differed considerably between groups. A summary of the results from the study of Pfeiffer and Francis (1986) is provided in Fig. 6.3.

There is less information about the trainability of absolute strength; four studies have reported lower absolute strength trainability in pre-adolescents compared with adolescents (Hakkinen *et al.* 1989) and adults (Sailors & Berg 1987; Sale 1989; Fukunga *et al.* 1992), whereas a fifth study, which may be criticized because of its small sample size (Westcott 1979), reported greater absolute strength gains in pre-adolescent girls compared with adolescent and adult females. Whether or not there is a sex difference in strength trainability remains to be established; one study (Lillegard *et al.* 1997) reported a trend towards larger strength gains in pre- and early post-pubescent males compared with maturity-matched groups of females, but these findings remain to be confirmed.

Based on the available information, however limited, it appears that pre-adolescents are probably less trainable in terms of absolute strength gains, but equally if not more trainable in a relative or proportional sense (percentage improvement) compared to adolescents and young adults. Additional studies that include distinct maturity groups, identical training programs across levels of maturity, and that also control for age- and sex-associated differences in background level of physical activity and training are required, however, before the question of comparative strength trainability is unequivocally resolved.

Persistence of strength gains

After having begun a strength training program, the child will, for various reasons (e.g., disinterest, injury, illness, time constraints), probably discontinue training sometime afterwards. Because training appears to be effective in increasing strength, the question arises whether prior training induced strength gains will be maintained or lost (will they persist or desist?) during periods of partial or complete withdrawal from training (detraining). The answer to this question is not as straightforward as it first appears, because any loss in strength brought about by a partial or complete reduction in training may be masked by the growth-related increase in strength that will occur concomitantly during the detraining period. The growth-related strength increase may wholly or partially mask the effect of the withdrawal of the training stimulus on the strength gain achieved through prior training. A simple model of the potential interactions between growth and training–detraining during childhood is presented in Fig. 6.4.

Only a few studies have investigated the question of the persistence of strength gains during detraining in children; all involved pre-adolescents, and all have design limitations (Sewall & Micheli 1986; Blimkie *et al.* 1989a; Faigenbaum *et al.* 1996; Sadres *et al.* 2001; Tsolakis *et al.* 2004). If strength gains are maintained, one would expect strength for a previously trained group to increase by the same magnitude as the change in a control group (simple additive effect of the growth-related increase in

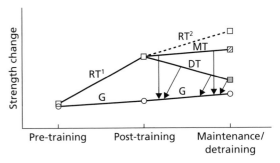

Fig. 6.4 Model of expected strength changes with growth (G), resistance training (RT), maintenance training (MT), and detraining (DT) during childhood. Section G, strength increases resulting from growth and maturation—serves as a control for growth and maturation in training studies during childhood. Rates may vary depending on developmental stage; Section RT^1, strength increases rapidly during the initial stage of training because of growth and training effects—assumes that learning effects are controlled; RT_2, strength increases more slowly during the later stages of training and is a result of growth and a dampened training effect; MT, strength increases beyond the post-training level caused solely by growth—the post-training difference in strength is sustained during this period as indicated by the equal length long arrows; DT, strength decreases below the post-training level resulting from the complete withdrawal of training—the post-training strength difference is lost progressively with time and may converge with the control level (G), as indicated by the diagonal arrows of diminishing length.

strength) during the detraining period, and persistence of the strength difference that had been established at the end of training. If strength gains are not permanent, and there is a loss in strength because of detraining, then there will be a gradual regression in the strength curve of the previously trained group, and a convergence with the strength curve for the control group at a level below the peak strength achieved at the end of training (Fig. 6.4).

In three of the studies that included control groups (Blimkie *et al.* 1989a; Faigenbaum *et al.* 1996; Tsolakis *et al.* 2004), the majority of strength measures in the previously trained group converged over periods ranging from several weeks to several months toward the control values, suggesting that training induced strength gains during pre-adolescence were probably impermanent. In another study, strength training induced gains appeared to be maintained over a 12-week period of relative detraining for a specific exercise (bench press) in groups that performed either one or two maintenance training sessions per week, but lost for leg press and pull-up strength measures, regardless of the number of maintenance training sessions (DeRenne *et al.* 1996). In the most recent study of this issue, strength gains elicited by prior training were sustained over the summer holiday period (duration unspecified) even without a specific strength maintenance program (Sadres *et al.* 2001); there was no control, however, over the amount or intensity of activity and sports participation in the trained or control groups during the detraining period, making it difficult to unequivocally address this issue. Whether the strength gains will revert fully to the growth-adjusted control levels will probably depend upon the magnitude of the initial strength gains, the duration of the detraining period, and the amount and types of physical activity that the previously trained child is exposed to during the detraining period. If level of physical activity is high, involves a high level of general muscle strength, and isolates muscle groups that were previously targeted in the training program, then the probability of persistence of strength gains is likely.

Only two studies have investigated the question of maintenance strength training during childhood. In the earliest study (Blimkie *et al.* 1989a), a once weekly high-intensity strength training session was not sufficient to conserve prior training induced strength gains in a group of pre-adolescent boys. The training induced strength gains regressed toward the growth-adjusted control level in a manner identical to that for a totally detrained group. In the more recent study (DeRenne *et al.* 1996), bench press strength gains were maintained with one relatively high intensity strength training session over a 12-week period, whereas neither 1 or 2 weekly high intensity maintenance sessions were sufficient to sustain strength gains for the leg press or pull-up strength measures over the same period.

Clearly, no firm conclusions can be drawn about the persistence of strength training induced strength gains or the requirements for maintenance training during either pre-adolescence or adolescence based on the available literature. Nevertheless, it appears

from the few studies that have investigated these questions that training induced strength gains are probably impermanent, and that one high intensity training session per week is probably insufficient for maintenance training to fully conserve prior training induced strength gains, at least during pre-adolescence.

Mechanisms underlying strength changes

What are the physiologic adaptations, and the mechanisms underlying training and detraining induced strength changes during childhood? Are the adaptations and mechanisms similar during pre-adolescence and adolescence, and in comparison to adulthood?

Morphologic adaptations during training

The possibility of strength training induced morphologic adaptations in muscle size during pre-adolescence has been assessed using both indirect and direct measurement techniques. Training induced changes in gross limb morphology and, by inference, changes in muscle size, have been assessed mostly using indirect anthropometric measurement techniques. In brief, there is no evidence based on these indirect techniques from any of the studies that reported significant increases in strength, of resistance training induced muscle hypertrophy during pre-adolescence (Siegel *et al.* 1989; McGovern 1984; Weltman *et al.* 1986; Sailors & Berg 1987; Blimkie *et al.* 1989b; Hakkinen *et al.* 1989; Ramsay *et al.* 1990; Hassan 1991; Ozmun *et al.* 1991).

However, the effect of strength training on muscle size in pre-adolescents has also been studied using more sensitive imaging techniques, including soft-tissue roentgenography, ultrasound, computerized axial tomography, dual energy X-ray absorptiometry (DEXA), and magnetic resonance imaging (Vrijens 1978; Mersch & Stoboy 1989; Ramsay *et al.* 1990; Fukunga *et al.* 1992; Morris *et al.* 1997). Despite demonstrating significant improvements in muscle strength, Ramsay *et al.* (1990) found no evidence of upper arm or thigh muscle hypertrophy measured by computerized tomography in pre-adolescent boys following 20 weeks of high intensity strength training. Vrijens (1978), using roentgenography, likewise found no evidence of strength training induced muscle hypertrophy in the upper arm or thigh in pre-adolescent boys. This is perhaps not all that surprising, because this study failed to demonstrate a significant training induced strength improvement.

Two other studies, however, have reported resistance training induced muscle hypertrophy in pre-adolescents. Mersch and Stoboy (1989) reported significant strength training induced increases in both knee extension isometric strength and quadriceps muscle cross-sectional area determined by magnetic resonance imaging in two pre-adolescent twin boys. This is the first study to report muscle hypertrophy resulting from strength training in pre-adolescents. Likewise, Fukunga *et al.* (1992) reported significant increases in upper arm isometric and isokinetic strength and lean (muscle and bone) cross-sectional area determined by ultrasound in pre-adolescent Japanese girls and boys. The absolute increase in muscle size, however, was only half of the typical change observed in adults in response to similar training. It is difficult given the small sample and other peculiarities in the data of Mersch and Stoboy (1989), and the imprecision inherent in the ultrasound technique employed by Fukunga *et al.* (1992), to totally discount the largely negative results from all the other studies in this area. Nevertheless, these results leave open the possibility of strength training induced muscle hypertrophy even during pre-adolescence.

At the whole body level, a recent study involving a 10-month exercise program, including a component of resistance exercise, reported a significant increase in lean tissue mass (a proxy measure of muscle) by DEXA in pre-menarcheal girls, also supporting the possibility of gross morphologic adaptation to training even prior to full puberty (Morris *et al.* 1997). In an even more recent study, strength training gains in prepubertal boys were associated with increased levels of testosterone, considered by the investigators to be a marker of protein anabolism (Tsolakis *et al.* 2004). However, there were no direct measures of changes in protein or muscle mass in this study to support the inference of increased anabolism as a potential mechanism underlying the training related strength adaptations.

Skeletal muscle clearly is capable of hypertrophy even during pre-adolescence, as evidenced by increased muscle size in children with the rare congenital disease myotonia congenita (Israel 1992). Whether resistance training in the context of recreational, fitness, or sport-based programs provides sufficient additional mechanical strain beyond normal levels of generally high background muscular activity to induce muscle hypertrophy in otherwise healthy pre-adolescent children remains to be unequivocally established.

Surprisingly few studies have investigated the mechanisms underlying strength gains with resistance training in adolescents. Strength training induced increases in muscle size have been inferred both from indirect anthropometric measures of increased arm and thigh girths (DeLorme *et al.* 1952; Kusinitz & Keeney 1958; Hakkinen *et al.* 1989) and from roentgenographically determined increases in arm and thigh muscle cross-sectional areas (Vrijens 1978) in adolescent boys. Only two studies have investigated this issue in adolescent females. Fukunaga (1976) reported an 8.3% increase in upper arm lean area (bone and muscle) determined by ultrasound in a group of 13-year-old Japanese girls following a 3-month program of isometric training which elicited a 93.4% increase in absolute isometric strength. In another study (Blimkie *et al.*, unpublished results), 26 weeks of heavy resistance training, which resulted in significant strength increases, failed to cause any increase in anthropometrically determined upper arm girth or quadriceps muscle cross-sectional area determined by computerized axial tomography in adolescent females.

It appears from these studies that training induced muscle hypertrophy may be possible, but is probably unlikely during pre-adolescence. By comparison, muscle hypertrophy appears to be a more consistent outcome of strength or resistance training during adolescence, especially for males. Although based on only two studies, it appears that the hypertrophy response may be more variable and of a smaller (absolute) magnitude in adolescent females compared to males. However, there are no studies to date that permit a valid comparison between sexes of the relative hypertrophy responses to identical training programs during adolescence, or between adolescence and adulthood. Whatever the hypertrophy response, it is evident from the results of all of these studies, regardless of developmental status, that the magnitude of this morphologic adaptation is small in comparison to the reported strength gains. Other factors besides changes in muscle size must also contribute to the strength gains observed.

Neurologic adaptations during training

Only a few studies have investigated the contribution of neurologic adaptations to training induced strength gains in pre-adolescents. By inference, and based solely on the lack of evidence for muscle hypertrophy, training induced strength increases in pre-adolescent boys have been attributed to undefined neurologic and neuromotor adaptations (Weltman et al. 1986; Hakkinen et al. 1989; Hassan 1991). These studies provide only weak indirect support for unspecified neurologic and motor coordination contributions to strength training induced strength gains in pre-adolescents.

A more direct means of neurologic assessment, the twitch interpolation technique (Belanger & McComas 1981), has been used by Blimkie et al. (1989b) and Ramsay et al. (1990) to assess the contribution of changes in motor unit activation (MUA) to training induced strength increases in pre-adolescent boys. MUA of the elbow flexors and knee extensors increased by 9% and 12%, respectively, after 10 weeks of training, and an additional 10 weeks of training resulted in much smaller increases of only 3% and 2%, respectively. The percentage increases in MUA were less than the increases in strength for both muscle groups. Most recently, Ozmun et al. (1991) used electromyography to measure strength training induced changes in neuromuscular activation of the elbow flexors in pre-adolescent boys and girls. Eight weeks of training resulted in significant increases in both integrated electromyographic (EMG) amplitude (16.8%) and maximal isokinetic strength (27.8%). Results from these studies provide direct evidence that training induced strength gains in pre-adolescents, especially during the early stages of strength training,

are attributable at least in part to increases in neuro-muscular activation.

Likewise, the contributions of neurologic adaptations to training induced strength gains have not been extensively studied in adolescents. Concomitant increases in isometric strength and maximum integrated electromyographic activity (IEMG), a direct measure of maximal voluntary neural activation, have been reported for the vastus lateralis and vastus medialis muscles in adolescent males (Hakkinen et al. 1989), and the rectus femoris muscle (Komi et al. 1978) in adolescent males and females. In both studies, the increase in IEMG activity was greater than the observed strength increase (8.9% vs. 5.2 %, Hakkinen et al. 1989; 38% vs. 20%, Komi et al. 1978). In a recent study of adolescent females, training induced knee extensor strength gains (23.3%) were accompanied by a smaller increase (9.5%) in knee extensor motor unit activation (Blimkie et al., unpublished results).

It appears from these studies that resistance training induced strength gains both during pre-adolescence and adolescence are achieved in part from increased voluntary neuromuscular activation. The magnitude of the changes in neuromuscular activation are generally smaller than the observed increases in strength during pre-adolescence, but appear to be more proportional to strength gains, at least in males, during adolescence. These findings suggest differences in the relative importance of neurologic adaptations in relation to strength gains between pre-adolescents and adolescents. Alternatively, these observations may simply reflect differences in measurement techniques and muscle groups used to assess neuromuscular activation between studies, and differences in the nature and intensity of the resistance training programs.

Based on the magnitude of the neurologic responses, at least for the pre-adolescents, it appears that other factors besides increased neuromuscular drive may also have an important role in the determination of training induced strength gains. It is likely that part of the strength gain may also be attributed to improved motor coordination. Improved movement coordination is probably a more important contributor to strength gains in more complex, multijoint exercises (e.g., the 1 RM arm curl or leg press exercises) than in less complex and more isolated actions such as those involved in isometric strength assessment of the elbow flexors or knee extensors. Results from the studies by Blimkie *et al.* (1989b) and Ramsay *et al.* (1990) indirectly support this contention, because training resulted in larger percent improvements in 1 RM arm curl and leg press strength (specific exercises performed during training) than in non-specific isometric elbow flexion and knee extension strength. Improved motor coordination is also probably a contributing factor to increased strength gains in adolescent females, because gains measured on the training devices were recently shown to be larger than gains assessed with non-specific strength testing dynamometers (Blimkie *et al.*, unpublished results).

Intrinsic adaptations during training

Training induced changes in the intrinsic contractile characteristics of muscle could also account for part of the observed increase in strength in pre-adolescents following strength training. In the only study to investigate this issue in pre-adolescents (Ramsay *et al.* 1990), twitch torque, a measure of intrinsic muscle strength, increased significantly for both the elbow flexors and knee extensors after 20 weeks of strength training. Because there were no corresponding increases in muscle size, these results indicate an improvement in twitch specific tension (strength per cross-sectional area). If this adaptation in twitch-specific tension persists, and transfers to maximal voluntary efforts, it may account for some of the unexplained increase in training induced maximal voluntary strength gains evident in pre-adolescents. This finding suggests that undefined qualitative adaptations in muscle may account in part for the training induced strength gains evident during pre-adolescence following strength training. Whether resistance or strength training induces intrinsic muscle adaptations during adolescence remains to be determined.

Adaptations during detraining

In adults, strength training induced increases in muscle size and neural drive decay during detraining at about the same rate as they increase during training (Narici *et al.* 1989). Detraining in adults is apparently characterized by a relatively rapid reduction in neuromuscular activation and a more gradual reduction in muscle size (Narici *et al.* 1989). Because strength training appears to have little if any effect on muscle size during pre-adolescence, it is probable that the decrement in training induced strength gains in this group during detraining are attributable predominantly to changes in level of neuromuscular activation and motor coordination.

Only one study has investigated the physiologic adaptations during maintenance (reduced) training during pre-adolescence (Blimkie *et al.* 1989a). Eight weeks of detraining had no significant effect on the magnitude of change in estimated (by anthropometry) lean upper arm or thigh cross-sectional areas among groups of maintenance trained, detrained, and control pre-adolescent boys. The maintenance trained and detrained groups had completed 20 weeks of heavy strength training prior to detraining. However, the lack of change in muscle size with detraining in this study was not surprising because, in contrast to adults, there was no evidence of muscle hypertrophy at the end of the training program. Results from this single study suggest that any loss in strength during reduced training or total detraining in pre-adolescents is probably not attributable to a reduction in muscle size.

In the same study (Blimkie *et al.* 1989a), there was a trend towards reduced neuromuscular drive (reduced MUA) in both the maintenance trained and totally detrained groups; the reductions were considerably larger in the totally detrained than in the maintenance trained group. These results suggest that the loss of strength gains during detraining in pre-adolescents is, as it is also in adults, attributable in part to a reduction in neuromuscular activation. Although it has never been assessed directly, it is likely that part of the decrement in strength during detraining, especially for more complex, multijoint strength maneuvers, may also be attributed to a loss in motor coordination. There are no studies of the detraining response to resistance or strength training involving adolescents. Clearly, more information is required about detraining and the physiologic adaptations that accompany this process during both pre-adolescence and adolescence. Table 6.1 provides a summary of the probable physiologic adaptations underlying strength

Table 6.1 Probable physiological adaptations underlying strength changes with resistance training and detraining during preadolescence and adolescence—relative responses.

	Relative response
Training phase	
Absolute strength	Greater gains in the adolescent compared to the preadolescent
Relative strength	Equal or greater gains in the preadolescent compared to the adolescent
Muscle hypertrophy	Smaller gains in muscle size in the preadolescent compared to the adolescent
Neuromuscular activation	Possible greater potential for increased activation in the preadolescent compared to the adolescent due to a lower lifetime exposure to different types of activities
Motor skill	Possible greater potential for improvement in skill in the preadolescent compared to the adolescent due to lower lifetime exposure to skilled activities
Detraining phase	
Absolute strength	Probably a smaller loss in strength in the preadolescent compared to the adolescent due to a greater degree of compensation from growth
Relative strength	Same as for absolute strength
Muscle hypertrophy	Muscle size will probably continue to increase during preadolescence due to growth, but may decrease or remain unchanged in the adolescent depending on the magnitude of the weaker (compared to preadolescence) but still present growth effect
Neuromuscular activation	Will probably decrease in both the preadolescent and adolescent stages by an equal magnitude
Motor skill	Will probably decrease more in the preadolescents than in the adolescent due to relative inexperience with related types of skilled activities which may transfer to strength

training and detraining induced strength changes during childhood.

Strength training—benefits and risks

Strength training has the potential of improving sports performance, enhancing body composition, and reducing sports injury rate and rehabilitation time following injury. However, these potential beneficial effects of strength training remain largely unproven for both the pre-adolescent (Blimkie 1993a,b) and, with the exception of the potential positive impact on injury rate and rehabilitation time, the adolescent. Strength training is also a potentially risky activity in that it may induce temporary or permanent musculoskeletal injury, and have detrimental effects on cardiorespiratory fitness and cardiovascular function. With appropriate technique instruction, and proper exercise prescription and supervision, strength training does not appear to be a particularly risky activity for either pre-adolescents or adolescents in terms of injury, and it seems to have no detrimental effect on either cardiorespiratory fitness or blood pressure (Blimkie 1993a,b).

Whereas it may be an effective and relatively low risk activity for most healthy children, strength training should be recommended cautiously, and then only under close medical supervision and monitoring for children with physical, mental, and medical disabilities. Position statements or opinions regarding the trainability of strength in children and other closely related concerns have been published by several professional bodies (Faigenbaum *et al.* 1996; Washington *et al.* 2001; Lavallee 2002; Strong *et al.* 2005). Because it is such a highly specialized type of exercise, strength training should be recommended as only one of a variety of physical activities and sport pursuits for younger children.

Lastly, a distinction must be made between strength training and participation in the sports of competitive and Olympic weight lifting and power-lifting. Strength training, if performed under supervision and with appropriate technique instruction and prescription of loads, can be an enjoyable and relatively low-risk activity for most children. However, competitive and Olympic weight lifting,

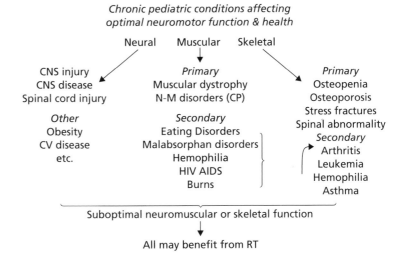

Fig. 6.5 Summary of pediatric conditions, diseases, or disabilities that may be associated with compromised muscle strength or may benefit from strength training.

powerlifting, and body building may prove riskier activities for children, and according to some professional bodies should not be recommended for pre-adolescents (American Academy of Pediatrics 1990; American Orthopaedic Society For Sports Medicine—see Cahill 1988).

Strength training in special populations

Approximately 10–20% of the pediatric population is afflicted with a chronic disease or disability that may limit participation in physical activity, sport, and even specialized exercise programs such as strength training (Gortmaker & Sappenfield 1984). Examples of subclasses of primarily neural, muscular, and skeletal conditions that may be associated with compromised strength in children are provided in Fig. 6.5. Strength training may be a useful and effective adjunct treatment in attenuating disease or disability progression in these conditions, in the rehabilitation of muscle mass and strength to more normal levels, and in many cases in the preparation of these children for participation in recreational or high level competitive sport. The rational for strength training among the myriad conditions afflicting children are summarized in Table 6.2. They are as varied in terms of their goals as the conditions themselves, and they are not solely targeted for strength or muscle mass improvement.

With regards to the effectiveness of strength or resistance training to improve strength, there is ample evidence from adequately designed and well-controlled clinical studies to support the conclusion that strength training is effective in this regard in children with cystic fibrosis (Selvadurai

Table 6.2 Summary of stated rational for incorporation of strength training in selected published studies involving children with a chronic medical illness, disease, or disability.

Illness specific rationale for resistance training in pediatric populations (past 10 years)

Neural
No studies to date

Muscular
To improve residual muscle strength: MD, CP, burns, AN
To slow disease progression: MD
To attenuate muscle loss & weakness: burns, AN
To improve performance of ADL: CP
To improve gait mechanics & efficiency: CP, obesity
To normalize strength asymmetry: CP
To increase LTM-metab. & improve BC: burns, AN, obesity
To improve self-efficacy: AN, obesity, hemophilia

Skeletal
To decease risk of osteoporosis: AN
To normalize spinal alignment: CP, scoliosis
To stabilize & strengthen joint capsule: hemophilia
To increase activities of daily living: hemophilia

ADL, activities of daily living; AN, anorexia nervosa; BC, body composition; CP, cerebral palsy; LTM, lean tissue mass; MD, muscular dystrophy; RT, resistance training—same as strength training.

et al. 2002; Orenstein *et al.* 2004), cerebral palsy (Blundell *et al.* 2003), obesity (Treuth *et al.* 1998a,b; Lazzer *et al.* 2005), and those recovering from burns (Suman *et al.* 2001). Regrettably, there are no published data on the effectiveness or efficacy of strength training among young disabled athletes. Experience and anecdotal evidence, however, suggest that this type of specialized training is routinely incorporated into training programs for sports preparation by many young disabled athletes. Programs are usually modified according to the physical constraints imposed by the disability, but in general they are based on the same principles and approaches used for able-bodied athletes. Clearly, more research is required in this area to establish the effectiveness and risks associated with this type of training in these groups and to determine optimal training regimens.

Strength training guidelines

The following guidelines are provided to ensure the safety, effectiveness, and enjoyment of strength training in a non-competitive recreational, fitness, or sports context for children:

General guidelines

- Preclude physical and medical contraindications
- Provide detailed instructions, and demand proper technique
- Warm-up with calisthenics and stretches
- Begin with exercises that use body weight as resistance before progressing to free weights or weight training machines
- Individualize training loads when using free weights and training machines
- Train all major muscle groups, and both flexors and extensors
- Exercise muscles through their entire range of motion
- Alternate days of training with rest days, and do not train more than 3 times per week
- When using free weights or machines, progress gradually from light loads, high repetitions (>15), and few sets (2–3), to heavier loads, fewer repetitions (6–8), and moderate numbers of sets (3–4)
- Cool down after training with stretching exercises for major joints and muscle groups

- When selecting equipment, check for durability, stability, sturdiness, and safety
- Heed sharp or persistent pain as a warning, and seek medical advice

Developmental considerations

- Encourage resistance training as only one of a variety of normal recreational and sport activities, especially during pre-adolescence
- Encourage using a variety of different training modalities (e.g., free weights, springs, machines, and body weight)
- Discourage interindividual competition, and stress the importance of personal improvement, especially during pre-adolescence
- Discourage extremely high intensity (loading) efforts (e.g., maximal or near-maximal lifts with free weights or weight machines), especially during pre-adolescence
- Avoid isolated eccentric training until the latter stages of adolescence
- Encourage a circuit system approach to capitalize on possible cardiorespiratory benefits
- If using weight training machines, select those that have either been designed for children or those for which the loads and levers can be easily adjusted to accommodate the reduced strength capacity and size of the child
- Ensure experienced supervision, preferably by an adult, when free weights or training machines are used in training

Trainability of muscle power and local muscle endurance

Much less information is available on the trainability of muscle power and endurance in children and adolescents compared with trainability of their muscle strength. One reason for such a paucity of information is that the equipment and protocols needed for testing power and changes in power are more complex than those available for strength testing. While the latter requires measurement of force only, the former calls for the simultaneous measurement of force and velocity over time (Fig. 6.1). Another difference between the study of muscle strength on the one hand and muscle power and endurance on the other is that the latter must include the analysis of anaerobic energy turnover, in addition to mechanical and neurologic considerations. In this section, muscle power denotes the peak mechanical power generated by one or more muscle groups over a brief period (e.g., 1–5 s), whereas muscle endurance denotes the ability to sustain high mechanical power over time (e.g., 30–60 s) (for details of methods used for testing muscle power and muscle endurance see Chapter 33 and Inbar *et al.* 1995).

Effectiveness of training programs

In adults, numerous intervention studies have demonstrated trainability of muscle power and endurance, as reviewed by Skinner and Morgan (1985) and by Inbar *et al.* (1995). Training regimens have spanned various approaches, but the common denominator has been the use of repetitions of short-term (e.g., 5–30 s) activities such as cycling or running at maximal or near-maximal intensity.

Cross-sectional comparisons among children and adolescents have demonstrated higher muscle power and muscle endurance among trained individuals than among untrained controls. An example is a study of 13- to 16-year-old Chinese girls and boys (Weijang & Juxiang 1988), which compared performance in the Wingate anaerobic test (for test description see Chapter 33) of track and field athletes (*n* = 47) with that of non-athletes (*n* = 126). When expressed per kilogram of body mass, peak power and mean power of the girl athletes were 21% and 28%, respectively, higher than in the non-athletes. Somewhat lower differences (14% and 15%, respectively) were observed among the boys. A similar pattern emerged when performance was calculated per kilogram of lean body mass. While the above differences could, in part, reflect a training effect, they could also result from preselection.

Few intervention studies assessed the trainability of muscle power and endurance (for review see Bar-Or 1989). Clarke and Vaccaro (1979) tested fifteen 9- to 11-year-old American girls and boys before and after a 7-months intense 4 times per week swimming program. Fifteen girls and boys served as controls. A combined score of pull-ups and push-ups served as an index of arm and shoulder girdle muscle

endurance. As shown in Fig. 6.6, muscle endurance increased more than 100% in the swimmers, but not in the controls. To study the effects of sprint training, Grodjinovsky *et al.* (1980) compared the effects of sprint running (40 and 150 m) and sprint cycling (8- and 30-s all-out bouts) in a 6-week, 3 times per week program on 11- to 13-year-old Israeli boys. Using the Wingate test, peak power and the mean power over 30 s (taken as muscle endurance) increased by about 3–5% in the two training groups, but not in the controls (Fig. 6.7). Such a small training effect may reflect the mild nature of the intervention, which was held during a 10–15 min segment of regular physical education classes.

Indeed, a greater training effect was observed when the program was more intense and prolonged: 10.2- to 11.6-year-old Israeli boys underwent a 9-week (three 45-min sessions per week) interval running program (Cadefeau *et al.* 1990). Distances ranged from 150 to 600 m per interval. As determined by the Wingate test, the program induced a 14% increase in the peak power and 10% increase in mean power. There were no changes in

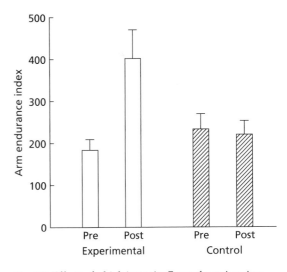

Fig. 6.6 Effects of a high intensity 7-months swimming program on muscle endurance of 15 9- to 11-year-old girls and boys. A combined index (mean and SEM) of push-ups, pull-ups, and body mass was taken to represent the endurance of the arm and shoulder girdle muscles. Both the training and the control group included 13 girls and two boys. After Clarke and Vaccaro (1979).

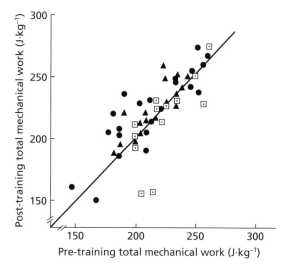

Fig. 6.7 Effects of moderately intense 6-week sprint running and sprint cycling programs on the leg muscle endurance of 11- to 13-year-old boys. Total mechanical work per kilogram of body mass during the 30-s Wingate anaerobic test was taken as muscle endurance. Individual data of 50 boys were divided into sprint cycling (filled triangle), sprint running (filled dot), and control groups (open box with dot in centre), each representing a whole sixth grade class. The diagonal line denotes identity. After Grodjinovsky *et al.* (1980).

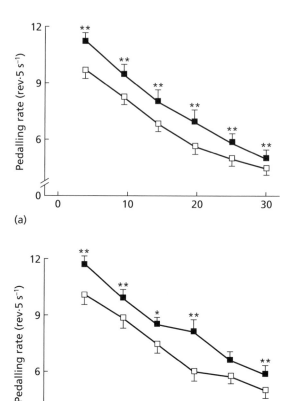

Fig. 6.8 Trainability of muscle power and endurance of: (a) 12- to 13-year-old girls ($n = 18$); and (b) boys ($n = 14$), who took part in a 7-month enhanced physical education program. The program included six periods per week, plus three European handball training sessions per week. The highest 5-s pedalling rate represents peak power, whereas the area under the curve reflects muscle endurance. Open square, pretraining; filled square, post-training. * $P < 0.05$; ** $P < 0.01$. From Grodjinovsky & Bar-Or (1984).

muscle performance of a control group of boys, matched for age and initial activity level. This program was not specific for muscle power and endurance, because it also yielded an increase in maximal oxygen uptake and in 1200-m running velocity. Such non-specificity may have resulted from the relatively long duration (approximately 2 min) of the 600-m intervals.

Ingle *et al.* (2006) reported a significant but small 4.0–5.5% increase in anaerobic peak and mean power, 40-m sprint running and vertical jump performance in pre- and early pubertal boys following a 12-week, 3 times per week combination of resistance training and plyometrics. No changes were observed in a control group. After 12 weeks of detraining, the benefits in the intervention group were lost. These studies show that a training program involving short-term high intensity exercises may improve muscle power and endurance in children.

Grodjinovsky and Bar-Or (1984) compared the responses of 12- to 13-year-old Israeli girls and boys to a 7-month program of six physical education classes per week, plus three practices per week of European handball. As seen in Fig. 6.8, this non-specific program was accompanied by similar increases in the anaerobic performance of both genders. Control girls and boys, attending two physical education classes per week, also had an increase in performance, but less than the experimental groups.

More recently, the effects of a 13-week, twice per week aerobic running program on muscle power have been investigated in 10- to 11-year old boys and girls (Obert *et al*. 2001). The training group increased maximal power during a force–velocity test (for details of the test see Chapter 33) by 23% in absolute terms or 18% when related to fat free mass, while the control group did not show any changes. Furthermore, a series of recent studies (Baquet *et al*. 2001, 2004) reported significant increases in leg power (assessed indirectly by performance improvement for the standing long jump) among prepubertal children and adolescents, following 7–10 weeks of maximal and supramaximal high intensity aerobic training, supporting the idea that anaerobic performance is indeed trainable across the pediatric age range.

As is true for other fitness components (Katch 1983), muscle power and endurance trainability in children seems to depend on the fitness level prior to the start of the training program. Docherty *et al*. (1987) administered a three per week, 4-week program to 12-year-old Canadian boys who had just completed a competitive ice hockey or soccer season. The program comprised all-out repetitions of 20-s bouts of isokinetic activities with various muscle groups, including 20 s cycling at high intensity. Using a modified Wingate test, the authors found no training induced differences in performance. There are no data to indicate whether a similar regimen would have been more effective for children who were not trained athletes.

Mechanisms for trainability of muscle power and endurance

Conceptually, neurologic changes, as described above for muscle strength trainability, can also explain improvement in peak power and, possibly, muscle endurance. However, there are no studies that have analyzed associations between improvements in the latter functions on the one hand, and EMG or MUA on the other, in children or adolescents.

Some data link the improvement in anaerobic power and muscle endurance to morphologic and histochemical changes. In a longitudinal study of 11- to 13-year-old Swedish boys who participated in a 4-year sprint training program (Jacobs *et al*. 1982), the improvement in muscle endurance (50 all-out repetitions of isokinetic knee extensions) was associated with an increase in muscle cross-sectional area, but without changes in muscle fiber-type composition. This study did not include a control group to tease out the effects of growth per se. In another uncontrolled intervention study, 15- to 17-year-old Spanish girls and boys were tested before and after a year of intense sprint, power, and strength training. Biopsies of the vastus lateralis muscle revealed an increase in the diameter of both type 1 and 2 fibers, the proportion of type 1 fibers, and the content of glycogen, as well as the activity of glycolytic (phosphofructokinase and primarily pyruvate kinase) and oxidative (succinate dehydrogenase and amino acid transferases) enzymes. Again, the lack of a control group does not allow differentiation of the contributions from growth per se from those attributed to training. However, similar changes in some muscle enzymes, as well as in muscle lactate, have been shown in young adult Swedish men and women following a 6-week "supramaximal" controlled training program (Jacobs *et al*. 1987). This suggests that an increase in glycolytic enzymes can result directly from high intensity power training. An increase in "anaerobic" substrates (creatine phosphate, adenosine triphosphate, and glycogen), as well as in phosphofructokinase, may result also from a non-specific mix of aerobic and anaerobic training, as shown for 11- to 13-year-old Swedish boys (Eriksson *et al*. 1973).

In summary, there is some, albeit inconclusive, evidence that an increase in glycolytic flux is one factor that may contribute to training induced changes in peak muscle power and muscle endurance of children and adolescents. More research is needed regarding the respective contribution of enhanced muscle contractility and other neurologic factors.

Challenges for future research

• Establish the minimal effective training load (intensity, volume, frequency) required for significant strength, power, and endurance gains at different stages of development.

• Establish the minimal effective training loads for maintenance of strength, power, and endurance gains at different developmental stages.

• Determine whether it is possible to induce muscle hypertrophy with tolerable (without injury and pain) resistance training programs during pre-adolescence.

• Clarify the neurologic adaptations and establish their relative importance and temporal sequence in relation to strength, power, and endurance changes with training and detraining at different stages of development.

• Determine the degree, nature, and relative importance of intrinsic muscle adaptations to strength, power, and endurance changes with training and detraining at different stages of development.

• Compare the effectiveness and safety of different resistance training modes (e.g., free weights, isokinetic, accommodating) and methods (e.g., Berger, DeLorme, pyramid) on strength gains and other physiologic outcomes at different stages of development.

• Determine the importance of neuroendocrine adaptions for training induced strength, power, and endurance, and muscle morphologic adaptations at different stages of development and between the sexes.

• Determine the optimal training regimen for specific improvement of strength, power, and endurance in children and adolescents.

References

Ainsworth, J.L. (1970) The effect of isometric-resistive exercises with the Exer-Genie on strength and speed in swimming. Unpublished doctoral thesis. University of Arkansas, Arkansas.

American Academy of Pediatrics (1990) Strength training, weight and power lifting, and body building by children and adolescents. *Pediatrics* **86**, 801–803.

American Academy of Pediatrics (2001) Strength training by children and adolescents. *Pediatrics* **107**, 1470–1472.

Baquet, G., Berthoin, S., Gerbeaux, M. & Van Praagh, E. (2001). High-intensity aerobic training during a 10 week one-hour physical education cycle: effects on physical fitness of adolescents aged 11 to 16. *International Journal of Sports Medicine* **22**, 295–300.

Baquet, G., Guinhouya, C., Dupont, G., Nourry, C. & Berthoin, S. (2004) Effects of a short-term interval training program on physical fitness in prepubertal children. *Journal of Strength and Conditioning Research* **18**, 708–713.

Bar-Or, O. (1989) Trainability of the prepubescent child. *Physician and Sportsmedicine* **17**, 65–82.

Belanger, A.Y. & McComas, A.J. (1981) Extent of motor unit activation during effort. *Journal of Applied Physiology* **51**, 1131–1135.

Blimkie, C.J.R. (1989) Age- and sex-associated variation in strength during childhood: anthropometric, morphologic, neurologic, and biomechanical correlates. In: *Perspectives in Exercise Science and Sports Medicine*, Vol. 2, *Youth, Exercise and Sport* (Gisolfi, C.V. & Lamb, D.R., eds.) Benchmark Press, Indianapolis: 99–163.

Blimkie, C.J.R. (1992) Resistance training during pre- and early puberty: efficacy, trainability, mechanisms, and persistence. *Canadian Journal of Sport Sciences* **17**, 264–279.

Blimkie, C.J.R. (1993a) Benefits and risks of resistance training in children. In: *Intensive Participation in Children's Sports* (Cahill, B.R. & Pearl, A.J., eds.) Human Kinetics, Champaign, IL: 133–165.

Blimkie, C.J.R. (1993b) Resistance training during preadolescence. Issues and controversies. *Sports Medicine* **15**, 1–18.

Blimkie, C.J.R. & Bar-Or, O. (1996) Trainability of muscle strength, power and endurance during childhood. In: *The Encyclopaedia of Sports Medicine*. Vol. VI. *The Child and Adolescent Athlete.* (Bar-Or, O., ed.) Blackwell Science, Oxford, UK: 113–129.

Blimkie, C.J.R., Martin, J., Ramsay, J., Sale, D. & MacDougall, D. (1989a) The effects of detraining and maintenance weight training on strength development in prepubertal boys. *Canadian Journal of Sport Sciences* **14**, 102P (Abstract).

Blimkie, C.J.R., Ramsay, J., Sale, D., MacDougall, D., Smith, K. & Garner, S. (1989b) Effects of 10 weeks of resistance training on strength development in prepubertal boys. In: *Children and Exercise* Vol. XIII (Oseid, S. & Carlsen, K-H., eds.) Human Kinetics, Champaign, IL: 183–197.

Blimkie, C.J.R., Rice, S., Webber, C.E., Martin, J., Levy, D. & Gordon, C.L. (1993) Effects of resistance training on bone mass and density in adolescent females. *Medicine and Science in Sports and Exercise* **25** (Supplement 48), Abstract 266.

Blundell, S.W., Shepherd, R.B., Dean, C.M. & Adams, R.D. (2003) Functional strength training in cerebral palsy: a pilot study of a group circuit training class for children aged 4–8 years. *Clinical Rehabilitation* **17**, 48–57.

Cadefau, J., Casademont, J., Grau, J.M., et al. (1990) Biochemical and histochemical adaptations to sprint training in young athletes. *Acta Physiologica Scandinavica* **140**, 341–351.

Cahill, B.R., ed. (1988) Proceedings of the Conference on Strength Training and the Prepubescent. American Orthopaedic Society for Sports Medicine, Chicago.

Clarke, D.H. & Vaccaro, P. (1979) The effect of swimming training on muscular performance and body composition in children. *Research Quarterly* **50**, 9–17.

DeKoning, F.L., Binkhorst, R.A., Vissers, A.C.A. & Vos, J.A. (1984) The influence of static strength training on the force–velocity relationship of the arm flexors of 16-year-old boys. In: *Pediatric Work Physiology* (Ilamarian, J. &

Vilimaki, I., eds.) Springer-Verlag, New York: 201–205.

DeLorme, T.L., Ferris, B.G. & Gallagher, J.R. (1952) Effect of progressive resistance exercise on muscle contraction time. *Archives of Physical Medicine and Rehabilitation* **33**, 86–92.

DeRenne, C., Hetzler, R.K., Buxton, B.P. & Ho, K.W. (1996) Effects of training frequency on strength maintenance in pubescent baseball players. *Journal of Strength and Conditioning Research* **10**, 8–14.

Docherty, D., Wenger, H.A., Collis, M.L. & Quinney, H.A. (1987) The effects of variable speed resistance training on strength development in prepubertal boys. *Journal of Human Movement Studies* **13**, 377–382.

Eriksson, B.O., Gollnick, P.D. & Saltin, B. (1973) Muscle metabolism and enzyme activities after training in boys 11–13 years old. *Acta Physiologica Scandinavica* **87**, 485–497.

Faigenbaum, A. (2001) Strength training and children's health. *Journal of Physical Education, Recreation and Dance* **72**, 24–30.

Faigenbaum, A., Kraemer, W., Cahill, B., *et al.* (1996) Youth resistance training: Position statement paper and literature review. *Strength and Conditioning Journal* **18**, 62–75.

Faigenbaum, A.D., Milliken, L., Moulton, L. & Westcott, W.L. (2005) Early muscular fitness adaptations in children in response to two different resistance training regimens. *Pediatric Exercise Science* **17**, 237–248.

Falk, B. & Mor, G. (1996) The effects of resistance and martial arts training in 6–8-year-old boys. *Pediatric Exercise Science* **8**, 48–56.

Falk, B. & Tenenbaum, G. (1996) The effectiveness of resistance training in children. A meta-analysis. *Sports Medicine* **22**, 176–186.

Fleck, S.J. & Kraemer, W.J. (1987) *Designing Resistance Training Programs*. Human Kinetics, Champaign, IL.

Fleck, S.J. & Kraemer, W.J. (1988) Resistance training: physiological responses and adaptations (Part 3 of 4). *Physician and Sportsmedicine* **16**, 63–66, 69, 72–74.

Freedson, P.S., Ward, A. & Rippe, J.M. (1990) Resistance training for youth. *Advances in Sport Medicine and Fitness* **3**, 57–65.

Froberg, K. & Lammert, O. (1996) In: *The Encyclopaedia of Sports Medicine*, Vol. VI, *The Child and Adolescent Athlete* (Bar-Or,

O., ed.) Blackwell Science, Oxford: 25–41.

Fukunaga, T. (1976) Die absolute muskelkraft und das muskelkrafttraining. *Sportarzt und Sportmedizin* **11**, 255–266.

Fukunga, T., Funato, K. & Ikegawa, S. (1992) The effects of resistance training on muscle area and strength in prepubescent age. *Annals of Physiological Anthropology* **11**, 357–364.

Gallagher, J.R. & DeLorme, T.L. (1949) The use of the technique of progressive-resistance exercise in adolescence. *Journal of Bone and Joint Surgery* **31-A**, 847–858.

Gillam, G.M. (1981) Effects of frequency of weight training on muscle strength enhancement. *Journal of Sports Medicine* **21**, 432–436.

Gortmaker S.L. & Sappenfield, W. (1984) Chronic childhood disorders: prevalence and impact. *Pediatric Clinics of North America* **31**, 3–18.

Green, H.J. (1991) What do tests measure? In: *Physiological Testing of the High-Performance Athlete*, 2nd edn. (MacDougall, J.D., Wenger, H.A. & Green, H.J., eds.) Human Kinetics, Champaign, IL: 7–19.

Grodjinovksy, A. & Bar-Or, O. (1984) Influence of added physical education hours upon anaerobic capacity, adiposity and grip strength in 12- to 13-year-old children enrolled in a sports class. In: *Children and Sport* (Ilmarinen, J. & Valimaki, I., eds.) Springer-Verlag, New York: 162–169.

Grodjinovsky, A., Inbar, O., Dotan, R. & Bar-Or, O. (1980) Training effect on the anaerobic performance of children as measured by the Wingate anaerobic test. In: *Children and Exercise* Vol. IX. (Berg, K. & Eriksson, B.G., eds.) University Park Press, Baltimore: 139–145.

Guy, J.A. & Micheli, L.J. (2001) Strength training for children and adolescents. *Journal of the American Academy of Orthopedic Surgery* **9**, 29–36.

Hakkinen, K., Mero, A. & Kauhanen, H. (1989) Specificity of endurance, sprint and strength training on physical performance capacity in young athletes. *Journal of Sports Medicine* **29**, 27–35.

Hassan, S.E.A. (1991) Die Trainierbarkeit der Maximalkraft bei 7-bis 13 jährigen Kindern. *Leistungssport* **5**, 17–24.

Hettinger, T.H. (1958) Die Trainierbarkeit menschlicher Muskeln in Abhängigkeit vom Alter und Geschlecht. *Internationale Zeitschrift fur angewandte Physiologie*

einschliesslich Arbeitsphysiologie **17**, 371–377.

Inbar, O., Bar-Or, O. & Skinner, J.S. (1995) *The Wingate Anaerobic Test: Development, Characteristics and Applications*. Human Kinetics, Champaign, IL.

Ingle, L., Sleap, M. & Tolfrey, K. (2006) The effect of a complex training and detraining programme on selected strength and power variables in early pubertal boys. *Journal of Sports Sciences* **24**, 987–997.

Israel, S. (1992) Age-related changes in strength and special groups. In: *Encyclopedia of Sports Medicine* Vol. III, *Strength and Power in Sport* (Komi, P.V., ed.) Blackwell Scientific Publications, Oxford: 319–328.

Jacobs, I., Esbjornsson, M., Sylven, C., Holm, I. & Jansson, E. (1987) Sprint training effects on muscle myoglobin enzymes, fiber types, and blood lactate. *Medicine and Science in Sports and Exercise* **19**, 368–374.

Jacobs, I., Sjodin, B. & Svane, B. (1982) Muscle fiber type, cross-sectional area and strength in boys after 4 years' endurance training. *Medicine and Science in Sports and Exercise* **14**, 123.

Katch, V.L. (1983) Physical conditioning for children. *Journal of Adolescent Health Care* **3**, 241–246.

Kirsten, G. (1963) Der Einfluß isometrischen Muskeltrainings auf die Entwicklung der Muskelkraft Jugendlicher. *Internationale Zeitschrift fur angewandte Physiologie einschliesslich Arbeitsphysiologie* **19**, 387–402.

Komi, P.V., ed. (1992) Strength and power in sport. *Encyclopedia of Sports Medicine* Vol. III. Blackwell Scientific Publications, Oxford.

Komi, P.V., Viitasalo, J.T., Rauramaa, R. & Vihko, V. (1978) Effect of isometric strength training on mechanical, electrical, and metabolic aspects of muscle function. *European Journal of Applied Physiology* **40**, 45–55.

Kraemer, W.J., Fry, A.C., Frykman, P.N., Conroy, B. & Hoffman, J. (1989) Resistance training and youth. *Pediatric Exercise Science* **1**, 336–350.

Kusinitz, I. & Keeney, C.E. (1958) Effects of progressive weight training on health and physical fitness of adolescent boys. *Research Quarterly* **29**, 294–301.

Lavallee, M. (2002) Strength training in children and adolescents. Current Comment, American College of Sports Medicine, September 2002. www.acsm.org

Lazzer, S., Boirie, Y., Poissonnier, C., *et al.* (2005) Longitudinal changes in activity patterns, physical capacities, energy expenditure, and body composition in severely obese adolescents during a multidisciplinary weight-reduction program. *International Journal of Obesity* **29**, 37–46.

Lillegard, W., Brown, E., Wilson, D., Henderson, R. & Lewis, E. (1997) Efficacy of strength training in prepubescent to early postpubescent boys and girls: effects of gender and maturity. *Pediatric Rehabilitation* **1**, 147–157.

McCubbin, J.A. & Shasby, G.B. (1985) Effects of isokinetic exercise on adolescents with cerebral palsy. *Adapted Physical Activity Quarterly* **2**, 56–64.

McGovern, M.B. (1984) Effects of circuit weight training on the physical fitness of prepubescent children. *Dissertation Abstracts International* **45**, 452A–453A.

Mersch, F. & Stoboy, H. (1989) Strength training and muscle hypertrophy in children. In: *Children and Exercise*, Vol. XIII (Oseid, S. & Carlsen, K.-H., eds.) Human Kinetics, Champaign IL: 165–182.

Morris, F., Naughton, G., Gibbs, J., Carlson, J. & Wark, J. (1997) Prospective ten-month exercise intervention in premenarcheal girls: positive effects on bone and lean mass. *Journal of Bone and Mineral Research* **12**, 1453–1462.

Munson, W.W., Baker, S.B. & Lundegren, H.M. (1985) strength training and leisure counselling as treatments for institutionalized juvenile delinquents. *Adapted Physical Activity Quarterly* **2**, 65–75.

Narici, M.V., Roi, G.S., Landoni, L., Minetti, A.E. & Cerretteli, P. (1989) Changes in force, cross-sectional area and neural activation during strength training and detraining of the human quadriceps. *European Journal of Applied Physiology* **59**, 310–319.

Nielsen, B., Nielsen, K., Behrendt-Hansen, M. & Asmussen, E. (1980) Training of "functional muscular strength" in girls 7–19 years old. In: *Children and Exercise* Vol. IX (Berg, K. & Eriksson, B.D., eds.) Human Kinetics Publishers, Champaign, IL: 69–78.

Obert, P., Mandigout, M., Vinet, A. & Courteix, D. (2001) Effect of a 13-week aerobic training programme on the maximal power developed during a force-velocity test in prepubertal boys

and girls. *International Journal of Sports Medicine* **22**, 442–446.

Orenstein, D.M., Hovel, M.F., Mulvihill, M., *et al.* (2004) Strength vs aerobic training in children with cystic fibrosis. *Chest* **126**, 1204–1214.

Ozmun, J.C., Mikesky, A.E. & Surburg, P.R. (1991) Neuromuscular adaptations during prepubescent strength training. *Medicine and Science in Sports and Exercise* **23**, 186 (Abstract).

Payne, V.G., Morrow, J.R., Johnson, L.L. & Dalton, S.N. (1997) Resistance training in children and youth: a meta-analysis. *Research Quarterly for Exercise and Sport* **68**, 80–88.

Pfeiffer, R.D. & Francis, R.S. (1986) Effects of strength training on muscle development in prepubescent, pubescent, and postpubescent males. *Physician and Sportsmedicine* **14**, 134–143.

Ramsay, J.A., Blimkie, C.J.R., Smith, K., Garner, S., MacDougall, J.D. & Sale, D.G. (1990) Strength training effects in prepubescent boys. *Medicine and Science in Sports and Exercise* **22**, 605–614.

Rarick, G.L. & Larsen, G.L. (1958) Observations on frequency and intensity of isometric muscular effort in developing static muscular strength in postpubescent males. *Research Quarterly* **29**, 333–341.

Sadres, E., Eliakim, A., Constantini, N., Lidor, R. & Falk, B. (2001) The effect of long-term resistance training on anthropometric measures, muscle strength, and self-concept in pre-pubertal boys. *Pediatric Exercise Science* **13**, 357–372.

Sailors, M. & Berg, K. (1987) Comparison of responses to weight training in pubescent boys and men. *Journal of Sports Medicine* **27**, 30–36.

Sale, D.G. (1989) Strength training in children. In: *Perspectives in Exercise Science and Sports Medicine*, Vol. 2, *Youth, Exercise and Sport* (Gisolfi, C.V. & Lamb, D.R., eds.) Benchmark Press, Indianapolis: 165–222.

Sale, D.G. (1991) Testing strength and power. In: *Physiological Testing of the High-Performance Athlete*, 2nd edn. (MacDougall, J.D., Wenger, H.A. & Green, H.J., eds.) Human Kinetics, Champaign, IL: 21–106.

Selvadurai, H.C., Blimkie, C.J., Meyers, N., Mellis, C.M., Cooper, P.J. & Van Asperen, P.P. (2002) Radomized controlled study of in-hospital exercise training programs in children with cystic fibrosis. *Pediatric Pulmonology* **33**, 194–200.

Sewall, L. & Micheli, L.J. (1986) Strength training for children. *Journal of Pediatric Orthopedics* **6**, 143–146.

Siegel, J.A., Camaione, D.N. & Manfredi, T.G. (1989) The effects of upper body resistance training on prepubescent children. *Pediatric Exercise Science* **1**, 145–154.

Skinner, J.S. & Morgan, D. (1985) Aspects of anaerobic performance. In: *Limits of Human Performance* (Clarke, D. & Eckert, H., eds.) Human Kinetics, Champaign, IL: 31–44.

Strong, W.B., Malina, R.M., Blimkie, C.J.R., *et al.* (2005) Physical activity recommendations for school-age youth. *Journal of Pediatrics* **146**, 732–737.

Suman, O.E., Spies, R.J., Celis, M.M., Mlcak, R.P. & Herndon, D.N. (2001) Effects of a 12-week resistance exercise program on skeletal muscle strength in children with burn injuries. *Journal of Applied Physiology* **91**, 1168–1175.

Treuth, M.S., Hunter, G.R., Figueroa-Colon, R. & Goran, I. (1998a) Effects of strength training on intra-abdominal adipose tissue in obese prepubertal girls. *Medicine and Science in Sports and Exercise* **30**, 1738–1743.

Treuth, M.S., Hunter, G.R., Pichon, C., Figueroa-Colon, R. & Goran, M.I. (1998b) Fitness and energy expenditure after strength training in obese prepubertal girls. *Medicine and Science in Sports and Exercise* **30**, 1130–1136.

Tsolakis, C.K., Vagenas, G.K. & Dessypris, A.G. (2004) Strength adaptations and hormonal responses to resistance training and detraining in preadolescent males. *Journal of Strength and Conditioning Research* **18**, 625–629.

Vrijens, J. (1978) Muscle strength development in the pre- and post-pubescent age. *Medicine and Sport* **11**, 152–158.

Washington, R.L., Bernhardt, D.T., Gomez, J.G., *et al.* (2001) Strength training by children and adolescents. *Pediatrics* **107**, 1470–1472.

Webb, D.R. (1990) Strength training in children and adolescents. *Pediatric Clinics of North America* **37**, 1187–1210.

Weijang, D. & Juxiang, Q. (1988) Anaerobic performance of Chinese untrained and trained 11–18 year-old boys and girls. *Medicine and Sports Science* **28**, 52–60.

Weltman, A. (1989) Weight training in prepubertal children: physiologic benefit and potential damage. In:

Advances in Pediatric Sport Sciences,
Vol. 3 (Bar-Or, O., ed.) Human Kinetics,
Champaign, IL: 101–129.

Weltman, A., Janny, C., Rians, C.B., *et al.*
(1986) The effects of hydraulic resistance
strength training in pre-pubertal males.
Medicine and Science in Sports and Exercise
18, 629–638.

Westcott, W.L. (1979) Female response to
weight training. *Journal of Physical
Education* **77**, 31–33.

Westcott, W.L. (1991) Safe and sane
strength training for teenagers. *Scholastic
Coach* **Oct**, 42–44.

Witzke, K.A. & Snow , C.M. (2000) Effects
of plyometric jump training on bone

mass in adolescent girls. *Medicine and
Science in Sports and Exercise* **32**,
1051–1057.

Wolbers, C.P. & Sills, F.S. (1956)
Development of strength in high
school boys by static muscle
contractions. *Research Quarterly*
27, 446–450.

Chapter 7

Endurance Trainability of Children and Youth

KARIN A. PFEIFFER, FELIPE LOBELO,
DIANNE S. WARD, AND RUSSELL R. PATE

Regular participation in adequate amounts of moderate to vigorous physical activity is a key component of a healthy lifestyle and is known to protect against many chronic diseases (World Health Organization 2005). Nonetheless, most adults in industrialized nations do not participate in physical activity at recommended levels (Lindstrom *et al.* 2003; Centers for Disease Control and Prevention 2005). While physical activity levels tend to be higher in children and adolescents than in adults, numerous medical and public health authorities have expressed concern that many youth are less active than recommended (Centers for Disease Control and Prevention 2004b). In addition, it has been demonstrated that many children and youth fail to meet health-related standards for physical fitness (Corbin & Pangrazi 1992; Chatrath *et al.* 2002; Wedderkopp *et al.* 2004; Pate *et al.* 2006).

The consequences of such inactivity and low fitness levels are readily apparent in recent increases in the prevalence of childhood obesity and type 2 diabetes mellitus and the appearance of cardiovascular risk clustering (Steinberger & Daniels 2003; Wedderkopp *et al.* 2003, 2004). For this reason and to promote overall health and prevent chronic disease, experts agree that all youth should be able to participate in systematic exercise programs (Institute of Medicine 2005). In general, experts have indicated that these programs should be designed to accomplish two major goals: (i) in the short term, to enhance physical fitness; and (ii) in the long term, to promote adoption of a physically active lifestyle, which in turn can be expected to maintain physical fitness into and throughout adulthood (Telama *et al.* 2005).

Although some children and youth are less active than desirable, others participate regularly in organized sports. In addition, in recent decades organized sport programs for children and youth have become increasingly common. These programs also have become increasingly competitive. Endurance sport programs (e.g., swimming, distance running) for youth have become quite popular, and often involve long-term exposure to heavy training. Some experts have raised concerns about the health consequences of such a training regime, including risk of sport injuries, overuse syndromes, and abnormal physiologic reactions (Bar-Or & Rowland 2004). However, training itself does not appear to adversely affect growth and maturation in young athletes (Malina *et al.* 2004).

Because endurance exercise training is frequently used with children and youth for the purpose of promoting health-related fitness and for enhancing sport performance, pediatric exercise scientists have been interested in the physiologic adaptations that result from the training process. In particular, scientists have studied "trainability" (i.e., the extent to which the physiologic markers of endurance fitness change as a result of regular participation in endurance exercise). Accordingly, the major purpose of this chapter is to review the scientific literature pertinent to trainability in children and youth. The chapter also evaluates the extent to which research directions proposed in previous reviews of this topic have been addressed. These directions included studying gender and maturational differences in the aerobic trainability of youth, and changes in performance measures and related physiologic correlates after the training stimulus. Finally, the authors present important directions for future research on this issue.

Physiology of endurance exercise performance

In the sport setting, exercise training is designed to enhance exercise tolerance and ultimately to improve sport performance. If a training program succeeds in enhancing performance or health-related endurance fitness, it is likely that it will do so largely by enhancing one or more of the key physiologic factors that are known to limit tolerance for endurance exercise. Therefore, it is logical to begin a discussion of trainability with a brief review of the physiologic determinants of endurance performance.

Three physiologic variables, operating in combination, are thought to determine endurance exercise performance (Sjodin & Svedenhag 1985; Pate & Branch 1992). Maximal aerobic power, also described as maximal oxygen consumption ($\dot{V}O_{2max}$), is the greatest rate at which the individual can use oxygen in the aerobic metabolic process. This is a key determinant of endurance performance because endurance exercise must depend primarily on aerobic oxidation of carbohydrates and lipids (Maughan *et al.* 1997). Hence, the individual with the higher $\dot{V}O_{2max}$ is capable of a higher maximal rate of aerobic energy expenditure (although it should be noted that this maximal rate typically can be sustained for no more than a few minutes without involving anaerobic pathways of energy production).

The ability to sustain a high rate of aerobic energy expenditure for a prolonged period of time is a function of $\dot{V}O_{2max}$ and a second important physiologic variable—lactate threshold. Lactate threshold is the rate of aerobic expenditure at which the fatiguing byproduct of anaerobic metabolism, lactic acid, begins to accumulate in the blood. Lactate threshold is often expressed as the percentage of the $\dot{V}O_{2max}$ at which it is observed (i.e., the relative exercise intensity). This percentage varies markedly between individuals, even among endurance-trained athletes, which indicates that it is, at least partially, genetically determined (Weston *et al.* 1999). Athletes typically perform long-duration sport events at intensities approximating the lactate threshold, and this performance $\dot{V}O_2$ is linked primarily to adaptations in muscles resulting from prolonged endurance training (Holloszy & Coyle 1984). Therefore, the ability to sustain a high rate of aerobic energy expenditure can be enhanced by increasing $\dot{V}O_{2max}$, thus setting up a higher limit for endurance exercise, or by increasing lactate threshold, allowing a better performance $\dot{V}O_2$ (Bassett & Howley 2000).

A third important physiologic variable, economy, sets the ratio between the rate of aerobic energy expenditure and the pace of endurance exercise. Economy is typically quantified as the rate of oxygen consumption observed at a specified movement pace (e.g., running, cycling, or swimming speed). The more economical an individual is, he or she will be able to perform at a given speed with a lower rate of oxygen consumption (and hence lower rate of energy expenditure) than a less economical counterpart. In adults, running economy is highly correlated with endurance performance and, in conjunction with lactate threshold, may be a better indicator of running times than $\dot{V}O_{2max}$ values (Bassett & Howley 2000).

Training enhances endurance performance by increasing maximal aerobic power, lactate threshold, and/or economy. Of the three, maximal aerobic power is best understood, because its relationship to endurance performance has been recognized for longer and the biologic mechanisms explaining the relationship have been studied in greater detail. Several factors are thought to limit $\dot{V}O_{2max}$ and have been typically divided into those limiting the oxygen transport to the muscles by the cardiorespiratory system (central factors) and those constraints created by the limits of aerobic enzyme activity and the skeletal muscle environment (peripheral factors) (Rowland 2005). The following discussion focuses on the changes in maximal aerobic power that have been shown to result from endurance training in children and youth. It should be remembered that training could enhance endurance performance in at least some individuals by increasing lactate threshold and/or economy. (For more details about the development of maximal aerobic power during childhood and adolescence, see Chapter 4.)

Factors related to trainability of youth

Exercise scientists have been interested in the effects of physical training on the functional capacity of children and youth for over 75 years (Schwartz *et al.* 1928). Researchers have published several scientific reviews on this issue (Vaccaro & Mahon 1987; Pate & Ward 1990; Baquet *et al.* 2003; Bar-Or & Rowland 2004; Rowland 2005). In general, most concluded that children and youth are physiologically adaptive to endurance exercise training, if the training stimulus is adequate. Additionally, investigators have identified several factors related to aerobic trainability in children and youth.

Over time, the conclusions regarding aerobic trainability and factors associated with trainability of children and youth have not changed significantly. Earlier reviews indicated that the following major issues were of particular interest: trainability of prepubescent youth; initial fitness values of youth; and effects of growth and development. Recent investigations have highlighted other topics, including determination of underlying mechanisms for training adaptations and effects of the interaction between frequency, intensity, and duration of training (i.e., dosage). In the past, researchers hypothesized that prepubescent children may be less adaptive to endurance exercise training than older youth and adults. Results from recent studies refute that hypothesis, indicating that an increase of 1–14% in $\dot{V}o_{2max}$ is seen in prepubescent children (Table 7.1). This is similar to the results from a meta-analysis performed by Payne and Morrow (1993), which cited an average increase in $\dot{V}o_{2max}$ of 5% in 23 endurance training studies of children.

It is well known that maximal aerobic power tends to be relatively high in children compared to adults (Rowland 2005). This may be a result of genetic programming, and it may also be explained by the fact that children tend to be more physically active than adults (environmental factors) (Centers for Disease Control and Prevention 2004a,b); however, there is no evidence to support a high correlation between fitness and physical activity in childhood (Morrow & Freedson 1994). It is difficult to differentiate any effects that genes or environ-

ment may separately exert on aerobic trainability, and it is difficult to quantify the combined effect of genes and environment together. Regardless of the source of potential effects, the typical child's relatively high baseline fitness level may tend to limit his or her functional adaptation to training.

Children and youth, particularly at certain critical periods, experience rapid growth and development. These phenomena certainly operate as complicating factors for scientists studying the physiology of exercise in pediatric populations. This is because some of the changes associated with growth and development are also associated with exercise training. Researchers have used allometric scaling in attempts to attenuate the effects of growth on performance. When allometry is used, comparison across studies can be difficult because each population is likely to require a different exponential factor for energy expenditure values. Beyond this, it is possible that trainability in children and youth may vary with developmental status (Malina *et al.* 2004). It is also possible that during certain developmental periods children and youth are highly adaptive to training. Based on the available evidence, it is not possible to determine the impact of growth and maturation on aerobic training. In any case, both growth and development are factors to consider whenever exercise training is studied in children and youth.

Several underlying mechanisms for differences in training adaptations between children/youth and adults have been proposed. Some of these differences were previously discussed (e.g., growth and maturation). One variable that has received attention over time is arteriovenous oxygen difference. An increase in $\dot{V}o_{2max}$ requires an increase in maximal cardiac output and/or maximal arteriovenous oxygen difference. Bar-Or & Rowland (2004) noted that maximal arteriovenous oxygen difference already tends to be high in prepubescent children in the absence of training. This observation led investigators to theorize that the overall adaptation to endurance training could be limited in children by a "ceiling effect" in maximal arteriovenous oxygen difference. Rowland (2005) recently suggested that two other potential mechanisms for differences in training adaptations between children and adults

Table 7.1 Procedures and findings of high and moderate quality studies addressing the trainability of youth.

Subjects	Age (years)	Training stimulus	Change $\dot{V}O_{2max}$ (%)	Reference
High quality I: 20 boys C: 20 boys	8–9	I1: 85% HRmax I2: 68% HRmax All: 3 days/week* 10 weeks of walking, jogging, running	I1: 6.7%* I2: 4.0% C: <0%	Savage *et al.* (1986)
I: 23 girls C: 7 girls	9–10	Cycle: 25 min Interval running: 15 min All 160–170 bpm* 3 days/week* 8 weeks	Cycle: 10.0%* Sprint: 8.5%* C: <0%	McManus *et al.* (1997)
I: 35 girls C: 16 girls	10	Cycle: 25 min Aerobics: 40 min All: 160–170 bpm* 3 days/week* 8 weeks	Cycle: 1.7% Aerobics: 1.7% C: 0%	Welsman *et al.* (1997)
I: 25 boys C: 14 boys	10	Cycle: 20 min Interval running: 15 min Both 160–170 bpm* 3 days/week* 8 weeks	Intervals: <0% Cycle: 5.1% C: 0.1%	Williams *et al.* (2000)
I: 11 boys C: 11 boys	9–11	3 days/week 40 min at 85% HRmax* 3 days/week* 8 weeks of cycling	I: 20.0% C: 10.0%	Becker & Vaccaro (1983)
I: 27 boys C: 9 boys	11–13	I1: 91% HRmax I2: 78% HRmax I3: 70% HRmax All: 12 min* 3 days/week* 6 weeks of cycling	I1: 10.9%* I2: 1.0% I3: 3.0% C: <0	Massicotte & MacNab (1979)
I: 9 boys C: 9 boys	11–14	60–90 min at 75–97% $\dot{V}O_{2max}$* 3 monozygotic twins days/week* 24 weeks of running	I: 10.6%* C: 2.5%	Danis *et al.* (2003)
I: 6 boys C: 5 boys	11	Interval running* 2 days/week* 26 weeks	E: 10.2%* C: 0.6%	Ekblom (1969)
I: 20 obese youth C: 61 obese youth	13–16	5 days/week 30–45 min at 55–80% $\dot{V}O_{2max}$* 5 days/week* 32 weeks of aerobic training	I: 14.0%* C: <0%	Mitchell *et al.* (2002)
I: 22 girls C: 22 girls	15–17	5 days/week* 120 min* 5 weeks of running, team sports and aerobic dancing	Ex: 10.0%* C: <0%	Eliakim *et al.* (1996)
I: 9 boys C: 10 boys	18	4 min sessions at 90–95% HRmax* 2 days/week* 8 weeks of interval running	I: 10.6%* C: 0.2%	Helgerud *et al.* (2001)
Moderate quality I: 8 girls C: 8 girls	4	915 m runs* 6 days/week* 54 weeks	I: 19.4%* C: 8.3%	Yoshisawa *et al.* (1997)
I: 20 C: 10	5	I1: 1 to 3 days/week I2: 1 day/week All 28 weeks of running	I1: 2.0% I2: 2.0% C: 8.0%	Yoshida *et al.* (1980)
I: 18 (8 girls) C: 10 (4) girls	8–11	Running/aerobics at 160–170 bpm* 3 days/week* 60 mins* 10 weeks	I: <0% C: 0.5%	Ignicio & Mahon (1995)
I: 26 C: 10	8–12	Running at 75–80% $\dot{V}O_{2max}$* 4 days/week* 10–35 mins* 12 weeks	I: 6.8%* C: 1.5%	Lussier & Buskirk (1977)

Continued on p. 88

Table 7.1 (*Cont'd*)

Subjects	Age (years)	Training stimulus	Change $\dot{V}_{O_{2max}}$ (%)	Reference
I: 19 (10 girls) C: 16 (7 girls)	10–11	Aerobic exercise at >80% HRmax* 3 days/week* 60–90 mins* 13 weeks	I Boys: 15.0%* I girls: 8.0%* C Boys: <0% C Girls: <0%	Obert *et al.* (2003)
I: 35 (17 girls) C: 50 (22 girls)	10–11	Aerobic exercise at >80% HRmax* 3 days/week* 60–90 mins* 13 weeks	I Boys: 4.2%* I Girls: 8.5%* C Boys: <0% C Girls: < 0%	Mandigout *et al.* (2001)
I: 26 (14 girls) C: 19 (9 girls)	10–11	Stationary cycle at >80% Peak HR* 3 days/week* 30 mins* 12 weeks	I Boys: 1.3%* I Girls: 8.0%* C Boys: <0% C Girls: <0%	Tolfrey *et al.* (1998)
I: 14 boys C: 14 boys	10–11	Interval running: 3 days/week* 45 mins* 9 weeks	I: 8.0%* C: 2.0%	Rotstein *et al.* (1986)
I: 13 boys C: 13 boys	8–12	Continuous running at 70–80%* 15 mins $\dot{V}_{O_{2max}}$ and interval running at 90–100% $\dot{V}_{O_{2max}}$* 15–35 mins* 3 days/week* 14 weeks	I: 12.9%* C: <0%	Mahon & Vaccaro (1994)
I: 5 girls C: 9 girls	9–10	Swimming at 170–180 bpm* 60–90 mins* 5 days/week* 40 weeks	I: 29.0%* C: 0.8%	Obert *et al.* (1996)
I: 20 (10 boys) C: 33 (13 boys)	9–10	Running at 100–130% Max aerobic speed* 10–20 s* 30 mins* 2 days/week* 7 weeks	I: 9.0%* C: <0%	Baquet *et al.* (2002)
I: 12 boys C: 5 boys	12	Aerobic exercise* 3 days/week* 15 weeks	I: 10.0%* C: 0%;	Williford *et al.* (1996)
I: 31 (20 girls) C: 37 (24 girls)	10–12	Endurance exercise* 25 mins* 3 days/week	I: 5.4%* C: 0%	Rowland *et al.* (1996)
I: 37 (24 girls) C: 37 (24 girls)	10–12	Aerobic exercise at mean HR of 166 bpm* 30 mins* 3 days/week* 12 weeks	I: 6.5%* C: 0%	Rowland & Boyajian (1995)
I: 8 boys C: 8 boys	10–14	Running 100–800 m at 70–80% $\dot{V}_{O_{2max}}$ and interval running 10–30 m at 90–100% $\dot{V}_{O_{2max}}$* 4 days/week* 30 mins* 8 weeks	I: 7.5%* C: 1.1%	Mahon & Vaccaro (1989)
I: 8 girls C: 8 girls	12–14	Running and bench stepping* 3 days/week* 14 weeks	I: 16.2%* C: <0%	Eisenman & Golding (1975)
I: 12 boys C: 12 boys	10, 13, and 16 pairs of twins	Running, step bench and cycle intervals* 4 days/week* 10 weeks	10 years I: 19.0%* C: 6.0% 13 years I: 11.0% C: 10.0% 16 years I: 17.0% C: 2.0%	Weber *et al.* (1976)
I: 12 girls C: 12 girls	15	Swimming* 4 days/week* 7 weeks	I: 16.1%* C: 0%	Stransky *et al.* (1979)

High quality studies: Randomized design, accurate description of training stimulus, objective assessment of $\dot{V}_{O_{2max}}$.
Moderate quality studies: Non-randomized design, accurate description of training stimulus, objective assessment of $\dot{V}_{O_{2max}}$.
* Statistically significant difference from the control group, based on reported data.
I, intervention group; C, control group; HR, heart rate; bpm, beats per minute; C: <0% indicates a decrease in $\dot{V}_{O_{2max}}$ in the control group.

may be increased plasma volume and cellular aerobic capacity in the young population. Eriksson (1972) and Eriksson and Koch (1973) have examined both variables in a small number of studies. However, very little information is available regarding either variable, and it is too soon to comment definitively. Investigating mechanisms of aerobic trainability in children and youth is challenging, and study protocols examining cellular level variables are not likely to pass easily through institutional review boards.

Dosage of training is an important variable to consider, yet it is difficult to differentiate the effects of type, frequency, intensity, and duration of training. Even when researchers carefully control these factors, there is considerable variation across studies. Some studies have set an exercise dosage according to percent of heart rate maximum or absolute heart rate value, while others may set an exercise dosage to percent of maximal aerobic capacity. Even if the intensity is similar across studies, the duration of training sessions (e.g., 30 vs. 40 min per session), frequency of sessions (e.g., three vs. four per week), type of exercise (cycling vs. running), or duration of the exercise intervention itself (e.g., 8 vs. 12 weeks) may differ. This makes it difficult to establish concrete conclusions regarding the effects of endurance training by dosage.

Although the conclusions regarding aerobic trainability and factors associated with trainability have not changed much over time, some questions that previously existed have not yet been answered. In addition, new research continues to generate new questions related to trainability and its related correlates in children and youth. Future research should focus on growth and development, physiologic mechanisms, and dosage in the area of child and adolescent aerobic trainability.

Functional adaptations to endurance training

In a previous review article (Pate & Ward 1990), the authors examined trainability in children and youth by applying a stringent set of criteria for inclusion of primary research studies:

1 Use of a control group (random or pair-matched);

2 Provision of a clear description of the training protocol;

3 Application of physiologic measures as indicators of training outcomes;

4 Use of appropriate statistical procedures; and

5 Publication in a peer-reviewed research journal.

In a chapter published in a previous volume of this encyclopedia, *The Child and Adolescent Athlete* (Pate & Ward 1995), more stringent inclusion criteria were added, including use of:

1 Training protocol administered outside the physical education class setting;

2 Subjects with no known health problems; and

3 Endurance training without any supplementary modes of training, such as weight-training.

Since 1996, scientists have expanded the body of knowledge on trainability in youth. Thus, our intention for this chapter is to go beyond both earlier reviews and draw conclusions about trainability in youth based on the best research available. For this review we categorized studies based on design quality, and employed a rigorous search strategy to identify articles. Studies included in the previous chapter were published between 1969 and 1989 (Pate & Ward 1995). For this chapter we performed additional literature searches in order to include quality experiments published between 1990 and 2005. A literature review was conducted in the electronic National Library of Medicine (PubMed) using the subject's age (0–18 years) and publication date (1990–2005) limits. Search keywords included a combination of MesH (physical fitness, physical endurance, exercise) and non-Mesh (training, $\dot{V}o_{2max}$) terms. We also examined book chapters and articles published in *Pediatric Exercise Science*. In the preparation of this chapter a total of 67 published studies were reviewed, but studies that did not meet the inclusion criteria were excluded from the set of papers on which conclusions were based. This chapter summarizes the available evidence regarding the endurance trainability of children and youth, citing 29 studies published between 1969 and 2003.

The 29 studies included in this review are summarized in Table 7.1. Studies were subdivided in two categories based on their design quality. In the first 11 studies, investigators randomly assigned youth to control or exercise training groups, provided detailed and accurate descriptions of the exercise stimulus implemented, and used objective measures to detect changes in cardiorespiratory fitness. These are considered "high quality" studies. The remaining 18 studies were not randomized protocols and are considered to be of "moderate quality." Most studies used only male subjects (12) or a combination of males and females (11). Of the 11 "high quality" studies, 10 found a net increase in $\dot{V}O_{2max}$ in the exercise-trained group(s) over the control group, but only seven of those reported that difference to be statistically significant. Similarly, among the 18 "moderate quality" studies, 16 found a net increase in $\dot{V}O_{2max}$ in the trained group(s) over the control group and 15 reported that difference to be statistically significant. The range of net increases in $\dot{V}O_{2max}$ was large, extending from a high of 29.0% (Obert *et al.* 1996) to a low of 1.0% (Massicotte & MacNab 1979). The average net increase in $\dot{V}O_{2max}$ across the 29 studies was 8.6%. The average net increase in the "high quality" and "moderate quality" studies was 6.7% and 9.7%, respectively.

Differences in the net $\dot{V}O_{2max}$ increase were seen when studies were divided by training mode. Upright exercise (running, sprint or interval training, aerobics) was associated with an 8.1% net increase in $\dot{V}O_{2max}$, while those using cycling (six studies) or swimming (two studies) as the primary exercise training stimulus showed a net increase in $\dot{V}O_{2max}$ of 6.8% and 22.6%, respectively. In one study employing a running program, a greater increase in $\dot{V}O_{2max}$ was seen in the control group compared to the two training groups (Yoshida *et al.* 1980).

Figures 7.1 and 7.2 provide graphic comparison of intervention and control groups in terms of the observed changes in $\dot{V}O_{2max}$ as measured before and after the training period. For the high quality group of studies (Fig. 7.1), a total of nine comparisons drawn from six studies are presented. For the moderate quality group of studies (Fig. 7.2), a total of 11 comparisons drawn from eight studies are presented. Studies that did not provide values for pre- and post-training in both the intervention and control groups are not included in either figure. A wide range of variability exists in the degree of $\dot{V}O_{2max}$ change after the training stimulus between studies

and within studies based on the exercise type or dose of training. Overall, the high quality studies showed a more consistent pattern of the effects of training than those of moderate quality. This may be related to heterogeneity in the groups of subjects who participated in the randomized studies. Figure 7.3 provides a graphic comparison between genders and by intervention vs. control status with respect to the average change in aerobic power after the exercise stimulus. These studies suggest that, in general, boys and girls respond to endurance training programs in a similar fashion.

Measures of functional status other than $\dot{V}O_{2max}$ were used in only a few of the studies included in this chapter. Four studies (Becker & Vaccaro 1983; Mahon & Vaccaro 1989; Helgerud *et al.* 2001; Danis *et al.* 2003) reported measures of lactate threshold (LT) or its related correlate, ventilatory threshold (VT). In all of them, the increases in LT or VT in the training group(s) over the control group were much larger than those observed for $\dot{V}O_{2max}$ (15–20% change in LT or VT vs. 7–10% change in $\dot{V}O_{2max}$). Other studies measured physiologic variables in relation to exercise training such as left ventricular function (Mitchell *et al.* 2002), maximal arteriovenous oxygen difference (Yoshisawa *et al.* 1997), and total energy expenditure (Eliakim *et al.* 1996). Pure performance measures (e.g., run times or distances; time to fatigue at submaximal power outputs) are rarely used as outcome measures in training studies with children. In the present review chapter, only one study (Ignicio & Mahon 1995) reported field performance measures (run times) and, interestingly, these investigators found significant changes after the training program in the intervention group for run times but not for $\dot{V}O_{2max}$. It is possible that our strict criteria for selecting studies to be incorporated in this review did not capture studies that used performance measures as indicators of change in fitness after exercise training. Because the purpose of the training process is to enhance fitness (i.e., exercise performance or tolerance), it seems logical to use both physiologic and performance measures as outcome variables because both reflect changes that are mechanistically related to the improvement of fitness.

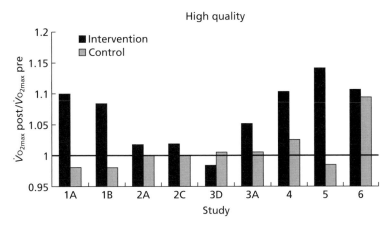

Fig. 7.1 Comparison of pre- to post-test changes in $\dot{V}o_{2max}$ as observed in training and control groups in selected studies of trainability in youth. High quality refers to the design rigor including randomization of the intervention. Data points represent mean effect in each study; data from some studies that were considered high quality were not included in this table because of unavailability of numbers to calculate changes in $\dot{V}o_{2max}$. Studies are ordered from left to right based on the participants' ages (mean age for study 1 was 9.5 years and for study 6 was 18 years; exact ages for each study can be found in Table 7.1). Mean change in $\dot{V}o_{2max}$ for the intervention and control group were 6.7% and 0.8%, respectively. Studies: 1, McManus *et al.* (1997); 2, Welsman *et al.* (1997); 3, Williams *et al.* (2000); 4, Danis *et al.* (2003); 5, Mitchell *et al.* (2002); 6, Helgerud *et al.* (2001). A, cycle; B, sprint running; C, aerobics; D, interval training.

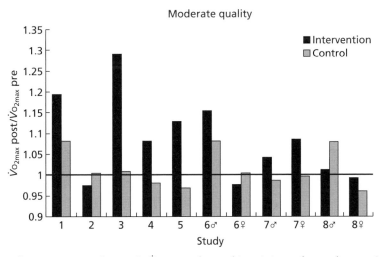

Fig. 7.2 Comparison of pre- to post-test changes in $\dot{V}o_{2max}$ as observed in training and control groups in selected studies of trainability in youth. Moderate quality refers to the design rigor excluding randomization of the intervention. Data points represent mean effect in each study; data from some studies that were considered moderate quality were not included in this table because of unavailability of numbers to calculate changes in $\dot{V}o_{2max}$. Studies are ordered from left to right based on the participants' ages (mean age for study 1 was 4 years and for study 8 was 10.5 years; exact ages for each study can be found in Table 7.1). For studies 6–8, ♂ = males and ♀ = females. Mean change in $\dot{V}o_{2max}$ for the intervention and control group were 9.7% and 2.3%, respectively. Studies: 1, Yoshisawa *et al.* (1997); 2, Ignico and Mahon (1965); 3, Obert *et al.* (1996); 4, Baquest *et al.* (2003); 5, Mahon and Vaccuro (1994); 6, Obert *et al.* (2003); 7, Mandigout *et al.* (2001); 8, Tolfrey *et al.* (1998).

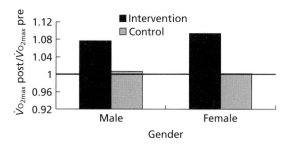

Fig. 7.3 Comparison of pre- to post-test changes in $\dot{V}o_{2max}$ as observed in training and control groups by gender in selected studies of trainability in youth. Mean change in $\dot{V}o_{2max}$ for the intervention group in males and females were 9.5% and 10.5%, respectively. Data are presented for studies in which amount of change was provided in the text of the manuscript or calculable based on information presented in the manuscript.

Gender and developmental age

Over the past 15 years there has been a fivefold increase in the number of training studies that included female participants and presented their data analyzed separately. In the 1996 chapter in the encyclopedia, only two studies that met the strict inclusion criteria reported data separately for female participants (Eisenman & Golding 1975; Stransky *et al.* 1979). In both cases the subjects were adolescents in the 15–16 year age range, and in both studies $\dot{V}o_{2max}$ was observed to increase by 15–16% in the training group. Although a very limited number of studies were available, adolescent girls appeared to be at least as adaptive to endurance training as boys. Based on Fig. 7.3, it is evident that this conclusion remains confirmed. Eleven studies reviewed for this current chapter analyzed data from female subjects separately. The age range of female participants was 4–17 years, with 10–11 years as the predominate age. Improvement at post-training ranged from 0 (–0.02%) to 29.0% (mean = 11.5 ± 8.2%).

Developmental age has often been hypothesized as a factor that could affect endurance exercise trainability. Child development is typically divided into three periods: (i) prepubescence; (ii) pubescence (circumpubertal stage); and (iii) post-pubescence (adolescence). The period of most rapid linear growth (peak height velocity) is considered the best marker of pubescence, with prepubescence and post-pubescence falling before and after this period. Unfortunately, no exercise training studies have been designed to examine comprehensively the trainability in children and youth in the three developmental stages. Also, most of the relevant studies have used chronologic age, not developmental status, as the basis for categorizing the subjects. The available data from these studies do not indicate periods of enhanced aerobic trainability during childhood and/or youth (Figs 7.1 & 7.2). (For more details about the relevance of developmental age to fitness see Chapters 1 and 4.)

Conclusions

The overall conclusion of this chapter is that children and youth are physiologically adaptive to endurance exercise training. Specifically, it appears that both male and female, prepubescent and post-pubescent youth are trainable and that increases in $\dot{V}o_{2max}$ (with training) of approximately 5–10% are typical.

Children and youth are often exposed to endurance exercise training for the purpose of promoting their health and fitness. This can occur in the context of school-based physical education classes or in other settings. The conclusion that children and youth are trainable indicates that, if the exercise program meets the criteria for intensity, frequency, and duration as applied in the available studies, improvements in physiologic function and performance should be attained. However, a word of caution should be added. In settings such as physical education classes, a goal is to promote long-term development of an active lifestyle while providing for short-term enhancement of physical fitness. Dealing effectively with both of these goals is a challenge because, with some children and youth, it is difficult to provide the relatively heavy dose of exercise needed to generate a training effect in a manner that is enjoyable and psychologically reinforcing.

An increasing number of children and youth participate in endurance sport competitions. The conclusion of this review, when applied to the youth sport setting, is that young athletes are trainable and should manifest improved performance with regular participation in endurance exercise. These improvements would be above and beyond those that are expected to occur with normal growth and development. Unfortunately, few of the controlled exercise training studies in children and youth have used pure performance measures (e.g., run, swim, or cycling time) as outcome variables. Consequently, based on the available studies, it is not possible to characterize the expected levels of improvement in endurance performance that should be expected with endurance training.

Challenges for future research

Many pertinent issues require further investigation.
1 Scientists should replicate the studies that have examined, in a precise and well-controlled manner, the effects of endurance training on $\dot{V}o_{2max}$ in pre-pubescent, pubescent, and post-pubescent boys and girls (preferably using longitudinal design). Such studies would provide an enhanced understanding of the effects of developmental status and gender on endurance trainability.
2 Future studies should include measures of lactate (or ventilatory) threshold and economy and pure performance measures such as distance run times. Including these measures would improve the understanding of relationships between endurance training, $\dot{V}o_{2max}$, and performance outcomes in children and youth.

3 More work is necessary regarding the underlying mechanisms of aerobic trainability in children and youth. Knowledge of these constructs (e.g., cellular activity) would also assist in understanding the effects of growth and maturation.
4 Scientists should conduct precise and well-controlled studies of exercise dose. This type of research would provide indications of potential threshold or dosage effects for a desired training response and will make comparison among studies more feasible. Such studies would also indicate the effects of subtle differences in frequency, intensity, duration, and mode.
5 It is likely that physically active or athletic children and adolescents have been participants in most studies thus far, which may be a limitation in our knowledge base (e.g., overweight or unfit children or adolescents may respond differently to endurance training than those of normal weight or fitness). Future studies should involve representative samples whenever possible in order to broaden generalizability.

Acknowledgments

The authors thank Jenny Thompson for word processing assistance, Rachel Tabak for assisting in the preparation of the figures, and Gaye Groover Christmus for editing the manuscript.

References

Baquet, G., Berthoin, S., Dupont, G., Blondel, N., Fabre, C. & van Praagh E. (2002) Effects of high intensity intermittent training on peak $\dot{V}o_{2max}$ in prepubertal children. *International Journal of Sports Medicine* **23**, 439–444.

Baquet, G., van Praag, E. & Berthoin, S. (2003) Endurance training and aerobic fitness in young people. *Sports Medicine* **33**, 1127–1143.

Bar-Or, O. & Rowland, T.W. (2004) *Pediatric Exercise Medicine: From Physiologic Principles to Health Care Applications.* Human Kinetics, Champaign, IL.

Bassett, D.R. Jr. & Howley, E.T. (2000) Limiting factors for maximum oxygen uptake and determinants of endurance performance. *Medicine and Science in Sports and Exercise* **32**, 70–84.

Becker, D.M. & Vaccaro, P. (1983) Anaerobic threshold alterations caused by endurance training in young children. *Journal of Sports Medicine and Physical Fitness* **23**, 445–449.

Centers for Disease Control and Prevention (2004a) Behavioral Risk Factor Surveillance System. Physical Activity, 2003. http://apps.nccd.cdc.gov/brfss/page.asp?yr=2003&state=All&cat=PA#P A [Announcement posted on the World Wide Web].

Centers for Disease Control and Prevention (2004b) Youth Risk Behavior

Surveillance: United States, 2003. *Morbidity and Mortality Weekly Report* **53**, 1–96.

Centers for Disease Control and Prevention (2005) Trends in leisure-time physical inactivity by age, sex, and race/ethnicity: United States, 1994–2004. *Morbidity and Mortality Weekly Report* **54**, 991–994.

Chatrath, R., Shenoy, R., Serratto, M. & Thoele, D.G. (2002) Physical fitness of urban American children. *Pediatric Cardiology* **23**, 608–612.

Corbin, C.B. & Pangrazi, R.P. (1992) Are American children and youth fit? *Research Quarterly for Exercise and Sport* **63**, 96–106.

Danis, A., Kryiazisy, Y. & Klissouras, V. (2003) The effect of training in male prepubertal and pubertal monozygotic twins. *European Journal of Applied Physiology* **89**, 309–318.

Eisenman, P.A. & Golding, L.A. (1975) Comparison of effects of training on $\dot{V}o_{2max}$ in girls and young women. *Medicine and Science in Sports and Exercise* **7**, 136–138.

Ekblom, B. (1969) Effect of physical training in adolescent boys. *Journal of Applied Physiology* **27**, 350–355.

Eliakim, A., Barstow, T.J., Brasel, J.A., *et al.* (1996) Effect of exercise training on energy expenditure, muscle volume, and maximal oxygen uptake in female adolescents. *Journal of Pediatrics* **129**, 537–543.

Eriksson, B.O. (1972) Physical training, oxygen supply and muscle metabolism in 11–13-year-old boys. *Acta Physiologica Scandanavia Supplement* 1–48.

Eriksson, B.O. & Koch, G.G. (1973) Effect of physical training on hemodynamic response during submaximal and maximal exercise in 11–13-year-old boys. *Acta Physiologica Scandanavia* **87**, 27–39.

Helgerud, J., Engen, L.C., Wisloff, U. & Hoff, J. (2001) Aerobic endurance training improves soccer performance. *Medicine and Science in Sports and Exercise* **33**, 1925–1931.

Holloszy, J.O. & Coyle, E.F. (1984) Adaptations of skeletal muscle to endurance exercise and their metabolic consequences. *Journal of Applied Physiology* **56**, 831–838.

Ignicio, A.A. & Mahon, A.D. (1995) The effects of a physical fitness program on low-fit children. *Research Quarterly for Exercise and Sport* **66**, 85–90.

Institute of Medicine (2005) *Preventing Childhood Obesity: Health in the Balance.* National Academies Press, Washington, DC.

Lindstrom, M., Isacsson, S.O. & Merlo, J. (2003) Increasing prevalence of overweight, obesity and physical inactivity: Two population-based studies, 1986 and 1994. *European Journal of Public Health* **13**, 306–312.

Lussier, L. & Buskirk, E.R. (1977) Effects of an endurance training regimen on assessment of work capacity in prepubertal children. *Annals of New York Academy of Science* **301**, 734–747.

Mahon, A.D. & Vaccaro, P. (1989) Ventilatory threshold and $\dot{V}o_{2max}$ changes in children following endurance training. *Medicine and*

Science in Sports and Exercise **21**, 425–431.

Mahon, A.D. & Vaccaro, P. (1994) Cardiovascular adaptations in 8- to 12-year-old boys following a 14-week running program. *Canadian Journal of Applied Physiology* **19**, 139–150.

Malina, R.M., Bouchard, C. & Bar-Or, O. (2004) *Growth, Maturation and Physical Activity*, 2nd edn. Human Kinetics, Champaign, IL.

Mandigout, S., Lecoq, A.M., Courteix, D., Guenon, P. & Obert, P. (2001) Effect of gender in response to an aerobic training programme in prepubertal children. *Acta Paediatrica* **90**, 9–15.

Massicotte, D.R. & MacNab, R.B. (1979) Cardio-respiratory adaptation to training at specified intensities in children. *Medicine and Science in Sports and Exercise* **6**, 242–246.

Maughan, R., Gleeson, M. & Greenhaf, P.L. (1997) *Biochemistry of Exercise and Training*. Oxford University Press, Oxford.

McManus, A.M., Armstrong, N. & Williams, C.A. (1997) Effect of training on the aerobic power and anaerobic performance of prepubertal girls. *Acta Paediatrica* **86**, 456–459.

Mitchell, B.M., Gutin, B., Kapuku, G., *et al.* (2002) Left ventricular structure and function in obese adolescents: relations to cardiovascular fitness, percent body fat, and visceral adiposity, and effects of physical training. *Pediatrics* **109**, E73.

Morrow, J.R. & Freedson, P.S. (1994) Relationship between habitual physical activity and aerobic fitness in adolescents. *Pediatric Exercise Science* **6**, 315–329.

Obert, P., Courteix, D., Lecoq, A.M. & Guenon, P. (1996) Effect of long-term intense swimming training on the upper body peak oxygen uptake of prepubertal girls. *European Journal of Applied Physiology and Occupational Physiology* **73**, 136–143.

Obert, P., Mandigouts, S., Nottin, S., Vinet, A., N'Guyen, L.D. & Lecoq, A.M. (2003) Cardiovascular responses to endurance training in children: Effect of gender. *European Journal of Clinical Investigation* **33**, 199–208.

Pate, R.R. & Branch, J.D. (1992) Training for endurance sport. *Medicine and Science in Sports and Exercise* **24**, S340–S343.

Pate, R.R. & Ward, D.S. (1990) Endurance exercise trainability in children and youth. In: *Advances in Sports Medicine and Fitness* (Grana, W.A., *et al.*, eds.) Year Book Medical, Chicago: 37–55.

Pate, R.R. & Ward, D.S. (1995) Endurance trainability in children and youth. In: *The Child and Adolescent Athlete* (Bar-Or, O., ed.) Blackwell Publishing, Oxford: 130–137.

Pate, R.R., Wang, C.Y., Dowda, M., Farrell, S.W. & O'Neill, J.R. (2006) Cardiorespiratory fitness levels among US youth 12 to 19 years of age: findings from the 1999–2002 National Health and Nutrition Examination Survey. *Archives of Pediatric and Adolescent Medicine* **160**, 1005–1012.

Payne, V.G. & Morrow, J.R. (1993) Exercise and $\dot{V}o_{2max}$ in children: a meta-analysis. *Research Quarterly for Exercise and Sport* **64**, 305–313.

Rotstein, A., Dotan, R., Bar-Or, O. & Tenenbaum, G. (1986) Effect of training on anaerobic threshold, maximal aerobic power and anaerobic performance of preadolescent boys. *International Journal of Sports Medicine* **7**, 281–286.

Rowland, T.W. (2005) *Children's Exercise Physiology*, 2nd edn. Human Kinetics, Champaign, IL.

Rowland, T.W. & Boyajian, A. (1995) Aerobic response to endurance exercise training in children. *Pediatrics* **96**, 654–658.

Rowland, T.W., Martel, L., Vanderburgh, P., Manos, T. & Charkoudian, N. (1996) The influence of short-term aerobic training on blood lipids in healthy 10–12 year old children. *International Journal of Sports Medicine* **17**, 487–492.

Savage, M.P., Petratis, M.M., Thomson, W.H., Berg, K., Smith, J.L. & Sady, S.P. (1986) Exercise training effects on serum lipids of prepubescent boys and adult men. *Medicine and Science in Sports and Exercise* **18**, 197–204.

Schwartz, L., Britten, R.H. & Thompson, L.R. (1928) The effect of exercise on the physical condition and development of adolescent boys. *Public Health Bulletin* **179**, 1–124.

Sjodin, B. & Svedenhag, J. (1985) Applied physiology of marathon running. *Sports Medicine* **2**, 83–99.

Steinberger, J. & Daniels, S.R. (2003) Obesity, insulin resistance, diabetes, and cardiovascular risk in children: an American Heart Association scientific statement from the Atherosclerosis, Hypertension, and Obesity in the Young Committee (Council on Cardiovascular Disease in the Young) and the Diabetes Committee (Council on Nutrition,

Physical Activity, and Metabolism). *Circulation* **107**, 1448–1453.

Stransky, A.W., Mickelson, R.J., van Fleet, C. & Davis, R. (1979) Effects of a swimming training regimen on hematological, cardiorespiratory and body composition changes in young females. *Journal of Sports Medicine and Physical Fitness* **19**, 347–354.

Telama, R., Yang, X., Viikari, J., Valimaki, I., Wanne, O. & Raitakari, O. (2005) Physical activity from childhood to adulthood: A 21-year tracking study. *American Journal of Preventive Medicine* **28**, 267–273.

Tolfrey, K., Campbell, I.G. & Batterham, A.M. (1998) Aerobic trainability of prepubertal boys and girls. *Pediatric Exercise Science* **10**, 248–263.

Vaccaro, P. & Mahon, A. (1987) Cardiorespiratory responses to endurance training in children. *Sports Medicine* **4**, 352–363.

Weber, G., Kartodihardjo, W. & Klissouras, V. (1976) Growth and physical training with reference to heredity. *Journal of Applied Physiology* **40**, 211–215.

Wedderkopp, N., Froberg, K., Hansen, H.S. & Andersen, L.B. (2004) Secular trends in physical fitness and obesity in Danish 9-year-old girls and boys: Odense School Child Study and Danish substudy of the European Youth Heart Study. *Scandanavian Journal of Medicine and Science in Sports* **14**, 150–155.

Wedderkopp, N., Froberg, K., Hansen, H.S., Riddoch, C. & Andersen, L.B. (2003) Cardiovascular risk factors cluster in children and adolescents with low physical fitness: The European Youth Heart Study (EYHS). *Pediatric Exercise Science* **15**, 419–427.

Welsman, J.R., Armstrong, N. & Withers, S. (1997) Responses of young girls to two modes of aerobic training. *British Journal of Sports Medicine* **31**, 139–142.

Weston, A.R., Karamizrak, O., Smith, A., Noakes, T.D. & Myburgh, K.H. (1999) African runners exhibit greater fatigue resistance, lower lactate accumulation, and higher oxidative enzyme activity. *Journal of Applied Physiology* **86**, 915–923.

Williams, C.A., Armstrong, N. & Powell, J. (2000) Aerobic responses of prepubertal boys to two modes of training. *British Journal of Sports Medicine* **34**, 168–173.

Williford H.N., Blessing, D.L., Duey, W.J., et al. (1996) Exercise training in black adolescents: changes in blood lipids and $\dot{V}O_{2max}$. *Ethnicity and Disease* **6**, 279–285.

World Health Organization (2005) *Preventing Chronic Diseases: A Vital Investment:* WHO global report. WHO, Geneva.

Yoshida, T., Ishiko, I. & Muraoka, I. (1980) Effect of endurance training on cardiorespiratory function of 5 year old children. *International Journal of Sports Medicine* **1**, 91–94.

Yoshisawa, S., Honda, H., Nakamura, N., Itoh, K. & Watanabe, N. (1997) Effects of an 18-month endurance run training program on maximal aerobic power in 4–6-year-old girls. *Pediatric Exercise Science* **9**, 33–43.

Chapter 8

Skill Acquisition in Childhood and Adolescence

ROBERT M. MALINA

Systematic instruction, practice, and training are basic to youth sport programs and to athlete development. Such programs are important for several essential components of athletic performance—general motor skills, sport-specific skills, muscular strength, cardiovascular and muscular endurance, and anaerobic capacity. Specific instruction, practice, and training for young sport participants are often discussed in the context of trainability and two related concepts—readiness and critical periods. This chapter initially discusses the concepts of trainability, readiness, and critical periods, and then the perspectives of dynamical systems and cognitive psychology in the context of skill acquisition. It briefly reviews the development of movement patterns and trends in motor performance, and then addresses skill acquisition.

Basic concepts

Trainability

Trainability refers to the responsiveness of an individual to a specific instructional, practice, and/or training stimulus. Two related but somewhat different issues are relevant:

1 What are the responses of children and adolescents to such programs?
2 How responsive are children and adolescents to specific programs?

The responsiveness of children and adolescents to such programs probably varies at different stages of growth and maturation and behavioral develop-

ment, and with different instructional and practice environments.

The issue of trainability in the context of sport has been discussed primarily for muscular strength and aerobic power, and to a lesser extent anaerobic power (Malina *et al.* 2004a). The approach is experimental (e.g., the response of youth to progressive resistance exercises at set loads two or three times per week for several weeks, or training at 80% $\dot{V}o_{2max}$ for 30–45 min, three or more times per week for several weeks) (Malina & Eisenmann 2003; Strong *et al.* 2005). The issue of trainability also applies to the development of proficiency in general and sport-specific motor skills (e.g., responses of youth to instruction and practice protocols). The issue of age- and/or sex-associated variation in the responsiveness of youth to such protocols needs consideration. Because the development of proficiency in skills depends to a large extent on feedback from teachers and coaches (e.g., corrective statements or demonstrations by instructors, knowledge of results), the effectiveness of different instructional and practice strategies needs evaluation. These issues have received relatively little emphasis in the context of youth sport.

Readiness

The concept of trainability is related to the concepts of readiness and critical periods. Readiness relates to the ability of the individual to handle successfully the demands of a structured learning situation (e.g., specific instruction and practice of sport skills). Discussions of readiness have been generally set in the context of school and some visual and performance arts. The concept is implicit in youth sport, specifically the readiness of a child to handle the demands of a competitive sport and in some cases selection for training in a sport at a relatively early age.

Broadly speaking, readiness can be viewed as including two components: the characteristics of the child and the demands of the instructional or practice setting. Readiness is the match between characteristics and demands. Characteristics of the child include his or her growth (size attained, physique, body composition), maturation (timing and tempo of progress towards the biologically mature state), and developmental features (cognitive, social, emotional, motor behaviors) at a given point in time. Growth, maturation, and development occur simultaneously and interact, and show considerable interindividual variability (Malina *et al.* 2004a). Demands of instructional and practice situations depend on many factors (e.g., the skill per se, the style and quality of teaching or coaching, individual or group activity, and general conditions).

Critical periods

The concept of critical periods implies the presence of specific times during which a youngster may be maximally sensitive to environmental influences, both positive and negative, during growth and maturation and the development of behaviors and skills. It assumes that changes underlying growth, maturation, and development occur rapidly during a specific time period and that organizational processes can be modified most easily at this time (Scott 1986; Bornstein 1989). Critical periods, if they can be established with certainty, may thus represent times of maximal readiness. Evidence dealing with the application of critical periods to the development of motor and sport-specific skills is limited and not convincing (Anderson 2002; Haubenstricker & Seefeldt 2002).

Nevertheless, the concept of critical periods appears to be implicit in sport talent identification and development programs (Bompa 1985, 1995; Petiot *et al.* 1987; Hartley 1988). Such programs include an initial phase beginning at about 6–7

years of age, especially in early entry sport—artistic gymnastics, figure skating, and diving. Focus at this time is on general skill development, especially overall dexterity and coordination. There is a balance between general and sport-specific skills with age during childhood, and focus on sport-specific skill development (i.e., specialization) emerges during the transition into adolescence. Procedures and timing of screening for other sports vary, but the underlying principles are similar. Early selection criteria focus on motor performance, in addition to body size and physique. Primary selection for sport in Romania, for example, occurred at 3–8 years for gymnastics, figure skating, and swimming, and at 10–15 years in girls and 10–17 years in boys for other sports (Bompa 1985). Selection of potential rowers, basketball players, and weight lifters in the former USSR and East Germany was not carried out until after puberty (Hartley 1988).

Movement patterns and skills

The development of proficiency in movement behaviors is a major developmental task of childhood. Discussion of skill acquisition and trainability requires an understanding of motor development and corresponding age- and sex-associated variation in outcomes of developmental processes. For the sake of convenience, movement activities can be viewed as patterns and skills. Pattern refers to the basic elements of specific movement behaviors (e.g., walking, running, jumping, throwing patterns). It is a global concept capturing general features of the movement. Skill refers to the accuracy, economy, and efficiency of movements and combinations of movements as in sports skills. All children eventually learn to run, jump, throw, skip, hop, and so on; however, all do not perform these movements with the same degree of skill. As might be expected, definitions of patterns and skill vary. Fundamental movement patterns are occasionally described as basic movement skills (Seefeldt & Haubenstricker 1982). The term skill may have a different meaning applied to specific demands of a sport, for example, ". . . skill refers to a player's ability to select, organize, and execute an action, appropriate to a given situation in an effective, consistent and efficient manner" (Williams *et al.* 2003, p. 198). In this context, skill is different from technique, which is more akin to a movement pattern.

Dynamical systems perspective

The framework that currently holds a dominant position in studies of motor development, and to some extent motor learning, is dynamical systems (Thelen & Smith 1994; Lewis 2000). This approach emphasizes the ongoing interactions between the child, the environment, and the motor task. Dynamical systems are complex and interconnected, have many different components, and are characterized by self-organization. Dynamical systems, as the name implies, continuously change; they operate in different timescales and levels such that there is variation in temporal–spatial patterns. Behavior emerges from self-organization in the context of constraints associated with the child, environment, and movement task, so that it is difficult to describe emerging behaviors in advance.

Motor development and skill acquisition are thus viewed as emerging from interactions between:

1 *The child* Performer: size, proportions, body composition, biologic maturation, cognitive abilities, behaviors, etc.;

2 *The environment* Rearing atmosphere, opportunities, stimulation, object size in manipulative tasks, instruction and practice, quality of adult instruction and supervision, rules, etc.; and

3 *The specific movement task.*

The child, environment, and task are labeled constraints. Changes in the constraints per se and their interactions function to guide the individual or channel the motor system in the development and refinement movement skills (Newell 1986). From the perspective of understanding dynamic systems, how can variance in skill acquisition be partitioned among the performer, environments and task, and interactions? To what extent does the structure of variance change as skills become finely tuned or approach expert levels?

Specific applications of dynamical systems concepts to the development of movement patterns of young children are somewhat limited. In an interesting example, six 3- and two 7-month-old infants were "trained" daily to step on a slowly moving treadmill. The "training" resulted in improved stepping, and infants whose stepping behavior was unstable at the start seemed to benefit more from the practice on the treadmill. The results of this experiment suggest that the developing motor system can be influenced by "training" and that infants have their own preferred stepping patterns which interacted with the "training" on the treadmill (Vereijken & Thelen 1997). The results were interpreted as indicating that the neuromuscular pathway for stepping is in place in infancy and that stepping emerges in the context of practice on the treadmill. (For a more detailed discussion of treadmill stepping in the context of treadmill speed and coordination between the legs during the first year of life see Thelen & Ulrich 1991.) The dynamical systems approach to the transition from independent walking to running has been applied to four children observed at about 6, 8, and 10 months after the onset of independent walking and then at 3 years of age (Whitall & Getschell 1995; see also Whitall & Clarke 1994). Changes in control parameters or constraints were described (stride characteristics: length, time, velocity, center of mass, intralimb coupling, and knee and ankle actions). With the exception of intralimb coupling, all parameters showed continuous change. Although interesting, the results are limited to small samples, are largely descriptive and basically qualitative, and indicate a need to include other potential control parameters associated with the child and the environment.

Specific instruction and practice represent a manipulation of environmental constraints in an effort to channel a motor behavior into a finely tuned, controlled system (i.e., skill). Motor development and skill acquisition are thus the outcome of the interaction of the growing and maturing child, demands of specific motor tasks, and the environment. Child–environment interactions are most often viewed in the context of changing body dimensions and proportions (body scaling) and improving levels of motor competence (action scaling). Body size, proportions, and composition change as the child grows, and levels of motor proficiency change as the child develops. These influence the nature of the interactions between the child and his or her environments. Children are themselves dynamic beings, who, as they learn to behave within their respective cultures, become capable of making decisions on how they interact with the environment even when presented with specific environmental opportunities or stimulation. The child's perceptions of the environment in the context of his or her abilities are related but important factors affecting motor development that are not ordinarily considered.

Cognitive psychology perspective

In contrast to dynamical systems, most of the literature on motor skill acquisition is derived from cognitive psychology. The literature is to a large extent laboratory based and experimental, and is limited to non-sport skills (e.g., tracking and aiming tasks, joy stick manipulation and lever displacement, juggling, ball tossing, stabilometer, and assorted manipulative tasks). Focus of studies is on different aspects of the learning process; for example, motivation, instruction, and practice protocols (distribution of sessions, whole versus part instruction), speed–accuracy trade-off, mental practice, imagery, intertask transfer, bilateral transfer, information processing, feedback and knowledge of results, associated cognitive skills (e.g., perception, attention, memory) (Singer *et al.* 2001; Magill 2004). Moreover, the vast majority of the research is conducted on adults, especially college age students. Detailed consideration of specific issues related to skill acquisition is beyond the scope of this chapter (Magill 2004).

Development of basic movement patterns

During the preschool years and extending into middle childhood, children develop competence in a variety of basic or fundamental movements. These are the foundation upon which other movement patterns, skills, and sport-specific skills are built. The temporal, spatial, and sequential elements of several basic movement patterns as they develop during childhood have been described. The specific elements for each fundamental movement have

been summarized in a sequence of stages or steps from an immature to a mature pattern. The definition and delineation of stages are to some extent arbitrary as they are superimposed on an ongoing process of development, which is not necessarily continuous. There is considerable inter- and intraindividual variability. Some children may show relatively long periods of stability or minimal change followed by a burst of progress; others may regress to less mature stages before progressing to a more advanced stage; and still others may show seemingly continuous progress.

Although stages are somewhat arbitrary and have limitations, they have facilitated the observation and understanding of the motor development of young children and have provided insights into the understanding of movement patterns. The development of nine fundamental movement patterns has been described for children in the mixed-longitudinal Motor Performance Study at Michigan State University (Roberton 1982, 1984; Seefeldt & Haubenstricker 1982; Wickstrom 1983; Haubenstricker *et al.* 1999; Payne & Isaacs 1999; Haywood & Getchell 2001). Ages at which 60% of children met the criteria for specific developmental stages for each of the nine fundamental motor patterns in the Motor Performance Study are shown in Table 8.1. Development apparently progresses rapidly during early childhood and continues well into middle childhood for some movement patterns. Boys tend to attain each stage of overhand throwing and kicking earlier than girls, whereas girls tend to attain each stage of hopping and skipping earlier than boys, which may be related to perceptions of the cultural appropriateness of activities that involve these movement patterns. The attainment of early stages, especially stages 2 and 3, of the other fundamental skills (running, jumping, catching, and striking) shows considerable similarity between boys and girls, but there is more variation between boys and girls in ages at which the final or mature stages are attained. For example, girls attain the final two stages of catching earlier than boys, although they do not differ in ages at attaining the earlier stages. In contrast, the difference between boys and girls for attaining the mature form of the standing long jump is small.

Table 8.1 Estimated ages (months) at which 60% of children attained defined stages performed for several fundamental motor skills in the Motor Performance Study at Michigan State University. The number of stages from immature (Stage 1) to mature varies for each skill. The last stage indicated is the mature stages; other stages indicate intermediate levels. The data were provided by courtesy of Dr. Vern Seefeldt, Michigan State University (see also Seefeldt & Haubenstricker 1982).

| Fundamental skill | Stages | | | | | | | | | |
| | 1 | | 2 | | 3 | | 4 | | 5 | |
	Boys	Girls	Boys	Girls	Boys	Girls	Boys	Girls	Boys	Girls
Run	23	20	27	25	40	40	51	62	–	–
Standing long jump	23	24	47	48	76	76	117	120	–	–
Overhand throw	10	10	40	44	45	56	50	73	63	102
Hop	34	28	46	41	64	58	90	86	–	–
Skip	59	56	65	63	78	70	–	–	–	–
Catch	24	23	41	40	51	50	73	61	80	77
Strike	24	23	32	34	44	46	88	101	–	–
Kick	22	20	40	47	56	73	90	99	–	–

Variation in the intervals between ages at the attainment of specific stages for the fundamental movement patterns should be noted. For example, the intervals between each of the four stages of jumping are quite large, whereas the interval between stages 3 and 4 for striking appears to be quite large compared with those between stages 1 and 2, and 2 and 3 (Table 8.1). Variation in intervals between stages is both real (i.e., inter- and intraindividual variation in the timing of mastery of each stage of a specific movement pattern) and methodologic (i.e., the time between observations in a longitudinal series), or the defined changes from one stage to the next may be too great or the stage demands may be too difficult. The stages of movement pattern development during childhood need to be addressed in the context of several questions (Malina *et al.* 2004a), but one is of particular relevance to the current discussion. What is the influence of specific instruction and practice, adult modeling, and/or entry into a sport on progress through specific movement patterns and their integration into more complex movement sequences?

Mature patterns of most fundamental movements are ordinarily attained by 6–7 years in 60% of the children in the Motor Performance Study (Table 8.1), although some are not attained until later (e.g., standing long jump in both sexes, overhand throw in girls). However, 40% of the children have not attained the specific developmental levels by these ages. In other words, many 6- to 9-year-old boys and girls have not developed sufficient motor control to successfully accomplish the mature patterns of fundamental movements.

Motor performance

The development of proficiency in basic movement patterns is accompanied by improved levels of performance which are routinely quantified in tasks performed under standardized conditions; for example, the distance or height jumped, the distance a ball is thrown, the time elapsed in completing a 30-m dash (speed) or a shuttle run (speed and agility), or sport-specific skills; for example, time elapsed while dribbling a soccer ball, accuracy of baseball pitches, football (American) passes or soccer passes. In sports where the body is projected, as in gymnastics and diving, outcome measures are ratings of judges and as such have a degree of subjectivity.

Performances on some standardized tests are often introduced as early as 3–4 years of age although many children may not have sufficiently mature movement patterns to perform the task as described in the test protocols. Allowing for these caveats, performances of children aged 3–6 years on standardized tests of motor proficiency tend to improve, on average, more or less linearly with age during early childhood and there is considerable overlap between boys and girls. Performances continue to improve with age through childhood. Although, on average, boys tend to perform better than girls, there is considerable overlap between the sexes. The improvement with age during middle childhood is largely the result of growth (e.g., changes in size, proportions, body composition) and general use and activity (experience). With the onset of adolescence, the performances of boys improve considerably, while those of girls improve to about 13–14 years of age and then level off or improve only slightly. Performances during adolescence are influenced by individual differences in the timing of the adolescent growth spurt in height and other body dimensions and growth spurts in motor abilities (Malina *et al.* 2004a). Although data that span adolescence are limited to boys, performance in the vertical jump (power) shows peak gains, on average, after peak height velocity (PHV), while performance on a shuttle run (speed and agility) and plate tapping (speed of arm movement) show peak gains before PHV (Beunen *et al.* 1988). Observations from a short-term mixed-longitudinal study suggest similar trends in peak gains for the standing long jump and medicine ball throw (power) and the shuttle run in boys and the standing long jump in girls. However, other observations in this short-term study are not consistent (e.g., a peak gain after PHV for the shuttle run and no peak in the medicine ball throw in girls) and no clear pattern for a 40-m dash during the interval of PHV (Heras Yague & de la Fuente 1998).

Trainability of motor skills

Improvement of motor skills in general and sport-specific skills is often a primary objective of youth sports programs ranging from those at the community level to more advanced sports schools and academies that ordinarily focus on a single sport. Improvement in sport skills is also a major motivation of children and adolescents for participation in sport. Given the importance placed upon skill acquisition, improvement, and refinement in youth sports programs, it is somewhat surprising that the

literature in the area that deals with children and adolescents is not more extensive.

Early skill acquisition

Most neural structures are near adult form and most fundamental movement patterns are reasonably well established by 6–8 years of age (Malina *et al.* 2004a). It might be expected therefore that these ages would be ideal for specific instruction and practice in the basic motor skills. Children refine established motor patterns and learn new motor skills and sequences of skills as they grow and mature with the experience and practice associated with everyday activities. Specific instruction and practice experiences such as those associated with developmental programs (e.g., preschool gymnastics) and with some youth sports are additional factors in the development and refinement of movement patterns and skills.

Although the vertical jump is a basic movement pattern common to many sports, development of the standing long jump has received more attention (Wickstrom 1983). Children 2–3 years of age will attempt a vertical jump, but with little success. However, if provided with an overhead target, the children will perform a vertical jump, albeit with considerable inter- and intraindividual variability in jumping patterns (Poe 1976). With age and practice during early childhood, the vertical jumping pattern improves as reflected in a deeper preparatory crouch, a more forceful arm lift or thrust (upward instead of out to the sides), and more extension at take-off and when in flight (Poe 1976; Wickstrom 1983).

Evidence indicates that planned instructional programs can enhance the development of basic movement patterns in children 4–5 years of age and more complex skills in older children. Guided instruction by specialists, trained parents, or qualified coaches, appropriate motor task sequences, and adequate time for practice are essential components of successful instructional programs at young ages (Haubenstricker & Seefeldt 1986).

Overhand throwing is a skill that has historically received considerable attention in the context of instruction and practice at young ages. Specific practice of the throw for distance resulted in little improvement in children aged less than 5 years and significant improvement in children 5–7 years of age (Dusenberry 1952). A combination of instruction and guided practice contributed to improvements in throwing distance and velocity of kindergarten children (Hanson 1961), whereas other observations with kindergarten children indicated no effect of practice on throwing velocity (Halverson et al. 1977).

Generally, similar results have been reported for the standing long jump with specific practice programs in young children (Sparks 1950; Dusenberry 1952). A guided instruction program resulted in improvements in the movement patterns for the standing long jump, soccer kick (volley), and ball bounce in preschool children (Werner 1974). Other data suggest similar improvements in motor proficiency of preschool children with guided instruction provided by motor development specialists or trained parents (Miller 1978).

The studies summarized in the preceding discussion were conducted prior to the emergence of the dynamical systems perspective. More recent studies have applied dynamical systems concepts to the development of the overhand throwing pattern, highlighting variation in constraints. For example, a basic motor skill intervention program with preschool children 4.5 years of age resulted in improvements in specific components (e.g., trunk rotation, elbow-humeral flexion, stride) of the throwing pattern (Goodway et al. 2005). Of interest, boys attained a more advanced throwing profile than girls, suggesting perhaps sex differences in response to the motor intervention program. Features of the overhand throwing pattern (e.g., linear and angular velocities of the trunk, trunk tilt, and stride characteristics) and ball velocity varied by developmental level and were identified as "important kinematic constraints" (Stodden et al. 2005). The results and technology of these more recent studies complement the earlier studies in showing that systematic instruction and practice favorably influenced components of the overhand throwing pattern in kindergarten children (Hansen 1961; Halverson & Roberton 1979). Advances in technology permit better definition of

"constraints" which are modified by the instruction and practice.

Overall, evidence indicates a beneficial role for instruction and practice on skill acquisition in early childhood and during the transition into middle childhood (about 3–7 years). More data are necessary in this area, and other variables need consideration, especially those related to environmental constraints. For example, the role of parental, sibling, or peer modeling in the development of motor proficiency merits consideration given the amount of time that these individuals spend with each other in a variety of settings and activities.

Motor skill acquisition during childhood and adolescence

There is relatively little systematic information on the role of specific instruction and practice in sport skills at these ages. The responsiveness of children and adolescents to instruction and practice associated with school physical education programs provides some general insights. Improvements in a variety of motor abilities are generally associated with physical education programs, although there is variation among studies (Vogel 1986). Motor abilities evaluated included agility (shuttle run, obstacle course), power (standing long and vertical jumps), speed (dashes), balance (stabilometer, stork stand), and a variety of manipulative skills (ball throw, ball handling, basketball foul shooting, volleyball wall volley and serve).

Studies of strength/resistance training occasionally include motor performance items. For example, three groups of girls aged 7–19 years trained (three times per week for 5 weeks) in isometric knee extension, vertical jumping, or sprint running (Nielsen et al. 1980). Responses were specific to the type of training, particularly for isometric knee extension and vertical jumping, whereas responses to the sprint running protocol were small. However, girls who trained in isometric knee extension made significant gains in vertical jumping and run acceleration, while those who trained in vertical jumping made significant gains in knee extension strength and run acceleration. Gains in run acceleration associated with run training, on the other hand, were negligible; corresponding gains in knee strength and the vertical jump associated with run training were relatively larger. Although maturity status and size of the girls was not controlled in the analysis, shorter (<155 cm) and younger (<13.5 years) girls made relatively greater domain-specific gains in isometric knee extension strength and the vertical jump, but not in acceleration of sprint running.

These observations have implications for the transfer of gains with one mode of training to other aspects of performance. In boys aged 6–11 years, 14 weeks of resistance training were associated with improvements in the vertical jump (Weltman *et al.* 1986), whereas in boys and girls aged 7–12 years, 8 weeks of strength training were associated with negligible changes in the vertical jump (Faigenbaum *et al.* 1996). The variable results may be related to difficulty in partitioning the effects of a training program from expected changes associated with normal growth. Given the age range of the samples, they also indicate a need to consider age per se and body size, and perhaps other characteristics in analyses of changes in performance associated with training.

With few exceptions, most of the experimental data set within the framework of cognitive psychology relates to relatively simple and discrete movement skills in young adults. Many of the studies focus on speed and accuracy of movements or projected objects under different experimental conditions. Interest in the speed–accuracy trade-off in motor skill acquisition has a long history in psychology (Malina 1972; Magill 2004). Baseball pitching requires the ability to throw the ball with high velocity and accuracy in addition to the ability to modify velocity and maintain accuracy. Similarly, fielders must be able to throw the ball with a high degree of accuracy (to a fielder at a specific base), although the required velocity may vary with position, distance, game situation, and so on. Football (American) quarterbacks routinely throw an oval-shaped ball (with rather sharply pointed ends) with a high degree of accuracy and with variable velocity, depending on distance and game situation, to a moving target (receiver). Soccer requires accurate and forceful passes and shots on goal. Other projection skills such as golf putting place a premium on accuracy.

The influence of different feedback (knowledge of results, KR) conditions on the speed and accuracy of a thrown baseball in 14- to 16-year-old boys is an example of the application of the experimental approach to a sport-related skill in youth (Malina 1969). After an initial test, four randomly assigned groups practiced (20 throws per session, three times per week for 4 weeks) under different feedback conditions: speed only, accuracy only, speed and accuracy, neither. The groups that received speed KR improved in throwing velocity while the groups that did not receive speed KR showed an initial decline in velocity followed by moderately stable albeit reduced levels. The groups that received accuracy KR maintained stable levels of accuracy during the first half of the practice program and increased in accuracy during the second half of the program. The groups that did not receive accuracy KR declined markedly in throwing accuracy during the first three sessions, followed by variable levels, and then a gradual improvement (although not reaching pre-test levels) in accuracy during the final part of the practice program. The final test actually represented a restoration of KR for three of the groups, and each responded to the restored KR with increased performances in the respective variables compared with the last (12th) practice session. Observations on the group that received both speed and accuracy KR suggested that the boys experienced difficulty combining the KR effectively early in the practice protocol when speed improved and accuracy was relatively stable. As practice continued, the boys apparently learned to combine both factors effectively into the throw and showed improvement in accuracy with a moderately stable velocity.

As with any sample of adolescent boys, there was considerable variation in body size and proportions. Unfortunately, these were not considered in the analysis. Spatial ability, based on a paper and pencil test, was significantly related to throwing accuracy in this sample (Kolakowski & Malina 1974). Accuracy was scored in five dimensions (Malina 1968): concentric circle score, horizontal direction (differentiating right from left of the center), horizontal deviation (absolute distance from the center in either direction), vertical direction (differentiating above from below the center), and vertical deviation (absolute distance from the center in either direction). Spatial ability was related to accuracy scored as vertical deviations and concentric circle scores. Controlling for vertical deviation accuracy eliminated the association between spatial ability and concentric circle accuracy; however, the converse was not true. What is the relevance of vertical deviation accuracy and spatial ability? Vertical deviations on an upright target would translate into skill and judgment with respect to distance if the target was laid on the ground (i.e., under- or overshooting the target).

Accuracy and trajectory of passes to ground level targets in soccer (i.e., players some distance away from the passer) present a situation that requires both kicking skill and judgment with respect to distance. The accuracy of a specialized kick under three conditions: full vision, and no vision following ball contact with and without KR, was considered in two experiments, one with skilled soccer players only and the other in which novice, intermediate, and skilled players were compared (P. Ford, N.J. Hodges, A.M. Williams, S.J. Hayes & N. Smeeton, 2005, personal communication). The task required the young adult subjects to kick the ball over a height barrier to a near or far target on the ground. The accuracy of skilled players did not differ under conditions with and without visual information (experiment 1). The accuracy of skilled players measured as radial error relative to the target was better compared with novice and intermediate level players (experiment 2), and withholding of vision of ball flight resulted in a decline in accuracy of the kick. Dependence on vision of ball trajectory was greater in less skilled players. The decline in accuracy when vision of ball trajectory was removed was associated with reduced variation in knee–ankle coordination. Although limited to young adults, the evidence indicates an important role for information of ball trajectory on kicking accuracy among individuals of different skill levels. Ball trajectory information was important for novice and intermediate level, but not for skilled soccer players. It may be inferred from this and other similar studies (e.g., Beilock et al. 2002) that different instructional and practice strategies are needed for individuals at different stages of the learning process for specific skills.

Three stages in acquiring a skill are commonly recognized (Williams et al. 2003, based on Fitts & Posner 1967): cognitive, associative, and autonomous. In the first stage, the basic mechanics of the performance of a skill are learned, and conscious evaluation and information processing are primary. With the establishment of the basic mechanics, issues related to methods of improving performance highlight the associative stage. Variability declines and consistency characterizes performance as the individual progresses through the second stage. In the final stage, the essentials of the skill are in place and performance becomes largely automatic or autonomous; the individual performs the skill either without thinking or with a different manner of thinking compared to the novice (Williams et al. 2003).

General guidelines for instruction in soccer skills in the framework of the three stages of the learning process are summarized in Table 8.2. They highlight the needs of learners at different stages of the sport skill learning process (Williams et al. 2003; see also Williams & Hodges 2005). Individual differences in age, size, maturity status, fitness, skill, and motivation of young athletes (internal constraints) present a challenge in applying the principles to youth players. In adolescent soccer players 13–15 years of age, for example, age, experience, body size, and stage of puberty contribute significantly to indicators of functional capacity (aerobic, power, speed), but relatively little to indicators of soccer-specific skills (Malina et al. 2004b, 2005). The challenge is to incorporate individual differences in internal constraints into the instructional and practice situations (environmental constraints) to facilitate the acquisition and refinement of soccer skills.

Expert performance

The development of expert performance in a variety of domains including sport is currently a major topic in sport psychology. From the perspective of youth, child prodigies are not necessarily successful performers as adults. Conversely, most successful adult performers were not child prodigies; rather, they had sustained instruction beginning at an early age. Detailed study of talented individuals in sport (Olympic swimmers, internationally ranked

Table 8.2 Instructional suggestions for soccer across different stages of skill learning. After Williams *et al.* (2003).

Cognitive
DO
Provide a general idea of the movement by using verbal instructions and demonstrations
Break skills down into constituent parts to simplify the task and then reintroduce them in a logical sequence or order
(i.e., easy to difficult progressions such as initially learning to control the ball before concentrating on passing or
introducing opponents gradually)
Provide prescriptive feedback for error correction and motivation purposes
Employ specific practice drills and low contextual interference conditions initially (i.e., only practice one skill per session)

DO NOT
Emphasize the outcome (i.e., stress the process of striking the ball well rather than where it goes)
Concentrate too much on errors (i.e., reinforce those components of the task that are correct)
Overload players with too much information

Associative
DO
Encourage performers to evaluate their own performance
Increase progressively the complexity of the task (e.g., introduce opponents, restrict time and space)
Increase variability in practice as well as the amount of functional or contextual interference by practicing more than one
skill in a session (e.g., passing and shooting)

DO NOT
Give too much feedback

Autonomous
DO
Use minimal intervention (i.e., encourage the player to evaluate his or her own feedback; use demonstration frequently)
Deal only with highly specific components of the task
Present the learner with complex, realistic, and challenging practice (e.g., further restrict time and space available to perform)
Practice under realistic match conditions and encourage improvisation and adaptability through variety in practice
Employ highly variable practice conditions and high contextual interference practice sessions (i.e., practice more than
one skill in each session)

DO NOT
Assume that learning has stopped, continued intensive practice still remains essential to further develop skills
(i.e., encourage overlearning)

tennis players), science (research mathematicians and neurologists), and the arts (concert pianists and sculptors) indicated three stages common to the three domains: initiation during which the youngster showed promise, development which was highlighted by significant deliberate practice, and perfection (Bloom 1985).

Interest in understanding the characteristics and development of highly talented individuals has increased, with a good deal of the information derived from studies of world class chess players and musicians. The theoretical framework of expert performance proposed by Ericsson *et al.* (1993; see also Ericsson 2003) is perhaps most dominant. The

framework "that explains expert performance in terms of acquired characteristics resulting from extended deliberate practice and that limits the role of innate (inherited) characteristics to general levels of activity and emotionality" (Ericsson *et al.* 1993, p. 363). Evidence from a variety of sources suggests, in general, that at least 10 years of experience and 10,000 hours of practice are needed to reach international levels of performance in music and chess. This has spurred interest in the development of expertise per se and comparisons of elites with amateurs and novices (Starkes & Ericsson 2003).

The research on expertise is relevant to youth sports. Elite athletes most likely have their initial experiences in childhood and in some cases are products of talent identification and development programs or specific sports schools (state run or private—fee for services), especially female artistic gymnastics, figure skating, tennis, swimming. Other forms of talent identification and development programs include the highly developed interscholastic sport programs in the USA which provide a regular flow of athletes to the university and professional ranks, specifically in basketball and American football. Baseball schools in the Caribbean and some Latin American countries provide a large pool of potentially talented players (about 40% of current players in the two professional baseball leagues in the USA are of Caribbean or Latin American origin). Similarly, soccer schools and academies affiliated with professional clubs provide a ready supply of talented youth.

Girls often specialize in gymnastics in middle childhood and the careers of those who are successful are generally concluded by the mid- to late-teens. Programs for gymnasts often begin in the preschool years with developmental programs, and at these ages coaches are already screening for potentially talented youngsters. Given the success of female gymnasts from the former Socialist countries of Eastern Europe at relatively young ages, youngsters identified at early ages were obviously quite responsive to the highly selective, structured, and intensive instruction and practice programs of sports schools. Unfortunately, specific data on individual progress in specific movement patterns and accomplishments are not available so that individual or group trajectories cannot be objectively reconstructed. Only the accomplishments of successful young gymnasts are highlighted, specifically in the media. It is thus difficult to document the relative success rate as well as the subsequent careers of those who did not successfully make it through the rigorous instruction and practice programs.

In the former Soviet Union in the 1980s (USSR), for example, coaches routinely visited kindergartens (3–7 years) to observe 5-year-old children and identify those having a "suitable build" for gymnastics. Subsequently, parents of identified children were invited to have them participate in a trial training session at the local sports school. Several standardized motor performance tests were administered at the trial session, including the 20-m dash and standing long jump. Training in the USSR gymnastics schools included general and special physical preparation, technical preparation—tumbling, choreography, apparatus work, judging and instruction training, and control tests. Time devoted to each component varied with age. Between 5–6 and 18 years of age, time spent in gymnastics instruction and practice for those who were successful in the program totaled about 11,000 h (Hartley 1988).

Hours provide limited information about the nature of instruction and practice. Details of practice programs are needed. For example, the practice protocols of four female (11–12 years) and four male (12–14 years) gymnasts in a select school in Poland were followed for 19 and 22 weeks, respectively, in the early 1970s (Ziemilska 1981). Data for four members of the female national team were also included. Results are summarized in Table 8.3. Demands of the sport vary by sex. Events for males place a premium on upper body muscular strength and endurance: pommel horse, parallel bars, rings, horizontal bar, in addition to the vault and floor exercise. Events for females do not include an event that places primary stress on upper body muscular strength and endurance: uneven bars, balance beam, vault, floor exercise.

Expressing the observations on a weekly basis, young female gymnasts have more practice sessions and do more repetitions, while young male gymnasts train more hours. Expressing repetitions per training session, there is overlap between young females (420–497) and males (426–571), but expressing repetitions per hour indicates more repetitions in females. Young females spend more hours training (~2 times), have more training sessions (~1.5 times), and do more repetitions (>2 times) than members of the national team. Trends are similar for males. The number of repetitions per week and estimated intensity of training in the young Polish male gymnasts were about double the estimates reported for first class youth gymnasts in the former USSR (Ziemilska 1981). Although the observations are limited to small numbers, they provide insights into the nature of gymnastics training at young ages. The variation in training protocols for young and more

Table 8.3 Training program for individual artistic gymnasts. Observations are summed over 19 weeks in girls, 19 weeks in members of the national team, 22 weeks in boys. Calculated from data reported in Ziemilska (1981).

	Individual gymnasts				
	1	2	3	4	Average
Girls 11–12 years, 19 weeks					
Practice sessions (*n*)	152	141	139	147	145
Hours (*n*)	491	411	419	436	439
Repetitions* (*n*)	63,793	60,974	69,057	65,212	64,759
Women's National Team members, 19 weeks†					
Practice sessions (*n*)	96	81	105	99	95
Hours (*n*)	222	203	245	232	225
Repetitions (*n*)	33,065	26,777	25,899	26,421	28,040
Boys, 12–14 years, 22 weeks					
Practice sessions (*n*)	143	138	115	115	128
Hours (*n*)	713	703	631	543	647
Repetitions (*n*)	72,894	68,704	65,699	49,001	64,074

* Repetitions refer to the number of gymnastic elements performed.
† Data for national team members are reported for 40 weeks; 19 weeks in the mid-portion of the distribution (weeks 12–30) were selected for comparison with younger gymnasts.

elite gymnasts is consistent with observations that different instructional and practice strategies are needed for individuals at different stages of the learning process for specific skills (see above).

Assuming the observation period represented about half of a gymnastics season, doubling the values provides an annual estimate of hours of training: 822–982 hours per year for the four girls and 1086–1426 per year for the four boys. If this time commitment is maintained over 9 or 10 years, the hypothesized 10,000 h of practice to reach international levels of performance would be approached. Note, however, hours of training of national team members were a bit more than half of the hours of the four young gymnasts.

The issue of tracking of size, physique, body composition, and performance is inherent in talent selection programs and also relevant to the development of expertise in sport. Tracking attempts to establish the stability of a characteristic over time, specifically the maintenance of relative rank within a group. After 2–3 years of age, height, weight, and skeletal lengths and breadths are quite stable over time. Tracking data are less extensive for physique and body composition. Somatotype and fat-free mass

are moderately stable from late childhood on, while fat mass and percentage fat are less stable. Indicators of size, physique, and body composition show some degree of instability during the adolescent spurt, which reflects individual differences in the timing and tempo of the growth spurt and sexual maturation. Indicators of strength, motor performance and skill, aerobic power and field tests of aerobic capacity are generally less stable characteristics than size, physique, and fat-free mass during childhood and adolescence. These functional variables are related in part to variation in size, physique, and body composition and are also influenced by motivation, opportunity for practice, and systematic instruction, practice, and training (Malina *et al.* 2004a).

Genetic considerations in skill acquisition

Genotype and genotype–environment interactions are not ordinarily considered in discussions of motor development, performance, and skill acquisition as potential constraints in the context of dynamical systems, or in the development of expertise. Both genetic and shared environment effects are apparent in familial studies of motor development and performance, although they are limited largely to twins and siblings. More data are available for motor performance in contrast to early motor development. Performance variables include standard measures of dashes, jumps and throws, balance, speed of limb movement, and fine motor skills (Malina & Bouchard 1989; Bouchard *et al.* 1997).

Although considerable effort has been devoted to documenting developmental stages for a variety of fundamental movements, little is known about the contribution of inherited characteristics to the development of movement patterns. Evidence for twins, 6–9 years (Goya *et al.* 1991, 1993) and 11–15 years (Skład 1972), suggests a significant genetic contribution to variance in the kinematic structure of running a dash. Among the older youth, differences in features of the dash were smaller between female monozygotic (MZ) and dizygotic (DZ) twins compared with male MZ and DZ twins (Skład 1972), suggesting perhaps that the running performance of girls is more amenable to environmental influences. In contrast to the dash, intrapair differences in the kinematic features of a throw and swimming crawl were similar in the MZ and DZ twins 6–9 years of age (Goya *et al.* 1991, 1993), suggesting an important role for environmental influences related to instruction, practice, and experiences in these two motor skills.

The potential role of genotype in motor skill acquisition needs attention. Several relatively dated experimental studies have considered the pattern of learning motor skills in adolescent twins (Bouchard *et al.* 1997). Except for a stabilometer task, which places a premium on dynamic balance and coordination, tasks used in the experimental studies were largely fine motor skills that stressed manual dexterity and precision of movement. Results suggest similar rates of learning motor skills in MZ compared with DZ twins, but estimates of the genetic contribution vary from task to task and during the time course of learning (i.e., over practice trials or training sessions). Detailed genetic analyses of learning curves for motor skills are limited. Parameters of the learning curves of four tasks—plate tapping with the hand, tapping with one foot,

mirror tracing, and a ball toss for accuracy—in twins 9–13 years of age give variable results (Skład 1975). Two parameters, level and rate of learning, were more similar in MZ than in DZ twins, and intrapair correlations tended to be higher in male than in female MZ twins. The third parameter, the final level of skill attained, was quite variable between twin types and sexes and among the four tasks. The results, although limited, suggest genetic contributions to the learning process and potential sex differences.

Genotype may be an important determinant of the ease or difficulty with which new motor skills are learned, or of improvement in performance that occurs with practice. It is also possible that prolonged practice may influence gene expression. There is a need for more detailed study of the individuality of responses to instruction and regular practice of motor tasks during childhood and adolescence, and interactions of the characteristics of the learner (which may be in part genetic) and the instruction or practice (learning) environment.

Implications for youth sports

Many children enter organized youth sport programs at 5–6 years of age, even though a significant number of children have not yet developed mature movement patterns by these ages. However, one of the objectives of youth sports programs is to teach skills, so that it is imperative that coaches of young children have an understanding of developmental sequences and how to provide an environment in which the developing movement patterns can be nurtured and improved.

Movement patterns and performance can be refined through appropriate instruction and practice. Subsequently, the basic patterns must be integrated into more complex movement sequences and skills required for specific games and sports. The transition from basic movement patterns to more complex sports skills depends, in part, upon individual differences in growth and maturation, earlier experiences and opportunities, and the quality of instruction and practice.

A key player in skill development is the coach, who should be able to meet the developmental needs of young athletes through appropriate instructional sequences and guided practice opportunities. In order for a coach to teach motor skills effectively, he or she should have a sound knowledge of the developmental sequences for particular skills and should be able to identify different stages of development among youngsters involved in a specific sport. It is important in this context for coaches to know how to observe the movements of a child, evaluate technique, and be able to provide accurate feedback to improve performance. All too often, individuals tend to focus on the end product or outcome of a movement. As a corollary, a coach should have a sound knowledge of activities and experiences that will help the young athlete progress in the development of basic and more specialized skills in a given sport. Central to these processes is the ability of the coach to communicate with young athletes.

The role of coach education and coaching style in skill development of children enrolled in sport programs at young ages needs careful study and evaluation. The majority of youth sport coaches, specifically in North America, are volunteers, most of whom have little background in motor development and methods of instruction in general and sport-specific skills.

Future directions

• The growth, maturation, and behavioral characteristics of subjects are generally not incorporated into studies of skill acquisition and response to training programs. As a result, it is difficult to partition training effects from those associated with normal growth, maturation, and development.
• Appropriate and effective instructional and practice protocols for the development and maintenance of skills at different stages of growth and maturation should be established. How, for example, should practice or instructional schedules with associated feedback be adjusted to youth in different stages of the adolescent growth spurt?
• Individuals differ in their ability to learn and in learning styles (e.g., observation model, verbal instruction, ability to combine the two). Variation in learning styles for motor skills merits study.
• Intraindividual variation in responses to the instructional and practice programs for motor skill are not ordinarily considered or reported. Individual differences in response to instruction and practice need study. Are there specific age- and maturity-related effects on the responses?
• There is a need for further longitudinal study of the development of specific movement skills and also sport-specific skills during adolescence in both sexes. Does sport-specific training modify the magnitude and timing of adolescent spurts in movement skills?
• There is a need to extend studies of expertise to youth including practice protocols, mechanisms of deliberate practice, sensitive periods for practice, and behavioral correlates.
• There is a need for study of the estimated contribution of genotype in the acquisition of movement patterns and skills in children and adolescents as well as expertise at relatively young ages.
• Early specialization is often cited as a problem of youth sports. Evidence from studies of expertise, including elite athletes, highlights the importance of early exposure and practice. The issue of early specialization is thus two-edged: in some cases it may lead to expertise in a sport; in other cases it may eliminate other options and may potentially lead to frustration, burnout, and other personal problems.

References

Anderson, D.I. (2002) Do critical periods determine when to initiate sport skill training? In: *Children and Youth in Sport: A Biopsychosocial Perspective*, 2nd edn. (Smoll, F.L. & Smith, R.E., eds.) Kendall/Hunt, Dubuque, IA: 105–148.

Beilock, S.L., Carr, T.H., MacMahon, C. & Starkes, J.L. (2002) When paying attention becomes counterproductive: Impact of divided versus well-focused attention on novice and experienced performance of sensorimotor skills. *Journal of Experimental Psychology: Applied* **8**, 6–16.

Beunen, G.P., Malina, R.M., Van't Hof, M.A., *et al.* (1988) *Adolescent Growth and Motor Performance: A Longitudinal Study of Belgian Boys*. Human Kinetics, Champaign, IL.

Bloom, B.S., ed. (1985) *Developing Talent in Young People*. Ballantine Books, New York.

Bompa, T.O. (1985) *Talent identification*. Sports Science Periodical on Research and Technology in Sport: Physical Testing GN-1. Coaching Association of Canada, Ottawa.

Bompa, T.O. (1995) *From Childhood to Champion Athlete*. Veritas Publishing, Toronto.

Bornstein, M.H. (1989) Sensitive periods in development: Structural characteristics and causal interpretations. *Psychological Bulletin* **105**, 1–19.

Bouchard, C., Malina, R.M. & Perusse, L. (1997) *Genetics of Fitness and Physical Performance*. Human Kinetics, Champaign, IL.

Dusenberry, L. (1952) A study of the effects of training in ball throwing by children ages three to seven. *Research Quarterly* **23**, 9–14.

Ericsson, K.A. (2003) The development of elite performance and deliberate practice: An update from the perspective of the expert-performance approach. In: *Expert Performance in Sport: Recent Advances in Research on Sport Expertise* (Starkes, J. & Ericsson, K.A., eds.) Human Kinetics, Champaign, IL: 49–81.

Ericsson, K.A., Krampe, R.T. & Tesch-Römer, C. (1993) The role of deliberate practice in the acquisition of expert performance. *Psychological Review* **100**, 363–406.

Faigenbaum, A.D., Westcott, W.L., Micheli, L.J. *et al.* (1996) The effects of strength training and detraining on children. *Journal of Strength and Conditioning Research* **10**, 109–114.

Fitts, P.M. & Posner, M.I. (1967) *Human Performance*. Brooks/Cole, Belmont, CA.

Goodway, J.D., Quinones-Padovani, C., Segarra-Roman, A., Robinson, L. & Hugo, J. (2005) Developmental trajectories in the throwing profiles of Hispanic preschoolers. *Journal of Sport and Exercise Psychology* **27**, S25–S26 (Abstract).

Goya, T., Amano, Y., Hoshikawa, T. & Matsui, H. (1991) Longitudinal study on selected sports performance related with the physical growth and development of twins. *XIIIth International Congress of Biomechanics, Book of Abstracts*. University of Western Australia, Perth: 139–141.

Goya, T., Amano, Y., Hoshikawa, T. & Matsui, H. (1993) Longitudinal study on the variation and development of selected sports performance in twins: Case study for one pair of female monozygous (MZ) and dizygous (DZ) twins. *Sports Science* **14**, 151–168.

Halverson, L.E. & Roberton, M.A. (1979) The effects of instruction on overhand throwing development in children. In: *Psychology of Motor Behavior and Sport – 1978* (Newell, K. & Roberts, G., eds.) Human Kinetics, Champaign, IL: 258–269.

Halverson, L.E., Roberton, M.A., Safrit, M.J. & Roberts, T.W. (1977) Effect of guided practice on overhand throw ball velocities of kindergarten children. *Research Quarterly* **48**, 311–318.

Hanson, S.K. (1961) A comparison of the overhand throw performance of instructed and non-instructed kindergarten boys and girls. Master's thesis, University of Wisconsin, Madison.

Hartley, G.L. (1988) A comparative view of talent selection for sport in two socialist states—the USSR and the GDR—with particular reference to gymnastics. In: *The Growing Child in Competitive Sport*: The 1987 BANC International Proceedings. National Coaching Foundation, Leeds, UK: 50–56.

Haubenstricker, J.L., Branta, C.F. & Seefeldt, V.D. (1999) History of the Motor Performance Study and related programs. In: *100 Years of Kinesiology: History, Research, and Reflections* (Haubenstricker, J.L. & Feltz, D.L., eds.) Department of Kinesiology, Michigan State University, East Lansing, MI: 103–125.

Haubenstricker, J. & Seefeldt, V. (1986) Acquisition of motor skills during childhood. In: *Physical Activity and Well-Being* (Seefeldt, V., ed.) American Alliance for Health, Physical Education, Recreation and Dance, Reston, VA: 41–101.

Haubenstricker, J.L. & Seefeldt, V. (2002) The concept of readiness applied to the acquisition of motor skills. In: *Children and Youth in Sport: A Biopsychosocial Perspective*, 2nd edn. (Smoll, F.L. & Smith, R.E. eds.) Kendall/Hunt, Dubuque, IA: 61–81.

Haywood, K.M. & Getchell, N. (2001) *Life Span Motor Development*, 3rd edn. Human Kinetics, Champaign, IL.

Heras Yague, P. & de la Fuente, J.M. (1998) Changes in height and motor performance relative to peak height velocity: A mixed-longitudinal study of Spanish boys and girls. *American Journal of Human Biology* **10**, 647–660.

Kolakowski, D. & Malina, R.M. (1974) Spatial ability, throwing accuracy and man's hunting heritage. *Nature* **251**, 410–412.

Lewis, M.C. (2000) The promise of dynamic systems approaches for an integrated account of human development. *Child Development* **71**, 36–43.

Magill, R.A. (2004) *Motor Learning and Control: Concepts and Applications*, 7th edn. McGraw-Hill, New York.

Malina, R.M. (1968) Reliability of different methods of scoring throwing accuracy. *Research Quarterly* **39**, 149–160.

Malina, R.M. (1969) Effects of varied information feedback practice conditions on throwing speed and accuracy. *Research Quarterly* **40**, 134–145.

Malina, R.M. (1972) Information feedback. In: *Ergogenic Aids and Muscular Performance* (Morgan, W.P., ed.) Academic Press, New York: 67–91.

Malina, R.M. & Bouchard, C. (1989) Genetic considerations in physical fitness. In: *Assessing Physical Fitness and Physical Activity in Population-Based Surveys* (Drury, T.F., ed.) Public Health Service, DHHS Pub No (PHS) 89-1253. US Government Printing Office, Washington, DC: 453–473.

Malina, R.M., Bouchard, C. & Bar-Or, O. (2004a) *Growth, Maturation, and Physical Activity*, 2nd edn. Human Kinetics, Champaign, IL.

Malina, R.M., Cumming, S.P., Kontos, A.P., Eisenmann, J.C., Ribeiro, B. & Aroso, J. (2005) Maturity-associated variation in sport-specific skills of youth soccer players aged 13–15 years. *Journal of Sports Sciences* **23**, 515–522.

Malina, R.M. & Eisenmann, J.C. (2003) Trainability during childhood and adolescence. In: *Youth Sports: Perspectives for a New Century* (Malina, R.M. & Clark, M.A., eds.) Coaches Choice, Monterey, CA: 76–93.

Malina, R.M., Eisenmann, J.C., Cumming, S.P., Ribeiro, B. & Aroso, J. (2004b) Maturity-associated variation in the growth and functional capacities of youth football (soccer) players 13–15 years. *European Journal of Applied Physiology* **91**, 555–562.

Miller, S. (1978) The facilitation of fundamental motor skill learning in young children. Doctoral dissertation, Michigan State University, East Lansing.

Newell, K.M. (1986) Constraints on the development of coordination. In: *Motor Development in Children: Aspects of Coordination Control* (Wade, M.G. & Whiting, H.T.A., eds.) Martinus Nijhoff, Dordecht, The Netherlands: 341–359.

Nielsen, B., Nielsen, K., Behrendt Hansen, M. & Asmussen, E. (1980) Training of "functional muscular strength" in girls 7–19 years old. In: *Children and Exercise* Vol. IX (Berg, K. & Eriksson, B.O., eds.) University Park Press, Baltimore: 69–78.

Payne, V.G. & Isaacs, L.D. (1999) *Human Motor Development: A Lifespan Approach*, 4th edn. Mayfield, Mountain View, CA.

Petiot, B., Salmela, J.H. & Hoshizaki, T.B., eds. (1987) *World Identification Systems for Gymnastics Talent*. Sport Psyche Editions, Montreal.

Poe, A. (1976) Description of the movement characteristics of 2-year-old children performing the jump and reach. *Research Quarterly* **47**, 260–268.

Roberton, M.A. (1982) Describing "stages" within and across motor tasks. In: *The Development of Movement Control and Co-ordination* (Kelso, J.A.S. & Clark, J.E., eds.) Wiley, New York: 293–307.

Roberton, M.A. (1984) Changing motor patterns during childhood. In: *Motor Development During Childhood and Adolescence* (Thomas, J.R., ed.) Burgess, Minneapolis: 48–90.

Scott, J.P. (1986) Critical periods in organization processes. In: *Human Growth*, Vol. 1, *Developmental Biology, Prenatal Growth* (Falkner, F. & Tanner, J.M., eds.) Plenum, New York: 181–196.

Seefeldt, V. & Haubenstricker, J. (1982) Patterns, phases, or stages: an analytical model for the study of developmental movement. In: *The Development of Movement Control and Co-ordination* (Kelso, J.A.S. & Clark, J.E., eds.) Wiley, New York: 309–319.

Singer, R.N., Hausenblaus, H.A. & Janelle, C.M., eds. (2001) *Handbook of Research on Sport Psychology*, 2nd edn. John Wiley & Sons, New York.

Skład, M. (1972) Similarity of movement in twins. *Wychowanie Fizycznie i Sport* **16**, 119–141.

Skład, M. (1975) The genetic determination of the rate of learning of motor skills.

Studies in Physical Anthropology **1**, 3–19.

Sparks, N.E. (1950) *A study of the effectiveness of practice in the development of certain motor skills in first grade children*. Studies in Education, Illinois State Normal University, No. 158.

Starkes, J. & Ericsson, K.A., eds. (2003) *Expert Performance in Sport: Recent Advances in Research on Sport Expertise*. Human Kinetics, Champaign, IL.

Stodden, D., Langendorfer, S.J. & Robinson, R.R. (2005) Kinematic constraints associated with the acquisition of overarm throwing. *Journal of Sport and Exercise Psychology* **27**, S24–S25 (Abstract).

Strong, W.B., Malina, R.M., Blimkie, C.J.R., et al. (2005) Evidence based physical activity for school youth. *Journal of Pediatrics* **146**, 732–737.

Thelen, E. & Smith, L.B. (1994) *A Dynamic Systems Approach to the Development of Cognition and Action*. MIT Press, Cambridge, MA.

Thelen, E. & Ulrich, B.D. (1991) Hidden skills. *Monographs of the Society for Research in Child Development*, No. 223.

Vereijken, B. & Thelen, E. (1997) Training infant treadmill stepping: The role of individual pattern stability. *Developmental Psychobiology* **30**, 89–102.

Vogel, P.G. (1986) Effects of physical education programs on children. In: *Physical Activity and Well-Being* (Seefeldt, V., ed.) American Alliance for Health, Physical Education, Recreation and Dance, Reston, VA: 455–509.

Weltman, A., Janney, C., Rians, C.B. et al. (1986) The effects of hydraulic resistance strength training in pre-pubertal males.

Medicine and Science in Sports and Exercise **18**, 629–638.

Werner, P. (1974) Education of selected movement patterns of preschool children. *Perceptual and Motor Skills* **39**, 975–978.

Whitall, J. & Clark, J.E. (1994) The development of bipedal interlimb coordination. In: *Interlimb Coordination: Neural, Dynamical, and Cognitive Constraints* (Swinnen, S.P., ed.) Academic Press, San Diego, CA: 391–411.

Whitall, J. & Getchell, N. (1995) From walking to running: Applying a dynamical systems approach to the development of locomotor skills. *Child Development* **66**, 1541–1553.

Wickstrom, R.L. (1983) *Fundamental Motor Patterns*, 3rd edn. Lea and Febiger, Philadelphia.

Williams, A.M. & Hodges, N.J. (2005) Practice, instruction and skill acquisition in soccer: Challenging tradition. *Journal of Sports Sciences* **23**, 637–650.

Williams, A.M., Horn, R.R. & Hodges, N.J. (2003) Skill acquisition. In: *Science and Soccer*, 2nd edn (Reilly, T. & Williams, A.M., eds.) Routledge, London: 198–213.

Ziemilska, A. (1981) Wpływ intensywnego treningu gimnastycznego na rozwój somatyczny I dojrzewanie dzieci (influence of intensive gymnastics training on growth and sexual maturation of children). *Studia i Monografie Akademia Wychowania Fizycznego (Studies and Monographs of the Academy of Physical Education)* Warsaw, Poland.

Chapter 9

Growing a Healthy Skeleton: Exercise— the Primary Driving Force

SHONA L. BASS, ROBIN M. DALY, AND CAMERON J.R. BLIMKIE

Osteoporosis is a major public health problem for both men and women because of the morbidity and mortality associated with fragility fractures. Although considered to be a disease affecting the elderly, the pathogenesis of osteoporosis may have its origins in childhood. The amount of bone that is gained during growth is believed to be an important determinant of future fracture risk. It is estimated that a 10% increase in peak bone mineral content (BMC) may delay the development of osteoporosis by 13 years (Cumming *et al.* 1993; Hernandez *et al.* 2003).

Childhood and adolescence is a critical time for the skeleton as the growth-related increases in bone length and mass are sculptured into a shape that is best suited for its function and the lifetime demands placed on it. The body builds a skeleton that is light and strong; the results of the perfect combination of stiffness and flexibility to enable bone to absorb energy and resist deformation. The genetic map of bone provides the template for the defining characteristics of each individual bone which in turn requires the presence of mechanical loading to fulfill the structural phenotype designed for its unique function within the body. Thus, this development of bone during growth is influenced by forces associated with gravity and physical activity (Burr 1997; Frost 1997; Turner 2000); it is the muscle forces, however, that create the peak forces (load) acting on bone during physical activity.

Understanding how loading during growth results in greater peak bone strength in adulthood requires an understanding of the cellular, tissue, and structural responses, and the interaction between these processes with other factors that influence bone

growth. For instance, research at the cellular and tissue level has revealed much about the mechanism(s) of the bones' adaptive responses to different components of loading. The importance of these studies, however, can only be realized when the data can be translated to inform practice in humans.

In this chapter, the role of exercise for improved bone health during growth is presented through understanding the response to loading at the cellular, tissue, and organ level. The first section of this chapter is devoted to an explanation of how the skeleton responds to loading at the cellular level. This is followed by a synopsis of the results from animal studies that have provided the evidential basis for human intervention studies. Next, we review the different techniques used to assess the strength of the skeleton, which is important to understand and interpret the results from human trials. The final section provides a critical summary of what we know about the skeletal adaptations to exercise during growth in humans.

The skeleton as a dynamic organ

Bone is a dynamic organ which adjusts its mass and architecture to accommodate the loads (forces) placed on it. Bones are loaded from direct muscle action pulling on an origin or insertion region, from dispersed strains resulting from the combined muscle forces, or from external forces acting directly on a bone or joints. The two most important parameters related to bone loading are *stress* (defined as the force per unit area) and *strain* (defined as the change in length per unit length) which describes the deformation of a material. It is the unique cellular environment of bone that responds to the imparted strains that drive bone adaptation. This section presents an overview of how basic bone metabolism maintains bone in its active dynamic form and how the cells respond to loading (termed *mechanotransduction*). This is followed by a discussion on the mechanostat, a unifying model which proposes how the bone responds to loading in the presence of various environments.

Bone modeling and remodeling

Bone is an active organ that undergoes changes throughout life via the processes of modeling and remodeling. The driving forces behind bone modeling and remodeling are the activities of the bone resident cells: osteoblasts, osteoclasts, and osteocytes. Bone *modeling* refers to the sculpturing of bone (size, shape, and spatial location) through two independent mechanisms referred to as resorption and formation drifts. Modeling involves the addition of bone, without prior resorption, and therefore does not depend on any local biologic coupling between osteoclasts and osteoblasts (Baron 1990). It can affect cortical, periosteal, endocortical, and trabecular surfaces; it can increase but rarely decreases the periosteal perimeter, cortical thickness, and cortical BMC; it can only thicken, but not reduce trabeculae. Modeling drifts are reported to operate via an "on–off" mechanism, regulated primarily by mechanical stimuli (Frost 1987). The majority of bone modeling occurs during the growing years, with limited modeling occurring following skeletal maturation (Burr *et al.* 1989).

Bone *remodeling* represents a lifelong renewal process that involves the continual replacement or "turnover" of fatigue-damaged bone in small packets referred to as basic multicellular units (BMUs), which consist of osteoclasts and osteoblasts. The remodeling sequence is always one of activation–resorption–formation, during which, under normal conditions, the processes of bone resorption and formation are tightly coupled. Remodeling acts throughout life on periosteal, Haversian, endocortical, and trabecular surfaces. Except on the periosteal surface, remodeling does not usually make more

bone than is resorbed—bone is either removed or is conserved (Frost 1992). In middle age there is an uncoupling of the action of the osteoclast and osteoblasts leading to more bone being resorbed than is formed. This is the basis of bone loss during menopause in women and the age-related bone loss that occurs in both men and women.

Mechanotransduction

Mechanotranduction is the term used to describe the process by which cells sense a stimulus created by mechanical loading and translate this information into a signal that leads to a change in cellular activity and thus a physiologic skeletal response. In bone, this process consists of four distinct phases:

1 *Mechanocoupling* The detection of the mechanical signal by sensory cells which, in turn, produce a local mechanical signal.

2 *Biochemical coupling* Transformation of the mechanical signal into a biochemical signal.

3 *Signal transmission* Sensory cells communicate with the effector cells; these are the cells that remove or form bone (osteoclasts and osteoblasts).

4 *Effector cell response* Tissue response (i.e., bone formation) (Duncan & Turner 1995).

For this process to occur, the mechanical signal(s) must be presented with specific physical loading characteristics that will be detected by the cells, and bone cells must be in a receptive state to detect the stimulus. Stimulation of bone cells via mechanical loading is not only the direct result of the physical deformation of the bone tissue, but also the indirect effect of the pressure-induced movement of extracellular fluid through the bones' lacuno-canalicular network. For instance, strain-induced fluid flow may stimulate streaming potentials, wall shear stress, or chemotransport-related effects that can be detected by effector cells to stimulate a response (Burr *et al.* 2002; Ehrlich & Lanyon 2002).

It is proposed that the predominant mechanosensors in bone are the osteocytes, which are osteoblasts that have become trapped and embedded throughout the mineralized bone matrix (lacuna). These mechanosensor cells communicate with other osteocytes through a complex connected network of fluid-filled canaliculi (Huiskes *et al.*

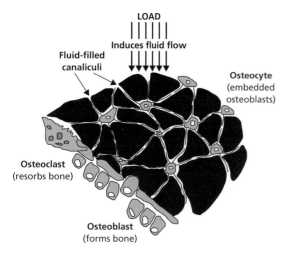

LOAD

Induces fluid flow

Fluid-filled canaliculi

Osteocyte (embedded osteoblasts)

Osteoclast (resorbs bone)

Osteoblast (forms bone)

Fig. 9.1 Stimulation of bone cells via mechanical loading is not only the direct result of the physical deformation of the bone tissue, but also the indirect effect of the pressure-induced movement of extracellular fluid through the bones' lacuno-canalicular network. It is proposed that the predominant mechanosensors in bone are the osteocytes which communicate with other osteocytes through a complex connected network of fluid-filled canaliculi. This network also extends to cells along the periosteal and endosteal membranes, and bone lining cells. Osteocytes communicate with neighboring bone cells via specialized gap junctions, and it is this network of osteoblasts, osteocytes, and lining cells that form a syncytium which is well equipped for signal transduction.

2000). This network also extends to cells along the periosteal and endosteal membranes, and bone lining cells, which are derived from osteoblasts that line the bone surface in the periosteum. Osteocytes communicate with neighboring bone cells via specialized gap junctions, and it is this network of osteoblasts, osteocytes, and lining cells that form a syncytium which is well equipped for signal transduction (Fig. 9.1) (Huiskes *et al.* 2000; Ehrlich & Lanyon 2002).

Does estrogen influence the osteogenic response to loading?

Traditionally, estrogen and androgens were thought to be responsible for the sexual dimorphism of skeletal geometry; that is, estrogen was considered

the key regulator of the female skeleton whereas androgens were considered critical for the male skeleton. However, it is now evident that this is not the case; the presentation of an unusual case study of an adult male with an estrogen receptor defect who presented with open epiphyses and osteoporosis (Smith *et al.* 1994) was the first hint that estrogen has a dominant role in regulating bone metabolism in males as well as females. Several subsequent follow-up case studies of males with aromatase deficiency (aromatase is an important enzyme for the conversion of androgens to estrogen) further identified the important role of estrogen for growth in bone length and BMC accrual in males (Morishima *et al.* 1995; Smith & Korach 1996). These clinical case findings demonstrated clearly that estrogen was an important regulator of longitudinal growth in both sexes by controlling closure of the epiphysis. Estrogen also suppresses bone remodeling and maintains BMC in both men and women. Interestingly, estrogen and androgens are thought to have differing surface specific effects; it has been hypothesized that androgens enhance periosteal bone formation in males but have no effect on the endocortical surface. In females, estrogen inhibits periosteal bone formation but enhances endocortical contraction.

In addition to estrogen being a major regulator of skeletal development during growth and responsible for maintenance of bone in old age, it also appears to regulate how the skeleton responds to loading. For instance, the results of studies comparing pre- and post-menopausal women and post-menopausal women with and without hormonal replacement therapy show that the effect of exercise may be enhanced in the presence of estrogen (Prince *et al.* 1991; Kohrt *et al.* 1995; Heikkinen *et al.* 1997; Cheng *et al.* 2002). However, the relationship between estrogen and loading is complex and often inconsistent. The apparent interaction between estrogen, mechanical strain, and an effective loading response has led to the proposal that strain and estrogen share common transduction pathways. However, this interaction is complex and while recent research has led to a greater understanding of how estrogen and strain interact, there remain many unanswered questions.

The action of estrogen on bone occurs predominantly through two receptors: estrogen receptor alpha (ERα) and beta (ERβ). It has recently been proposed that these two receptors may result in opposing responses to loading (Saxon & Turner 2005). This may help to explain some of the complex and sometimes inconsistent interactions reported between estrogen and loading. Saxon and Turner (2005) propose that estrogen interacts with exercise on the endocortical surface via ERα, whereas estrogen inhibits exercise-induced gains at the periosteum via ERβ. They also propose that exercise enhances osteoblast proliferation on the periosteal surface, and because these cells express ERβ they provide a pathway in females by which estrogen can suppress exercise-induced activation of osteoblasts (and thus periosteal apposition). However, this area remains controversial and further research is needed to elucidate the role of estrogen, and the specific roles of ERα, ERβ, and exercise (Khosla et al. 2006; Saxon & Turner 2005).

Gene–environment interactions

Advances in knowledge about gene–environment interactions in bone responses to exercise are relatively recent and are often difficult to elucidate because most gene interactions are polygenic (or complex traits) and thus large-scale human studies are required to provide the necessary power to detect gene–environment interactions. Despite this, there is some indication that variation in several specific genes may influence an individual's response to loading. That is, the same loads may engender a different osteogenic response in individuals with similar prior loading backgrounds. Variation in the vitamin D receptor genotype has been associated with variance in the osteogenic responses to hours of physical activity in children (Nakamura et al. 2002; Omasu et al. 2004) and bone metabolism responses following strenuous resistance training in young male adults (Tajima et al. 2000). Recently, a modulating role of the PvuII polymorphism in the ERα gene was identified in an investigation of the effect of hours of habitual activity on bone density and structure in children (Suuriniemi et al. 2004). The osteogenic response of femoral cortical bone resorption

following 10 weeks of basic fitness training was also recently linked to a functional polymorphism in the interleukin-6 gene (Dhamrait et al. 2003). Additional information on gene modulation of prospective bone adaptations in response to exercise in well-controlled intervention studies with pre- and peripubertal children is currently unknown.

Investigating gene modulation of long-term bone adaptations in response to exercise during growth will increase our understanding of the normal variation in the skeletal responses to environmental factors. Furthermore, assessing gene–environmental interactions may help to identify those individuals at greatest risk of osteoporosis and could lead to the identification of individuals in whom exercise could be expected to be most efficacious. For instance, there is preliminary evidence showing that there may be a *high BMC gene* that results in a greater than expected response to loading. The high BMC mutation in the *Lrp5* gene results in a "high BMC" mouse that is the same size and weight as the wild type but has bigger and stronger bones (Little et al. 2002). When subjected to loading, the change in periosteal formation rates was almost double the response in the wild type. This result is particularly impressive given that one would expect the response to loading to have been less in the high BMC animals because of the relatively lower strain per bone size. Whether similar mutations exist in humans and lead to similar responses to exercise remains to be determined.

Adaptation of bone to loading

Bone is constantly adapting to changes in its loading environment via modeling and remodeling through a controlled mechanical feedback system in which bone cells detect and alter the structure and strength of bone in response to its loading requirements. This intrinsic feedback relationship is encapsulated by Frost's "mechanostat" theory, which predicts that BMC, structure, and strength will increase predictably and correspondingly in response to increasing maximal muscle force brought about by growth or loading to ensure that peak strains do not exceed a certain threshold level or set-point referred to as the *minimum effective strain* (MES) (Frost & Schonau 2000) (Fig. 9.2). If customary mechanical strains

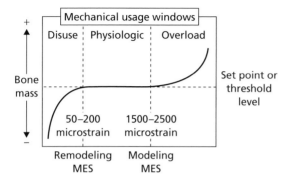

Fig. 9.2 The skeleton maintains its strength and structure by an intrinsic feedback relationship encapsulated by Frost's "mechanostat" which predicts that bone mineral content (BMC), structure, and strength will increase predictably and correspondingly in response to increasing maximal muscle force resulting from growth or loading to ensure that peak strains do not exceed a certain threshold level or set-point. MES, minimum effective strain. After Burr (1995).

(200–2500 microstrains) remain within a "normal physiologic" window, bone structure will be maintained. However, if local mechanical strains exceed the upper boundary of the physiologic window or set-point (1500–3000 microstrains), bone will undergo modeling and change its structure to reduce local strains below the MES. Conversely, unloading (disuse or immobilization) will reduce mechanical strains on bone leading to BMU-based remodeling and a reduction in the mass, size, and strength of bone. Central to Frost's mechanostat theory is the notion that there are different threshold levels or set-points for modeling and remodeling. While these set-points establish an appropriate sensitivity for skeletal adaptation to mechanical stimuli, the proper functioning of the mechanostat depends on the normal state of all its cells (osteocytes, osteoblasts, and osteoclasts), the customary mechanical usage of the skeleton, and the endocrine–metabolic environment (Cointry *et al.* 2004). While these set-points appear to be genetically controlled, they vary depending on the skeletal site, loading history, and several hormonal and local agents, including estrogen (Frost 1987). For instance, estrogen is thought to be a key regulator of MES in bone; lower estrogen levels result in a decrease in the sensitivity of the MES

in bone and consequently a greater load is required to elicit an adaptive bone response. Other theories have been proposed to explain the adaptive bone responses to loading that "extend" the mechanostat theory. The "Principle of Cellular Accommodation" proposed by Turner (1999) is based on the assumption that bone cells respond strongly to changes in the mechanical environment, but the response will eventually phase out as the cells "accommodate" to the steady state signals.

Characteristics of loading for optimizing the osteogenic response—the results of animal studies provide the platform for human studies

While Frost's mechanostat theory proposes a model of mechanical feedback, how mechanical loads are perceived by the skeleton is dependent on the characteristics of the loading. For instance, to achieve an optimal osteogenic response the loading must result in fluid flow within the bone's fluid-filled lacuno-canalicular network, which either induces local deformation of cells, or coupling via an electrical effect related to streaming potentials. There is also some evidence that bone cells could respond directly to small deformations induced by external forces (Weinbaum *et al.* 1994; Hsieh & Turner 2001). The importance of fluid flow is clearly demonstrated by comparing the osteogenic response that occurs in dynamic compared with static loading. The results of animal studies have convincingly shown that the rate of bone formation is reduced when loads are applied statically. In contrast, large positive skeletal changes have been observed when bone cells are subjected to loads similar in magnitude but applied in a dynamic nature (Turner 1998). While these and other data clearly demonstrate the importance of dynamic loading, there are many other characteristics of dynamic loads that influence the adaptation by bone to loading. For instance, there is strong evidence to support the notion that bone cells respond preferentially to high magnitude strains that are applied rapidly (high strain rate) and are presented in an unusual or diverse loading distribution (i.e., differing from that to which the bone is typically accustomed).

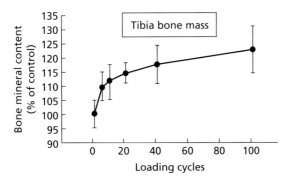

Fig. 9.3 The number of loading cycles required to stimulate osteogenesis is an important determinant of the adaptive process. The osteogenic response to load is not proportional to the loading duration. For instance, in this study rats jumped down from a height of 40 cm; an osteogenic response was achieved with as few as five loading cycles and there was limited benefit of additional loading beyond 40 jumps per day. After Umemura *et al.* (1997).

The number of loading cycles required to stimulate osteogenesis is also an important determinant of the adaptive process (Fig. 9.3). Early work by Rubin and Lanyon (1984) using a controlled external loading regimen (i.e., functionally isolated avian ulnar model) demonstrated that the osteogenic response to relatively high magnitude loading became saturated after only a few loading cycles (i.e., 36 consecutive cycles per day). No further benefits were obtained by increasing the number of loading cycles up to 1800 per day. In another study mimicking more normal behavior, in which rats jumped down from a height of 40 cm, an osteogenic response was achieved with as few as five loading cycles; there was limited benefit of additional loading beyond 40 jumps per day (Umemura *et al.* 1997). In this study, however, the animals did not undergo typical loading during the non-loading period. Furthermore, in both these studies it is likely that the levels of strain exceeded those typically encountered during human physical activities, and thus it is not known whether these findings are relevant to humans.

While relatively few loading cycles may be required to elicit an osteogenic response, the minimum number of cycles may be influenced by strain magnitude. For instance, Cullen *et al.* (2001) compared the adaptation skeletal responses of the rat tibia to different loading cycles and strain magnitudes. While total bone formation rate (BFR) increased in response to 400 cycles at 25 N, at 30 N only 120 cycles were required to significantly increase BFR. These results suggest the minimum number of cycles needed for activation of bone formation depends on the magnitude of the load. The required mechanical load necessary to stimulate osteogenesis also decreases as the strain frequency increases. For instance, a study examining the influence of different strain magnitudes (4.3–18 N) and frequencies (1, 5, and 10 Hz) on bone formation reported that the strain threshold (magnitude) needed to stimulate osteogenesis decreased with increasing load frequency (Hsieh & Turner 2001). Similarly, when small loads were applied to the hind limbs of sheep (30 Hz for 20 min per day, 5 days per week) for 1 year, trabecular bone volume was increased by over 30% in the femur (Rubin *et al.* 2002). This was the result of an increased trabecular number and reduced trabecular spacing. Interestingly, the strain applied to the hind limb of the sheep was similar to vertical oscillation applied at 30 Hz producing 5 microstrains. It is thought that this type of loading (vibration) is typical of the stimulus associated with muscle contraction against gravity (i.e., as during standing) and has been associated with increased bone mineral density (BMD) in older adults with low BMD and poor muscle function (Rubin *et al.* 2002).

The finding that the osteogenic response to loading becomes saturated after relatively few loading cycles has also led to the notion that bone cells become desensitized to prolonged mechanical stimulation (Fig. 9.4). For instance, it is hypothesized that bone cell mechanosensitivity will recover following a period of no loading, and thus short periods of rest may resensitize bone cells to the next bout of loading (Turner & Robling 2003). This has been demonstrated in an experiment in rats where the osteogenic response to loading was increased when loading was separated into short bouts (Robling *et al.* 2002a,b). For instance, applying the same loading stimuli 360 times per day in a single session was less osteogenic than 90 loading cycles delivered over four bouts (Robling *et al.* 2002a,b). Lengthening the rest period also appeared to enhance the osteogenic response; 4 h of rest between loading

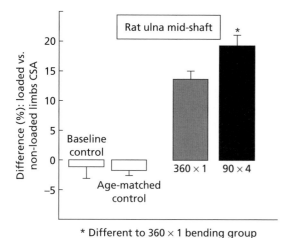

* Different to 360 × 1 bending group

Fig. 9.4 The finding that the osteogenic response to loading becomes saturated after relatively few loading cycles has led to the notion that bone cells become desensitized to prolonged mechanical stimulation. This has been demonstrated in an experiment in rats where the osteogenic response to loading (as assessed by the side-to-side difference in total cross-sectional area (CSA) of the ulna) was increased when loading was separated into short bouts (Robling *et al.* 2002a,b). For instance, applying the same loading stimuli 360 times per day in a single session was less osteogenic than 90 loading cycles delivered in four bouts (Robling *et al.* 2002a,b) .

bouts doubled the osteogenic response and there was almost complete restoration of sensitivity to loading regained after 8 h of recovery (Robling *et al.* 2001). More recent evidence indicates that prolonged periods of rest (i.e., weeks between loading bouts) may be just as effective for enhancing BMC and geometry as continuous training (Saxon & Turner 2005; Saxon *et al.* 2005). Similarly, a low magnitude loading regime that would not normally be considered to be osteogenic appears to be more effective when interspersed with rest. For instance, 10 cycles of low magnitude loading per day interspersed with 10 s rest induced equivalent bone formation as a regimen of 100 cycles per day involving double the strain magnitude and strain rate (Srinivasan *et al.* 2002). The insertion of the 10-s rest interval between each load cycle transformed the low magnitude minimally osteogenic loading regime into a potent osteogenic stimulus.

In summary, the mechanostat explains the feedback mechanism by which bones respond to

loading, but the actual characteristics of a loading regime have important implications of how the bone cell responds. How bone cells respond to dynamic load is dependent on the magnitude, rate, distribution, and frequency of the load, how much rest is given between loading cycles, and the previous loading history. However, the precise characteristics of the strain environment to which bone cells are actually responsive remain undefined, and may be very different from the overall strain data from *in vivo* environments (Ehrlich & Lanyon 2002). The concept that bone cells become desensitized to prolonged loading and that the introduction of rest periods may enhance the osteogenic response has changed the way we think about how the skeleton should be loaded to maximize the mass, structure, and strength of bone.

Assessing bone strength: the clinically important outcome

In lieu of measuring fracture risk reduction directly, whole bone strength, which is influenced by a combination of bone structural and tissue material properties, is the next most important clinical outcome when investigating the efficacy of any exercise intervention on bone. In the absence of non-invasive methods to measure "bone strength" directly, we rely on other indirect measures to provide a surrogate for the breaking strength of bone. In clinical practice, dual energy X-ray absorptiometry (DEXA) is considered the "gold standard" for assessing BMC and areal bone mineral density (aBMD) to diagnose osteoporosis and predict fracture risk in adults. Although aBMD has been shown to be a good predictor of whole bone strength and fracture risk, the measurement of aBMD alone provides little information on other biologically relevant parameters of skeletal health (bone size, shape, and geometry). The importance of these structural parameters is highlighted by data showing that small changes in bone size (i.e., periosteal apposition) can lead to large increases in bone strength with or without a corresponding change in aBMD, because the resistance of bone to bending or torsional forces is related exponentially to its diameter (Orwoll 2003).

Advanced and high precision technology for assessing bone micro-architecture and geometry can be obtained from devices such as magnetic resonance imaging (MRI) and quantitative computed tomography (QCT) or peripheral QCT (pQCT). MRI has the advantage of being non-invasive and can provide precise measures of cortical bone geometry, but is limited by prohibitive costs and accessibility. The advantage of pQCT is its ability to assess the cross-sectional size, shape, and geometry of bone and the apparent volumetric BMD (vBMD) of both cortical and trabecular bone, which can be used to provide an estimate of bone strength. Although the relatively high radiation dose, cost, and inaccessibility of QCT scanners limit their practical application for bone measurements, the introduction of pQCT with a lower radiation dose and cost means that it is suitable for use in young populations. Furthermore, pQCT can provide an assessment of muscle cross-sectional area, which is highly correlated with muscle strength and is often used as a surrogate measure of muscle strength. The latter provides an opportunity to investigate the role of muscle forces and action on skeletal adaptation to exercise, particularly given that muscle forces provide the largest natural strain load to the skeleton in humans during exercise.

Effect of exercise on bone strength during growth

The results of *in vitro* and animal studies provide important links to advance our understanding of the mechanisms involved in the skeletal response to loading—particularly when intrusive procedures are not appropriate in humans. The clinical importance of *in vitro* and animal research, however, is only realized when studies in humans can confirm or validate the findings. *In vitro* studies are limited by the outcome measure being isolated to a change in cell culture (rather than an actual change in skeletal tissue), and the results of animal studies are limited because loading applied is often supraphysiologic and is not applied in a similar direction as expected from locomotion, and bone metabolism in some animals is different to humans. Skeletal research in children has additional problems to

overcome and well-designed and controlled studies are required before any substantial conclusions can be reached.

How does exercise during growth affect bone mineral content, size, and strength?

Paradoxically, during human growth, the only constant is change: change in stature, mass, proportionality, body composition, and shape. These changes at the somatic level induce changes in biomechanical conditions which, coupled with changing patterns of physical activity, provide the growing skeleton with a continually varying mechanical strain environment. Mechanical strains or forces are needed to deform bone, and these forces are predominantly created by muscle contractions, and in weight bearing bones gravitational forces associated with body weight. During growth, bones are continually challenged to adapt to increases in bone length and muscle force. Longitudinal growth increases lever arms and bending moments, which create greater loads on bone (Rauch & Schoenau 2001). Body weight also increases and muscle forces parallel these changes in weight in order to allow effective movement. Thus, growing bone has to adjust its strength continually to keep strains (bone deformation) within the threshold range for modeling and remodeling. The magnitude of deformation will be determined by the characteristics of the deformed object (e.g., material properties, size, and architecture of the bone) and the force acting on it (mass times acceleration). Exercise training can increase muscle force and subsequently subject the skeleton to higher loads. Exercise may also increase muscle mass, thus further increasing gravitational forces acting on the weight-bearing bones. Thus, during growth the increase in bone length and muscle mass (and strength) and body mass (only important for weight-bearing bones) all add to the maximal forces to which bones adapt their structure and strength. Exercise has the potential to further increase peak muscle forces acting on bones, which leads to a proportional adaptation of bone strength (predominantly resulting from periosteal apposition and increase in trabecular thickness).

In the long term, intense exercise training during growth has been shown to lead to large increases in peak BMC (5–40%) (Huddleston et al. 1980; Bass et al. 1998). Large increases in cortical thickness as a result of lifelong exercise were first demonstrated by comparing the playing with the non-playing arm of tennis players (Huddleston et al. 1980). Higher BMC of similar magnitudes has also been reported in young elite athletes (Bass et al. 1998). Selection bias is unlikely to explain the higher aBMD because the benefits were specific to the site being loaded, and greater changes were observed in prospectively derived data. These data in elite athletes provide us with a model of what is possible rather than probable in normally active children. The results of prospective and retrospective cohort studies are supportive of these studies of elite athletes (Slemenda et al. 1994). Children and adolescents who were physically active (but not elite athletes) accrued more BMC than their sedentary peers (Cooper et al. 1995; Bailey et al. 1999). However, there may be selection bias in these studies; children who are bigger and stronger are likely to be more successful in sport. Intervention studies in pre- and peri-pubertal girls and boys have been mostly of short duration (8–11 months) (Morris et al. 1997; Bradney et al. 1998; Heinonen et al. 2000; McKay et al. 2000; Petit et al. 2002; Van Langendonck et al. 2003); most were controlled but not all were randomized. The interventions included either extra physical education classes or exercise additional to physical education classes. These interventions resulted in a 1.3–5% greater increase in aBMD in the legs. Findings were equivocal in the spine, with only two studies reporting an increase in BMC at this site. More recently, several studies have shown that higher frequency and/or shorter bouts of exercise appear to result in a similar osteogenic effect to previous studies (Saxon et al. 2000; Iuliano-Burns et al. 2003; McKay et al. 2005).

The osteogenic benefit achieved from exercise during growth appears to be dependent on the stage of maturation of the individual. For instance, up to four times greater skeletal benefits were observed in girls who exercised before, rather than after menarche (Kannus et al. 1995). However, in this study it could not be determined whether the skeletal benefits were achieved during the pre- or peripubertal years or were the combination of both stages of puberty (Bass 2000; MacKelvie et al. 2002). While large gains in aBMD were achieved in elite prepubertal gymnasts relative to controls, a study comparing differences in the playing and the non-playing arm of non-elite female tennis players reported that no differences between arms were evident until Tanner stage 3 (Haapasalo et al. 1998). In this study, the older players had been involved in tennis longer and were training more, which suggests that this difference was more a result of sampling bias rather than stage of puberty. Further research is required where carefully designed and well-controlled studies are conducted specifically to assess the osteogenic response in response to exercise at different stages of puberty in girls and boys.

In addition to increases in BMC, exercise before puberty is important because of the associated changes in bone geometry that translate to much greater increases in bone strength than an increase in BMC alone. The effects of physical loading on bone geometry in humans were first determined from the analysis of X-rays of the arms of tennis players (Ruff et al. 1994). In this study, the pattern of humeral hypertrophy was different between the players. Some showed an increase in all cortical dimensions, others had a narrowed medullary cavity, while others had enlarged periosteal and endocortical diameters. These characteristics of the cortical dimensions—periosteal and endocortical diameters, and the cross-sectional bone shape—may have been determined by the time in life when the players began their training. Analysis of three players showed that the player who started training at an early age had greater periosteal expansion than the two who had started later (Ruff et al. 1994). Limitations of this study include the retrospective study design, there was an overlap in playing years between the players, males and females were grouped together, and no assessments were made during childhood or adolescence.

From these data, Ruff proposed that loading increases bone apposition at the surfaces undergoing apposition because of growth. Consistent with Ruff's proposal is the finding that prepubertal gymnasts had a larger total bone area (periosteal expansion) of the forearm despite a smaller stature (Dyson *et al.* 1997). While exercise in adult tennis players resulted in no detectable change to the total bone area of the radius, it did result in thicker trabeculae (Ashizawa *et al.* 1999). Exercise also led to medullary contraction at the tibia in military recruits (Margulies *et al.* 1986). Data in competitive female tennis players also support this hypothesis (Bass *et al.* 2002); loading resulted in increased bone formation at both the periosteal and the endocortical surfaces when apposition was occurring at these surfaces as a result of growth (Fig. 9.5). However, there was heterogeneity in the response to loading at the endocortical surface along the length of the bone when growth-related resorption was occurring at this surface; at the mid-humerus, loading resulted in increased expansion but there was no detectable effect at the distal humerus (Bass *et al.* 2002).

It is thought that exercise may preferentially affect the surface of bone that is undergoing apposition during growth. Periosteal apposition dominates during the prepubertal years in boys and girls. During puberty, periosteal expansion continues in boys but ceases in girls as estrogen reduces periosteal apposition (Turner *et al.* 1989). Endocortical contraction occurs late in puberty in girls; in contrast, there is little or no endosteal contraction evident in boys (Garn 1970). Therefore, exercise should enhance bone size when undertaken before puberty in boys and girls. During puberty, exercise should enhance periosteal apposition in boys and in girls. Exercise late in puberty (and post-puberty) should increase endocortical contraction in girls and periosteal apposition in boys. These hypotheses have not been rigorously tested in humans as studies to test these hypotheses are difficult to undertake. However, the outcomes are important because apposition of bone on the periosteal (outer) surface of cortical bone is a more effective means of increasing the bending and torsional strength of bone than acquisition of bone on the endocortical (inner) surface (i.e., a greater external bone size increases load-bearing capacity) (Turner & Burr 1993). Furthermore, the implications are that there may be a much smaller window of opportunity in girls compared to boys if the change in the external bone size resulting from exercise is limited to pubertal growth in girls but not boys.

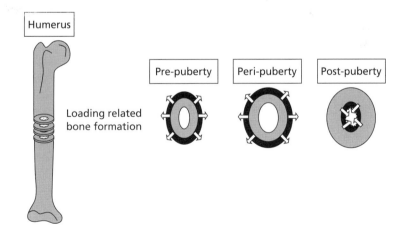

Fig. 9.5 The characteristics of the cortical bone dimensions in adulthood—periosteal and endocortical diameters, and the cross-sectional bone shape—is likely to be a reflection of the timing and duration of exposure to exercise. For instance, it has been hypothesized that loading during growth will result in increased adult bone mineral content (BMC) at the surface undergoing accrual during childhood. Data in competitive pre-, peri-, and post-pubertal female tennis players show that loading resulted in increased bone formation (shown in black) at the periosteal surface in the pre- and peri-pubertal years and at the endocortical surface in the post-pubertal years. After Bass *et al.* (2002).

Difficulties measuring the osteogenic response in children

The effects of exercise on skeletal development during growth are difficult to study because of the complex interaction between genetic, hormonal, and lifestyle factors on bone metabolism during growth, and the sometimes narrow time-frame for study between stages of maturation. Heterogeneity in the way bone develops from region to region and between sites also complicates the interpretation of studies in children. Children of a similar chronologic age may not be at a similar stage of skeletal or sexual maturation. Children from different ethnic origins may also have different temporal patterns of growth and maturation (Wong *et al.* 1996; Huen *et al.* 1997). Thus, when investigating the effect of exercise in children, it is important they are matched by gender, ethnicity, bone age, chronologic age, and stage of maturation of the site being studied (e.g., axial or appendicular skeleton). As the changes in skeletal size and mass occur rapidly during growth, even a slight difference in age (4–5 months) between controls and exercise groups may produce marked differences between the groups attributable to mismatching rather than exercise. Further, it is difficult if not impossible to account for the effects on bone in children with different loading histories associated with exercise among different developmental or maturity groups. These effects are most pronounced in the transition between pubertal stages, making it difficult to detect a critical or sensitive developmental stage for the introduction of exercise.

In addition to the aforementioned difficulties encountered with matching children, it is also difficult to equate the exercise-related mechanical loads on skeletons of different sizes during infancy, childhood, or adolescence. If the hypothesis is that exercise has a greater effect on bone before than during puberty, what load should be imposed in the two groups who differ by age and bone size to test this hypothesis? It is also difficult to determine how changes should be expressed. If there is a change, should this be expressed in absolute terms, percentage terms, or as standardized deviations? An absolute increase in an older child will be less in percentage terms than the same increase in a younger child

with a smaller skeleton. In studies comparing boys and girls, if matching is carried out by pubertal stage, chronologic age will differ; if matching is carried out by chronologic age then pubertal staging and skeletal maturation will differ. The correct approach will depend on the question being asked concerning gender differences in response to exercise, but this issue needs to be considered in the study design. The same issues arise in comparison of ethnic groups in whom the age at onset of puberty, duration of pubertal stages, and skeletal maturation patterns may differ (Wong *et al.* 1996; Huen *et al.* 1997). Furthermore, changes reported as an aBMD may be the result of changes in bone size, BMC, or both. Thus, while changes during growth are large and easy to detect, the variability in skeletal growth and maturation necessitate the need for large sample sizes and meticulous attention to matching for stage of maturation and development.

In summary, the challenges in studying the skeletal response to exercise in growing humans result from the length of time required to detect a change in BMC or structure (compared with cellular studies), the ability to maintain compliance to exercise, difficulty in estimating the load placed on bones, and accounting for different background loading histories (all while matching for the age, gender, and hormonal status of the individuals). Few studies in children or adults have attempted to record loading history accurately, and little is known about the typical loading history of children involved in their everyday activities.

Are benefits maintained into later life— when fractures occur?

A 10% increase in peak BMC is estimated to halve the risk of fracture and delay the development of osteoporosis by 13 years (Cumming *et al.* 1993; Hernandez *et al.* 2003). There is ample evidence that intense exercise during growth (but not adulthood) could potentially lead to increases in aBMD of 10% or more. However, there is a paucity of evidence that demonstrates that this adaptation is maintained throughout growth or even into adulthood, let alone into old age when fractures occur. Thus, while a goal of a 10% increase in peak BMC is achievable with exercise during growth, these benefits could not be considered to be clinically important unless they are maintained into adulthood. The site-specific higher bone density of gymnasts retired for up to 20 years suggests that this may be the case (Bass *et al.* 1998). Whether these residual benefits are maintained into later life when fractures occur is not known. The study to test this question will never be carried out because of the long time interval between exposure (exercise during growth) and outcome (fracture in the elderly). However, the limited data in 70- to 80-year-old retired athletes suggests that the effects may be eroded in those who have substantially decreased their training volumes (Karlsson *et al.* 2000).

The level of activity during growth and adulthood may be the key factor influencing the maintenance of any residual skeletal benefits. Lifetime tennis players aged 70–84 years who continued to play at a lower level of intensity than during youth were reported to have 4–7% higher radial BMC than controls (Huddleston *et al.* 1980). Retired soccer players also have higher aBMD during the first 10–20 years after cessation of sport, but aBMD lower than active soccer players (Karlsson *et al.* 2000). The correlation between proximal femoral aBMD in retired male soccer players and current activity (r = ~0.25) suggests continued exercise may maintain some of the skeletal benefits from sports participation during youth (Karlsson *et al.* 2000). There is also evidence suggesting that while exercise-induced gains in aBMD are reduced after retirement from sports, some benefit may be maintained as former male older athletes have fewer fractures than matched controls (Nordstrom *et al.* 2005).

The effects of exercise during growth may be more permanent than adaptive changes in adulthood. For instance, modeling changes during growth (i.e., changes in bone size and shape achieved by exercise) may be permanent whereas those derived by remodeling, such as endocortical accrual, or perhaps trabecular thickening, may be lost. Slowing of bone loss or modest increments in aBMD induced by exercise started in adulthood are likely to be the result of filling remodeling transients which reverse entirely when exercise is stopped. Evidence of a larger bone size (humerus, radius shafts, and distal humerus) resulting from exercise during growth was demonstrated in adult tennis players (Haapasalo *et al.* 2000); this was not accompanied by a change in vBMD. These observations fit with the notion that exercise produces enlargement of bone size that is permanent after retirement but any associated endocortical or trabecular apposition may be lost or partly lost. Further research is required to determine how exercise affects bone architecture (particularly bone size) in females and males during different stages of growth. It also needs to be determined if a change in bone architecture achieved during growth is maintained into adulthood.

In summary, an elevated aBMD is retained for many years after cessation of high intensity exercise during growth; it is not known if the benefits are maintained three to five decades after retirement. Continued activity at lower levels after retirement may preserve skeletal benefits likely to be lost with sedentary behavior. Changes in bone size may be preserved despite reduced levels of activity. Thus, further studies in this area are needed to define the distinct structural changes produced by exercise during growth and their persistence once exercise is stopped. As a corollary, if the effects of exercise during youth can be maintained, in part or totally, by lesser levels of exercise in later life, then information is needed to define the level of exercise needed to sustain a biologically worthwhile skeletal benefit. This is a pivotal area of research that underpins future decisions regarding the role of exercise during growth for improved bone health in the individual and in the community.

Conclusions and future directions

Childhood and adolescence is a critical time when the skeleton develops and its shape and mass is sculptured to be suitable to meet the long-term needs of life. Exercise is the primary driving force behind these adaptive changes in the skeleton during growth. Research in athletes shows that intense exercise during growth can lead to clinically important increases in aBMD and bone strength. Residual benefits appear to be maintained into older age when fractures occur. Research into normally active children has shown that only small benefits are obtained from short-term exercise programs. More research is required to investigate the effect of exercise on the structural properties of bone during growth before precise exercise prescription can be recommended for exercise during growth for improved bone strength in adulthood and older age. Specific areas of research that are needed to contribute to the knowledge base underpinning these recommendations include the following:

• Clarification of whether or not there is a developmentally sensitive period for optimization of the skeleton to exercise.

• Clarification of the characteristically important features of exercise that may be osteogenic for children and whether these vary by developmental stage.

• Clarification of the role of muscle forces and the biomechanical sequella of these forces in the generation of bone strain and thus their importance for osteogenic adaptation—is it all related to muscle forces or are other forces just as important?

• Refinement of measurement techniques to noninvasively assess gross and microstructural adaptations more precisely

• Determination of how the muscle–joint–bone unit responds to exercise—is what is good for bone equally good for muscle and joint development?

References

Ashizawa, N., Nonaka, K., Michikami, S., et al. (1999) Tomographical description of tennis-loaded radius: reciprocal relation between bone size and volumetric BMD. *Journal of Applied Physiology* **86**, 1347–1351.

Bailey, D., McKay, H., Mirwald, R.L., Crocker, P.R.E. & Faulkner, R.A. (1999) A six year longitudinal study of the relationship of physical activity to bone mineral accrual in growing children. The University of Saskatchewan Bone Mineral Accrual Study. *Journal of Bone and Mineral Research* **14**, 1672–1679.

Baron, R. (1990) Anatomy and ultrastructure of bone. In: *Primer on Metabolic Bone Diseases and Disorders of Mineral Metabolism* (Favus, M.J., ed.) American Society for Bone and Mineral Research, CA: 3–7.

Bass, S., Pearce, G., Bradney, M., et al. (1998) Exercise before puberty may confer residual benefits in bone density in adulthood: studies in active prepubertal and retired female gymnasts. *Journal of Bone and Mineral Research* **13**, 500–507.

Bass, S., Saxon, L., Daly, R., et al. (2002) The effect of mechanical loading on the size and shape of cortical bone in pre-, peri and post pubertal girls: A study in tennis players. *Journal of Bone and Mineral Research* **17**, 2274–2280.

Bass, S.L. (2000) The prepubertal years: a uniquely opportune stage of growth when the skeleton is most responsive to exercise? *Sports Medicine* **30**, 73–78.

Bradney, M., Pearce, G., Naughton, G., et al. (1998) Moderate exercise during growth in prepubertal boys: changes in BMC, size, volumetric density, and bone strength: a controlled prospective study. *Journal of Bone and Mineral Research* **13**, 1814–1821.

Burr, D.B. (1992) Orthopedic principles of skeletal growth, modeling and remodeling. In: Carlson, D.S. and Goldstein, S.A. (eds.) *Bone Biodynamics in Orthodontic and Orthopedic Treatment.* Center for Human Growth and Development, Ann Arbor, USA: University of Michigan: 15–49.

Burr, D., Schaffler, M., Yang, K.H., et al. (1989) Skeletal change in response to altered strain environments: Is woven bone a response to elevated strain? *Bone* **10**, 223–233.

Burr, D.B. (1997) Muscle strength, BMC, and age-related bone loss. *Journal of Bone and Mineral Research* **12**, 1547–1551.

Burr, D.B., Robling, A.G. & Turner, C.H. (2002) Effects of biomechanical stress on bones in animals. *Bone* **30**, 781–786.

Cheng, S., Sipla, S., Taffe, D., Puolakka, J. & Suominen, H. (2002) Change in BMC distribution induced by hormone replacement therapy and high impact physical exercise in post-menopausal women. *Bone* **31**, 126–135.

Cointry, G.R., Capozza, R.F., Negri, A.L., Roldan, E.J. & Ferretti, J.L. (2004) Biomechanical background for a noninvasive assessment of bone strength and muscle-bone interactions. *Journal of Musculoskeletal and Neuronal Interactions* **4**, 1–11.

Cooper, C., Cawley, M., Bhalla, A., et al. (1995) Childhood growth, physical activity, and peak BMC in women. *Journal of Bone and Mineral Research* **10**, 940–947.

Cullen, D.M., Smith, R.T. & Akhter, M.P. (2001) Bone-loading response varies with strain magnitude and cycle number. *Journal of Applied Physiology* **91**, 1971–1976.

Cumming, S.R., Black, D.M., Nevitt, M.C., et al. (1993) Bone density at various sites for prediction of hip fracture. The Study of Osteoporotic Fracture Research Group. *Lancet* **341**, 962–963.

Dhamrait, S.S., James, L., Brull, D.J., et al. (2003) Cortical bone resorption during exercise is interleukin-6 genotype-dependent. *European Journal of Applied Physiology* **89**, 21–25.

Duncan, R.L. & Turner, C.H. (1995) Mechanotransduction and the functional response of bone to mechanical strain. *Calcified Tissue International* **57**, 344–358.

Dyson, K., Blimkie, C.J.R., Davison, S., Webber, C.E. & Adachi, J.D. (1997) Gymnastic training and bone density in pre-adolescent females. *Medicine and Science in Sports and Exercise* **29**, 443–450.

Ehrlich, P.J. & Lanyon, L.E. (2002) Mechanical strain and bone cell function: a review. *Osteoporosis International* **13**, 688–700.

Frost, H.M. (1987) Bone "mass" and the "mechanostat": a proposal. *Anatomical Record* **219**, 1–9.

Frost, H.M. (1992) Perspectives: the role of changes in mechanical usage set points in the pathogenesis of osteoporosis. *Journal of Bone and Mineral Research* **7**, 253–262.

Frost, H.M. (1997) On our age-related bone loss: insights from a new paradigm. *Journal of Bone and Mineral Research* **12**, 1539–1546.

Frost, H.M. & Schonau, E. (2000) The "muscle-bone unit" in children and adolescents: a 2000 overview. *Journal of Pediatric Endocrinology and Metabolism* **13**, 571–590.

Garn, S. (1970) *The Earlier Gain and Later Loss of Cortical Bone.* Charles C. Thomas, Spingfield, IL.

Haapasalo, H., Kannus, P., Sievanen, H., *et al.* (1998) Effect of long-term unilateral activity on bone mineral density of female junior tennis players. *Journal of Bone and Mineral Research* **13**, 310–319.

Haapasalo, H., Kontulainen, S., Sievanen, H., Kannus, P., Jarvinen, M. & Vuori, I. (2000) Exercise-induced bone gain is due to enlargement in bone size without a change in volumetric bone density: a peripheral quantitative computed tomography study of the upper arms of male tennis players. *Bone* **27**, 351–357.

Heikkinen, J., Kyllonen, E., Kurttila-Matero, E., *et al.* (1997) HRT and exercise: effects on bone density, muscle strength and lipid metabolism. A placebo controlled 2-year prospective trial on two estrogen-progestin regimes in healthy premenopausal women. *Maturitas* **26**, 139–149.

Heinonen, A., Sievanen, H., Kannus, P., Oja, P., Pasanen, M. & Vuori, I. (2000) High-impact exercise and bones of growing girls: a 9-month controlled trial. *Osteoporosis International* **11**, 1010–1017.

Hernandez, C.J., Beaupre, G.S. & Carter, D.R. (2003) A theoretical analysis of the relative influences of peak BMD, age-related bone loss and menopause on the development of osteoporosis. *Osteoporosis International* **14**, 843–847.

Hsieh, Y.F. & Turner, C.H. (2001) Effects of loading frequency on mechanically induced bone formation. *Journal of Bone and Mineral Research* **16**, 918–924.

Huddleston, A.L., Rockwell, D., Kulund, D.N. & Harrison, R.B. (1980) BMC in lifetime tennis athletes. *Journal of the American Medical Association* **244**, 1107–1109.

Huen, K., Leung, S., Lau, J., Cheung, A., Leung, N. & Chiu, M. (1997) Secular trend in the sexual maturation of Southern Chinese girls. *Acta Paediatrica* **86**, 1121–1124.

Huiskes, R., Ruimerman, R., van Lenthe, G.H. & Janssen, J.D. (2000) Effects of mechanical forces on maintenance and adaptation of form in trabecular bone. *Nature* **405**, 704–706.

Iuliano-Burns, S., Saxon, L., Naughton, G., Gibbons, K. & Bass, S.L. (2003) Regional specificity of exercise and calcium during skeletal growth in girls: a randomized controlled trial. *Journal of Bone and Mineral Research* **18**, 156–162.

Kannus, P., Haapasalo, H., Sankelo, M., *et al.* (1995) Effect of starting age of physical activity on BMC in the dominant arm of tennis and squash players. *Annals of Internal Medicine* **123**, 27–31.

Karlsson, M., Linden, C., Karlsson, C., Johnell, O., Obrant, K. & Seeman, E. (2000) Exercise during growth and bone mineral density and fractures in old age. *Lancet* **355**, 469–470.

Khosla, S., Moedder, U.I. & Syed, F.A. (2006) Estrogen receptor beta: the antimechanostat? *Bone* **38**, 289.

Kohrt, W.M., Snead, D.B., Slatopolsky, E. & Birge, S.J. (1995) Additive effects of weight-bearing exercise and estrogen on mineral density in older women. *Journal of Bone and Mineral Research* **10**, 1303–1311.

Little, R., Carulli, J., Del Mastro, R., *et al.* (2002) A mutation in the LDL receptor-related protein 5 gene results in the autosomal dominant high-bone-mass trait. *American Journal of Human Genetics* **70**, 11–19.

MacKelvie, K., Khan, K. & McKay, H. (2002) Is there a critical period for bone response to weight-bearing exercise in children and adolescents? A systematic review. *British Journal of Sports Medicine* **36**, 250–257.

Margulies, J.Y., Simkin, A., Leichter, I., *et al.* (1986) Effect of intense physical activity on the bone-mineral content in the lower limbes of young adults. *Journal of Bone and Joint Surgery* **68-A**, 1090–1093.

McKay, H., Petit, M.A., Schutz, R.W., Prior, J.C., Barr, S.I. & Khan, K.M. (2000) Augmented trochanteric bone mineral density after modified physical education classes: A randomised school-based exercise intervention study in prepubescent and early pubescent children. *Journal of Pediatrics* **136**, 156–162.

McKay, H.A., Maclean, L., Petit, M.A., *et al.* (2005) "Bounce at the Bell": a novel program of short bouts of exercise improves proximal femur BMC in early pubertal children. *British Journal of Sports Medicine* **39**, 521–526.

Morishima, A., Grumbach, M.M., Simpson, E.R., Fisher, C. & Qin, K. (1995) Aromatase deficiency in male and female siblings caused by a novel mutation and the physiological role of estrogens. *Journal of Clinical Endocrinology and Metabolism* **80**, 3689–3698.

Morris, F.L., Naughton, G.A., Gibbs, J.L., Carlson, J.S. & Wark, J.D. (1997) Prospective ten-month exercise intervention in premenarcheal girls: positive effects on bone and lean mass. *Journal of Bone and Mineral Research* **12**, 1453–1462.

Nakamura, O., Ishii, T., Ando, Y., *et al.* (2002) Potential role of vitamin D receptor gene polymorphism in determining bone phenotype in young male athletes. *Journal of Applied Physiology* **93**, 1973–1979.

Nordstrom, A., Karlsson, C., Nyquist, F., Olsson, T., Nordstrom, P. & Karlsson, M. (2005) Bone loss and fracture risk after reduced physical activity. *Journal of Bone and Mineral Research* **20**, 202–207.

Omasu, F., Kitagawa, J., Koyama, K., *et al.* (2004) The influence of VDR genotype and exercise on ultrasound parameters in young adult Japanese women. *Journal of Physiological Anthropology and Applied Human Science* **23**, 49–55.

Orwoll, E.S. (2003) Toward an expanded understanding of the role of the periosteum in skeletal health. *Journal of Bone and Mineral Research* **18**, 949–954.

Petit, M.A., McKay, H.A., MacKelvie, K.J., Heinonen, A., Khan, K.M. & Beck, T.J. (2002) A randomized school-based jumping intervention confers site and maturity-specific benefits on bone structural properties in girls: a hip structural analysis study. *Journal of Bone and Mineral Research* **17**, 363–372.

Prince, R., Smith, M., Dick, I.M., *et al.* (1991) Prevention of postmenopausal osteoporosis. A comparative study of exercise, calcium supplementation, and hormone-replacement therapy. *New England Journal of Medicine* **325**, 1189–1195.

Rauch, F. & Schoenau, E. (2001) The developing bone: slave or master of its cells and molecules? *Pediatric Research* **50**, 309–314.

Robling, A.G., Burr, D.B. & Turner, C.H. (2001) Recovery periods restore mechanosensitivity to dynamically loaded bone. *Journal of Experimental Biology* **204**, 3389–3399.

Robling, A.G., Hinant, F.M., Burr, D.B. & Turner, C.H. (2002a) Improved bone structure and strength after long-term mechanical loading is greatest if loading is separated into short bouts. *Journal of Bone and Mineral Research* **17**, 1545–1554.

Robling, A.G., Hinant, F.M., Burr, D.B. & Turner, C.H. (2002b) Shorter, more frequent mechanical loading sessions enhance BMC. *Medicine and Science in Sports and Exercise* **34**, 196–202.

Rubin, C., Turner, A.S., Muller, R., *et al.* (2002) Quantity and quality of trabecular bone in the femur are enhanced by a strongly anabolic, noninvasive mechanical intervention. *Journal of Bone and Mineral Research* **17**, 349–357.

Rubin, C.T. & Lanyon, L.E. (1984) Regulation of bone formation by applied dynamic loads. *Journal of Bone and Joint Surgery* **66-A**, 397–402.

Ruff, C.B., Walker, A. & Trinkaus, E. (1994) Postcranial robusticity in Homo. III: Ontogeny. *American Journal of Physical Anthropology* **93**, 35–54.

Saxon, L., Iuliano-Bruns, S., Naughton, G. & Bass, S. (2000) The osteotrophic response to different mechanical loading regimes in pre and early pubertal girls. *Journal of Bone and Mineral Research* **17** (Supplement 1), S295.

Saxon, L.K., Robling, A.G., Alam, I. & Turner, C.H. (2005) Mechanosensitivity of the rat skeleton decreases after a long period of loading, but is improved with time off. *Bone* **36**, 454–464.

Saxon, L.K. & Turner, C.H. (2005) Estrogen receptor beta: the antimechanostat? *Bone* **36**, 185–192.

Slemenda, C.W., Reister, T.K., Hui, S.L., Miller, J.Z., Christian, J.C. & Johnston, C.C. (1994) Influences of skeletal mineralization in children and adolescents: Evidence for varying effects of sexual maturation and physical activity. *Journal of Pediatrics* **125**, 201–207.

Smith, E.P., Boyd, J., Frank, G.R., *et al.* (1994) Estrogen resistance caused by a mutation in the estrogen-receptor gene in a man. *New England Journal of Medicine* **331**, 1056–1061.

Smith, E.P. & Korach, K.S. (1996) Oestrogen receptor deficiency: consequences for growth. *Acta Paediatrica Supplement* **417**, 39–43.

Srinivasan, S., Weimer, D.A., Agans, S.C., Bain, S.D. & Gross, T.S. (2002) Low-magnitude mechanical loading becomes osteogenic when rest is inserted between each load cycle. *Journal of Bone and Mineral Research* **17**, 1613–1620.

Suuriniemi, M., Mahonen, A., Kovanen, V., *et al.* (2004) Association between exercise and pubertal BMD is modulated by estrogen receptor alpha genotype. *Journal of Bone and Mineral Research* **19**, 1758–1765.

Tajima, O., Ashizawa, N., Ishii, T., *et al.* (2000) Interaction of the effects between vitamin D receptor polymorphism and exercise training on bone metabolism. *Journal of Applied Physiology* **88**, 1271–1276.

Turner, C.H. (1998) Three rules for bone adaptation to mechanical stimuli. *Bone* **23**, 399–407.

Turner, C.H. (1999) Toward a mathematical description of bone biology: the principle of cellular accommodation. *Calcified Tissue International* **65**, 466–71.

Turner, C.H. (2000) Muscle–bone interactions, revisited. *Bone* **27**, 339–340.

Turner, C.H. & Burr, D.B. (1993) Basic biomechanical measurements of bone: a tutorial. *Bone* **14**, 595–608.

Turner, C.H. & Robling, A.G. (2003) Designing exercise regimens to increase bone strength. *Exercise and Sport Sciences Reviews* **31**, 45–50.

Turner, R.T., Hannon, K.S., Demers, L.M., Buchanan, J. & Bell, N.H. (1989) Differential effects of gonadal function on bone histomorphometry in male and female rats. *Journal of Bone and Mineral Research* **4**, 557–563.

Umemura, Y., Ishiko, T., Yamauchi, T., Kurono, M. & Mashiko, S. (1997) Five jumps per day increase BMC and breaking force in rats. *Journal of Bone and Mineral Research* **12**, 1480–1485.

Van Langendonck, L., Claessens, A.L., Vlietinck, R., Derom, C. & Beunen, G. (2003) Influence of weight-bearing exercises on bone acquisition in prepubertal monozygotic female twins: a randomized controlled prospective study. *Calcified Tissue International* **72**, 666–674.

Weinbaum, S., Cowin, S.C. & Zeng, Y. (1994) A model for the excitation of osteocytes by mechanical loading-induced bone fluid shear stresses. *Journal of Biomechanics* **27**, 339–360.

Wong, G., Leung, S., Law, W., Yeung, V., Lau, J. & Yeung, W. (1996) Secular trend in the sexual maturation of southern Chinese boys. *Acta Paediatrica* **85**, 620–621.

Chapter 10

Physical Activity in Youth: Health Implications for the Future

HAN C.G. KEMPER

In 1994, the American College of Sport Medicine (ACSM) organized an international consensus conference on physical activity and developed guidelines for youth based on scientific evidence related to the amount of physical activity needed to affect selected health variables. Nine review papers were used to examine the dose–response relationship between physical activity and health variables, and to identify a level or amount of physical activity that reliably improved health outcomes. The conference participants published two recommendations for the general youth population (Sallis 1994):

1 All children and adolescents should be physically active daily, or nearly every day, as part of play, sports, work, transportation, recreation, physical education, or planned exercise, in the context of family, school, and community activities. The activities should be enjoyable, involve a variety of muscle groups, and include some weight-bearing activities. The intensity or duration of the physical activity is probably less important than the fact the energy is expended and a habit of daily activity is established.

2 Children and adolescents should engage in three or more sessions per week of physical activities that last 20 min or more and require physical activities of moderate to vigorous intensity. These activities are those that require large muscle groups.

Since then, guidelines were issued also in Europe to propose recommendations for the minimal amount of physical activity in youth. Biddle *et al.* (1998) published a policy framework for young people and health-enhancing physical activity. Based on the North American and British guidelines,

in the Netherlands a consensus was reached in a recommendation for healthy physical activity in youth (Kemper *et al.* 2000). New in this guideline was the definition of the intensity of the physical activities in terms of metabolic rate expressed in multiples of resting metabolic rate (METs). The following guidelines were proposed:

1 All children and adolescents should be physically active on a daily base for 1 h with moderate intensive physical activities (5–8 MET). Examples are: walking, biking, climbing stairs (5 MET), swimming and running (6–7 MET), and team games such as basket ball, soccer, and field hockey (8 MET).

2 At least two times per week these physical activities should to be directed to enhance physical fitness (muscle force, flexibility, endurance, and coordination). Examples are: callisthenics, judo, athletics (jumping, throwing) for muscle force; rowing, cycling long distances, running for endurance; yoga, gymnastics, taekwondo for flexibility; all ball games for coordination.

All these guidelines and norms are based on consensus from experts in the field of pediatric exercise, but—naturally—consensus is not as valid as conclusions drawn from randomized controlled trials.

In all existing guidelines the notion of daily duration and the indicated minimal intensity of the proposed physical activities suggest a threshold of daily physical activity for a healthy life. This threshold has never been proven in experimental studies (Twisk 2001). In addition, most of the expected health effects are related to the prevention of cardiovascular and respiratory diseases but not cancer, obesity, or osteoporosis.

In this chapter the following issues are addressed:
1 Current physical activity patterns of youth (see also Bar-Or & Rowland 2004);
2 Stability of physical activity patterns during youth;
3 Methods of objective measurements of physical activities that can be used in youth (Trost 2001);
4 Feasibility and effectiveness of interventions and promotion programs to increase the daily physical activity patterns of youth (Kahn *et al.* 2002); and
5 New directions to change the inactivity patterns of youth in the future (for review see Epstein & Roemmich 2001).

Physical activity in youth

It has long been recognized that physical activity is important during the growing years if normal growth and development of children and adolescents are to be maintained (Bar-Or 1983). Children are generally thought to be naturally physically active. Indeed, up to one or two generations ago, physical activity was a natural part of daily life for most children. However, this is no longer true. One may well ask whether children and adolescents now get the physical activity required for a healthy development. The necessity for physical activity has been greatly reduced, owing to mechanization and automation in daily life (school, work, leisure, transport).

In recent years, the physical activity of youngsters has been a subject of great concern to health officials (Gezondheidsraad 2003). The prevalence of overweight and obesity in children is increasing alarmingly which is connected to a positive energy balance caused by a decrease in physical activity while energy intake remains constant.

Furthermore, physical inactivity is an important risk factor for coronary heart disease. Atherosclerosis starts soon after birth (Montoye 1985). It is often suggested that a sufficient amount and intensity of regular physical activity could decelerate this process (Powel *et al.* 1987). However, a prospective intervention study comparing a large number of physically active children with a randomized group of physically inactive children over a very long period into the adult age at which chronic cardiovascular diseases can be expected, has never been

conducted and apparently cannot be carried out for ethical reasons (Mednick & Baert 1981).

One way out of this dilemma is to measure habitual physical activity on a longitudinal basis in a large population of youth and to group individual subjects according to their observed physical activity patterns (Rutenfranz *et al.* 1974; Mirwald *et al.* 1981; Kemper 2004a). Another possibility is an experimental longitudinal study such as the Trois Rivieres Physical Education Study by Jequier *et al.* (1977) in Canada in which the effects of additional physical education on health and fitness were measured in comparison to control classes over a couple of years.

These studies show inconsistent results. Kemper (2004b) showed in his Amsterdam Growth and Health Longitudinal Study (AGAHLS) small (body composition, bone density) or non-significant "effects" ($\dot{V}o_{2max}$) in youth aged 13–36 years, while most of the effects in the Trois Rivieres Physical Education Study are damped at adult age (Shepard *et al.* 2005). So, there is—up till now—no strong scientific proof that physical activity in youth enhances health at adult age.

It has been proposed that critical developmental periods exist that determine whether individuals will later lead a physically active life (Masironi & Denolin 1985):

• At the age of 4–12 years, children first enter school and lose a considerable amount of playing time;

• At about age 12 years, children enter secondary school with further restriction of free time by homework, computer games, and the Internet;

• At the age of 15–16 years, adolescents in industrialized countries shift from bicycles to motorcycles and use mobile telephones instead of visits to their friends;

• From age 18 years on, young people further change to automobiles.

The consequence of the development described above is a gradual age-dependent decrease of the daily energy expenditure from physical activities. This is illustrated by cross-sectional data from total daily energy expenditure of boys and girls from different studies in youth from 6 to 18 years (Fig. 10.1) (Rowland 1990).

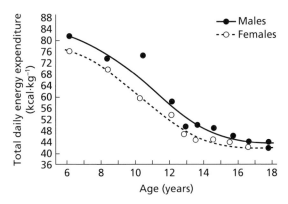

Fig. 10.1 Total daily energy expenditure of boys and girls aged 6–18 years; the data are from different studies in different countries. Redrawn after Rowland (1990).

Total daily energy expenditure (in kcal·kg body weight^{-1}) diminishes by almost 50% between 6 and 15 years in both sexes. Figure 10.1 also illustrates that, at all ages, boys are 10% more physically active than girls. Although these data are from different populations in the world and also cross-sectional in nature, this trend is very clear. The sex differences in physical activity are seen in all studies and they cannot simply be explained by differences in body mass, body build, or body composition before the age of puberty, because boys and girls do not differ in that respect. Differences in the type of physical activities may explain part of the gender differences because boys choose more sports with a higher intensity (e.g., ball games) than girls (e.g., gymnastics, dance).

Evaluating the natural history of physical activity in children and adolescents requires valid and accurate measurement methods. Daily physical activity, however, is a difficult lifestyle parameter to measure, because the measurement itself interferes with the normal physical activity pattern of the child. Also, children's activities change from day to day, week to week, and season to season.

Physical activity epidemiology in youth

Studies of the epidemiology of physical activity in youth address research questions such as the description of the level of physical activity in a young population, comparison of levels of physical activity among youth populations, determination of factors that are associated with participation in physical activity, and the investigation of the association between youth physical activity and the risk for adult chronic diseases such as coronary heart disease, stroke, diabetes, cancer, osteoporosis, and obesity.

The randomized controlled trial (RCT) is the gold standard of research designs for testing a research hypothesis about the possible relationship between physical activity and health. Although the RCT is the optimal research design, actually conducting these trials poses a number of challenging problems. For example, potential subjects (children and their parents) in a RCT must agree to participate without knowing whether they will be assigned to the exercise intervention or control group. Furthermore, a double-blind approach—although preferred for intervention studies in other areas—is not possible for obvious reasons. Only single-blind trials can be performed (the data collection personnel but not the subjects are unaware of group assignments). Biases can be introduced by poor compliance with the intervention and by dropouts in either the intervention or control group. Because of the difficulty in recruiting participants for large RCTs, these trials are often conducted using highly select samples and this reduces external validity. Therefore, longitudinal observational studies in larger representative groups such as the Amsterdam Growth and Health Longitudinal Study (AGAHLS) are extremely important to gather representative information in a population.

To understand the role of physical activity on health in youth, it is necessary to view these factors in the context of three epidemiologic models:

1 The first and most simple (unifactoral) one is the triangle consisting of host (i.e., child), the environment (e.g., physical, social), and the agent (i.e., physical activity).

2 A second and more recent model, called the "Web of Causation," is multifactorial and includes more factors with effects on health outcome in addition to physical activity (e.g., diet, stress, smoking) and their interactions with respect to health.

3 The third and most valid model approach nowadays is the "Wheel" model, because it views the

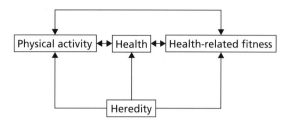

Fig. 10.2 Integration of traditional epidemiologic models illustrating how plausible causal paths for physical activity and heredity act on health and health-related fitness. Redrawn from Bouchard & Shephard (1994).

development of the child as intertwined with the environment, and it recognizes that the child develops from a genetic core that is modifiable to varying degrees by the biologic, physical, and social environments to which the child is exposed (Dishman *et al.* 2004).

The exercise scientists Bouchard and Shephard (1994) have integrated the traditional epidemiologic models to illustrate how the independent and interactive effects of heredity, habits other than physical activity, the physical and social environment, and personal attributes on health might be conceptualized. In Fig. 10.2 their model is illustrated and simplified.

Heredity, or genetic factors, is directly associated with all other parts of the model indicating that youth differ widely in genetic makeup and genetic predisposition. Thus, this model explains why individual children respond differently in health and health-related fitness to the same physical activity.

There is equally wide variation in the physical and social environments to which youth are exposed among and within societies (climate, population density, educational level). Even among identical twins, biologic adaptations to physical activity can vary by as much 50%. Hence, the environment apparently influences even gene expression in response to physical activity during the whole lifespan.

When a statistical association between physical activity and health outcome can be demonstrated, and the results of confounding (other causes than physical activity) and effect modification (interaction of other factors) have been accounted for, the question of a cause–effect relationship arises. In the 19th century, John Stuart Mill provided five criteria

that increase the probability that the association between physical activity and health or health-related fitness is causal:

1 *Temporal sequence:* physical activity must precede development of health-related fitness;

2 *Strength of the association:* there is a strong and meaningful difference in the health-related fitness between the children exposed to the high and low physical activity;

3 *Consistency:* the association is always observed regardless of sex, age, or methods of measurement;

4 *Dose–response:* the health effects are greater with more and more intensive physical activity;

5 *Biologic plausibility:* the observed effects of physical activity can be explained by existing knowledge about the possible biologic mechanisms of physical activity on health-related fitness.

Objective measurement of physical activity in youth

Public health authorities, including the Centers for Disease Control and Prevention (CDC), the National Institutes of Health (NIH), and the World Health Organization (WHO), agree that children and adolescents must become more physically active and maintain higher levels of physical activity throughout adulthood if they are to enjoy healthy and productive lives. However, to help children and adolescents become more active, researchers and practitioners need valid and reliable measures of youth physical activity (Trost 2001).

Montoye *et al.* (1996) summarized methods to assess physical activity and energy expenditure. Because the law of conservation of energy also applies to humans, measurements of physical activity are often expressed in terms of energy expenditure. Alternatively, physical activity can also be expressed as the amount of work performed (W), as the duration of activity (hours, minutes), as units of movements (counts), or even as a numerical score derived from responses to a questionnaire.

The term energy expenditure is not synonymous with physical activity: a child may expend the same amount of energy in a short burst of strenuous exercise (sprinting) as in a less intense endurance type activity (walking, jogging). It is also essential to remember that the energy expenditure is related to body size: a very active child may have a similar energy expenditure over 24 h as a large sedentary adult. Therefore, if physical activity is expressed as energy expenditure (J) body size must be taken into account. The use of MET (metabolic equivalents) is a valuable approach to correct for differences in body weight in growing youth. A MET score represents the ratio of energy expended for a specific physical activity divided by the individual's resting energy expenditure.

Laboratory methods (e.g., direct measurement of energy expenditure from heat production in a sealed, insulated chamber; and indirect measurement of energy expenditure from oxygen consumption with closed and open circuit methods using hood, face mask, or nose clip with mouthpiece) are complex and for the most part not useful for measuring habitual physical activity and do not apply to epidemiologic studies in children and adolescents (Saris 1986).

Field methods can be categorized into six different methods:

1 Observation works particularly well with small children, when most other assessment methods are unsuitable; with training, observers can be quite accurate and electronic devices facilitate the observation approach of assessing physical activity.
2 The diary method requires complete cooperation and precision from the subject so that it is not practical in young children.
3 Questionnaires and interviews are widely used, but validity and reproducibility have not been adequately studied and are usually inappropriate for use in children under 12 years of age.
4 Movement assessment devices such as pedometers or step-counters and accelerometers can quantify free-living physical activity in children and adolescents, because they are simple, small, and do not interfere with habitual free-living physical activities.
5 Estimation of energy expenditure from heart rate monitors can be carried out because of the linear relationship between heart rate and energy expenditure ($\dot{V}o_2$) during several steady state exercises of varying intensities.
6 A newer procedure, the double-labeled water (DLW) method, bridges the gap between precise laboratory measurements and field measurements

(Schoeller 1983). The method measures integral CO_2 production for up to 3 weeks from the difference in elimination rates of the stable isotopes deuterium and ^{18}O from double-labeled water, after ingestion of a volume of water enriched with these isotopes. This DLW method is considered the gold standard for assessing the average daily energy expenditure and thus total daily physical activity because it is not constrictive and ideally suited for use with youth. Any of the abovementioned assessment techniques, however, measures only one part of the habitual physical activity.

In Fig. 10.3 the same decline with age in daily energy expenditure per kilogram body weight in healthy children and adolescents from age 1 to 19 years appears as in Fig. 10.1. However, these cross-sectional data are of particular importance because they are based on several studies from various countries, in which energy expenditure was measured by DLW (Torun *et al.* 1996), the "gold standard" for the measurement of total daily energy expenditure.

Because children and adolescents have difficulties in recalling their past physical activity behavior accurately, new objective measures are being used with increasing regularity, but in using them in

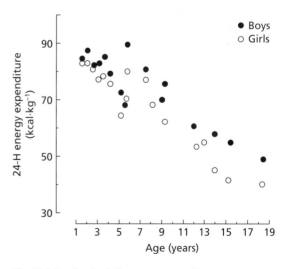

Fig. 10.3 Decline in daily energy expenditure per kilogram body weight in healthy children and adolescents between 1 and 18 years of age. Data are from several studies in various countries. Redrawn from Torun *et al.* (1996).

field-based research, new methodologic dilemmas arise (Trost 2001).

Heart rate monitoring remains an attractive approach to assess physical activity but there are several problems. First, heart rate is influenced not only by physical activity, but also by age, emotional stress, and cardiorespiratory fitness. Second, the heart rate response tends to lag behind changes in physical activity level and tends to remain elevated after cessation of a physical activity. Third, young children were found through direct observation to engage in physical activities with short bursts of activities: the median duration of light to moderate intensity activities was 6 s, and of high intensity activities less than 3 s. A total of 95% of the high intensity activities had a duration of less than 15 s (Bailey *et al.* 1995). The consequences of this activity behavior are that heart rate monitoring with averaging over 15 s, 1, or 5 min greatly underestimates the energy expenditure (Fig. 10.4).

A somewhat burdensome approach to assess physical activity with heart rate (HR) is to calibrate the HR–$\dot{V}o_2$ relationship on an individual basis (e.g., by applying the HR FLEX method). This approach uses the linear relationship of HR and $\dot{V}o_2$ above a given intensity threshold—the HR FLEX point—and a constant $\dot{V}o_2$ value for heart rate values below the HR FLEX point. Livingstone *et al.* (1992) and Emons *et al.* (1992) evaluated the accuracy of the HR FLEX method in children with the DLW method and found reasonable results.

Relative to heart rate monitors, accelerometers present fewer burdens to subjects and are capable of detecting the intermittent activity patterns characteristic of small children. On the other hand, they are insensitive to many forms of physical activity such as bicycling and stair climbing, and sensitive for passive movements of the body such as driving on a bumpy road.

Three-dimensional accelerometers were developed under the assumption that multiaxial monitoring of body accelerations would be advantageous compared with unidirectional assessments. However, it appears that uniaxial and triaxial accelerometers provide comparable assessments of physical activity in children (Eston *et al.* 1998; Ott *et al.* 2000; Welk *et al.* 2000).

Although accelerometers have been shown to be valid tools for quantifying physical activity in children, their relatively high cost prohibits their usage in large-scale epidemiologic studies. Electronic pedometers can be an alternative. Pedometers are similar to uniaxial accelerometers but are unable to record the intensity of movements and usually do not allow the measurement of activity profiles. Consequently, pedometers can only provide an estimate of the relative amount of physical activity totalized over a specified time period. Studies evaluating the concurrent validity of electronic pedometers in children aged 8–12 years have yielded positive results (Eston *et al.* 1998; Kilanowski *et al.* 1999), with high correlation coefficients between pedometer count and $\dot{V}o_{2peak}$ (0.95) and observation (0.92), respectively.

Measuring physical activity with objective instruments seems more valid than measurements with self-report methods, but the optimal sampling duration and frequency remains to be determined. Recently, Trost (2000) studied the day-to-day variability of physical activity by accelerometry in children and adolescents. It was estimated that 4–5 days of monitoring in children and 7 days in

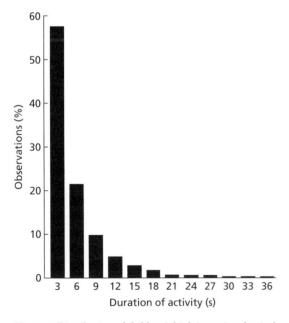

Fig. 10.4 Distribution of children's high intensity physical activities (percentage of observations) by the duration of the activity (in seconds). Redrawn from Bailey *et al.* (1995).

adolescents produced acceptable estimates of daily moderate-to-vigorous activity with correlations of 0.76–0.86. These time periods also accounted for significant differences in weekday and weekend physical activities.

Tracking of physical activity in youth

Tracking is defined as a measure of the stability of a certain variable over time, or the maintenance over time of a relative position within a population. Body height, for example, tracks well during the growing years, because a child whose height is at a certain percentile is likely to remain close to that percentile throughout childhood and adolescence. To determine tracking of physical activity, one must measure the variable in the same individual repeatedly over time, at least twice.

Tracking can be reported simply as the correlation between the two measurements. If there are more than two measurements, more interperiod correlations can be calculated over the same period and also over longer or shorter periods available. The disadvantage of calculating this interperiod correlation is that as much correlation coefficients result as there are interperiods. Computing an overall stability coefficient as suggested by Twisk (2003) can solve this problem.

How well does physical activity behavior track from childhood, or adolescence, into adulthood years? This is an important question if one assumes that physically active children, compared to sedentary children, have greater potential to become active adults.

A number of studies, mostly from Europe and the USA, have addressed tracking of physical activity from early to mid-childhood or from adolescence to young adulthood (for review see Bar-Or & Rowland 2004). There is a great variability among reported data, which reflects the variety of methods used to assess physical activity as well as cultural and societal differences. As expected, short-term (over 2–3 years) tracking of physical activity is stronger than long-term tracking. Physical activity tracks moderately during childhood and during transition into adolescence over a span of 2–3 years (correlations >0.50). However, the correlation

coefficients are lower over spans of 5–6 years (correlations of 0.30–0.50), and they further diminish when one compares physical activity between early adolescence and young adulthood (correlations <0.30).

In the AGAHLS, for example, interperiod correlations for boys were 0.44 for age 13–16 years, 0.20 for age 13–21 years, and 0.05 for age 13–27 years. The same general pattern was apparent for females (van Mechelen & Kemper 1994b). However, if one calculates the overall stability coefficient, taking into account all nine measurement points over a period of 23 years, the stability is 0.21 in males and 0.27 in females for age 13–36 years (Kemper 2004b). A stability coefficient of a variable over a period of 20 years of 0.50 would be assumed to show relative stability. Thus, compared to fitness parameters such as body fatness or aerobic fitness, physical activity shows considerably lower tracking. A similar trend has been found in youth in Finland, Belgium, Denmark, and the USA.

The poor tracking of physical activity in childhood and adolescence shown by several studies is in line with individual observations. Physical activity in most boys and girls is not stable over the youth period; children start to be active but may discontinue activity for a while and restart later in their adolescence. Other children are not active in the beginning but start to be active in adolescence; the reverse may also occur. Nevertheless, the relative low tracking of physical activity as shown above was observed in general populations with youth of both high and low physical activity. If one measures at the extremes of the physical activity spectrum (i.e., the most active and the least active), tracking seems stronger (Malina 1996).

Summarizing all available information, it appears that physical activity in youth is not a very stable behavior and is probably not very genetically determined, but can also be influenced by social and environmental factors.

Factors that affect physical activity in youth

Various biologic, psychologic, social or cultural, and physical environmental factors are shown or suggested to affect physical activity behavior and energy expenditure of children and adolescents. Most of the studies in this area are based on correlational analyses, which reflect only associations but no cause and effect relationships (Bar-Or & Rowland 2004).

Biologic factors

Physical activity is a behavior. It is difficult to establish that a behavior has a molecular basis and, in other words, is imprinted in the genes, especially in human beings.

However, even in fruit flies (*Drosophila melangaster*) the naturally occurring polymorphisms of behavior are difficult to map. One exception is the foraging gene "for." This food-searching gene has two naturally occurring variants that determine food search behavior of fruit flies: type "rover" and type "sitter". The "rover" type has a higher protein kinase (PKG) activity and flies will travel over far greater distances to collect their food compared with the "sitters." With the help of PKG, the "sitters" can be transformed into "rovers" (Osborne *et al*. 1997). It is possible that comparable activity genes may be discovered and identified in humans in the near future, and this would clarify why there are such big differences between humans when it comes to physical activity levels over time (Kemper 2004a).

Heredity also appears to have some influence on habitual physical activity pattern in youth. Several studies computed associations for pairs that included biologic relatives (parent/child, di-/monozygotic siblings) and non-biologic relatives (spouse, uncle/nephew or niece) (Perusse *et al*. 1988, 1989). From them it can be concluded that physical activity is significantly influenced by heredity (29% heritability index), but that environmental influences are stronger.

Social and cultural factors

Social and cultural factors such as parents' and peers' attitudes and behaviors, socioeconomic status, and cultural and ethnic values are also of importance for a child's or adolescent's physical activity.

Results from the Dutch Twin Research confirmed in teenage twins that the importance of the genetic element is relatively low (Koopmans 1997). Furthermore, the impact of parents and siblings on an adolescent's physical activity appears to be relatively low compared with that of peers (Koopmans 1997). In younger children (4–7 years), however, the parents are of importance. In children with physically active fathers or mothers, the odds are 2–3.5 times higher that their children are also active compared with children whose parents are not physically active (Moore *et al*. 1991). In children with both parents active, the odds are over 6 times higher.

Ecologic models are now used to understand the complex arrays that influence physical activity, resulting in a greater emphasis on environmental correlates. Within a multilevel ecologic framework, complex interactions between the multitude of individual, cultural, and social factors are studied in settings in which people live, go to school, work, and play (Giles-Cort *et al*. 2005). The setting in which the physical activity behavior takes place is probably important because people are likely to differ in their active transport behavior dependent on their local neighborhood. Similarly, children's physical activity at school is likely to be different from that at home. Unfortunately, little information is available on this topic.

Over the past decades enormous progress has been made in measuring physical activity. It will take a similar time period to develop valid measures of sociocultural correlates of physical activity behavior to get a good insight into the effects of sociocultural factors on physical activity.

Psychologic factors

A wellspring of short- and long-term benefits from regular physical activity has been demonstrated, yet over half to three-quarters of the population does not engage in enough physical activity, although most people are aware that regular physical activity is indeed beneficial. This suggests that physical activity promotion interventions and an understanding of the factors that facilitate or impair regular physical activity are warranted. Physical activity determinants and promotion research have focused on the role of the environment. An alternative to that approach is the assumption that the built-in environment (personality) facilitates or impairs an active lifestyle (Rhodes 2006). In his review, Rhodes (2006) evaluates evidence for the hypothesis that personality traits are related to physical activity. Current evidence has demonstrated that personality is heritable, structured similarly over cultures, has a high temporal stability, and does not relate strongly to parental rearing style. The most convincing evidence for physical activity and personality relations comes from Eysenck's three-factor taxonomy of extraversion, neuroticism, and psychoticism (integration of agreeableness and conscientiousness). The existing evidence suggests that people higher in extraversion and conscientiousness are more likely to be physically active and that neuroticism is a relative consistent negative correlate of physical activity.

Physical activity preferences differ by personality: for example, extravert individuals prefer group-based and high-intensity activities compared to introvert individuals; similarly, individuals higher on neuroticism may benefit from normative-based interventions (involving friends and family) more than less neurotic counterparts.

Future research is warranted to evaluate if these association can also be demonstrated in youth and whether personality channeled physical activity interventions hold utility for children and adolescents.

Physical environment

There is a long-running debate in urban planning about the degree to which the physical environment determines human behavior. The theory of environmental or architectural determinism ascribes great importance to the physical environment as a shaper of activity behavior. The counter view is that social and economic factors are the main determinants of activity behavior. Nearly all evidence of associations between the physical environment and physical activity is based on cross-sectional data. Depending on the point of view, the documented relationship between walking (or cycling) and the built environment might as well be caused by individuals who want to be physically active selecting

of pedestrian/cyclist friendly environments, as caused by pedestrian/cyclist environments making individuals more physically active than they would be otherwise (Ewing 2005).

The first studies linking the built environment to health outcomes appeared late in 2003 and show relative strong evidence of association between compact development patterns and the use of active travel modes such as walking, bicycling, and/or in combination with the use of public transport. Whether the physical environment is actually determining children's and adolescents' travel choices and their activity in playgrounds remain issues for future research.

Reducing sedentary behavior

Studies of physical activity determinants have tended to focus on biologic, psychologic, and sociocultural influences. The Behavioral Choice Theory (BCT) describes interactions between the individual and his or her environment and can help to understand the process of choosing to be physically active or sedentary (Owen *et al.* 2000). Environmental contexts can promote or discourage a range of behaviors that do have important consequences for overall energy expenditure. For example, it is quite apparent that sport fields, gymnasiums, public playgrounds, and bicycle trails promote physical activity. Others have functional attributes that discourage, restrict, or prohibit physical activity such as computer workstations, TV rooms, highways, and domestic living areas. There are also less obvious functional and socially defined attributes that influence physical activity; for example, access to stairs in public buildings, availability of public transport, safe and pleasant walking and cycling opportunities.

Although sedentary behavior may arguably be conceptionalized as no more than the other side of the physical activity coin, it can also be seen as a behavior that can coexist and can also compete with physical activity. Three of the most common leisure-time sedentary behaviors—television viewing and computer and internet use—have been studied extensively in children. Findings suggest that these may have detrimental effects on overweight and

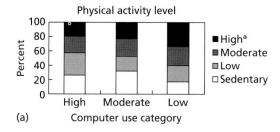

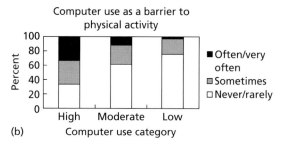

Fig. 10.5 (a) Categories of computer use and distributions of physical activity level; and (b) perception of computer use as a barrier to physical activity. Redrawn from Owen *et al.* (2000).

obesity which can act independently of leisure-time physical activity level. Physical activity may not be protective against prolonged periods of sedentary behavior; even those who were highly active, but reported TV watching more than 4 h·day^{-1}, were twice as likely to be overweight than those who watched less than 1 h·day^{-1} (Salmon *et al.* 2000). Higher levels of computer use were associated with increased likelihood of physical inactivity (Fig. 10.5) (Fotheringham *et al.* 2001).

Engaging in physical activity usually involves choosing exercise over a concurrent and powerful competing sedentary behavior. Epstein & Roemmich (2001) applied the BCT to the physical activity field in children:

• In the morning, do you exercise before breakfast or sleep in a little later and not exercise?
• At lunchtime, do you go for a swim and a fast lunch, or a more leisurely lunch without being physically active?
• On the weekend, do you watch sports or play sports?

These decisions are based in part on differences in access to active and sedentary alternatives and on the motivation to engage in the activities. If access to both activities is equal, people generally engage in the more reinforcing value of the activities. If the reinforcing values of the activities are equal, people generally engage in the most accessible activity. A main reason for choosing sedentary behaviors is easy acceptability, whereas physically active alternatives require more work to engage in them and are often accompanied by modest discomfort and sweating and the added cost of changing clothes and showering. Often the choice between being physically active or sedentary involves more than the immediateness of accessibility or reinforcing value of an activity. Many important health choices have delayed outcomes. A decreased intake of fatty foods (boiled potatoes instead of French fries) results in a loss of immediate pleasure but offers the potential for substantially delayed health benefits. It would not be surprising to find that children with poor impulse control choose the immediately gratifying sedentary or fatty alternative.

Pediatric obesity is related to increases in sedentary behavior, so it might be expected that obese children would find sedentary behaviors more reinforcing than physical activity, and it may therefore be harder to shift the choice from being sedentary to physically active in obese children. When provided the choice and equal access to sedentary or physical activity in a laboratory setting (variable ratio [VR] = 2/2), both obese and non-obese boys aged 8–12 years chose to be sedentary (Epstein *et al.* 1991). As increasing the work required to be sedentary reduced access to sedentary behaviors (variable ratio VR2/2-to-VR2/32), non-obese children quickly switched to working for the more easily obtained physical activity. After further increases in the amount of work required obtaining sedentary activity time, moderately obese children switched to working for physical activities, but very obese children did not (Fig. 10.6). This study (Epstein *et al.* 1991) suggests that the amount of obesity enhances the reinforcing value of sedentary behavior of these children.

Accessibility to sedentary behaviors is in general much easier than physical activity for most people. In a laboratory setting, physical and sedentary activities were located either near (immediate accessible; i.e., in the same room) or relatively far (5 min

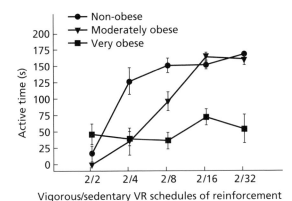

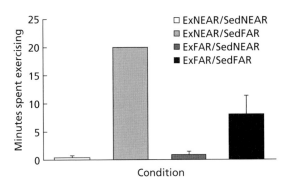

Fig. 10.6 Allocation of time working for vigorous physical activity (vertical axis) by non-obese, moderately obese, and very obese children in a choice situation. Accessability for vigorous activity and sedentary activities was varied from equal access at variable ratio 2/2 (VR2/2), till increasing work to get the higher rated sedentary activity ranging from VR2/2 to VR2/32 (horizontal axis). Redrawn from Epstein *et al.* (1991).

Fig. 10.7 Time spent in exercise activities (vertical axis) of young men under different experimental conditions (horizontal axis). Ex, exercise; Sed, sedentary; NEAR, in the same room; FAR, located 5 min walk away. Redrawn from Raynor *et al.* (1998).

walk away). If sedentary behaviors were near, subjects were sedentary, but if sedentary behaviors were far and physical activities were near, subjects spent the whole time being active. Reducing access by requiring subjects to walk 5 min to obtain access to sedentary activities shifted the choice from being sedentary to being physically active (Fig. 10.7) (Raynor *et al.* 1998). These data suggest that physical activity could increase if environments were changed to increase the proximity (bus stops) and convenience of playgrounds, and that access to sedentary activities (TV watching, snacking) could decrease physical activity.

Greater valued sedentary activities such as TV watching compete with physical activity more than lower valued sedentary activities such as reading. Klesges *et al.* (1993) found that the energy expenditure of children aged 8–12 years watching TV is 200 kcal·day^{-1} lower than their resting expenditure. The increase in the amount of time children nowadays spend watching TV could be a cause for the often-found positive relationship between obesity and the number of hours children view TV.

With respect to fitness and weight changes, studies reinforcing obese children to be less sedentary

show equal to or better success than studies promoting physical activity. Future research should aim on how to increase the reinforcing value of physical activity, so that more children and adolescents choose to be active: having a choice in different sport activities (non-weight-bearing for overweight children), competitive vs. non-competitive sports, individual vs. group exercise and activities that can be performed on the preferred time of the day.

Future directions

Although there is enough evidence that physical activity in youth and adult life reduces the risk of chronic disease, premature death, and improves quality of life, many youth and adults are not meeting public health standards. Leaders in health care, schools, government, and non-profit organizations are now investing time, money, and effort to promote physical activity. However, the effectiveness and sustainability of these promotion activities remain questionable (Dzewaltowski *et al.* 2004). There is also a lack of understanding why childhood physical activity interventions succeed or fail (Baranowski & Jago 2005).

There is a gap between physical activity intervention research and the delivery of evidence-based programs in practice. There is a large body of research evidence on "what works" to improve physical activity (Kahn *et al.* 2002), but there are problems in the delivery of prevention interventions to adults and to youth at schools. At both individual and setting levels, variables that likely moderate the uptake, impact, and sustainability of physical activity interventions are seldom studied or reported. To enhance the potential for translating research into practice, the Reach, Efficacy/Effectiveness-Adoption Implementation and Maintenance framework (RE-AIM) is introduced. Each element provides valuable information that may facilitate the translation:

• *Reach* (individual level): the number and representativeness of individuals who participate in a given intervention;
• *Efficacy/effectiveness* (individual level): the impact of an intervention on physical activity and other health outcomes;
• *Adoption* (setting level): the number and representativeness of settings that are willing to initiate a physical activity promotion program;
• *Implementation* (setting level): the quantity and quality of delivery of the intervention;
• *Maintenance* (setting level): the extent to which a physical activity promotion program becomes institutionalized;
• *Maintenance* (individual level): the long-term effect of a physical activity promotion program on behavior 6 or more months after the intervention.

A review of physical activity studies showed that results are seldom reported in respect to reach, representativeness, and adoption (Kahn *et al.* 2002). Only 14% of school-based physical activity interventions reported on any issue related to adoption. The Sports, Play and Active Recreation for Kids (SPARK) trial was an exception because it explained the selection and participation of the schools in the trial (Sallis *et al.* 1997).

The lack of reported data on the issues addressed above raises questions about the generalizability and feasibility of the physical activity interventions. Increase in translation of physical activity interventions into practice can improve future physical activity behavior change research into health promotion.

The mediating variable model (Fig. 10.8) has been proposed for understanding mechanisms of change in children's physical activity programs: it relates

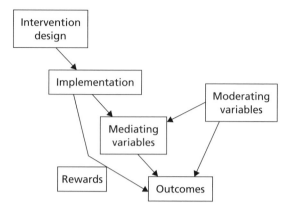

Fig. 10.8 The mediating variable model for a better understanding of how physical activity interventions programs in youth work. Redrawn from Baranowski *et al.* (2005).

program process to mediating variables and outcomes. This model suggests that changes in outcomes are the result of changes in mediating variables and changes in the mediating variables are induced by implementing programs. Moderating variables are those for which outcomes of the intervention are different (e.g., sex effect). Implementation could also have a direct effect on outcomes through rewards. The Child and Adolescent Trial for Cardiovascular Health (CATCH), was a 3-year multicenter field trial implemented in 96 schools. The physical education intervention focused on increasing time spent in moderate to vigorous intensity physical activity (McKenzie *et al.* 2001). The process measures indicated that the intervention was largely implemented as planned, but more detailed comparisons showed that the outcome was different between classroom and specialist teachers: specialist teachers were more likely to increase activity than classroom teachers, and increased activity was obtained more often among experienced classroom teachers compared to less experienced teachers.

It can be concluded that there is a gradual age-dependent decrease in both sexes in the daily energy expenditure from physical activity from age 1 to age 19 years. This is demonstrated by studies that are not flawed by self-reported activity but used valid meaurement methods such as DLW.

Although it is not fully proven that being physically active in youth is relevant for health as an adult, the few longitudinal studies that compare active with inactive youth at adult age show small effects that favor this hypothesis. This lack of proof is caused by the relative short duration of many studies, the non-interventional design, and the fact that many confounders other than physical activity are involved. The scientific knowledge from tracking studies of physical activity in youth indicates that activity behavior is not stable over time and probably not much genetically driven. Therefore, environmental influences (social, cultural, psychologic, and physical) can be used to turn the worldwide tendency of being more and more inactive.

In order to prevent the inevitable concomitent increase in chronic degenerative diseases as cardiorespiratory diseases, obesity, diabetes type 2, osteoporosis, and some cancers, much more emphasis has to be given to changes in environmental factors to reduce sedentary behavior.

The main challenge for future research for the next generation of youth is to develop effective and feasible physical activity interventions for youth that can improve their daily physical activity behavior including sports participation.

References

Bailey, R.C., Olson, J., Pepper, S.L., Porszasz, J., Barstow, T.J. & Cooper, D.M. (1995) The level and tempo of children's physical activities: an observational study. *Medicine and Science in Sports and Exercise* 27, 1033–1041.

Baranowski, T. & Jago, R. (2005) Understanding the mechanisms of change in children's physical activity programs. *Exercise and Sport Sciences Reviews* 33, 163–168.

Bar-Or, O. (1983) *Pediatric Sport Medicine for the Practitioner: From Physiologic Principles to Clinical Applications.* Springer, New York.

Bar-Or, O. & Rowland, T.W. (2004) *Pediatric Exercise Medicine, From Physiologic Principles to Health Care Application.* Human Kinetics, Champaign, IL.

Biddle, S., Sallis, J. & Cavill N., eds. (1998) *Young and Active? Policy framework for young people and health-enhancing physical activity.* Health Education Authority, London.

Bouchard, C. & Shephard, R.J. (1994) Physical activity, fitness, and health: the model and key concepts. In: *Physical Activity, Fitness and Health: International Proceedings and Consensus Statement* (Bouchard, C., Shephard, R.J. & Stephens, T., eds.) Human Kinetics, Champaign, IL: 77–88.

Dishman, R.K., Washburn, R.A. & Heath, G.W. (2004) *Physical Activity Epidemiology.* Human Kinetics, Champaign, IL.

Dzewaltowski, D.A., Eastbrooks, P.A. & Glasgow, R.E. (2004) The future of physical activity behaviour change

reseach: What is needed to improve translation of research into health promotion practice? *Exercise and Sport Sciences Reviews* 32, 57–63.

Emons, H.J.G., Groeneboom, D.C., Westerterp, K.R. & Saris, W.H.M. (1992) Comparison of heart rate monitoring with indirect calorimetry and the doubly labelled water (2H218O) method for the measurement of energy expenditure in children. *European Journal of Applied Physiology* 65, 99–103.

Epstein, L.H. & Roemmich, J.N. (2001) Reducing sedentary behaviour: Role in modifying physical activity. *Exercise and Sport Sciences Reviews* 29, 103–108.

Epstein, L.H., Smith, J.A., Vara, L.S. & Rodefer, J.S. (1991) Behavioral economic analysis of activity choice in obese children. *Health Psychology* 10, 311–316.

Eston, R.G., Rowlands, A.V. & Ingledew D.K. (1998) Validity of heart rate, pedometry, and accelerometry for predicting the energy cost of children's activities. *Journal of Applied Physiology* 84, 362–371.

Ewing, R. (2005) Can the physical environment determine physical activity levels? *Exercise and Sport Sciences Reviews* 33, 69–75.

Fotheringham, M.J., Wonnacot, R.L. & Owen, N. (2001) Computer use and physical inactivity in young adults: public health perils and potentials of new information technologies. *Annals of Behavioral Medicine* 22, 269–275.

Gezondheidsraad (Health Council of the Netherlands) (2003) *Overgewicht en Obesitas* [overweight and obesity]. The Hague publication no. 07.

Giles-Cort, B., Timperio, A., Bull, F. & Pikora, T. (2005) Understanding physical activity environmental correlates: increased specificity for ecological models. *Exercise and Sport Sciences Reviews* 33, 175–181.

Jequier, J.C., Lavallee, H., Rajic, M., Beaucage, L., Shephard, R.J. & Labarre, R. (1977) The longitudinal examination of growth and development: history and protocol of the Trois Riviere regional study. In: *Frontiers of Activity and Child Health* (Lavallee, H. & Shephard, R.J., eds.) Pelican, Ottawa: 49–54.

Kahn, E.B., Brownson, R.C., Heath, G.W., *et al.* (2002) The effectiveness of interventions to increase physical activity, a systematic review. *American Journal of Preventive Medicine* 22, 73–107.

Kemper, H.C.G. (2004a) *My e-motion(s).* Elsevier Gezondheidszorg, Maarssen.

Kemper H.C.G., ed. (2004b) Amsterdam Growth and Health Longitudinal study, a 23-year follow-up from teenager to adult about lifestyle and health. *Medicine and Sport Science*, Vol. 47. Karger, Basel.

Kemper, H.C.G., Ooijendijk, W.T.M. & Stiggelbout, M. (2000) Consensus over de Nederlandse Norm voor Gezond Bewegen [Dutch norm for healthy physical activity patterns]. *Tijdschrift voor Sociale Geneeskunde* 78, 180–183.

Kilanowski, C., Consalvi, A. & Epstein, L.H. (1999) Validation of an electronic pedometer for measurement of physical activity in children. *Pediatric Exercise Science* 11, 63–68.

Klesges, R.C., Shelton, M.L. & Klesges, L.M. (1993) Effects of television on metabolic rate: Potential implications for childhood obesity. *Pediatrics* **91**, 281–286.

Koopmans, J. (1997) The genetics of health-related behaviours, a study of adolescent twins and their parents. Thesis. Amsterdam Vrije Universiteit.

Livingstone, M.B.E., Coward, A.W., Prentice, A.M., *et al.* (1992) Dailey energy expenditure in free-living children: comparison of heart rate monitoring with the double labelled water (2H218O) method. *American Journal of Clinical Nutrition* **56**, 343–352.

Malina, R.M. (1996) Tracking of physical activity and physical fitness across the lifespan. *Research Quarterly for Exercise and Sport* **67**, 48–57.

Masironi, R. & Denolin, H. (1985) *Physical Activity in Disease, Prevention and Treatment*. Piccin, Padua.

McKenzie, T.L., Stone, E.J., Felman, H.A., *et al.* (2001) Effect of the Catch physical education intervention teacher types and lessons location. *American Journal of Preventive Medicine* **21**, 101–109.

Mednick, J.A. & Baert, A.E. (1981) *Prospective Longitudinal Research: an Empirical Basis for the Primary Prevention of Psychological Disorders*. Oxford University Press, Oxford.

Mirwald, R.L., Bailey, D.A., Cameron, N. & Rasmussen, R.L. (1981) Longitudinal comparison of aerobic power in active and active boys aged 7.0 to 17.0 years. *Annals of Human Biology* **8**, 405–414.

Montoye, H.J. (1985) Risk indicators for cardiovascular disease in relation to physical activity in youth. In: *Children and Exercise*, Vol. XI. (Binkhorst, R.A., Kemper, H.C.G., Saris, W.H.M., eds.) Human Kinetics, Champaign, IL: 3–25.

Montoye, H.J., Kemper, H.C.G., Washburn, R.A. & Saris, W.H.M. (1996) *Measurement of Energy Expenditure and Physical Activity*. Human Kinetics, Champaign, IL.

Moore, L.L., Lombardi, D.A., White, M.J., *et al.* (1991) Influence of parent's activity levels on activity levels of young children. *Journal of Pediatrics* **118**, 215–219.

Osborne, K.A., Robinson, A., Burgess, E., *et al.* (1997) Natural behaviour polymorphy due to a cGMP-dependent protein kinase of drosophila. *Science* **277**, 834–836.

Ott, A.E., Pate, R.R., Trost, S.G., Ward, D.S. & Saunders, R. (2000) The use of uniaxial and triaxial accelerometers to measure children's "free-play" physical activity. *Pediatric Exercise Science* **12**, 360–370.

Owen, N., Leslie, E., Salmon, J. & Fotheringham, M.J. (2000) Environmental determinants of physical activity and sedentary behaviour. *Exercise and Sport Sciences Reviews* **28**, 153–158.

Perusse, L., Leblanc, C. & Bouchard, C. (1988) Familial resemblance in lifestyle components: results from the Canada Fitness Survey. *Canadian Journal of Public Health* **79**, 201–205.

Perusse, L., Tremblay, A., Leblanc, C. & Bouchard, C. (1989) Genetic and environmental influences on habitual physical activity and exercise participation. *American Journal of Epidemiology* **129**, 1012–1022.

Powell, K.E., Thomson, P.D., Caspersen, C.J. & Kendrick, J.S. (1987) Physicality and the incidence of coronary heart disease. *Annual Review of Public Health* **8**, 253–287.

Raynor, D.A., Coleman, K.J. & Epstein, L.H. (1998) Effects of proximity on the choice of to be physically active or sedentary. *Research Quarterly for Exercise and Sport* **69**, 99–103.

Rhodes, R.E. (2006) The built-in environment: the role of personality and physical activity. *Exercise and Sport Sciences Reviews* **34**, 83–87.

Rowland, T.W. (1990) *Exercise and Children's Health*. Human Kinetics, Champaign, IL.

Rutenfranz, J., Berndt, I. & Knauth, P. (1974) Daily physical activity investigated by time budget studies and physical performance capacity of schoolboys. In: *Children and Exercise* (Borms, J., Hebbelinck, eds.) *Acta Paediatrica Belgica* **28** (Supplement), 79–86.

Sallis, J.F. (1994) Special issue. Physical activity guidelines for adolescents. *Pediatric Exercise Science* **6**, 299–463.

Sallis, J.F., McKenzie, T.L., Alcaraz, J.E., Kolody, B., Faucette, N. & Hovell, M.F. (1997) The effects of a 2-year physical education program (SPARK) on physical activity and fitness in elementary school students. *American Journal of Public Health* **87**, 1328–1334.

Salmon, J., Bauman, D., Crawford, A., Timperio, A. & Owen, N. (2000) The association between television viewing and overweight among Australian adults participating in varying levels of leisure-time activities. *International Journal of Obesity* **24**, 600–606.

Saris, W.H.M. (1986) Habitual physical activity in children: methodology and findings in health and disease. *Medicine and Science in Sports and Exercise* **18**, 253–263.

Schoeller, D.A. (1983) Energy expenditure from double labelled water: Some fundamental considerations in humans. *American Journal of Clinical Nutrition* **38**, 999–1005.

Shepard, R.J. & Trudeau, F. (2005) Lessons learned from the Trois-Rivieres physical education study: a retrospective. *Pediatric Exercise Science* **2**, 112–124.

Torun, B., Davies, P.S.W., Livingstone, M.B.E., Paolisso, M., Sackett, R. & Spurr, G.B. (1996) Energy requirements and dietary energy recommendations for children and adolescents 1 to 18 years old. *European Journal of Clinical Nutrition* **50**, 537–581.

Trost, S.G. (2001) Objective measurement of physical activity in youth: current issues, future directions. *Exercise and Sport Sciences Reviews* **29**, 32–36.

Twisk, J.W.H. (2001) Physical activity guidelines for children and adolescents: a critical review. *Sports Medicine* **31**, 617–627.

Twisk, J.W.R. (2003) *Applied Longitudinal Data Analysis for Epidemiology: a Practical Guide*. Cambridge University Press, Cambridge.

van Mechelen, W. & Kemper, H.C.G. (1995) Habitual physical activity in longitudinal perspective. In: *The Amsterdam Growth Study: a longitudinal analysis of health, fitness and lifestyle* (Kemper, H.C.G., ed.) Human Kinetics, Champaign, IL: 135–158.

Welk, G.J., Corbin, C.B. & Dale, D. (2000) Measurement issues in the assessment of physical activity in children. *Research Quarterly for Exercise and Sport* **71** (Supplement), 59–73.

Part 3

Injuries: Epidemiology, Prevention, Treatment, and Rehabilitation

Chapter 11

Epidemiology of Pediatric Sports-Related Injuries

EVERT VERHAGEN AND WILLEM VAN MECHELEN

A physically active lifestyle and active participation in sports is important, both for adults and children. There are many reasons to participate in sports and physical activity: pleasure and relaxation, competition, socialization, and maintenance and improvement of fitness and health. When compared with adults, in children the risk for injury resulting from participation in sports and free play is low (Van Mechelen 1997). However, with the current focus on a physically active lifestyle, an increasing number of sports and physical activity injuries are to be expected (Parkkari *et al.* 2001). In recent years, more and more children are undertaking intensive training at younger ages or participating in multiple sports, thereby exposing themselves to higher risk of injury (Adirim & Cheng 2003).

Consequently, in children, sports and physical activity injuries have become a major health problem. Given such unwanted side effects of a presumably healthy behavior, successful prevention of sports injuries in youth has great potential health gain: in the short-term, the absolute number of sports injuries falls and, in the longer term, the risk of injury recurrences and prolonged periods of impairment will be prevented. Prevention also promotes a physically active lifestyle from childhood into adulthood.

In general, measures to prevent sports injuries do not stand by themselves. They result from a series of four steps that form a sequence of prevention (Van Mechelen *et al.* 1992). First, the sports injury problem must be described in terms of incidence and severity. The second step identifies the etiologic risk factors and mechanisms underlying the occurrence

of injury. Based on this information, in the third step preventive measures that are likely to work can be developed and introduced. Finally, the (cost-)effectiveness of the introduced preventive measures should be evaluated by repeating the first step or by performing intervention trials.

The purpose of this chapter is to describe the epidemiology of pediatric sports-related injuries. This will be addressed along the sequence of prevention outlined above. However, a full epidemiologic overview of the injury problem in pediatric sports is beyond the scope of this chapter. Therefore, we first discuss some general methodologic problems in conjunction with the sequence of prevention. This will provide the reader with the ability to ascertain the methodologic quality and generalizability of any sports injury paper.

Methdologic problems in sports injury research

Definition of injury

When conducting (and also when interpreting the outcomes of) epidemiologic sports injury studies, one is confronted with a number of methodologic issues. The first issue of importance is the definition of sports injury. In general, sports injury is a collective term for all types of damage that can occur in relation to sporting activities. Various descriptive studies on sports injury incidence define the term sports injury in different ways. In some studies, a sports injury is defined as any injury sustained during sporting activities that causes (partial) absence from subsequent sports activities. In other studies the definition is confined to any injury sustained during sporting activities for which an insurance claim is submitted. These are only two examples of a wide array of sports injury definitions. A common observable fact is that in many studies the injury definition is restrained by the researcher's opportunity to collect accurate data. As an example, a hospital-based study is likely to define a sports injury as any injury sustained during sporting activities that is treated at a hospital casualty or other medical department.

This wide spectrum of available definitions of sports injury partly explains the differing sports injury incidences found in the literature. Therefore, the results of different sports injury surveys are not comparable. If sports injuries are recorded through medical channels (e.g., hospital emergency rooms), a fairly large percentage of serious, predominantly acute injuries will be observed, while less serious and/or overuse injuries will be underreported. If such a "limited" definition is used, only part of the sports injury problem is revealed. This so-called "tip-of-the-iceberg" phenomenon is often described in epidemiologic research (Walter et al. 1985). This is a commonly encountered problem in pediatric sports injury epidemiology, because there are many overuse and "minor" acute injuries in youth.

Sports injury incidence

The way the sports injury problem is described is the second methodologic issue that needs to be addressed. This is as important as the previous injury definition issue. One way of getting an impression of the size of the sports injury problem is by counting the absolute number of injuries. When these numbers are compared with, for instance, the number of road accidents or the number of injuries sustained during leisure time activities, the relative extent of the sports injury problem can be revealed. However, such a comparison fails to reveal the true risk of a certain activity. One can only sustain a road accident when in traffic. Even so, one can only sustain a sports injury when participating in sports. While the amount of time spent in leisure time activities or in traffic is usually greater than the amount of time spent participating in sports, a comparison of absolute injury numbers only sheds a dim light on the problem from a societal perspective.

However, the most appropriate indication of sports injury risk in a sporting population is the incidence rate. The incidence rate of sports injury is usually defined as the number of new sports injuries during a particular period (e.g., 1 year) divided by the total number of sports participants at the start of the period (i.e., population at risk). It should be realized that it is important, when interpreting and comparing the various incidence rates, to know what injury definition was used and how comparable the different samples were.

Another problem lies in the way incidence rates are expressed. In most cases, the number of injuries in a particular category of sports participants per season or per year is taken, or the number of injuries per player per match. In both examples no allowance is made for any differences in exposure (i.e., the number of hours during which the sports participant is actually at risk for being injured), despite the fact that this factor certainly influences the risk of injury. Incidence figures that do not take exposure into account are therefore not a good indication of the true extent of the injury problem, nor can the incidence rates for various sports or sporting populations be meaningfully compared. It would be better to calculate the incidence of sports injuries in relation to exposure time (hours).

We would like to give an example of the possible misinterpretations through improper reporting of injury numbers. The most recent count of sports injuries in the Netherlands (1997/1998) estimated that there was an absolute number of 2,300,000 acute sports injuries each year in a relatively small population of approximately 15 million inhabitants (Schmikli 2002). During this reference period almost half (48%) of the Dutch population participated in sports. A further in-depth study showed that annually 875,000 injuries (38%) required medical treatment. Therefore, it is reasonable to conclude that there is an injury problem in the Dutch sporting population. In Table 11.1 the 10 most injury-prone sports are given, based on the absolute number of injuries.

Table 11.1 The 10 sports with the highest absolute number of sports injuries, the corresponding injury incidence, and subsequent rank based on injury incidence. Data from Schmikli (2002).

Sport	Injury total (n)	Rank based on injury total	Injury incidence (n/1000 h)	Rank based on injury incidence
Soccer (outdoor)	620,000	1	2.0	6
Volleyball	142,000	2	2.4	3
Gymnastics	141,000	3	1.6	7
Soccer (indoor)	109,000	4	6.3	2
Field hockey	101,000	5	2.1	4
Swimming	92,000	6	0.6	9
Tennis (outdoor)	90,000	7	0.4	10
Skiing	79,000	8	10.1	1
Equestrian sports	77,000	9	0.9	8
Ice skating	68,000	10	2.1	4

According to the absolute number of injuries, outdoor soccer has the largest number of injuries (Schmikli 2002). However, this is not very surprising because in the Netherlands soccer is the sport with the most participants. This shows that one should be aware that absolute numbers of sports injuries might give an inaccurate view of the actual risk for injuries across sports. For instance, at the time of this study there were 1,066,000 soccer players, compared to 371,000 volleyball players (Schmikli 2002). Therefore, the absolute number of injuries is not the best measure to establish problem areas in sports. A better way to do this is by calculating the incidence of sports injuries (i.e., by assessing the number of injuries per 1000 hours of sports participation). As can been seen in Table 11.1, when sports participation is taken into account the order of the most injury-prone sports radically changes.

Research design

The extent to which sports injury incidence can be assessed depends upon: the definition of sports injury; the way in which incidence is expressed; the method used to count injuries; the method used to establish the population at risk; and the representativeness of the sample (Kranenborg 1982).

Injuries can be counted prospectively or retrospectively, using (paper or electronic) questionnaires or personal interviews. Exposure time can be quantified accurately in prospective studies. Therefore, this study design is appropriate to estimate the risk and incidence of injury according to the level and type of exposure of an athlete. Retrospective studies can also identify some risk factors, depending on the choice of research design (e.g., case–control studies) (Walter *et al.* 1985).

Depending upon the method of choice, the researcher will be confronted by phenomena such as recall bias, overestimation of hours of sports participation (Klesges *et al.* 1990), incomplete response, non-response, invalid injury descriptions, and problems related to the duration and cost of research.

Special attention has to be paid to the method of assessing the population at risk and to the representativeness of the study population. If the population at risk is not clearly identified, no reliable incidence data can be calculated. With regard to the representativeness of the study population, it has to be taken into consideration that the performance in sports (and therefore also the incidence of sports injuries) is highly determined by selection. Thereby, the results of any study are difficult to generalize and are mostly confined to the study population. Bol *et al.* (1991) set out four different types of selection with regard to sports injury epidemiology:

1 Self-selection (personal preferences) and/or selection by social environment (e.g., parents, friends, schools);

2 Selection by sports environment (e.g., trainer, coach);

3 Selection by sports organizations (e.g., organization of competitions by age and gender, the setting of participation standards); and

4 Selection by social, medical, and biologic factors (e.g., socioeconomic background, mortality, age, aging, gender).

For example, within a certain sport, competing at a high level increases sports injury incidence; in contrast to individual sports and team sports, more injuries are sustained during matches than during training; more injuries are sustained in contact sports than in non-contact sports; boys sustain more injuries during and shortly after the growth spurt.

Summary

The outcome of research on the extent of the sports injury problem is highly dependent upon the definition of "sports injury," "sports injury incidence," and "sports participation." The outcome of epidemiologic sports injury research depends on the research design and methodology, the representativeness of the sample, and whether or not exposure time was considered when calculating incidence.

The pediatric sports injury problem

As a result of the methodologic problems stated above, the injury problem in pediatric sports is difficult to grasp. The problem being that epidemiologic studies on sports injuries in youth are mostly restricted to a specific sport or to a limited number of sports. Although such studies can (to a certain extent) be used to determine the injury problem in a sport or population of predetermined choice, it might be clear that because of difficulties in comparability among studies, their findings cannot be combined to give a general overview of the pediatric sports injury problem. Therefore, in our attempt to obtain an impression of the pediatric sports injury problem in general, we are limited to studies that incorporate a wide array of sports, preferably in a general population. Such studies are expensive and are therefore limited in number. In addition, there is no such thing as "the injury problem." Different stakeholders have different views on this topic. For instance, a coach would see different injury prob-lems within his or her team than a ministry of sport would see within the sporting population. For this reason, we restrict ourselves in this chapter to a brief overview of descriptive studies on pediatric sports injuries.

Acute injuries

De Loës (1995) studied the sports injury incidence in a nationwide Swiss youth sporting organization. The number of injuries registered was limited by the injury definition used (i.e., medically treated sports injuries for which an insurance claim was made with the sports organization). During the period 1987–1989, a total of 16,120 injuries were registered, which was equal to an approximated annual 5,000 injuries in approximately 350,000 boys and girls aged 14–20 years. The overall injury incidence was 4.6 injuries per 10,000 h of sports participation. Major differences in injury incidence rates were found between the 32 included sports. The highest injury rates were found for contact sports (icehockey 8.6 injuries per 10,000 h; handball 7.2 injuries per 10,000 h; soccer 6.6 injuries per 10,000 h). In addition, differences were found between genders, where girls had higher incidences for basketball, alpine skiing, volleyball, and gymnastics. However, when data were standardized for differences in exposure time, no gender differences remained. Similar findings were previously reported by Macera and Wooten (1994) who reported no gender differences in a literature review on injuries among adolescents.

In the Netherlands, Backx *et al.* (1989) conducted a 6-week retrospective injury survey amongst 7468 school-aged children (8–17 years). They found an injury incidence of 10.6% over a period of 6 weeks. In this study, a sports injury was defined as any physical damage caused by a sports-related incident and reported as such. According to the authors, their broad injury definition led to a fairly high incidence figure for a 6-week recall period. They also reported a significant gender effect (girls having a 1.4 higher injury risk than boys), as well as a significant age effect (older children have more injuries), and a significant intensity effect (higher intensities are associated with higher injury risk). However, no exposure time was registered in this study, and therefore correction of possible exposure differences between genders, age groups, and intensities were not taken into account. In addition, only univariate statistics were applied to unravel a multicausal health problem. Thereby, any influence of interaction that may exist between for instance age, level of activity, and type of activity was not taken into account (perhaps younger children play at lower levels of intensity and in different sports than older children).

Baxter-Jones et al. (1993) studied a group of 453 elite 8- to 16-year-old athletes in the 2-year prospective TOYA study. In this study, a sports injury was defined as any injury resulting from sports participation with one or more of the following consequences: a reduction in the amount or level of sports activity and a need for medical treatment. The 1-year incidence was 40 injuries per 100 children. The authors were also able to collect training exposure and were able to determine injury incidence to be lower than 1 per 1000 h of training. While no gender differences were found, there were differences in injury incidence between sports and between training and competition (more injuries occurred during training). However, these differences were not corrected for exposure time. Thereby, it could well be that more training injuries were found because of the relatively large amount of training exposure as opposed to competition exposure.

In 2000, a TOYA follow-up study was conducted looking at the long-term injury effects of systematic training during or before adolescence (Maffulli et al. 2005). It was found that young elite athletes who continue training at a high level are at higher risk of injury than those who drop their level intensity to a lower level (e.g., competing at club level). From this study it remains uncertain whether intense training at a young age is associated with injury at later ages. However, it is more likely that injury risk at later ages is strongly associated with the current intensity and duration of training.

In addition to the abovementioned prospective studies, there are also a small number of continuous injury registration systems. The most commonly cited in the literature are the systems of the National Collegiate Athletic Association (NCAA; college sports) and the National Athletic Trainer's Association (NATA; high school sports). Table 11.2 shows the injury data for a variety of sports as registered between 1995 and 1997 by NATA (Powell & Barber-Foss 1999), as well as the injury data for 2003–2004 registered by the NCAA (2005). Although such ongoing systems suffer from their own methodologic problems and comparability depends on the mentioned methodologic issues, both systems clearly show higher injury rates during games compared to practice. In addition, a clear difference in gender and age (high school vs. college) cannot be seen.

Overuse injuries

Information on pediatric sports injuries comes from (prospective) epidemiologic studies such as the studies mentioned above. Because of difficulties in injury registration, most of these studies lack the ability to register overuse injuries. Our current knowledge of overuse injuries comes mostly from case studies and common clinical sense, with the exception of the study by Baxter-Jones et al. (1993). In this prospective study in elite athletes it was found that one-third of all injuries ($n = 148$) were of an overuse nature, where an overuse injury was defined as any injury for which the athlete was unable to remember a clear onset. A diagnosis could not be specified for 52% of these overuse injuries. The remaining injuries (48%) were diagnosed as osteochondrosis (26%), low back pain (13%), muscle strain (4%), stress fracture (3%), epiphyseal injury (1%), and spondylolysis (1%). No gender differences were found, but risk differences between sports were discovered (with swimmers being at highest risk). This finding is in line with the common belief that overuse injuries in children are caused by the repetitive training young athletes undergo in a single sports discipline (Micheli & Klein 1991; Gerrard 1993). In addition, it was found that overuse injuries were more severe than acute injuries. The mean absence from sport resulting from an overuse injury was 20 days compared to 13 days for acute injuries.

Summary

The studies discussed in this section do not give the reader a comprehensive view of the pediatric injury

	Injury rate (% of all injuries suffered in a specific sport) Injury rate expressed as the number of injuries per 1000 athlete exposures			
	NCAA		NATA	
Sport	Practice	Game	Practice	Game
Men				
Football	4.2 (58.2)	36.9 (41.8)	4.1 (59.1)	33.0 (40.9)
Wrestling	5.8 (66.8)	24.4 (33.2)	6.0 (69.1)	25.7 (30.9)
Soccer	4.1 (44.9)	20.1 (55.1)	4.4 (44.9)	18.8 (55.1)
Ice-hockey	2.0 (25.2)	19.7 (74.8)	1.9 (29.4)	15.9 (70.6)
Lacrosse	3.2 (61.8)	10.8 (38.2)	3.6 (66.3)	11.5 (33.7)
Basketball	4.0 (66.2)	8.6 (33.8)	3.9 (65.8)	9.0 (34.2)
Baseball	1.7 (40.8)	6.1 (59.2)	1.7 (44.3)	5.7 (56.7)
Women				
Soccer	4.9 (50.2)	17.2 (49.8)	5.2 (49.7)	15.5 (50.3)
Ice-hockey	4.3 (41.6)	17.2 (58.4)	2.3 (40.5)	10.4 (59.5)
Lacrosse	3.6 (67.0)	8.4 (33.0)	3.0 (70.8)	6.1 (29.2)
Basketball	3.8 (64.3)	8.0 (35.7)	4.0 (63.3)	~9 (36.7)
Gymnastics	6.2 (83.3)	13.9 (16.7)	3.5 (72.6)	14.0 (27.4)
Softball	2.1 (64.8)	4.7 (53.2)	2.2 (47.4)	4.0 (52.6)
Volleyball	3.5 (69.8)	3.9 (30.2)	3.2 (67.5)	3.9 (32.5)

Table 11.2 National Collegiate Athletic Association (NCAA; college) and National Athletic Trainer's Association (NATA; high school) pediatric injury rates by sport.

problem that may exist. However, one should keep in mind that at a younger age children are predominantly engaged in free play activities, school physical education lessons, and non-organized sports activities. As they grow older they move away from free play and become involved in organized sports. Obviously, in all these activities children sustain the risk of getting injured; nevertheless, there are differences. The younger child's free play activities, school physical education lessons, and non-organized sports activities tend to lead to acute (traumatic) sports injuries. Organized sports, on the other hand, may provide a greater risk of overuse injuries resulting from the repetitive strain placed upon tissues by the involvement in one or more specific sports and by advancing the duration and intensity of specialized training.

Preventing pediatric sports injuries

Preventive measures that are likely to work must be based upon proven risk factors and etiologic causes of injury. However, the information about the etiology of pediatric sports injuries is very limited, especially those that concern growth and growth spurt related overuse sports injuries. Nevertheless, a great number of measures to prevent pediatric sports injuries have been suggested. With respect to acute sports injuries, Smith *et al.* (1993) suggest the use of warm-up, the enhancement of compliance with (safety) rules, the improvement of adult knowledge about game rules (adults oversee pediatric sports participation), equipment and healthy sports behaviour, and the qualification of coaches and trainers. In addition, modification of the rules according to the physique of athletes, avoidance of excessive pressure from parents on winning, use and maintenance of certified safety equipment, and the supervision of all competitive sports are advocated preventive measures. Regarding prevention of overuse injuries, a reduction of training intensity (especially during periods of rapid growth) has been suggested (Baxter-Jones *et al.* 1993). Other suggested measures include the use of padded protective devices (Meyers 1993), matching children according to age, maturity, skill, weight, and height (Smith *et al.* 1993), and supervision of all competitive sports (Smith *et al.* 1993). Furthermore, it is advised that the 10% rule is followed, which indicates that in consecutive weeks the increase in training time, distance covered, or number of repetitions performed should not exceed 10% (Maffulli & Pintore 1990; Micheli & Klein 1991; Meyers 1993; Smith *et al.* 1993).

Although the preventive measures mentioned above seem logical and plausible, the "true" effects of many of these measures remain to be established in the pediatric sports setting. Nevertheless, despite this lack of etiologic information and lack of proven preventive measures, there is one crucial factor that has an important role in the prevention of sports injuries in children: understanding the behavior of children, their parents, and sports instructors.

In pediatric sports, behavior has a very important role in the etiology of injury (Van Mechelen & Verhagen 2005). It should be noted that, in this regard, risky behavior concerns not only the young athlete, but also all persons involved in the young athlete's activities (e.g., other athletes, parents, coaches, physical therapists). A young athlete is growing, learning, and developing his or her skills. During this process the youngest athletes (6–12 years) "evolve" from participants in joyful play to participants in competitive sports. Everything these athletes learn in this phase about preventive measures, listening to their own body, safe play, and fair play will reflect in sports participation at later ages. Especially during childhood, copying the behavior and techniques of professional role models (who are at the other side of the sports spectrum), may lead to risky situations in team sports where there are great differences between children in body size, skill level, and strength. Coaches and parents should remember that their "pupils" are not miniature Olympic athletes and should emphasize happy and safe play.

At later ages (12–18 years) the role of behavior in injury etiology changes, but does not diminish. At this stage, children enter competitive sports, where they are made responsible for their own sports behavior and preventive behavior. However, at these ages soccer players may not see the danger of a certain behavior on the field (e.g., certain forms of tackling or improper heading techniques). Although young athletes should assume responsibility for their own behavior, they need proper examples and education in their earlier childhood.

While the literature may provide "evidence-based" preventive measures that (potentially) reduce the risk of pediatric sports injuries, an intervention program aimed solely at changing or adapting behavior in children (an equally important preventive measure) has never been developed. Nevertheless, the current knowledge on (the etiology of) sports injuries is sufficient for the development of such an intervention program. The only randomized controlled trial in the area of pediatric sports injury prevention that incorporated behavioral change showed that in pupils of a secondary school (12–18 years) knowledge about injury prevention was improved (Backx 1991). This led to an improved attitude regarding sport injury prevention, which was suggested to have a favorable effect on injury incidence.

Conclusions

Pediatric athletes sustain both acute and overuse injuries. However, risk of sports-related injury appears to be lower than in adult athletes, although most previous research encounters methodologic problems that make it impossible to provide precise information. The current evidence suggests that acute injuries are more common than overuse injuries. However, it may well be that overuse injuries are largely underreported because of their self-limited nature. The risk of injury is linked with the type of sport, the amount of exposure time, and the quality of exposure (game vs. practice). Limited information is available on the etiology of pediatric sports injuries and most preventive measures are merely suggestions based on common sense. Nevertheless, many pediatric sports injuries are thought to be avoidable because behavioral causes might be tackled by proper education and adjustments during training and competitive play.

References

Adirim, T.A. & Cheng, T.L. (2003) Overview of injuries in the young athlete. *Sports Medicine* **33**, 75–81.

Backx, F.J.G. (1991) Sports injuries and youth. Etiology and prevention. Doctoral thesis, University of Utrecht, the Netherlands.

Backx, F.J.G., Erich, W.B.M., Kemper, A.B.A. & Verbeek, A.L.M. (1989) Sports injuries in school-aged children. An epidemiologic study. *American Journal of Sports Medicine* **17**, 234–240.

Baxter-Jones, A.D.G., Maffulli, N. & Helms, P. (1993) Low injury rates in elite athletes. *Archives of Disease in Childhood* **68**, 130–132.

Bol, E., Schmickli, S.L., Backx, F.J.G. & Van Mechelen, W. (1991) *Sportblessures onder de knie*. NISGZ publication 38, Papendal, the Netherlands.

De Loës, M. (1995) Epidemiology of sports injuries in the Swiss Organization "Youth and Sports" 1987–1989. Injuries, exposure and risks of main diagnosis. *International Journal of Sports Medicine* **16**, 134–138.

Gerrard, D.F. (1993) Overuse injury and growing bones: the young athlete at risk. *British Journal of Sports Medicine* **27**, 14–18.

Klesges, R.C., Eck, L.H., Mellon, M.W., Fulliton, W., Somes, G.W. & Hanson, C.L. (1990) The accuracy of self-reports of physical activity. *Medicine and Science in Sports and Exercise* **22**, 690–697.

Kranenborg, N. (1982) Sportbeofening en blessures. *Tijdschrift van de Socicale Geneeskunde* **60**, 224–227.

Macera, C.A. & Wooten, W. (1994) Epidemiology of sports and recreation injuries among adolescents. *Pediatric Exercise Science* **6**, 424–433.

Maffulli, N., Baxter-Jones, A.D.G. & Grieve, A. (2005) Long term sports involvement and sport injury rate in elite young athletes. *Archives of Disease in Childhood* **90**, 525–527.

Maffulli, N. & Pintore, E. (1990) Intensive training in young athletes. *British Journal of Sports Medicine* **24**, 237–239.

Meyers, J.F. (1993) The growing athlete. In: *Encyclopaedia of Sports Medicine*. Vol. IV, *Sports Injuries: Basic Principles of Prevention and Care* (Renstrom, P.O., ed.) Blackwell Scientific Publications, Oxford: 178–193.

Micheli, L.J. & Klein, J.D. (1991) Sports injuries in children and adolescents. *British Journal of Sports Medicine* **25**, 6–9.

National Collegiate Athletic Association Injury Surveillance System (2004) http://www1.ncaa.org/membership/ed_outreach/health-safety/iss/index.html. Accessed August 2005.

Parkkari, J., Kujala, U.M. & Kannus, P. (2001) Is it possible to prevent sports injuries? Review of controlled clinical trials and recommendations for future work. *Sports Medicine* **31**, 985–995.

Powell, J.W. & Barber-Foss, K.D. (1999) Injury patterns in selected high-school sports: a review of the 1995–1997 seasons. *Journal of Athletic Training* **34**, 277–284.

Schmikli, S.L. (2002) 97/98 Survey van sportblessures. In: *Trendrapport Bewegen en Gezondheid 2000/2001* (Ooijendijk, W.T.M., Hildebrandt, V.H. & Stiggelbout, M., eds.) TNO Arbeid, TNO PG. Hoofddorp, the Netherlands.

Smith, A.D., Andrish, J.T. & Micheli, L.J. (1993) The prevention of sports injuries of children and adolescents. *Medicine and Science in Sports and Exercise* **25**, 1–7.

van Mechelen, W. (1997) Etiology and prevention of sports injuries in youth. In: *Exercise and Fitness: Benfits and Risks* (Froberg, K., Lammert, O., St. Hansen, H. & Blimkie, C., eds.) Odense University Press, Finland: 209–228.

van Mechelen, W., Hlobil, H. & Kemper, H.C.G. (1992) Incidence, severity, aetiology and prevention of sports injuries. *Sports Medicine* **14**, 82–99.

van Mechelen, W. & Verhagen, E.A.L.M. (2005) Injury prevention in young people: time to accept responsibility. *Lancet* **366**, S46.

Walter, S.D., Sutton, J.R., McIntosh, J.M. & Connolly, C. (1985) The aetiology of sports injuries. A review of methodologies. *Sports Medicine* **12**, 65–71.

Chapter 12

Overuse Injuries in the Young Athlete: Stress Fractures

LYLE J. MICHELI AND JASON H. NIELSON

Over the last quarter century, children and adolescents have begun participating in organized sport training in growing numbers. As a result there has been an increase in stress fractures. This kind of overuse injury is caused by repetitive microtrauma from overhand throwing or foot impact in running and jumping. Annual incidence rates of stress fractures as high as 20% have been reported in prospective studies of young female athletes and military recruits (Brukner et al. 1999). Studies of collegiate athletes have estimated incidence of stress fractures among late adolescence and young adult female athletes to be between 2.7% and 6.9% (Goldberg & Pecora 1994; Johnson et al. 1994). Unfortunately, the details of the risk factors for overuse injuries such as stress fractures are as yet not well understood. In addition, the presentation of these injuries may sometimes cause confusion with neoplastic lesions because of the abundant callous present in the child or adolescent with stress fracture. What is currently known about risk factors for the occurrence of this overuse injury, as well as typical sites of stress fracture in young athletes, is the focus of this chapter.

Overuse injuries

Injuries sustained by young athletes in the course of athletic competition or training are well known to the coach, athletic administrator, and sports medicine physician. Sports-related injuries occur from two different mechanisms or combinations thereof:

1 Acute macrotraumatic injuries are those that occur as a result of a single application of major force to an area of the body, such as a twisting injury

of the ankle from a jump in basketball or a blow to the side of the leg in a football game.

2 Repetitive microtrauma results in so-called overuse injuries, which reflect repetitive microstress to areas of the body over a prolonged period of time, typically seen in the training regimen for sports.

One of the recent and healthy trends in sports medicine is to place special emphasis upon the prevention of injuries. Formerly, the great majority of physician attention in sport medicine was directed toward a proper diagnosis and appropriate treatment of sports-related injuries. This remains extremely important today, and the necessity for careful diagnosis and appropriate treatment cannot be overemphasized. In addition, however, prevention of sports-related injuries deserves equal emphasis in the armamentarium of the sports physician. Thus, the true sports medicine practitioner must assume responsibility for determining risk factors for the occurrence of injuries, particularly training-related overuse injuries, as a first step in injury prevention.

In recent years, we have gained more knowledge of the risk factors responsible for the occurrence of overuse injuries, particularly in young athletes (O'Neill & Micheli 1988; Hogan & Gross 2003). Overuse injuries in this age group are being seen with increasing frequency in sports medicine clinics. There are undoubtedly a variety of reasons for this, including:

1 Increased participation in organized sport by children and adolescents;

2 Tendency towards increased specialization in one or, at the most, two sports by growing numbers of children;

3 Growing emphasis upon increased duration and complexity of training at younger ages in a great variety of sports, particularly in gymnastics, figure skating, and swimming; and

4 Discrepancy between this increased activity and knowledge of coaches and parents.

Overuse injuries may occur in a variety of different tissues in the young athlete. They have in common a history of repetitive training or cyclic low level forces applied to an anatomic structure with the probable association of certain anatomic or physiologic susceptibilities in the affected individuals. These repetitive injuries can occur in articular cartilage, bone, muscle–tendon units, or fascia.

In addition to stress fractures occurring in long bones, tendon and apophyseal overuse injuries in the young athlete constitute an important subgroup of athletic injures in this age group. Chronic overuse or repetitive microtrauma in the pediatric and adolescent athlete or dancer has been described as etiology of injury at the tendon insertion of the traction apophysis (Micheli 1987; Micheli & Feghlandt 1996). Injury to the tendonitis secondary to repetitive microtrauma in the young athlete has also been recognized in the medical literature (Busch 1990). These injuries are similar to those in their adult counterpart. In this chapter, we limit our focus to actual bony stress fractures in the young athlete. However, it should be kept in mind that the young athlete may be more prone to all types of injury because of the immature nature of the skeleton.

Activity can not only be detrimental but can also be beneficial for bone health. Runners who participate during childhood and adolescence in ball sports may develop bone with greater and more symmetrically distributed bone mass, and with enhanced protection from future stress fractures (Fredericson *et al.* 2005). Despite the benefits of activity, there is a level of training at which the risk of stress fractures increases significantly (Loud *et al.* 2005). Stanitski (1993) has reported numerous stress fractures in young athletes. His hypothesis is that highly eccentric and concentric forces across a specific bone will produce repetitive muscle actions that predispose bone to failure.

Stress fracture

The overuse injury of bone (stress fracture) has attracted particular attention in medicine and, specifically, athletic medicine. The first report of a stress fracture in the medical literature was that of the German military surgeon Breithaupt (1855) who noted the occurrence of these lesions in young military recruits. These lesions were subsequently labeled as "march fractures" because of their propensity for occurrence with military training. This entity has been identified in subsequent literature by a variety of terms, including fatigue fracture, spontaneous fracture, pseudofracture, and insufficiency fracture.

Types of stress fracture

At the present time, stress fractures can be appropriately divided into two general categories: (i) insufficiency fractures; and (ii) fatigue fractures of bone. This division, first suggested by Pentecost *et al.* (1964), describes an insufficiency fracture as being produced by normal or physiologic stresses applied to bone with deficient structural characteristics, while a fatigue fracture occurs when excessive cyclical stress is applied to bone of normal structure.

Stress fractures in children: different sites from adults

While traditionally, and certainly in adults, stress fractures have been cataloged as those occurring in the metaphysis or diaphysis of bone and, in particular, long bones, it is appropriate at this time, particularly given additional information from the recent medical literature, to broaden the categories to include stress fractures occurring in the subchondral bone of the joint surface in children and adolescents and at the physeal plate of the child or adolescent (Song *et al.* 2004).

It is important to note that the response of the growing skeleton to repetitive training is quite different from that of the fully mature skeleton. Stress fractures in the child or growing adolescent occur in a different pattern of injury involving different sites, both throughout the body and within the very structures of the bones involved, and also have a different clinical and radiographic presentation and healing response (Devas 1963; Engh *et al.* 1970; Walter & Wolf 1977; Reeder *et al.* 1996). In cases with atypical location or presentation, magnetic resonance imaging (MRI) is reliable in detecting injury. MRI allows early detection of osseous changes and precise anatomic detail of the extent of injury. In addition, MRI is the preferred choice of imaging for evaluation the continuum of osseous manifestation of stress injuries (Spitz & Newberg 2002). In the lower extremity, the tibia appears to be much more commonly affected than the fibula or bones of the foot, similar to adults. However, fatigue fractures of the tibia in children tend to occur at the juncture of the diaphysis and metaphysis, while adult fractures more commonly occur in the diaphysis, in particular the distal third of the diaphysis of the tibia (Fig. 12.1).

Fibular fractures, which are much more common in the running adult or female ballet dancer, may also occur in the child. As opposed to tibial stress fractures, which are thought to be brought about by impact, fibular stress fractures may be related more to distraction and rotational forces occurring in the process of running or jumping.

Sports producing special risk

Additionally, there are different levels of risk between sports, which reflect the different patterns of forces involved in these activities. Running sports characteristically involve fatigue fractures of the lower extremity but, in particular, of the tibia, fibula, and foot (Devas & Sweetnam 1956; Devas 1958; Orava *et al.* 1978; Norfray *et al.* 1980; Orava & Hulkko 1984; McBryde 1985; Matheson *et al.* 1987a,b; Milgrom *et al.* 1994; Bennell *et al.* 1995). Certainly, stress fractures of the femur and pelvis can occur in runners (Major & Helms 1997), but these are less common. By contrast, the jumping sports, such as basketball, have been reported with a relatively higher incidence of stress fractures of the distal femur, pelvis, and patella (Devas 1960; Kaltsas 1981). Overhand throwing and racquet sports are associated with stress fractures of the humerus, first rib, and elbow (Miller 1960; Allen 1974; Belkin 1980;

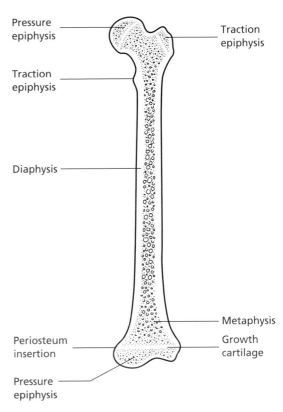

Fig. 12.1 A schematic long bone of a child with epiphysis, metaphysis, and diaphysis. Redrawn from Renström and Roux (1988).

Rettig 1983; Lankenner & Micheli 1985; Rettig & Beltz 1985; Brukner 1998). More recent reports have demonstrated repetitive overuse physeal stress fractures of the distal radius and ulna in gymnasts, and scaphoid stress fractures as well as articular surface osteochondral injuries of the elbow in gymnasts and throwers (Carter *et al.* 1988; Albanese *et al.* 1989; Krijnen *et al.* 2003).

Differential diagnoses

It is imperative for the sports physician dealing with a young athlete presenting with chronic pain always to include the possibility of stress fracture in the differential diagnoses. Fortunately, the clinical presentation in the child or adolescent with stress fracture may be more dramatic than that seen in the adult. In superficial bones, there may be an area of swelling or very localized tenderness and, by radiograph, healing callous may be evident in response to the repetitive microfracture and subsequent partial healing at the site (Devas 1963). This is less common in the adult. A very careful history, taking into account the exact details of training and the equipment used in training, can help determine with some certainty that: (i) an overuse injury is present; and (ii) what type of overuse injury and which tissue is most suspect. However, it is important to remember that infection or tumor may present chronically in the child or adolescent participating in organized sport competition or training. Because these entities are relatively more common in the musculoskeletal system of the child than in the adult, additional care must be taken when dealing with the young athlete presenting with extremity symptoms.

We have seen a fatigue fracture of the distal femur in a cross-country runner diagnosed unnecessarily late and initially confused with chronic patellofemoral stress syndrome and given treatment with exercise and icing to the knee. Additionally, we have seen a young athlete with pain at the knee treated again as patellofemoral stress syndrome with icing and exercise when the etiology was actually an osteogenic sarcoma of the distal femur.

Risk factors

It is useful when assessing the young athlete complaining of chronic or training-related pain of gradual onset to have in mind a specific category of risk factors for overuse injuries when beginning the history and physical examination. The risk factors for overuse injuries are listed in Table 12.1 (O'Neill & Micheli 1988; Gerrard 1993; Adirim & Cheng 2003).

Often, two or more of these risk factors will appear to be acting in the occurrence of a given overuse injury. For example, a young athlete rapidly increases the volume of training while training in inadequately cushioned, older shoes and on surfaces that have become harder because of climatic changes such as lack of rain.

Table 12.1 Risk factors for overuse injury. (Reproduced with permission from O'Neill & Micheli 1988.)

Training error/error of technique
Muscle–tendon imbalance
Anatomic malalignment
Footwear
Playing surface
Associated disease state
Gender factors
Cultural deconditioning
Growth

Training error

The most important risk factor for stress fracture is training error. It is the most frequently encountered risk factor in the development of overuse injuries in young athletes. The most important component of this appears to be an increase in the total volume and also the rate of progression of training (Nilsson & Westlin 1971; Mustajoki *et al.* 1983; Swissa *et al.* 1989; Adirim & Cheng 2003; Bergstrom 2004). Training error may be a risk factor in the highly skilled, elite athlete as well as the novice athlete just beginning training (Fig. 12.2). We have learned empirically that most athletes should not increase their training more than 10% per week. In effect then, a young runner who is running 20 min·day^{-1}, 5 days per week, can probably safely increase to

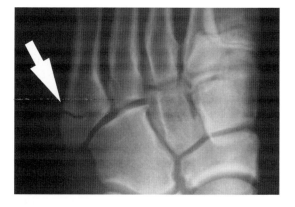

Fig. 12.2 An AP X-ray of the foot of a young football player who began experiencing pain after the onset of rigorous preseason conditioning under a new coach. He presented with bilateral proximal fifth metatarsal stress fractures.

22 min·day^{-1}, 5 days per week, the following week. Similarly, we have seen a case of an elite distance runner at college level who decreased his running training from 145 to 97 km·week^{-1} during a 3-week examination period. When he quickly resumed his previous training regimen of 145 km·week^{-1}, he developed a stress fracture of the tibia. Intensive summer sports camps specializing exclusively in one sport also increase the risk of overuse injury through training error. For example, youngsters intensely interested in soccer, who normally play a total of 8–10 h·week^{-1} of soccer, may suddenly be put in a summer camp situation in which they are training in soccer 6 h·day^{-1} for 5 days per week. This risk factor alone may be sufficient to precipitate the occurrence of a tibial or fibular stress fracture.

Muscle–tendon imbalance

Muscle–tendon imbalance is perhaps the second most important risk factor in overuse injury in this age group. Growth may contribute to changes in the relative strength and flexibility of agonist or antagonist muscle groups across major joints in the young athlete and, in particular, the adolescent growth spurt in this instance (Micheli 1983; Hawkins & Metheny 2001). A careful assessment of muscle–tendon characteristics should be carried out as a preparticipation assessment in young athletic candidates. This is particularly important with respect to the prevention of stress fractures. Matheson et al. (1987b) have proposed that muscle bulk and, in particular, the potential for muscle fatigue, may be an important contributory factor to the etiology of stress fractures. This hypothesis has been supported by others (Stanitski 1993). In young athletes in particular, four different characteristics of growth should be assessed:

1 Decreases in flexibility in association with growth and, in particular, growth spurts;
2 Strength increases with growth, which may not be uniform, additionally contribute to the imbalances about joints;
3 Sport-specific imbalances of muscle strength or flexibility that are related to the particular demands or training regimens of certain sports or activities;

4 Repetitive techniques, such as overhand throwing or swimming, which can result in joint contractures and secondary asymmetrical stresses upon the bones and joints involved.

Anatomic malalignment

Anatomic malalignment, particularly of the spine and lower extremities, has been suggested as a contributory factor in the occurrence of overuse injuries in young athletes (Krivickas 1997). The malalignments may include:

1 Discrepancies of leg length;
2 Abnormalities of hip rotation;
3 Coronal alignment of the femur and tibia, such as genu valgum or tibia vara; and
4 Excessive flattening of the arch or pronation of the foot.

Unfortunately, no specific studies on risk factors for stress fracture in young athletes have yet been performed. However, studies of military recruits have suggested a number of potential risk factors. Anatomic alignment of the hip, in particular, may contribute to the potential for stress fracture in the young athlete. Giladi et al. (1987) found that excessive external rotation of the hip in military recruits increased the risk of lower extremity stress fracture twofold compared with military recruits with less hip turnout or internal rotation. Similarly, there have been a number of clinical observations that tibia vara may increase the potential for tibial stress fracture in running athletes, particularly young female athletes (Engber 1977; Dickson & Kichline 1987). Excessive pronation has been discussed as a risk factor for overload of the entire lower extremity, including the potential for stress fractures (Dickson & Kichline 1987; Renstrom 1993). High-arched cavus feet, with their apparent decreased ability for impact absorption, have also been implicated in overuse injuries about the foot and lower leg in particular (Cornwell 1984).

Footwear

Impact-absorbing qualities as well as the mechanical stabilization potential of footwear use in sports, particularly the running sports, appear to be an important component in the prevention of overuse injury (Milgrom *et al.* 1985; Thacker *et al.* 2002). The importance of impact-absorbing materials not only in the hind foot and heel area of the shoe, but also in the forefoot, has been noted (Cavanagh 1980). A study of stress fractures of the foot in basketball players has also suggested that inadequately cushioned footwear may increase stress to these anatomic structures (Milgrom *et al.* 1992).

Playing surface

Clinical observation for a number of years has suggested that the relative hardness of the running or playing surface is a factor in the stress delivered to the lower extremities in sports. Observations of distance runners and dancers have suggested hardness of surface as a possible contributing factor in the occurrence of lower extremity stress fractures in particular (Washington 1978; McMahon & Greene 1979; Seals 1983).

Associated disease state

In assessing the potential for overuse injury and, in particular, stress fracture, the overall health of the child, including pre-existent illnesses, particularly viral illnesses, hormonal conditions, or any other factors that can affect the relative structural strength of the bones must be carefully assessed.

Gender factors

A number of recent studies have suggested deficient intake of calcium and vitamins in amenorrheic distance runners and ballet dancers. Prevention of stress injury to bone involves maximizing peak bone mass in the pediatric, adolescent, and young adult age groups. Maintaining adequate calcium nutrition and caloric intake, exercise, and hormonal balance are important in optimizing skeletal integrity and preventing overuse fractures (Nattiv & Armsay 1997). The combination of amenorrhea, osteopenia, and increased incidence of overuse injuries, particularly stress fractures, has been referred to as the "female athlete triad." Studies have shown significantly lower levels of bone mineral density in

amenorrheic vs. eumenorrheic female athletes matched by age, weight, sport, and training regimen (Drinkwater *et al.* 1984; Warren *et al.* 1986; Warren 1987; Warren & Goodman 2003). Barrow and Salia (1988) found a 2 : 1 ratio of occurrence of stress fractures in amenorrheic vs. menstruating runners, while another study of female athletes at Penn State University found 24% of the amenorrheic college athletes to have stress fractures, while the overall prevalence of stress fractures in female athletes was 9% (Cook *et al.* 1987). Despite this, more recently, Loud *et al.* (2005) reported that age at menarche, z-score of BMI, calcium intake, vitamin D intake, and daily dietary intake were all unrelated to stress fractures after controlling for age among young females. They did find that each hour of high-impact activity significantly increased the risk of a stress fracture among adolescent girls. In particular, running, gymnastics, and cheerleading were sports with greater odds of sustaining a stress fracture (Loud *et al.* 2005).

Cultural deconditioning

At the present time, there is a great deal of debate regarding the relative level of fitness or declining levels of fitness in children in industrialized nations, particularly in the USA. It can be hypothesized that the child who is physically inactive will show a decline and a decreased level of fitness in its most basic sense in all the tissues of the body, particularly in the musculoskeletal tissues. The responses of the musculoskeletal system, particularly the bones, to increased levels of physiologic stress are increases in bone size, density, and strength. These improved physical characteristics from general physical activity would exert a protective effect on the child who begins progressive sport-specific athletic training and decrease the potential for overuse injuries in general and stress fractures in particular in the face of increased levels of sport training. Conversely, the relatively inactive and culturally deconditioned child who does an excessive amount of sitting at school, travels in cars, and watches television not only has been demonstrated to have increased levels of obesity, but undoubtedly will demonstrate decreased levels of structural strength in bones and joints.

Growth

Growth is the unique characteristic of the child or young adolescent. With physeal closure, childhood ends; the adolescent approaches the adult stage of physical development and in turn the characteristics of the musculoskeletal system including bone changes dramatically.

Growth cartilage has been demonstrated to be more susceptible to repetitive trauma than adult cartilage, whether at the physis, articular surface, or the apophyseal sites of major muscle–tendon insertions. Repetitive microtrauma to the growth plate from athletic activities has been suggested as an etiologic factor in adult-onset arthritis at both the hip and knee (Murray & Duncan 1971; Bright et al. 1974; Stulberg et al. 1975).

There is a growing body of evidence demonstrating that repetitive microtrauma, particularly of floor work and vaulting activities, has resulted in an overuse injury of the physeal plate in young gymnasts (DiFiore et al. 1996, 1997; Koh et al. 2003). The gymnast complaining of wrist pain with repetitive activities, particularly on hand impact, must be assessed very carefully for the possibility of either scaphoid stress fracture or distal radial physeal injury (Gabel 1998). This, in turn, can result in relative overgrowth of the ulna and progression of serious joint derangement at the wrist in this athletic age group (Caine et al. 1997).

The articular cartilage in the child is also undergoing endochondral ossification and is, in effect, a growth plate. During more intense phases of growth, the columns of cartilage are the weakest portion of the extremity. This weakness is secondary to the influence of somatotropin and low levels of testosterone (Segesser et al. 1995). Repetitive impact or shear stresses to the adult articular cartilage can result in mechanical disruption and the development of "chondromalacia." In the child, the response to similar repetitive forces appears to result in a "stress fracture" of the subchondral bone. Osteochondritis dissecans of the capitellum in the child baseball pitcher (Klingele & Kocher 2002; Hang et al. 2004) or gymnast represents stress fractures of the subchondral bone in this age group. Similarly, osteochondritic defects at the knee, ankle, and

within the foot in runners, gymnasts, and field sport players, as well as young dancers, may reflect similar abnormal stress fractures at the joint surface (Conway 1937).

Osgood–Schlatter disease of the tibial tubercle is the best-known apophyseal stress fracture (Demirag et al. 2004). The general class of overuse injuries, entitled traction apophysitises, appears to be very similar in pattern of injury to stress fractures of long bone diaphysis and metaphysis (Ogden & Southwick 1976; Micheli 1987; Segesser et al. 1995). Similar injuries occur at the heel (Sever's disease) and in the foot at the tarsal accessory navicular (Micheli & Ireland 1987; Omey & Micheli 1999; Ogden et al. 2004).

During periods of accelerated growth rate, particularly occurring in the summer seasons and during the adolescent growth spurt, where primary sites of growth are within the long bones, a relative tightness of the muscle–tendon units spanning these bones and joints may occur. Periods of "growth spurt" may be followed by secondary transient increase in muscle–tendon tightness or imbalances of alignment, which may increase the chance of overuse injury in general, and stress fracture in particular. During these periods of rapid growth and increased susceptibility, supplemental exercises to combat these muscle imbalances as well as a decrease in the total volume of training is advisable.

Sites of stress fracture in young athletes

Low back

Young athletes involved in sport with repetitive flexion or, in particular, repetitive extension maneuvers of the back may have onset of back pain, which is often brought about by a stress fracture through the pars intra-articularis of the lumbar spine. Low back pain in young athletes has significant differences from their adult counterpart (Micheli & Wood 1995).

These injuries were once thought to be primarily genetic or congenital in origin, but this has been largely disproved. It is now widely recognized that these are acquired lesions, which result from repetitive stress to the lumbar spine. In most cases, fatigue failure occurs through the pars intra-articularis but, on occasion, this may also occur to the pedicle or facet of the spine.

Imaging advances, including single photon emission computerized tomography (SPECT) bone scan, have greatly aided the early diagnosis of this injury (Gregory *et al.* 2005), particularly before frank fracture has occurred through the pars. In addition, the sports physician must be alert to the occurrence of this injury and should have a very high index of suspicion for it based upon the history and physical examination. In a child involved in repetitive extension sports in particular, such as gymnastics, figure skating, or dance, who complains of insidious onset of pain and who, on physical examination, is found to have pain with provocative hyperextension testing, a posterior element failure of the stress type must be presumed until proven otherwise.

If these lesions are detected early before fibrous union or non-union has occurred, there is a good potential for healing with relative rest or immobilization in spinal orthotics (Cohen & Stuecker 2005). Unfortunately, because the environment for fracture is that of distraction rather than compression, once the frank bone lesions have occurred, particularly if they have occurred bilaterally in the posterior elements, attainment of ultimate union can be much more difficult.

Upper extremity

Stress fractures of the upper extremity in young athletes are relatively uncommon but certainly are to be suspected in the throwing sports or in sports involving repetitive overloading of the upper extremity (Brooks 2001). Stress fractures of the humerus and forearm occurring in the throwing sports appear to be brought about by repetitive torsional stress of the upper extremity. In the child athlete with open growth plates, this stress may be localized at the physeal plate and has been dubbed "Little League shoulder" (Fig. 12.3) (Cahill *et al.* 1974). Frank rotational fractures through the humerus have occurred from throwing, and fractures of the forearm have also been reported in young athletes.

Repetitive impacting at the elbow in young athletes, who have not yet reached full skeletal

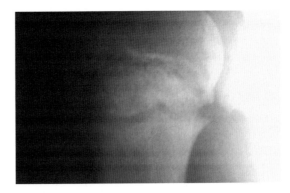

Fig. 12.3 An AP X-ray of the shoulder in a young baseball pitcher demonstrates a widened proximal humeral physis.

maturity, can result in osteochondral lesions of the capitellum or partial avulsion injuries at the medial epicondyle of the elbow as a result of repetitive traction in secondary fatigue failure through the cartilage bone junction of the epicondyle (Fig. 12.4). Fatigue fractures have also been reported across the olecranon from repetitive throwing in young athletes (Parr & Burns 2003).

Fatigue fractures at the wrist have been reported as a result of repetitive impacting of the upper extremity in young athletes. Most notable have been the recent reports of physeal injury of the distal radius and ulna in young gymnasts. Stress fractures of the os scaphoideum (Matzkin & Singer 2000) have also been reported in this group of athletes.

Pelvis and hip

Stress fractures about the pelvis and hip in young athletes are relatively unusual. These have been much more commonly reported in young female runners or athletes involved in jumping sports. Iliac crest stress injuries have been reported in young athletes as a result of repetitive training (Soyuncu & Gur 2004). Much more commonly in this age group, stresses about the pelvis will result in frank apophyseal avulsions (Micheli 1990).

Stress fractures of the femur in young athletes have certainly been reported (Walter & Wolf 1977; St Pierre *et al.* 1995). Distal stress fractures of the femur are much more common than proximal stress

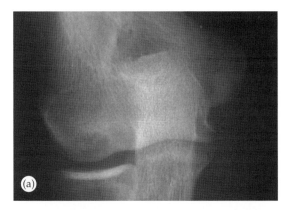

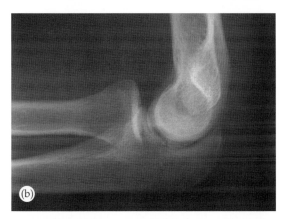

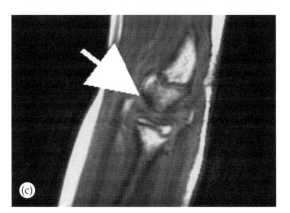

Fig. 12.4 (a,b) An AP and lateral X-ray; and (c) magnetic resonance image (MRI) of the elbow in young competitive baseball player demonstrating an osteochondral lesion of the capetellum.

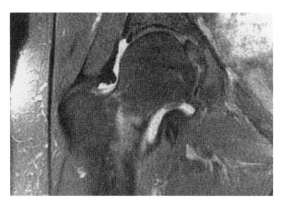

Fig. 12.5 A coronal T2 magnetic resonance image (MRI) of the hip demonstrating a stress fracture of the femur.

fractures. Occasionally, however, hip pain in the young athlete will ultimately be found to be caused by a fracture of the base of the neck of the femur (Fig. 12.5) (St Pierre *et al*. 1995). Unfortunately, these stress fractures in young athletes have often been confused with the reports of stress fractures of the hip in military recruits. In military recruits, these have typically been detected late with frank displacement of these fractures and a poor prognosis. In the young athlete, however, these are often compression-type stress fractures at the base of the femur and, if detected early enough, healing can be expected with relative rest and limited weight-bearing.

The stress fractures of the femur more commonly encountered in this age group are those of the distal femur. These can be encountered in the jumping sports but have also been seen in young runners. Very often the first complaint in this fracture is that of knee pain. The diagnosis may not be suspected early on. We have encountered cases of frank displacement of these fractures in this age group.

Ankle and foot

The complaint of ankle pain in young athlete undergoing repetitive training may be secondary to early signs of stress fractures occurring at this site. Stress fractures of the medial malleolus have been encountered in this age group and, again, partial avulsions of the medial malleolus in younger children engaged in repetitive training activities and running

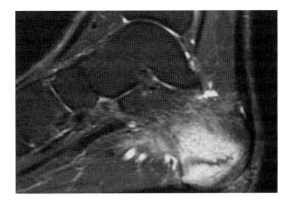

Fig. 12.6 A magnetic resonance image (MRI) of the calcaneous demonstrating a stress fracture.

have been reported (Stanitski & Micheli 1993; Shabat *et al.* 2002).

Stress fractures of the foot may also occur in young athletes. While stress fractures of the body of the os calcis are relatively rare in this age group (Fig. 12.6), apophyseal injury from repetitive training, such as Sever's apophysitis at the heel and painful accessory navicular in the midfoot, have been reported (Micheli 1987; Micheli & Ireland 1987).

Two stress fractures of the foot in young athletes bear special mention. Stress fractures of the tarsal navicular (Omey & Micheli 1999; Ostlie 2001) may present as low grade, aching midfoot pain and medial midfoot tenderness (Monteleone 1995). This is most commonly seen in basketball players and runners and particularly hurdlers (Keene & Lange 1986). Too often, the diagnosis is not made sufficiently early. This appears to be because these pains are often non-specific and associated with repetitive running in particular. Often plain radiographs are unremarkable early on, and the diagnosis is not made until frank fracture has occurred through the navicular. Early detection, of course, can be made with MRI or a bone scan. Detailed bony definition of the frank fracture is often possible only with computerized tomography (CT) scanning. Delayed detection of this fracture is doubly unfortunate because this is a bone with tenuous blood supply resulting in a slow rate of healing and a relatively high rate of complications develops from this fracture.

The second site of difficult stress fracture in the foot in young athletes is that of the base of the fifth metatarsal (Fig. 12.2). Once again, these stress fractures are often detected late after they have become fully established. This is a slow healing bone, sometimes requiring internal fixation to attain satisfactory union of the stress fractures in the proximal third of the fifth metatarsal.

Other special stress fractures have been encountered in young athletes undergoing repetitive training, including stress fractures of the proximal second metatarsal, as well as the shaft of the metatarsal, which is much better known.

Conclusions

This discussion of stress fractures in young athletes has emphasized early detection of risk factors for stress fracture in order to aid in the early diagnosis and the prevention of later complications when dealing with this entity. Early symptoms of pain, swelling, and limitation of motion accompany stress fractures. Ohta-Fukushima *et al.* (2002) found that continuous pain lasting over 3 weeks was a common finding in young athletes with stress fractures. In addition, young athletes who were diagnosed within 3 weeks of onset of symptoms had a significant decrease in time to return to play compared with those who were treated after the 3-week point (Ohta-Fukushima *et al.* 2002). In most of these stress fractures, early diagnosis results in a much simpler mechanism of treatment and, in many cases, ensures satisfactory union with ability to resume progressive athletic training without problem.

As our understanding of the risk factors for the occurrence of this serious overuse injury increases, it is hoped that it will be possible to detect individuals with a special propensity for stress fractures, particularly at certain sites of the body. Steps may then be taken to prevent the occurrence of these injuries by careful management of training regimens, protective footwear, and playing surfaces.

Challenges for future research

The major thrust of any repetitive or training injury in athletes of any age should be determination of risk factors for injury and steps to prevent the occurrence of these injuries. At the present time, there is growing knowledge about risk factors for the occurrence of both acute traumatic injuries and repetitive microtrauma overuse injuries in adults, particularly in such activities as military training, work activities, and sports.

All too little is known about the details of risk factors for overuse injury, particularly stress fractures in young athletes. The presence of physeal cartilage at the joint surface, epiphyseal plate, and apophyseal sites of major muscle–tendon insertions appears to alter the presentation and the occurrence of stress injuries to bone, but this has not been well studied or well researched in either animal models or human epidemiologic studies.

At the clinical level, much more information could be gained about these injuries by establishing a clinical registry of stress fractures in young athletes in which the occurrence of injury and the determination of associated risk factors could be recorded in addition to epidemiologic data of age,

gender, height and weight, and, if possible, pubertal stage.

Epidemiologic studies in sport-specific environments in which the population at risk is well known would add greatly to the understanding of the particular sport activities, which carry the greatest risk of the occurrence of overuse injuries, and stress fractures in particular.

More basic research is needed in the study of response of bone to repetitive training. Little is currently known about changes in tertiary structure, numbers of Haversian systems, bone mineral density, and size dimensions of long bones in response to repetitive training. The relationship of repetitive training to longitudinal transverse and circumferential bone growth in children and adolescents participating in repetitive training is now well known. Human studies of this phenomenon as well as the development of an animal model to study repetitive training and its effects upon the strength, dimensions, and "fitness" level of the musculoskeletal system remains to be developed.

References

Adirim, T.A. & Cheng, T.L. (2003) Overview of injuries in the young athlete. *Sports Medicine* **33**, 75–81.

Albanese, S.A., Plamer, A.K., Kerr, D.R., Carpenter, C.W., Lisi, D. & Levinsohn, E.M. (1989) Wrist pain and distal growth plate closure of the radius in gymnasts. *Journal of Pediatric Orthopedics* **9**, 23–28.

Allen, M.E. (1974) Stress fracture of the humerus: a case study. *American Journal of Sports Medicine* **12**, 244–245.

Barrow, G.W. & Saha, S. (1988) Menstrual irregularity and stress fractures in collegiate female distance runners. *American Journal of Sports Medicine* **16**, 209–216.

Belkin, S.C. (1980) Stress fractures in athletes. *Orthopaedic Clinics of North America* **11**, 735–742.

Bennell, K.L., Malcolm, S.A., Thomas, S.A., *et al.* (1995) Risk factors for stress fractures. I. Female track and field athletes: a retrospective analysis. *Clinical Journal of Sports Medicine* **5**, 229–235.

Bergstrom, K.A. (2004) Back injuries and pain in adolescents attending a ski high school. *Knee Surgery, Sports Traumatology, Arthroscopy* **12**, 80–85.

Breithaupt, M.D. (1855) Zur pathologie des mensch lichen Fusses [The pathology of human feet]. *Medicishche Zeitung* **24**, 169–171, 175–177.

Bright, R.W., Burstein, A.H. & Elmore, S.M. (1974) Epiphyseal plate-cartilage. A biomechanical and histological analysis and failure modes. *Journal of Bone and Joint Surgery* **56A**, 688–703.

Brooks, A.A. (2001) Stress fractures of the upper extremity. *Clinical Journal of Sports Medicine* **20**, 613–620.

Brukner, P. (1998) Stress fractures of the upper limb. *Sports Medicine* **26**, 415–424.

Brukner, P., Bennell, K. & Matheson, G. (1999) *Stress Fractures*. Blackwell Science, Victoria, Australia.

Busch, M.T. (1990) Sports medicine in children and adolescents In: *Lovell and Winter's Pediatric Orthopaedics*. Lippincott-Raven, Philadelphia, PA: 1273–1285.

Cahill, B.R., Tullos, H.S. & Fain, R.H. (1974) Little League shoulder. *Journal of Sports Medicine* **2**, 150–153.

Caine, D., Howe, W., Ross, W. & Bergman, G. (1997) Does repetitive physical loading inhibit radial growth in female

gymnasts? *Clinical Journal of Sports Medicine* **7**, 304–308.

Carter, S.R., Aldridge, M.J., Fitzgerald, R. & Davies, A.M. (1988) Stress changes of the wrist in adolescent gymnasts. *British Journal of Radiology* **61**, 109–112.

Cavanagh, P.R. (1980) *The Running Shoe Book*. Anderson World, Mountain View, CA.

Cohen, E. & Stuecker, R.D. (2005) Magnetic resonance imaging in diagnosis and follow-up of impending spondylolysis in children and adolescents: early treatment may prevent pars defects. *Journal of Pediatric Orthopedics B* **14**, 63–67.

Conway, F.M. (1937) Osteochondritis dissecans: description of the stages of the condition and its probable traumatic etiology. *American Journal of Surgery* **38**, 691.

Cook, S.D., Harding, A.F., Thomas, K.A., Morgan, E.L., Schnurpfeil, K.M. & Haddad, R.J. (1987) Trabecular bone density and menstrual function in women runners. *American Journal of Sports Medicine* **15**, 503–507.

Cornwell, G. (1984) Sports medicine and the pes cavus foot. *British Columbia Medical Journal* **26**, 573–574.

Demirag, B., Ozturk, C., Yazici, Z. &
Sarisozen, B. (2004) The
pathophysiology of Osgood–Schlatter
disease: a magnetic resonance
investigation. *Journal of Pediatric
Orthopedics B* **13**, 379–382.

Devas, M.B. (1958) Stress fractures of the
tibia in athletes or "shin soreness". 1.
Bone Joint Surgery **40B**, 227–239.

Devas, M.B. (1960) Stress fractures of the
patella. *Journal of Bone and Joint Surgery*
42B, 71–74.

Devas, M.B. (1963) Stress fractures in
children. *Journal of Bone and Joint Surgery*
45B, 528–541.

Devas, M.B. & Sweetnam, R. (1956) Stress
fractures of the fibula: a review of 50
cases in athletes. *Journal of Bone and Joint
Surgery* **38B**, 818–829.

Dickson, T.B. & Kichline, P.D. (1987)
Functional management of stress
fractures in female athletes using a
pneumatic leg brace. *American Journal of
Sports Medicine* **15**, 869.

DiFiore, J.P., Puffer, J.C., Mandelbaum,
B.R. & Dorey, F. (1997) Distal radial
growth plate injury and positive ulnar
variance in nonelite gymnasts.
American Journal of Sports Medicine
25, 763–768.

DiFiore, J.P., Puffer, J.C., Mandelbaum,
B.R. & Mar, S. (1996) Factors associated
with wrist pain in the young gymnast.
American Journal of Sports Medicine **24**,
9–14.

Drinkwater, B.L., Nilson, K., Chestnut,
C.M., *et al.* (1984) Bone mineral content
of amenorrheic and eumenorrheic
athletes. *New England Journal of Medicine*
311, 277–281.

Engber, W.D. (1977) Stress fractures of the
medial tibial plateau. *Journal of Bone and
Joint Surgery* **59A**, 767–769.

Engh, C.A., Robinson, R.A. & Milgram, J.
(1970) Stress fractures in children.
Journal of Trauma **10**, 532–541.

Fredericson, M., Ngo, J. & Cobb, K. (2005)
Effects of ball sports on future risk of
stress fracture in runners. *Clinical Journal
of Sports Medicine* **15**, 136–141.

Gabel, G.T. (1998) Gymnastic wrist
injuries. *Clinical Journal of Sports
Medicine* **17**, 611–621.

Gerrard, D.F. (1993) Overuse injury and
growing bones: the young athlete at risk.
British Journal of Sports Medicine **27**,
14–18.

Giladi, M., Milgrom, C., Stein, M., *et al.*
(1987) External rotation of the hip. A
predictor of risk for stress fractures.
Clinical Orthopaedics and Related Research
216, 131–134.

Goldberg, B. & Pecora, C. (1994) Stress
fractures: a risk of increased training in
freshman. *Physician and Sportsmedicine*
22, 68–78.

Gregory, P.L., Batt, M.E., Kerslake, R.W. &
Webb, J.K. (2005) Single photon
emission computerized tomography
and reverse gantry computerized
tomography findings in patients with
back pain investigated for
spondylolysis. *Clinical Journal of Sports
Medicine* **15**, 79–86.

Hang, D.W., Chao, C.M. & Hang, Y.S.
(2004) A clinical and roentgenographic
study of Little League elbow. *American
Journal of Sports Medicine* **32**, 79–84.

Hawkins, D. & Metheny, J. (2001) Overuse
injuries in youth sports: biomechanical
considerations. *Medicine and Science in
Sports and Exercise* **33**, 1701–1707.

Hogan, K.A. & Gross, R.H. (2003) Overuse
injuries in pediatric athletes. *Orthopaedic
Clinics of North America* **34**, 405–415.

Johnson, A.W., Weiss, C.B. Jr. &
Wheeler, D.L. (1994) Stress fractures of
the femoral shaft in athletes: more
common than expected: a new clinical
test. *American Journal of Sports Medicine*
22, 248–256.

Kaltas, D.S. (1981) Stress fractures of the
femoral neck in young adults. *Journal of
Bone and Joint Surgery* **63B**, 33–37.

Keene, J.S. & Lange, R.H. (1986) Diagnostic
dilemmas in foot and ankle injuries.
*Journal of the American Medical
Association* **256**, 247–251.

Klingele, K.E. & Kocher, M.S. (2002) Little
league elbow: valgus overload injury in
the paediatric athlete. *Sports Medicine* **32**,
1005–1015.

Koh, M., Jennings, L. & Elliott, B. (2003)
Role of joint torques generated in an
optimised Yurchenko layout vault.
Sports Biomechanics **2**, 177–190.

Krijnen, M.R., Lim, L. & Willems, W.J.
(2003) Arthroscopic treatment of
osteochondritis dissecans of the
capitellum: Report of 5 female athletes.
Arthroscopy **19**, 210–214.

Krivickas, L.S. (1997) Anatomical factors
associated with overuse sports injuries.
Sports Medicine **24**, 132–146.

Lankenner, P.A. & Micheli, L.J. (1985)
Stress fracture of the first rib. *Journal of
Bone and Joint Surgery* **67A**, 159–160.

Loud, J., Gordon, C.M. & Micheli, L.J.
(2005) Correlates of stress fractures
among preadolescent and adolescent
girls. *Pediatrics* **115**, 399–406.

Major, N.M. & Helms, C.A. (1997) Pelvic
stress injuries: the relationship between
osteitis pubis (symphysis pubis stress

injury) and sacroiliac abnormalities in
athletes. *Skeletal Radiology* **26**, 711–717.

Matheson, G.O., Clement, D.B., McKenzie,
D.C., *et al.* (1987a) Scintigraphic update
of 99Tc at non-painful sites in athletes
with stress fractures: the concept of bone
strength. *Sports Medicine* **4**, 65–75.

Matheson, G.O., Clement, D.B., McKenzie,
D.C., Taunton, J.E., Lloyd-Smith, D.R. &
MacIntyre, J.B. (1987b) Stress fractures in
athletes: A study of 320 cases. *American
Journal of Sports Medicine* **15**, 46–58.

Matzkin, E. & Singer, D.I. (2000) Scaphoid
stress fracture in a 13-year old gymnast:
a case report. *Journal of Hand Surgery
[Am]* **25**, 710–713.

McBryde, A.M. (1985) Stress fractures in
runners. *Clinical Journal of Sports
Medicine* **4**, 737–752.

McMahon, T.A. & Greene, P.R. (1979)
The influence of track compliance on
running. *Journal of Biomechanics* **12**,
893–904.

Micheli, L.J. (1983) Overuse injuries in
children's sports: the growth factor.
Orthopaedic Clinics of North America **14**,
337–360.

Micheli, L.J. (1987) The traction
apophysitises. *Clinical Journal of Sports
Medicine* **6**, 389–404.

Micheli, L.J. (1990) Injuries to the hip
and pelvis. In: *The Pediatric Athlete*
(Sulivan, J.A. & Grana, W.A., eds.)
American Academy of Orthopedic
Surgeons, Park Ridge, IL: 167–172.

Micheli, L.J. & Fehlandt, A.F. Jr. (1996)
Overuse tendon injuries in pediatric
sports medicine. *Sports Medicine and
Arthroscopy Review* **4**, 190–195.

Micheli, L.J. & Ireland, M.L. (1987)
Prevention and management of
calcaneal apophysitis in children: an
overuse syndrome. *Journal of Pediatric
Orthopedics* **7**, 34–38.

Micheli, L.J. & Wood, R. (1995) Back pain
in young athletes. Significant differences
from adults in causes and patterns.
*Archives of Pediatrics and Adolescent
Medicine* **149**, 15–18.

Milgrom, C., Finestone, A., Shlamkovitch,
N., *et al.* (1992) Prevention of overuse
injuries of the for by improved shoe
shock attenuation: A randomized
prospective study. *Clinical Orthopaedics
and Related Research* 189–192.

Milgrom, C., Finestone, A., Shlamkovitch,
N., *et al.* (1994) Youth is a risk factor for
stress fracture. A study of 783 infantry
recruits. *Journal of Bone and Joint Surgery*
76B, 20–22.

Milgrom, C., Giladi, M., Kashtan, H., *et al.*
(1985) A prospective study of the effect

of a shock absorbing orthotic device on the incidence of stress fractures in military recruits. *Foot & Ankle* **6**, 101–104.

Miller, J.E. (1960) Javeline thrower's elbow. *Journal of Bone and Joint Surgery* **42B**, 788–792.

Monteleone, G.P. (1995) Stress fractures in the athlete. *Orthopedic Clinics of North America* **26**, 423–432.

Murray, R.O. & Duncan, C. (1971) Athletic activity in adolescence as an etiologic factor in degenerative hip disease. *Journal of Bone and Joint Surgery* **53B**, 406–419.

Mustajoki, P., Laapio, H. & Meurmann, K. (1983) Calcium metabolism, physical activity, and stress fractures. *Lancet* **ii**, 797.

Nattiv, A. & Armsey, T.D. Jr. (1997) Stress injury to bone in the female athlete. *Clinical Journal of Sports Medicine* **16**, 197–224.

Nilsson, B.E. & Westlin, N.E. (1971) Bone density in athletes. *Clinical Orthopedics and Related Research* **77**, 179–182.

Norfray, J.F., Schlachter, L., Kernahan, W.T. Jr., *et al.* (1980) Early confirmation of stress fractures in joggers. *Journal of the American Medical Association* **243**, 164–179.

Ogden, J.A., Ganey, T.M., Hill, J.D. & Jaakkola, J.I. (2004) Sever's injury: a stress fracture of the immature calcaneal metaphysic. *Journal of Pediatric Orthopedics* **24**, 488–492.

Ogden, J.A. & Southwick, W.O. (1976) Osgood–Schlatter disease and tibial tuberosity development. *Clinical Orthopedics and Related Research* **116**, 180–189.

Ohta-Fukushima, M., Mutoh, Y., Takasugi, S., Iwata, H. & Ishii, S. (2002) Characteristics of stress fractures in young athletes under 20 years. *Journal of Sports Medicine and Physical Fitness* **42**, 198–206.

Omey, M.L. & Michlei, L.J. (1999) Foot and ankle problems in the young athlete. *Medicine and Science in Sports and Exercise* **31** (Supplement), S470–486.

O'Neill, D.B. & Micheli, L.J. (1988) Overuse injuries in the young athlete. *Clinical Journal of Sports Medicine* **7**, 591–610.

Orava, S. & Hulkko, A. (1984) Stress fracture of the mid-tibial shaft. *Acta Orthopaedica Scandinavica* **55**, 35–37.

Orava, S., Purenan, J. & AlaKetole, L. (1978) Stress fractures caused by physical exercise. *Acta Orthopaedica Scandinavica* **49**, 192–197.

Ostlie, D.K. & Simons, S.M. (2001) Tarsal navicular stress fracture in a young athlete: case report with clinical, radiologic, and pathophysiologic correlations. *Journal of the American Board of Family Practice* **14**, 381–385.

Parr, T.J. & Burns, T.C. (2003) Overuse injuries of the olecranon in adolescents. *Orthopedics* **26**, 1143–1146.

Pentecost, R.L., Murrav, R.A. & Brindley, H.H. (1964) Fatigue, insufficiency, and pathological fractures. *Journal of the American Medical Association* **187**, 1001–1004.

Reeder, M.T., Dick, B.H., Atkins, J.K., Pribis, A.B. & Martinez, J.M. (1996) Stress fractures. Current concepts of diagnosis and treatment. *Sports Medicine* **22**, 198–212.

Renstrom, A.F. (1993) Mechanism, diagnosis, and treatment of running injuries. *Instructional Course Lectures* **42**, 225–234.

Renström, P. & Roux, C. (1988) Clinical implications of youth participation in sports. In: *The Encyclopaedia of Sports Medicine*, Vol. 1. *The Olympic Book of Sports Medicine* (Dirix, A., Knuttgen, H.G. & Tittel, K., eds.) Blackwell Scientific Publications, Oxford: 474.

Rettig, A.C. (1983) Stress fracture of the ulna in an adolescent tournament tennis player. *American Journal of Sports Medicine* **11**, 103–109.

Rettig, A.C. & Beltz, M.F. (1985) Stress fracture in the humerus in an adolescent tournament tennis player. *American Journal of Sports Medicine* **13**, 55–58.

Seals, J.G. (1983) A study of dance surfaces. *Clinical Journal of Sports Medicine* **2**, 557–561.

Segesser, B., Morscher, E. & Goelsel, A. (1995) Lesions of the growth plate caused by sports stress. *Orthopade* **24**, 446–456.

Shabat, S., Sampson, K.B., Mann, G., *et al.* (2002) Stress fractures of the medial malleolus: review of the literature and report of a 15-year-old elite gymnast. *Foot & Ankle International* **23**, 647–650.

Song, W.S., Yoo, J.J., Koo, K.H., Yoon, K.S., Kim, Y.M. & Kim, H.J. (2004) Subchondral fatigue fracture of the femoral head in military recruits. *Journal of Bone and Joint Surgery* **86A**, 1917–1924.

Soyuncu, Y. & Gur, S. (2004) Avulsion injuries of the pelvis in adolescents. *Acta Orthopaedica et Traumatologica Turcica* **38** (Supplement 1), 88–92.

Spitz, D.J. & Newberg, A.H. (2002) Imaging of stress fractures in the athlete. *Radiologic Clinics of North America* **40**, 313–331.

St Pierre, P., Staheli, L.T., Smith, J.B. & Green, N.E. (1995) Femoral neck stress fractures in children and adolescents. *Journal of Pediatric Orthopedics* **15**, 470–473.

Stanitski, C.L. (1993) Combating overuse injuries: A focus on children and adolescents. *Physician and Sportsmedicine* **21**, 87–106.

Stanitski, C.L. & Micheli, L.J. (1993) Observations on symptomatic medial malleolar ossification centers. *Journal of Pediatric Orthopedics* **13**, 164–168.

Stulberg, S.D., Cordell, L.D., Harris, W.H., *et al.* (1975) Unrecognized childhood hip disease: a main course of idiopathic osteoarthritis of the hip. In: *The Hip: Proceedings of the Third Open Scientific Meeting of the Hip Society*. C.V. Mosby, St. Louis: 212–228.

Swissa, A., Milgrom, C., Giladi, M., *et al.* (1989) The effect of pretraining sports activity, on the incidence of stress fractures among military recruits. A prospective study. *Clinical Orthopaedics and Related Research* **245**, 256–260.

Thacker, S.B., Gilchrist, J., Stroup, D.F. & Kimsey, C.D. (2002) The prevention of shin splints in sports: a systematic review of literature. *Medicine and Science in Sports and Exercise* **34**, 32–40.

Walter, N.E. & Wolf, M.D. (1977) Stress fractures in young athletes. *American Journal of Sports Medicine* **5**, 165–170.

Warren, M.P. (1987) Excessive dieting and exercise. The dangers for young athletes. *Journal of Musculoskeletal Medicine* **4**, 31–40.

Warren, M.P., Brooks-Gunn, J., Hamilton, L.H., Warren, L.F. & Hamilton, W.G. (1986) Scoliosis and fractures in young ballet dancers: relation to delayed menarche and secondary amenorrhea. *New England Journal of Medicine* **314**, 1348–1353.

Warren, M.P. & Goodman, L.R. (2003) Exercise-induced endocrine pathologies. *Journal of Endocrinological Investigation* **26**, 873–878.

Washington, E.L. (1978) Musculoskeletal injuries in theatrical dancers: site, frequency, and severity. *American Journal of Sports Medicine* **6**, 75–98.

Chapter 13

Protective Sports Equipment

DAVID T. BERNHARDT

There are approximately 30 million young athletes participating in sports in the USA. Youth sports and recreational activities account for 35% of injuries on an annual basis, with the highest risk age group between 14 and 17 years of age (Bijur *et al.* 1995). Although there is inherent risk associated with almost any sport, contact and collision sports such as football, ice-hockey, wrestling, rugby, and soccer have the highest injury risk. Proposed models for reducing injury risk in youth sports include rule changes, sports participation in programs with appropriate age, maturation, size and skill level, injury reduction programs focusing on strength and proprioception, and the use of protective sports equipment. This chapter reviews the use of protective sports equipment in reducing risk of injury focusing on evidence relating to use.

Helmets

Both severe head injuries and mild traumatic brain injuries (concussions) are common in contact (i.e., football) and non-contact sports (baseball, bicycling, in-line skating). Mechanisms of head injury related to these sports include falls (bicycling, skiing or skating), collisions with others (football or soccer) or stationary pieces of equipment (goal posts), or being struck by a moving object (baseball or soccer). A study of urban youth showed sports of baseball/ softball, bicycling, and soccer to be associated with the highest risk of head injury (Cheng *et al.* 2000).

Helmets have been shown to be very effective in reducing the risk of injury in many different sports. In a study of two contact/collision sports, the use of

a helmet significantly reduced the risk of head injury in the sport requiring helmet use. When comparing New Zealand rugby with American collegiate football, the rate of head injuries per 1000 player-games is almost 10 times higher in the unhelmeted sport (rugby) (Marshall *et al.* 2002). Not only do the helmets reduce the risk of major head injury and concussions but they also reduced the risk of lacerations, contusions, and facial fractures.

Although football helmets offer protection from mild head and facial injuries along with protection from more severe head injuries, they are not foolproof. The improvement in helmet technology resulted in more players using their head at contact. Players using their head for contact resulted in axial loading and an increased risk of catastrophic injury to the cervical spine from spearing. To reduce the risk of neck injury, players must be taught to avoid head-down contact, using their head for initial contact, and leagues must enforce a penalty for spearing to discourage this type of contact. Players should be encouraged to make contact with their shoulder first and their head up to avoid serious neck injury.

Each year there is a substantial number of deaths, emergency room visits, and millions of dollars spent on the consequences of head injuries related to bicycle riding. Head trauma constitutes 33% of all bicycling injuries and is responsible for 80% of bicycle-related deaths (Center for Disease Control and Prevention 1987). Bicycling is a sport or recreational event where the use of helmets has been studied extensively with the intervention of helmet use resulting in a substantial decrease in the risk of head injury. A simple intervention of wearing a bicycle helmet can significantly reduce the risk of head injuries. A case–control study demonstrated an 85% reduction in the risk of head injury and an 88% reduction in the risk of brain injury when wearing a helmet (Thompson *et al.* 1989). Helmet use can be increased through legislation and education (Cote *et al.* 1992; Rivara *et al.* 1994). Helmet use is required for US Cycling Federation racing and triathalons. Primary care providers and sports medicine physicians can play a large part in advocating bicycle helmet use (American Academy of Pediatrics, Committee on Injury and Poison Prevention 2001).

Helmet use has been shown to reduce the risk of head injury in downhill skiing and snowboarding. A study of Norwegian skiers and snowboarders demonstrated a 60% reduction in head injuries among those wearing helmets compared to controls (Sulheim *et al.* 2006). Although head injuries may be prevented by helmet use in these sports, emphasis on skiing in areas appropriate for skill level and under control at all times must also be emphasized as ways of reducing injury risk.

Helmets have been shown to reduce the risk of head injury in equestrian sports. Although riders can still be fatally crushed when the horse rolls on the rider, the risk of head injury can be reduced for other mechanisms related to this sport (Whitlock 1999). Helmet modification and research are ongoing in the hope of reducing the fatality risk from head injury resulting from the crush mechanism.

Other sports where helmet use should be advocated include ice-hockey, bull riding, and baseball. Although football helmets have been shown to reduce the impact of a soccer ball when heading the ball (Lewis *et al.* 2001), a true helmet has not been accepted as part of the game by youth or adult programs. Soccer headbands have been shown to dampen the blow from head–head contact but do not make significant changes in ball–head impact (Withnall *et al.* 2005). Future research demonstrating a decreased risk of head injury in players wearing headbands is the next step in demonstrating their protective effect and increasing acceptance among players and organizations.

Mouth guards

Mouth guards have been classified into three types by the American Society for Testing and Materials:
1 *Stock:* ready made and purchased over the counter; does not require further modification.
2 *Mouth-formed:* boil-and-bite; made from a thermoplastic polyvinylacetate/polyethylene copolymer. There is no control over thickness of material which tends to thin over prominent teeth.
3 *Custom-fitted:* custom-made and fit by dentists. Thickness of mouthguard can be monitored. Made from polyvinylacetate/polyethylene copolymer.

A recent study of an intervention requiring mouthguard use among New Zealand rugby players demonstrated a rate of injury claims for non-mouthguard wearers that was 4.6 times higher than that in those who wore mouthguards (Quarrie *et al.* 2005). Any sport where there is a risk for dental trauma (soccer, basketball, boxing, rugby, and wrestling) should consider use of mouthguards to protect against dental injury.

Research into materials, shock absorption, and risk of concussion is ongoing. Continuing education of athletes, coaches, and parents needs to emphasize mouthguard use in decreasing risk of dental injury for at-risk sports.

Chest protectors

Commotio cordis is the second leading cause of sudden death in young athletes (Maron 2003). Sports involving trajectile objects (baseballs, hockey pucks, and lacrosse balls) increase the risk of the chest being struck during the vulnerable period of the cardiac cycle. Chest protectors have been advocated to decrease the risk of this rare but serious event. However, a report from the US Commotio Cordis Registry showed that more than 25% of cases involved children and adolescents who were wearing chest protectors at the time of the event (Maron *et al.* 2002). In an experimental animal model, neither lacrosse nor baseball chest protectors were particularly effective in reducing the risk of ventricular fibrillation caused by a traumatic blow to the chest in the laboratory setting (Weinstock *et al.* 2006). Further research into more protective materials and a proof of risk reduction in the laboratory and on the field needs to occur prior to advocating routine use of this equipment.

Wrist guards

Currently, over 20 million people participate in the growing sport of in-line skating. Falls on an outstretched hand are the common mechanism in most in-line skating injuries. Wrist injuries account for over 35% of the injuries related to this sport, with fractures making up the majority (Scheiber *et al.* 1994). A case–controlled study using the National Electronic Injury Surveillance System showed a 12.9 times higher likelihood of sustaining a wrist fracture in skaters who were not wearing wrist guards (Scheiber *et al.* 1996). Similar to other sports that require coordination, novice in-line skaters must learn to skate in safe areas, in controlled situations, and at a level appropriate for their level of expertise.

Snowboarding is another sport where falls result in frequent wrist injuries resulting from the same outstretched hand mechanism. A prospective study of novice snowboarders demonstrated a significantly reduced risk of injury in snowboarders using wrist guards (O'Neill 2003). Thus, regular use of wrist guards in snowboarders is recommended to decrease the risk of injury, especially among beginners.

Knee braces

A variety of functional knee braces specific to sport have been designed to protect different structures in the knee. One of the most studied are the functional anterior cruciate ligament (ACL) knee braces which have been prescribed to improve function and stability in ACL-deficient knees and postoperatively in ACL reconstructed knees. Because of the variety of different sports and mechanisms of injuries, it is difficult to ascertain the effectiveness of one uniform brace for all sports. A functional ACL brace should not only subjectively provide more stability to the knee, but there should be objective evidence supporting the effectiveness of the brace relating to anterior tibial translation, neuromuscular function, and isokinetic performance. In a study of five ACL-deficient patients and six different ACL functional braces, Wojtys *et al.* (1996) demonstrated an average decrease in tibial translation of 33% from baseline in a relaxed muscle test and 80% in a contracted muscle test when compared to baseline. Neuromuscular function also demonstrated improvement by the ACL brace compared to baseline. However, hamstring performance was decreased with ACL braces in this same study, which may decrease knee joint stability because the hamstring muscles are major stabilizers of the knee joint. Furthermore, this study was performed under low load conditions and it is unclear how this would compare to the higher loads that the knee experiences in the field or on the court.

In a more recent study of non-surgical acute ACL-deficient patients, patients subjectively sensed less instability when wearing the brace. However, the brace did not result in any improvement in terms of objective pain scales, ability to walk on uneven ground, regaining preinjury physical activity, climbing, twisting, or running (Swirtun *et al.* 2005). In postoperative brace use, there is some evidence suggesting improved performance and stability at 3 months postoperatively compared with the non-braced group. A non-significant improvement was also observed after 6 months, 1 year, and 2 years postoperatively (Risberg *et al.* 1999).

In terms of injury prevention, a study of football players starting high school showed almost equal injury rates between braced and non-braced groups over a 4-year study period (Deppen & Landfried 1994). In a study of army cadet football players over two seasons, there was no difference in the number of ACL and medial collateral ligament (MCL) injuries among brace versus non-brace wearers (Sitler *et al.* 1990). In a 3-year study of North Carolina high school sports (12 sports studied), there was an increased risk of knee injury among athletes wearing a brace compared with their non-braced counterparts. Athletes wearing an ankle brace in this study were also more likely to sustain a knee injury (Yang *et al.* 2005). Only one multicenter study of college football players showed a trend towards a reduced incidence of knee injuries in braced lineman, especially in the beginners compared to the skilled players (Albright *et al.* 1994).

Based on these studies and others, most functional ACL braces are mainly used for the initial postoperative period but are not meant to be a substitute for rehabilitation and are not routinely used for return to play in either the deficient or reconstructed knee.

Knee sleeves or patellar stabilization sleeves are routinely used in the management and prevention of recurrent patellar dislocations. However, in a study of 100 patients with a history of recurrent patellar dislocation, there was no evidence supporting their use for prevention of recurrent injury (Maenpaa & Lehto 1997). In consequence, patellar sleeves should mainly be used for initial subjective stability and for compression of swelling. In addition, there may be a proprioceptive benefit toward wearing the brace. At this time, there does not seem to be any added benefit toward reducing the risk of recurrent patellar dislocation.

Ankle bracing

Similar to other injured areas, the highest risk for spraining an ankle is seen in the person with a previous ankle sprain. Intrinsic (weakness and balance) and extrinsic factors (brace, tape, shoe type) may be associated with recurrent ankle sprains. Different types of ankle braces have been studied including an elastic support, stirrup, or lace-up.

In the acute setting, the stirrup-type brace has been shown to be more effective in improving joint function than an elastic support at both 10 days and 1 month after the initial injury (Boyce et al. 2005).

Injury prevention is the other common reason for prescribing ankle orthoses. Ankle braces do not appear to affect function in terms of ability to jump, run, and cut. In addition, ankle braces are subjectively fairly comfortable and give the athlete a feeling of increased stability. In terms of injury prevention, most studies support the use of tape or brace to prevent instability. A study of over 1600 intramural basketball players demonstrated an injury rate of 5.2 per 1000 athlete-exposures in an unbraced group vs. 1.6 per 1000 athlete-exposures in the braced group (Sitler et al. 1994). In a similar study of soccer players, a semi-rigid orthosis was found to reduce the risk of ankle injury among athletes with a history of a previous ankle sprain by 60–70%. Interestingly, in this study, there was no significant effect of bracing among those who had no previous injury (Surve et al. 1994). Based on the information provided above, many high schools and colleges promote the use of ankle orthoses to reduce the risk of injury and save cost on use of athletic tape. This practice is even more important in athletes rehabilitating from a previous injury and those returning to competition after completing physical therapy.

Genital cups

There is no scientific evidence demonstrating the effectiveness of a testicular cup in preventing testicular injury in any sport. When looking for evidence, keep in mind that the rate of testicular injury among athletes is exceedingly low and therefore demonstrating effectiveness may be quite difficult. Intuitively, some sports are at higher risk than others for possible testicular injury and expert opinion would advocate the use of genital cups in these "high-risk" sports. However, in a recent survey of Ohio athletes, 53% of all male athletes and 22% of baseball players do not wear a protective cup (Congeni et al. 2005). For sports where a fast trajectory is involved (ice-hockey and baseball), the use of protective cup and education regarding testicular injury should be advocated.

Directions for future research

There are millions of athletes involved a variety of sports around the world. Manufacturers of protective sporting equipment promote the use of this equipment in preventing injury and making sports safer. Most research on the use of this equipment has been carried out on older adolescents and adults. Extrapolating the research to the young athlete may be reasonable in some instances. Sports medicine physicians and primary care providers need to educate athletes regarding which of these devices are most effective in preventing injury and which do little to make their sport safer. More research needs to be carried out in this field as it relates to the effectiveness of these devices for the skeletally immature athlete.

References

Albright, J.P., Powell, J.W., Smith, W., *et al.* (1994) Medial collateral ligament knee sprains in college football. Effectiveness of preventive braces. *American Journal of Sports Medicine* **22**, 12–18.

American Academy of Pediatrics, Committee on Injury and Poison Prevention (2001) Bicycle helmets. *Pediatrics* **108**, 1030–1032.

Bijur, P.E., Trumble, A., Harel, Y., Overpeck, M.D., Jones, D. & Scheidt, P. (1995) Sports and recreation injuries in US children and adolescents. *Archives of Pediatric and Adolescent Medicine* **149**, 1009–1016.

Boyce, S.H., Quigley, M.A. & Campbell, S. (2005) Management of ankle sprains: a randomized controlled trial of the treatment of inversion injuries using an elastic support bandage or an Aircast ankle brace. *British Journal of Sports Medicine* **39**, 91–96.

Center for Disease Control and Prevention (1987) Bicycle-related injuries. *MMWR Morbidity and Mortality Weekly Report* **36**, 269–271.

Cheng, T.L., Fields, C.B., Brenner, R.A., Wright, J.L., Lomax, T., Scheidt, P.C. & the District of Columbia Child/Adolescent Injury Research Network (2000) Sports injuries: an important cause of morbidity in urban youth. *Pediatrics* **105**, 625–626.

Congeni, J., Miller, S.F. & Bennett, C.L. (2005) Awareness of genital health in young male athletes. *Clinical Journal of Sports Medicine* **15**, 22–26.

Cote, T.R., Sacks, J.J., Kresnow, M.J., *et al.* (1992) Bicycle helmet use among Maryland children: effect of legislation and education. *Pediatrics* **89**, 1216–1220.

Deppen, R.J. & Landfried, M.J. (1994) Efficacy of prophylactic knee bracing in high school football players. *Journal of Orthopaedic and Sports Physical Therapy* **20**, 243–246.

Lewis, L.M., Naunheim, R., Standeven, J., Lauryssen, C., Richter, C. & Jeffords, B. (2001) Do football helmets reduce acceleration of impact in blunt head injuries? *Academic Emergency Medicine* **8**, 604–609.

Maenpaa, H. & Lehto, M.U. (1997) Patellar dislocation. The long-term results of nonoperative management in 100 patients. *American Journal of Sports Medicine* **25**, 213–217.

Maron, B.J. (2003) Sudden death in young athletes. *New England Journal of Medicine* **349**, 1064–1075.

Maron, B.J., Gohman, T.E., Kyle, S.B., Estes, M.N.A. & Link, M.S. (2002) Clinical profile and spectrum of commotio cordis. *Journal of the American Medical Association* **287**, 1142–1146.

Marshall, S.W., Waller, A.E., Dick, R.W., Pugh, C.B., Loomis, D.P. & Chalmers, D.J. (2002) An ecologic study of protective equipment and injury in two contact sports. *International Journal of Epidemiology* **31**, 587–592.

O'Neill, D.F. (2003) Wrist injuries in guarded versus unguarded first time snowboarders. *Clinical Orthopaedics and Related Research* **409**, 91–95.

Quarrie, K.L., Gionnatti, S.M., Chalmers, D.J. & Hopkins, W.G. (2005) An evaluation of mouthguard requirements and dental injuries in New Zealand rugby union. *British Journal of Sports Medicine* **39**, 650–654.

Risberg, M.A., Holm, I., Steen, H., Eriksson, J. & Ekeland, A. (1999) The effect of knee bracing after anterior cruciate ligament reconstruction. A prospective, randomized study with two years' follow-up. *American Journal of Sports Medicine* **27**, 76–83.

Rivara, F.P., Thompson, D.C., Thompson, R.S., *et al.* (1994) The Seattle children's bicycle helmet campaign: changes in helmet use and head injury admissions. *Pediatrics* **93**, 567–569.

Scheiber, R.A., Branche-Dorsey, C.M. & Ryan, G.W. (1994) Comparison of in-line skating injuries with rollerskating and skateboarding injuries. *Journal of the American Medical Association* **271**, 856–858.

Scheiber, R.A., Branche-Dorsey, C.M., Ryan, G.W., Rutherford, G.W., Stevens, J.A. & O'Neil, J. (1996) Risk factors for injuries from in-line skating and the effectiveness of safety gear. *New England Journal of Medicine* **335**, 1630–1635.

Sitler, M., Ryan, J., Hopkinson, W., *et al.* (1990) The efficacy of a prophylactic knee brace to reduce knee injuries in football. A prospective, randomized study at West Point. *American Journal of Sports Medicine* **18**, 310–315.

Sitler, M., Ryan, J., Wheeler, B., *et al.* (1994) The efficacy of a semi-rigid ankle stabilizer to reduce acute ankle injuries in basketball: a randomized clinical study at West Point. *American Journal of Sports Medicine* **22**, 454–461.

Sulheim, S., Holme, I., Ekeland, A., & Bahr, R. (2006) Helmet use and risk of head injuries in alpine skiers and snowboarders. *Journal of the American Medical Association* **295**, 919–924.

Surve, I., Schwellnus, M.P., Noakes, T. & Lombard, C. (1994) A fivefold reduction in the incidence of recurrent ankle sprains in soccer players using the sport-stirrup orthosis. *American Journal of Sports Medicine* **22**, 601–606.

Swirtun, L.R., Jansson, A. & Renström, P. (2005) The effects of functional knee brace during early treatment of patients with nonoperated acute anterior cruciate ligament tear: a prospective randomized study. *Clinical Journal of Sport Medicine* **15**, 299–304.

Thompson, R.S., Rivara, F.P. & Thompson, D.C. (1989) A case–control study of the effectiveness of bicycle safety helmets. *New England Journal of Medicine* **320**, 1361–1367.

Weinstock, J., Maron, B.J. & Song, C. (2006) Failure of commercially available chest wall protectors to prevent sudden cardiac death induced by chest wall blows in an experimental model of commotio cordis. *Pediatrics* **117**, e656–e662.

Whitlock, M.R. (1999) Injuries to riders in the cross country phase of eventing: the importance of protective equipment. *British Journal of Sports Medicine* **33**, 212–216.

Withnall, C., Shewchenko, N., Wonnacott, M. & Dvorak, J. (2005) Effectiveness of headgear in football. *British Journal of Sports Medicine* **39** (Supplement 1), i40–i48.

Wojtys, E.M., Kothari, S.U. & Huston, L.J. (1996) Anterior cruciate ligament use in sports. *American Journal of Sports Medicine* **24**, 539–546.

Yang, J., Marshall, S.W., Bowling, J.M., Runyan, C.W., Mueller, F.O. & Lewis, M.A. (2005) Use of discretionary protective equipment and rate of lower extremity injury in high school athletes. *American Journal of Epidemiology* **161**, 511–519.

Chapter 14

Rehabilitation of Children Following Sport and Activity Related Injuries

ANTHONY LUKE, MICHELINA CASSELLA, AND KATHLEEN RICHARDS

Children are competing in organized activities (Pate *et al.* 2000) and specializing in sports at an early age. Excessive, repetitive training, and complicated, extreme sports maneuvers can lead to overuse and acute traumatic injuries, resulting in the rise of sports-related injuries in young athletes. In the last decades, sport has become the leading cause of injuries in children aged 5–17 years (Bijur *et al.* 1995; Chen *et al.* 2005).

This chapter highlights the principles of rehabilitation, the planning of injury recovery programs, as well as rehabilitation techniques. Unfortunately, the evidence for rehabilitation practices in sports medicine is often lacking proper research trials. Many of the rehabilitation programs recommended in practice are based on clinical experience and/or research with adult populations. When developing an individual plan of care for a young athlete presenting with a sports injury, one should consider the following:

1 The goals of rehabilitation;
2 Any injury-specific and age-specific factors; and
3 The rehabilitation techniques that can facilitate healing.

Appropriate management and education of athletes, parents, and coaches are crucial steps in assisting young people to recover from injury, so they may achieve their goals and enjoy physical activity.

Principles of rehabilitation

The major principle of rehabilitation is to safely maximize the child athlete's abilities despite an existing or a developing impairment. The goals of

rehabilitation following a sports-related injury (Table 14.1) include the following:

1 Control inflammation and pain;
2 Promote healing;
3 Restore function;
4 Safely return to activities and sports;
5 Prevent future injury; and
6 Enable competitive athletes to perform at their best.

Understanding the physiology of tissue healing, as well as the physical demands of rehabilitation and the athlete's sport can help the clinician guide the athlete, parents, and coaches through the recovery process.

Injury-specific considerations

Different injuries occur in the child athlete compared to an adult (Table 14.2). The growth plates or "physes" are vulnerable areas which are commonly injured, rather than the ligament tears or fractures that happen in adults. Injuries to connective tissues (bone, tendon, muscle, ligament, and cartilage) follow typical expected healing sequences. The initial healing process usually involves an inflammatory response by the body, with proliferation of cells and increased vascularity, triggered by chemical mediators. A remodeling phase occurs over weeks to months, as the healing tissues adapt in terms of strength, flexibility, and endurance to be capable of withstanding the stresses necessary to return the athlete to function and ultimately sports (Kannus *et al.* 2003). Healing rates are usually faster in children than adults because they have greater proliferative

169

Table 14.1 General guidelines for a rehabilitation program for a major soft connective tissue injury based on defined stages of healing. The timeline for the rehabilitation program would depend on the severity of injury and the type of tissue that is injured.

Time	Stages of healing	Therapeutic goals	Rehabilitation steps
Phase 1 Day 1–3	Acute inflammation	*1 Control inflammation and pain* Acute care management Protect affected area, (protective weight bearing in lower extremity injuries) Reduce swelling and inflammation Minimize hypoxic damage to tissue	Modified activities, ice, compression, elevation (MICE) Crutches, braces, supportive devices if needed
Day 4–7	Repair/substrate/inflammation	Limit further tissue damage Gradually increase "pain free" range	Isometric strength exercises Gentle "pain free" active range of motion of motion
Phase 2 Day 7–21	Proliferation	*2 Promote healing* Decrease protected status if indicated (i.e., increase weight bearing status) Reduce muscle atrophy Improve: • Range of motion • Flexibility • Strength	Restore full active range of motion Gentle progressive resistive exercises
Phase 3 Week 3–6	Healing and maturation	*3 Restore function* Continue to restore range of motion and strength Restore proper muscle activation and biomechanics Improve proprioception Improve endurance	Functional activities as tolerated More complex movements Progress loading (i.e., cycling, light weights)
Phase 4 Week 6 to 6 months	Tissue remodeling	*4 Return to activities and sports* Restore anatomic form, physiologic function Improve conditioning Return to play/sport *5 Prevent future injury* Protective equipment Injury prevention exercises/programs	Sport-specific training Simulate the demands of the sport/activity Coordination and balance exercises Eccentric loading exercises Consider training modifications and return to play/sports plans
Phase 5 6–12 months	"Complete" healing	*6 Performance training* Return to highest or previous level of performance Review training considerations	Strength and conditioning programs Plyometrics Cross-training Discuss nutrition and diet

Table 14.2 Common injuries and considerations for rehabilitation, based on tissue type.

Tissue	Common injuries	Age-specific considerations	Rehabilitation considerations
Bone	Physeal fractures Cortical fractures Stress injury and fractures Bone contusion Apophysitis	Presence of the growth plates Growth plates are often the area of weakness Check for physeal fractures Apophysites occur from traction injuries to growth plates at local tendon insertion Plastic deformation can occur due to thick periosteum rather than fracture Bone maturity can be assessed	Treatment aims to restore the anatomy Bone mineral density, area and shape can be influenced by a growing athlete's activities Consider if there is surgical hardware Protected stress loading required to the fracture site while healing, especially if physeal injury present Bone healing process takes from four to more than sixteen weeks (Frost 1989)
Tendon	Tendinitis Tenosynovitis Tendinosis (less common) Tendon rupture (rare)	Muscle–tendon flexibility may decrease during the growth spurt (Micheli 1987)	Tendons have viscoelastic properties Rest and modification of activities are often beneficial Therapeutic exercises to specifically eccentrically load the tendon without causing reinjury have shown promise (Khan *et al.* 1999) Assess biomechanics including flexibility and muscle strength/balance
Cartilage	Osteochondroses (osteochrondritis dissecans (OCD), avascular necrosis) Partial or full thickness defects Meniscal tears	Osteochondroses refer to conditions involving abnormal endochodral ossification of physeal growth (Canale *et al.* 1994) OCD involves microtrauma to the subchondral bone at the epiphysis, which can lead to avascular necrosis and subsequent loosening and separation of the fragment into the joint Meniscus tears have poor healing potential even at young ages and may require surgical attention Discoid lateral menisci may become symptomatic in young athletes	In prepubertal athletes, treatment of OCD can be conservative because there is potential for spontaneous healing of stable lesions (Sales de Gauzy *et al.* 1999) Weight bearing and impact activities should be reduced and protected in severe cases, during recovery of injuries involving the articular cartilage Early motion of the joint, even non- weightbearing activity, is essential for adequate nourishment and healing of the cartilage
Ligament	Sprain (complete, partial)	Avulsion fractures rather than ligament tears can occur as ligaments are stronger than associated growth plate (i.e., tibial spine avulsion rather than ACL tear) If the growth plates are open and ligament injury is suspected, check for associated physeal injury	Exercises to promote dynamic stabilization and enhance proprioception Function and sharing of the load of the damaged ligament needs to be replaced, usually through surgery or bracing
Muscle	Strain/tear Contusion Myositis ossificans	Less capacity for muscle strength and hypertrophy improvements with exercises	Higher grade muscle injuries require a short period of immobilization followed by early movement (Kannus *et al.* 2003) Muscle is kept under adequate tension to maximize healing response and limit contracture Avoid early return to athletic activities that involve maximal muscle contractions until fully recovered

Table 14.3 Developmental stages and suggestions in planning rehabilitation programs.

Chronologic age	Psychologic	Motor	Suggestions for rehabilitation
Preschool	Early play to gain mastery over environment Curious (Passer 1988)	Develop basic forms of motor patterns Hard to stay still (Passer 1988)	Use imitation to get the child to accomplish the necessary objectives Involve parents
Early primary school (5–7 years)	Formative years (imagination) Should introduce sport through play in order to stimulate imagination Activities must be intrinsically enjoyable Award schemes (and variations) are extremely valuable Teacher and coach have an important role	Begins combined movements (run and jump) Can carry out all-round exercise with variety Still exhibit slow movements (reaction time >0.5 s) (Dick 2002)	Can understand simple instructions Incorporate therapeutic goals into activities they enjoy Make each activity "fun" Design colorful daily activity chart for positive reinforcement for completing their daily program Consider reward/treat for completing exercises
Primary–secondary school (8 to 11–13 years of age)	Critical realism (logical thinking) Attention span is still short Seeks logical connections and generalizations Can understand other people's point of view Can understand team concepts (Passer 2002)	Most important "Best age for learning" Youngsters may develop keen interest in sports, love of activity Value learning athletic skills Want achievement and challenge	Can understand instructions and reasons for treatment and exercise Can start getting them to take responsibility for the exercise program under parental supervision (Passer 1988) Relate the benefit of the exercise to their sport
Adolescence (11–13 to 16)	Learning becomes an intellectual exercise and productive activity assumes a major role (Dick 2002) Social changes with heavy peer influence Concept of self (individualization) Understands the consequences of compliance, but focuses on the here and now (Patel 2002)	Strength increases from increased testosterone and estrogen Neuromuscular system reaches full capacity	Can start adult rehabilitation programs Exercises should be focused Noticeable, quick improvements can increase compliance Relate the benefits of the exercises to their sport Responds best to reaching performance goals rather than injury prevention

and remodeling potential because of remaining growth processes. Specific rehabilitation techniques may be implemented based on the tissue injury and stage of recovery, to facilitate healing and prevent complications, such as weakness, stiffness, and dysfunction.

Age-specific considerations

Careful analysis of the stages of growth and development must be performed when designing a rehabilitation program. One can divide participants into prepubertal, pubertal, and post-pubertal athletes. Post-pubertal athletes are physically adults. An individual's stage of maturation is usually more important than chronologic age when considering the child athlete's developmental level. Pratt (1989) found that assessing sexual maturity according to Tanner had greater predictive value than chronologic age for physical attributes, such as strength and flexibility. The stages defined by Tanner identify the individual's level of maturity based on the presence of specific physical and/or sexual characteristics, specifically, pubic hair, breast, penis, or testicular development (Tanner 1978). The physical, psychologic, and emotional maturity of the child or adolescent athlete should be considered to plan the best individual rehabilitation program (Table 14.3).

Prepubertal children should have different expectations and goals placed on rehabilitation. Young children have short attention spans and are still developing their motor skills, so rehabilitation exercises selected should emphasize fun and skill building. Strength gains and aerobic trainability are more limited in the prepubertal and pubertal child (Naughton *et al.* 2000), possibly based on a lack of circulating androgens in prepubertal children which results in less muscle hypertrophy after training than older populations (Fleck & Kramer 1997). Still, changes in neuromuscular recruitment and tissue quality contribute to improvements in strength, sport performance, and injury prevention. Prepubertal children are often more flexible than adolescents and adults, and regain range of motion well. They also have a good capacity for remodeling tissues after injury, especially bone, because of the amount of growth remaining.

During puberty athletes experience physical changes and often present with different injuries. Pubertal athletes are more likely to present with tendinopathies and apophysites, such as Osgood–Schlatter disease, brought about by muscle–tendon imbalances and eccentric loading forces that exceed the tissue's inherent capabilities to handle stress. Adolescents often demonstrate a generalized loss of flexibility especially in larger muscle units such as the hamstrings, hip flexors, quadriceps, and iliotibial band (Fig. 14.1). Especially during mid-puberty, there can be a loss of strength and flexibility which may predispose adolescents to injuries (Micheli 1987). The hypothesis has been proposed that during adolescence, the linear growth of the skeletal long bones and spine exceeds the rate of muscle–tendon unit lengthening (Micheli 1983). However, the evidence supporting an association between growth and changes in flexibility have yet to be clearly established (Feldman *et al.* 1999).

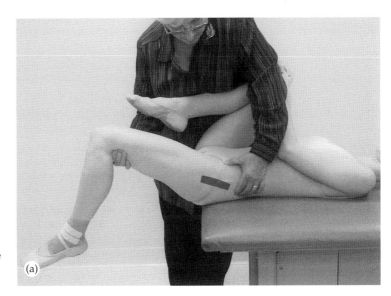

Fig. 14.1 (a) A positive Thomas test illustrating tightness in the hip flexors. The lower extremity is unable to assume a horizontal position with the pelvis in a neutral alignment.

(a)

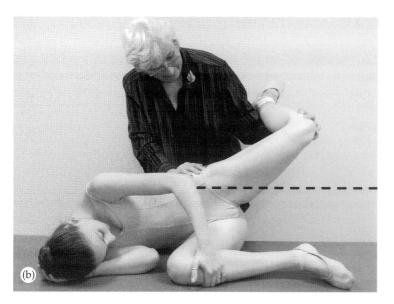

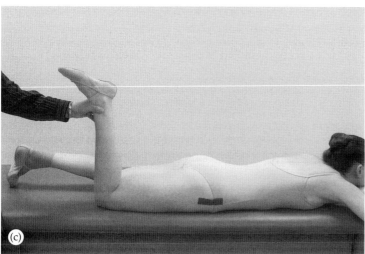

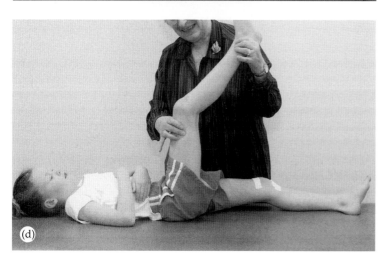

Fig. 14.1 (*cont'd*) (b) The Ober test (iliotibial band tightness) is positive if the knee does not drop to the horizontal position. (c) A negative Ely's test. The knee is passively flexed to 90° with the pelvis in neutral alignment. If the quadriceps muscles are tight, the pelvis may tilt, or there may be asymmetry from side to side in knee flexion in the prone position. (d) Popliteal angle (hamstring tightness) is positive if the knee cannot be extended when the hip is flexed to 90°. The angle from the long axis of thigh to the tibia is measured and can be compared from side to side (135° in this athlete).

Rehabilitation plan of care

When planning a rehabilitation program, the diagnosis, anticipated course of healing, short- and long-term goals of treatment, and the patient's expectations have to be considered, in addition to whether conservative or surgical management is chosen. A detailed history and appropriate physical examination lead the clinician to a working diagnosis. A comprehensive evaluation of the athlete includes assessments of posture, joint range of motion, muscle strength, and functional testing in order to establish an individual plan of care (Kendall & Kendall 1952; Kendall *et al.* 1983; Norkin & White 1985; Greens 1993; Hislop & Montgomery 1995). Accurate assessment using standardized measures can identify physical impairments and functional limitations.

Motivation and compliance

A successful rehabilitation program depends not only on physiologic factors, but also on the emotional and psychosocial attitudes of the athlete (Feltz & Ewing 1987). These factors have a profound influence on exercise performance, understanding, and the expectations of both the athlete and clinician regarding goals of rehabilitation.

Patient and parent education is a key component for promoting compliance (Fotheringham & Sawyer 1995). To reinforce the rationale for the safe performance of the rehabilitation program, it is helpful to describe the mechanism of injury, the roles of anatomic structures, how the exercises will aid healing, and any activity limitations the athlete should require. Teaching how the exercise program will complement the athlete's sports performance can make the program more applicable and acceptable to the individual. Clear, written exercise instructions and a daily exercise log will help the athlete perform a scheduled exercise program. Reviewing the log at each patient visit will allow an opportunity to provide positive, encouraging feedback to the athlete and to identify any problems with the program. The clinician should plan regular follow-up in order to assess improvements, to revise the rehabilitation program, and to review the expected

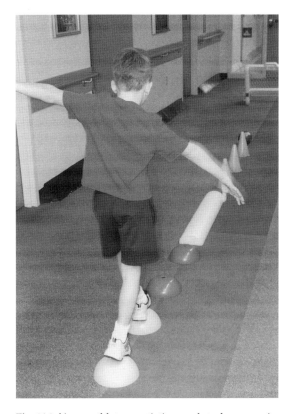

Fig. 14.2 Young athlete negotiating an obstacle course. A creative program to challenge balance.

schedule for healing. Failure to improve may suggest injury complications, an incorrect or underestimated diagnosis, or patient non-compliance.

A rehabilitation plan that prescribes the best exercises with the least effort and the most gains will lead to the most successful outcome (Sluijs *et al.* 1993). Young children usually need individual instruction for best results. A creative exercise program works best for very young athletes, aged 5–6 years (Fig. 14.2). Exercises should be fun, relatively easy to perform, and take no longer than 15–20 min to complete. If exercises are too easy, children may get bored; however, if the exercises are too hard, they can become discouraged. A proper balance between skill, challenge, and competence can improve compliance. Training programs should emphasize volumes and loads that stimulate positive physiologic changes (Stricker 2002). Parents should be encouraged to assist with the home exercise program.

Rehabilitation techniques

Implementation of various rehabilitation techniques should be based on the therapeutic goals and the stage of tissue healing for each particular injury (Table 14.1).

Control inflammation and pain

INITIAL MANAGEMENT

The popular adage of modified activity, ice, compression, and elevation (MICE) is applied empirically in most acute injuries involving inflammation. Self-treatment should ideally begin within the first 15–20 min after an injury. Anecdotally, the practice of MICE can shorten the duration of impairment after an injury by several days or weeks, depending on the type of injury. Initiating MICE in the first 24 h can significantly reduce disability (Micheli 1995). However, there is no randomized clinical trial to prove the effectiveness of this principle (Bleakley *et al.* 2004).

Modified activity (relative rest)

When an athlete can no longer participate in her or his activities after an injury, it is recommended that regular sport activities and all exercises cease for the first 24–72 h. As soon as possible the child should be evaluated by a physician, who will determine the appropriate level of activity depending on the severity of the injury.

Ice

Ice should be applied as soon as possible after the injury to decrease pain, swelling, and bleeding. Ice should never be applied directly to the skin, but should have a thin protective barrier, such as a moist towel, to prevent frostbite. An exception to this is the technique of ice massage, which should be applied under direction of a health professional. Cryotherapy should be applied for intermittent periods up to 10 min (MacAuley 2001), but care should be taken with icing the extremities or areas with large superficial nerves.

Compression

Compression is achieved by applying an elastic bandage with gentle pressure in order to reduce swelling. The bandage must never be applied too tightly in a circular fashion around an extremity to avoid circulatory impairment. The combination of ice and compression applied in shifts of 15–20 min duration, repeated at intervals of 30–60 min can result in a 3–7° decrease in the intramuscular temperature and a 50% reduction of blood flow (Michlovitz 1990).

Elevation

Elevation of the injured part is necessary to prevent pooling of blood. The rationale of raising the injured extremity above the heart results in a decrease in hydrostatic pressure and reduces the accumulation of interstitial fluid.

PAIN CONTROL

Pain needs to be controlled before a successful exercise program can proceed.

In the past, assessing pain in younger children was difficult. Currently, there are reliable and valid tools to assess pain in neonates, infants, toddlers, school age children, adolescents, and adults. The Wong–Baker Pain Scales (ages 3 years and up) is an example using a faces scale, allowing the child to discriminate degrees of pain intensity by facial expressions (Wong *et al.* 2001) (Fig. 14.3). For older children, Visual Analog Scales describe the pain level as a percentage or a number, where the child marks a point on a 10-cm long line with anchors, (0 no pain, 10 extreme pain) (Maxwell 1978).

The athlete and parents need to be able to differentiate between pain associated with an injury and mild discomfort that may result from therapeutic exercise. It is helpful to explain that pain is the body's signal that there is a problem. However, the athlete should be informed that delayed muscle soreness may be expected following stretching or strengthening exercises. If recurrent swelling, worsening stiffness, loss of motion, or severe discomfort occur at any time during the rehabilitation exercises,

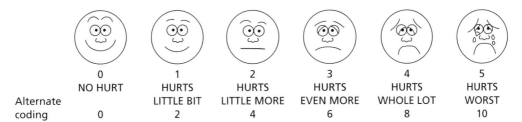

0	1	2	3	4	5
NO HURT	HURTS LITTLE BIT	HURTS LITTLE MORE	HURTS EVEN MORE	HURTS WHOLE LOT	HURTS WORST

Alternate coding: 0   2   4   6   8   10

Fig. 14.3 Wong–Baker FACES Pain Rating Scale. From Hockenberry *et al.* (2005).

the program should be discontinued until further consultation with the athlete's physician.

Medications

Medications should be used judiciously in young athletes, because their natural healing potential is good. Commonly used medications for sports injuries involve influencing the pathways of inflammation and pain, such as non-steroidal anti-inflammatory drugs (NSAIDs). Serious side effects from long-term NSAID use include gastrointestinal bleeding, acute renal failure, and hypertension, which are associated with inhibition of COX-1 enzymes that perform homeostatic functions in the body (Mukherjee *et al.* 2001). There has been some evidence that, when NSAIDs are used, cytokines involved in tissue healing are inhibited and muscle fiber recovery and regeneration may be delayed (Almekinders & Gilbert 1986; Mishra *et al.* 1995). Furthermore, bone healing may be prolonged (Dahners & Mullis 2004). Many medications have been tested in adults but not in children. It is recommended that medications should be used under the supervision of a physician, so the clinician can consider the known indications and side effects of any specific drug in children before it is prescribed.

Superficial heat and cold

Superficial heat and cold increase or decrease tissue temperature, at a depth up to 5 cm, depending on the method of delivery (Starkey 2004). The initial goal is to decrease pain and promote relaxation of the tissues. Applying pressure with cold reduces post-traumatic swelling and can further help to reduce metabolism and secondary hypoxic injury

(Bleakley *et al.* 2004). The physiologic response to heat causes vasodilatation and erythema, while the application of cold causes vasoconstriction followed by vasodilatation. Both heat and cold can reduce fast and slow nerve fiber sensation (Rennie & Michlovitz 1996). There is no clear evidence to demonstrate the effectiveness, indications, duration, and optimal mode of cryotherapy for closed soft tissue injuries (Bleakley *et al.* 2004). Also, the use of heat has not demonstrated long-term effects on pain (Curkovic *et al.* 1993). In any case, it is essential to have a proper barrier between the skin and the hot or cold pack in order to prevent skin irritation and/or damage.

Hydrotherapy

Hydrotherapy can increase or decrease tissue temperature in a large body part by immersing the body segment in water (e.g., a whirlpool). The main goals of hydrotherapy are to decrease swelling, relieve joint pain and stiffness, and promote relaxation. The child must be positioned safely and supervised by an adult at all times during the treatment (Walsh 1996).

Acupuncture

Acupuncture describes a family of procedures involving stimulation of anatomic points on the body using a variety of techniques (e.g., fine needles) in order to bring the body's systems into "balance." It has been used in China for over 2000 years in the treatment of many health problems including musculoskeletal injuries, headaches, gastrointestinal problems, and pain (Vickers & Zollman 1999). Some young children may have a fear of needles but acupuncture can be an effective treatment for pain management and is accepted by most pediatric patients (Kemper *et al.* 2000).

Transcutaneous Electrical Nerve Stimulation

Transcutaneous Electrical Nerve Stimulation (TENS) is the procedure of applying controlled, low voltage, electrical impulses to the nervous system by passing electricity through the skin. TENS is effective for the symptomatic acute and chronic pain. TENS is based on the theory that the peripheral stimulation of large diameter cutaneous afferent nerve fibers blocks transmission of sensoric information at the level of the spinal cord through the gate control mechanisms. Children should be old enough to understand the purpose of TENS use and demonstrate safety awareness (Smith & Madsen 2003).

Orthotic and assistive devices

Orthotic and assistive devices are prescribed to support or immobilize a body part, correct or prevent deformity, and/or to assist function. Devices include braces, foot orthotics, shoulder slings, splints, prosthetics, and crutches. The goal of device use is to apply appropriate forces to affect the movement about the skeletal joints. Some devices, such as braces, restrict, control, or eliminate joint movement, while others, such as prosthetics, assist movement (Redford 1980; Cordova *et al.* 2005). Other orthotic devices can help to reduce pain, decrease swelling, control and enhance movement, and improve proprioception. Proper selection, evaluation, and fit of the orthoses are critical to insure both safety and patient compliance. Patient and parent instruction on proper orthotic application and care is a key component to a successful outcome.

Promote healing

EARLY MOBILIZATION

Joint range of motion may be limited because of pain, swelling, internal joint derangement, scar tissue formation, and/or prolonged immobilization. In children, the period of immobilization for an injury can be longer than in adults, because children recover range of motion much better. However, prolonged immobilization can have negative effects including degenerative changes at the myotendinous junction, as well as the muscle spindles (Józsa & Kannus 1997). Muscle shortening and loss of sarcomeres can lead to atrophy and weakening of the muscle. Following some injuries, tightening of surrounding tissues from scarring can cause impaired movement. Further adverse effects that affect connective tissue can be observed with prolonged immobilization: tendons have decreased collagen synthesis and content of sulfated glycosaminoglycans following immobilization. Noyes (1977) found a decrease of 39% in load to failure in ligaments that were immobilized. Articular cartilage receives its nutrients through the synovial fluid dynamics. Joint movement, exercise, and load-bearing are essential to maintain cartilage health (Kannus *et al.* 2003), improve bone mineralization, and prevent bone loss.

Controlled, early mobilization of muscle, tendon, and ligament injuries is recommended in most cases before or during the proliferative phase of healing (Kannus *et al.* 2003), as opposed to suggesting rest only. The period of muscle–tendon immobilization should be short, usually less than 1 week in order to limit the extent of connective tissue proliferation at the site of injury (Jarvinen & Lehto 1993). However, sufficient time should be allowed for adequate granulation tissue to form in order to attain sufficient tensile strength to allow mobilization of the injured tissue. A series of carefully taught range of motion and isometric muscle strengthening exercises can help counteract the negative effects of immobilization early on in injury, until more active, loading exercises can be safely started.

PHYSICAL AGENTS AND ELECTROTHERAPY

The proper use of physical agents, including superficial heat and cold, deep heat modalities, and electrotherapy, can be used to enhance desired outcomes. These modalities can help to decrease swelling, relieve muscle spasm, increase or decrease blood flow, promote relaxation, and improve tissue extensibility.

Therapeutic ultrasound

Therapeutic ultrasound is produced by a transducer, which converts electrical energy into sound energy. Ultrasound produces a thermal effect by increasing tissue temperature 1–2° at a depth of 5 cm. Non-thermal positive effects include cavitations, mechanical, and chemical alterations (Michlovitz 1990). The main goals are to increase tissue extensibility, decrease inflammation, swelling, pain, and muscle spasm. In addition, ultrasound can help to reduce joint contractures and scar tissue. Extreme caution must be taken when administering ultrasound to children to avoid open epiphyses (Deforest *et al.* 1953; Gann 1991), even though there have not been any reported adverse effects on growth plates (Smith 1995). Although ultrasound is widely used, there is minimal evidence to date that it has long-term effectiveness on the outcomes of musculoskeletal injury (Baker *et al.* 2001; Robertson & Baker 2001).

Neuromuscular Electrical Nerve Stimulation

Neuromuscular Electrical Nerve Stimulation (NMES) is electrical current applied to the skin, which activates motor units causing an involuntary skeletal muscle contraction (Nelson & Currier 1991). The main goals are to provide biofeedback to the involved area and re-educate the muscles. Young children may not be able to tolerate NMES because of the irritant nature of electrical stimulation. If NMES is to be used on children, it is recommended that the child observe the NMES being applied to the therapist or to the parent prior to treatment in order to alleviate fear and apprehension. NMES has been shown to enhance muscle function postoperatively (Robertson & Ward 2002; Fitzgerald *et al.* 2003).

Iontophoresis

Iontophoresis is the transfer of topical medications in the form of applied active ions into the epidermis and mucous membranes of the body by direct current (Kahn 1985). Topical steroids are commonly administered using iontophoresis. The goals of iontophoresis include the reduction of inflammation and edema as well as the softening of scar tissue. The child should be old enough to understand the purpose of the treatment, to identify any irritating effects of the direct current, and to lie still during therapy.

Massage

Massage is the manipulation of soft tissues using the hands. Pressure, stretching, and compression of soft tissues can cause an increase in arterial blood and lymphatic circulation promoting better muscle nutrition and relaxation (Beard & Wook 1964). Massage prior to performing a series of exercises can promote better mobility, positive cardiovascular and neuromuscular relaxation, pain reduction, and psychologic benefits (Starkey 2004).

Restore function

The goal of restoring function is to regain maximum efficiency and effectiveness of the affected body part, in order to achieve full independence and ability in all activities, which in the case of the young athlete is sport. During movement, the interaction of each joint of the body influences and is dependent on the others, producing a "kinetic chain" of activity (Kibler 2000). Therefore, rehabilitation of areas along the chain that are associated with function of the injured joint must be considered. Exercises to improve flexibility, muscle strength, proprioception, neuromuscular control, and cardiovascular endurance are major components for full restoration of function. The rate of exercise progression is based on the athlete's abilities and the nature of the injury.

RANGE OF MOTION AND FLEXIBILITY

Restricted joint motion and limited muscle flexibility can hinder the overall rehabilitation program, as it is difficult to progress to proper strength and functional exercises. Stretching is needed, especially following a muscle or tendon injury or following a period of joint immobilization. Specific examination maneuvers can identify tight muscle–tendon groups (Fig. 14.1a–d). Restoring range of motion in a painful joint, such as postoperatively or after a fracture, may need to begin very slowly with passive exercises aided by a therapist. The athlete can then progress to active exercises carried out with gravity eliminated or with assistance. For example, the child with an acute knee injury may use a gentle "contract–relax" exercise technique to regain knee range of motion more quickly (Knott & Voss 1956). Non-weight-bearing active or passive motion exercises may be performed in the side-lying position, which is very comfortable and less stressful and painful, especially for the younger child, thus instilling confidence in the athlete about moving the knee. As the injury heals, more active, loading exercises can be performed.

The safest and most effective method of stretching appears to be static stretching, when the muscle is elongated to tolerance in a position and sustained for a length of time (Bandy et al. 1998). The optimal length of time, frequency, and the type of exercises to improve flexibility in children still need to be clearly established. In adults, static hamstring stretching has been shown to be ideally performed once a day for a period of 30 s, resulting in significant greater improvements in flexibility over protocols with shorter duration of stretches (Bandy & Irion 1994) or more frequent episodes of dynamic stretching (Bandy et al. 1998). Patients often feel less pain for the same force applied to the muscle as they become more tolerant to the stretch (Shrier & Gossal 2000).

Teaching the child how and when to stretch is the key to a successful outcome. Stretching before activities is best performed following a series of "warm-up" exercises. "Warm-up" exercises increase tissue elasticity, thus protecting the muscle–tendon units from further stretch injury (Safran et al. 1988). This will also help to increase the muscle and body core temperature (Alter 1986). A suggestion for "warming-up" is to start with global gentle movements over 3–5 min. As a rule, stretching exercises that involve elongation of muscle tendon units that cross one joint should be stretched first, followed by those that traverse two separate joints (Tippett 1997).

A subset of patients who have "hypermobility syndrome" present a different rehabilitation challenge (Klemp et al. 1984). Hypermobility is found more commonly in females than males, 22% vs. 6% ($P < 0.001$) (Decoster et al. 1997). "Hypermobile" children may have a variant of collagen disorder, such as Ehlers–Danlos syndrome, and can present with joint subluxations and dislocations, especially involving the patella and the glenohumeral joint. In addition, recurrent tendinopathies can occur around joints that have a high degree of motion, such as the shoulder, hip, and ankle. In these patients, strengthening and joint stabilization exercises should be focused on rather than stretching.

Manual therapies

Manual therapies have been used to increase range of motion. Manipulation is defined as a small amplitude, high velocity thrust technique involving a rapid movement beyond a joint's available range of motion. Mobilizations are low velocity techniques that can be performed in various parts of the available joint range based on the desired effect (Sran & Khan 2002). Mobilization techniques have been shown to produce concurrent effects on pain, sympathetic nervous system activity, and motor activity. Joint mobilizations are considered to be far safer than manipulations, because the patient participates in the techniques. The use of manipulation is not well described in young patients and should be considered with extreme caution in children with open physes (Simonian & Staheli 1995; McGuiness et al. 1997; Vicenzino et al. 1998; Sterling et al. 2001).

RESTORE AND IMPROVE STRENGTH

Resistive exercises

Resistive exercises are usually a major portion of the rehabilitation program. The aim of resistance exercises is to regain the strength, joint stability, and neuromuscular control to perform functional activities. Appropriate rehabilitation exercise programs should be designed to apply controlled but not excessive stress to healing structures, based on the underlying pathology. Following injuries, there can often be persistent weakness, muscle atrophy, and painful inhibition that need to be overcome.

The amount of resistance, repetitions, frequency, speed, and rest intervals can be varied during strength training exercises to optimize loading of the muscles. Other basic details include the following:

1 Whether the exercise is isometric, isotonic, or isokinetic;

2 If it involves concentric or eccentric muscle contractions; and

3 If it is an open or closed chain activity.

Simple exercises are started, followed by more complex activities involving more than one joint. Very young children require size-specific weights and machines in order to exercise the appropriate muscle groups safely and properly. Elastic bands and weighted balls are colorful and fun for children to use (Fig. 14.4).

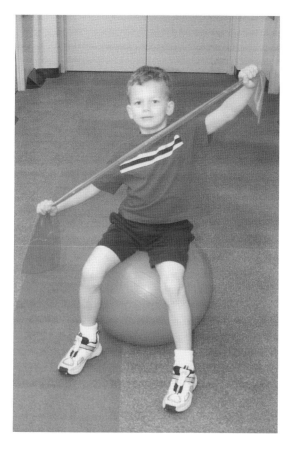

Fig. 14.4 A young athlete balances on a ball while strengthening his upper extremities with a band.

Eccentric loading

Eccentric loading involves the development of tension while the muscle is contracting yet lengthening (e.g., the biceps muscle contracts during the downward movement of a dumbbell biceps curl). The high forces produced from eccentric contractions can cause strain damage, particularly muscle and tendon tears, as well as overuse injuries (Archambault *et al.* 1995). During rehabilitation, eccentric contractions are specifically performed progressively and repeatedly during isolated exercises, in order to adapt the muscle–tendon unit to these high forces. The concept is to stress the collagen eccentrically along its longitudinal axis in order to align the collagen fibers and induce cross-link formation and remodeling. The goal is to improve the size, strength, and spring quality of the affected tissues (Lastayo *et al.* 2003). Eccentric loading exercises have been demonstrated through research to help in rehabilitation of chronic tendinopathies (e.g., heel drop programs in Achilles tendinosis) (Alfredson *et al.* 1998) and incline drop squats for athletes with patellar tendinosis (Young *et al.* 2005).

Core stabilization

Core stabilization of the central core (trunk) in sports has benefits for injuries as well as performance. The trunk is stabilized by the abdominal musculature and the deep and superficial muscle groups of the spine, providing stable foundation for movement of the extremities. The strength of the abdominal muscles is critical in maintaining optimal alignment of the trunk and pelvis in standing (Kendall *et al.* 1983). Dynamic lumbar muscular stabilization has become the most popular method of improving proprioception and strengthening the lower back, which facilitates control of intersegmental spinal motion and load on the spinal elements (O'Sullivan *et al.* 1997).

PROPRIOCEPTION AND NEUROMUSCULAR TRAINING

Proprioception is a somatic sense and is defined as "the afferent input of joint position sense or kinesthesia" (Lephart 1994). Two components of proprioception include the "static" sense or joint position sense, which provides the individual with an appreciation of the orientation of different body parts with respect to one another, and the "dynamic" sense, which gives the neuromuscular system feedback about the presence and rate of movement (Safran *et al*. 2001). The afferent input is created by different mechanoreceptors found in the soft tissues, including ligaments, muscles, and tendons, which convert mechanical deformation into a frequency modulated neural signal (Safran *et al*. 1999). When the mechanoreceptors are triggered, an involuntary protective reflex arc may be activated, which acts faster than pain nociceptors (Van-Duersen *et al*. 1998). This theory suggests that proprioception may have a more significant role than pain in preventing injury (Safran *et al*. 1999). In the case of a sports injury, proprioception can be diminished because of damage to mechanoreceptors, loss of the tensile properties of static structures such as ligaments or the joint capsule, and the latent response of muscles to provide reflex stabilization of a joint (Borsa *et al*. 1997).

Neuromuscular training describes a progressive exercise program that restores synergy and synchrony of muscle firing patterns required for dynamic stability and fine motor control. This is accomplished by enhancing the dynamic muscular stabilization of the joint and by increasing the cognitive awareness of both joint position and motion. Activities are designed to restore both functional stability about the joint and enhance motor control skills. Use of balance equipment such as a wobble board or therapeutic exercise balls can challenge the proprioceptive and balance systems to help restore dynamic stability and allow the control of abnormal joint translation during functional activities (Fig. 14.5) (Bahr & Lian 1997). Balance and proprioception training is important to improve performance (Myer *et al*. 2005) and enable the athlete to return to training.

Return to activities and sport

A program designed for sport-specific activities is initiated when the athlete has achieved full, pain-

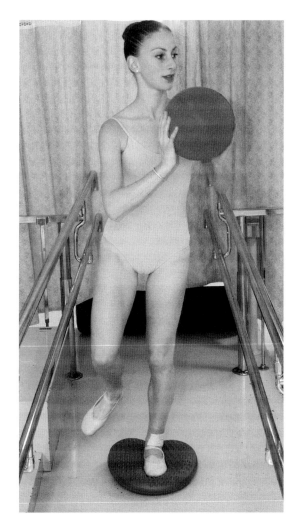

Fig. 14.5 Balancing on an inflatable disk while throwing a ball for proprioceptive training for the athlete with an ankle sprain.

free passive and active motion, adequate muscle strength and endurance, and return of normal movement patterns. The skills and movements of the sport are broken down into individual parts and performed in a controlled, progressive manner to build the athlete's confidence and decrease any fear and apprehension the individual may have.

The athlete will be able to return to play or sport and competition when the injury has healed adequately and their physical attributes are sufficient to withstand the physical demands of the sport. Additional factors that may influence return to play decisions include the nature of the sport (contact vs. non-contact), modifications in activity or technique that can protect the affected area, and the possible use of protective devices, such as braces or orthoses. Screening an athlete to return to sport includes clinical examination and testing, functional testing, and assessment for readiness to return. Functional testing assesses skill-related activities, including agility, balance, coordination, speed, power, and reaction time to test the site of the injury and evaluate the athlete's capacity to meet the specific demands of sport. Outcome questionnaires and scores can provide quantitative, more reliable, standardized measures to assess function and can be used as tools to determine the athlete's motivation and physical readiness (Paxton *et al.* 2003).

Communication between the physician, health care provider, athletic trainer, coach, parent, and athlete is essential to determine the athlete's readiness to return to sport. Return to play must be acceptable to the athlete and the family especially if there are regulations when dealing with patients who are under age for consent. The priority is to return the injured athlete safely without putting the athlete or others at risk for injury.

Preventive measures

Prevention is the ideal management for all sports injuries. However, because the nature of competitive sports involves risk-taking and pushing individuals to the limits of performance, injuries will continue to occur. The risk factor that is associated most with future injury is a previous history of similar injury (Lysens *et al.* 1984).

Preseason conditioning and warm-up can help to reduce injuries. Preseason conditioning (treadmill running on incline to 40° twice a week and plyometric sessions) reduced injuries in adolescent competitive female soccer players (14.3% vs. 33.7%) (Heidt *et al.* 2000). A structured program of warm-up exercises was shown to prevent knee and ankle injuries in young female handball players by approximately 50% (Olsen *et al.* 2005).

Proprioception and neuromuscular training continue to be areas of injury prevention research. A weekly 6-month home-based balance-training program using a wobble board showed improvements in static and dynamic balance for the intervention group but not in the control group (Emery *et al.* 2005a,b). The protective effect of balance training in over 6 months decreased the number of self-reported injuries (relative risk of injury 0.2; 95% confidence interval [CI], 0.05–0.88), with the number needed to treat to avoid one injury over 6 months being 8 (95% CI, 4–35). Balance training has been particularly important in the reduction of anterior cruciate ligament (ACL) injuries, especially for female athletes (Carraffa *et al.* 1996; Myklebust *et al.* 2003; Hewett *et al.* 2005). Female soccer players, aged 14–18 years, who underwent a neuromuscular training program (Preventative Injury and Enhance-ment Program [PEP] program) consisting of basic warm-up activities, stretching techniques for the trunk and lower extremity, strengthening exercises, plyometric activities, and soccer-specific agility drills had 88% less ACL injuries in the first year and 74% less injuries in the second year (Mandelbaum *et al.* 2005). Ankle sprains have also been shown to be reduced by half over three seasons in volleyball athletes involved in an injury prevention program with education on injury awareness, technical jumping training, and balance board training (Bahr & Lian 1997).

Protective equipment including helmets, braces, orthoses, padding, and taping have been used to prevent injuries. Bicycle, hockey, and football helmets are critical in reducing the number of head injuries (Parkkari *et al.* 2001). To reduce ankle sprains, braces have been demonstrated to be effective. Semi-rigid orthosis reduced the incidence of ankle injury (0.46 vs. 1.16 sprains per 1000 player hours) (Verhagen *et al.* 2000).

Performance training

The elite child athlete is typically involved in very intensive training starting at a young age. Examples include figure skaters, gymnasts, little league baseball, tennis, golf, hockey, and soccer players. Training can consist of as many as 6 h of practice each day (Smith 1995). Parents, coaches, and trainers must have an appreciation of the child athlete's developmental, physiologic, and emotional growth and a full understanding of the stages of healing so as not to put undue stress on the recovering athlete.

Sport-specific activities can be implemented during the rehabilitation period. Variables such as speed, directions, and timing are introduced to enhance agility. For example, a program for neuromuscular training in figure skating demonstrates the effective use of balance training exercises and objective sport-specific outcomes to improve postural control (Kovacs *et al.* 2004). The investigators used single-limb stance test, landing jump test, and single-limb stance with a skate on to test for improvements in neuromuscular and postural control. Dealing with the child athlete requires the clinician to be familiar, knowledgeable, careful and often creative, in order to navigate the player safely back to sport.

SWIFTER, HIGHER, STRONGER

In order to reduce the risk of reinjury, when returning to an intensive training schedule, the athlete must maintain a high level of fitness during the rehabilitation phase. Selection of an appropriate aerobic conditioning program in children must take into account the child's age, physical ability, cognition, and condition. A well-rounded, age-specific conditioning program that includes aerobic and strength building exercises, stretching and plyometrics is an excellent approach for a safe rehabilitation program. A study of female athletes ages 15.3 ± 0.9 years who underwent 6 weeks of training that included plyometric and movement, core strengthening and balance, resistance training, and speed training improved measures of performance and movement biomechanics (Myer *et al.* 2005). Activities such as swimming, low-impact exercises, and strengthening of the uninjured area will help to maintain this high level of fitness. Suggested increases for frequency, intensity, and duration are about 5–10% per week dependent on the child's level of fitness (Micheli 1995). The child should begin slowly and adequate periods of recovery should be planned between training sessions.

Cross-training

Cross-training involves different forms of exercise that are performed in the same workout or separate workouts. For example, the child may run and participate in a strengthening program on one day and on the next day, swim. Repetitive training in a specific sport can often cause overuse injuries in the child athlete (Pill *et al.* 2003). Because different exercises target different parts of the body, cross-training allows the benefits of many types of exercise without overstressing a particular muscle group or system. Participating in a variety of exercises can prevent boredom and improvements can be made in total body strength, endurance, and flexibility (Stamford 1996).

Plyometrics

Plyometrics is a natural event that occurs in jumping, hopping, skipping, and even walking. The principle of plyometric training is the stretch–shortening cycle, where the muscle is stretched eccentrically then contracted immediately, leading to an increase in the force of the contraction. Jumping power and running velocities were improved in prepubescent boys who performed plyometric exercises, and these improvements were maintained after a brief period of reduced training when compared with matched controls (Dialli *et al.* 2001). Carefully designed, safe, plyometric conditioning exercises can be incorporated into the athlete's functional programs (e.g., a set of 5–10 repetitions of low intensity drills, such as squat jumps, and medicine ball chest passes performed twice per week). Depending on the child's ability, the program may progress to multiple hops, jumps, and throws. Extreme caution should be used when initiating plyometric exercises in very young children as they can potentially lead to injury to the growth plates (Faigenbaum & Yap 2000).

Strength training

Strength training can be safe in young athletes (American Academy of Pediatrics Committee on Sports Medicine, 1990; Faigenbaum & Bradley 1998) and can improve performance. The child should be supervised by a qualified instructor in a safe environment, instructed in proper technique, participate in warm-up and cool-down periods, and follow proper spotting technique when required (Faigenbaum & Westcott 2004).

Future directions

More evidence-based research is required to determine appropriate, effective age-specific rehabilitation protocols for specific injuries in young athletes.

The epidemiology of sports injuries needs further investigation in children, including risk factors. The level of proper training and effects of early specialization in specific sports should be better established to avoid the numerous overuse injuries that occur. Developing useful outcome scores can establish more objective means of monitoring healing and determining return to play decisions. Educational programs must continue to be developed for athletes, as well as coaches and trainers. Especially in youth sports, injury prevention should be the focus, so that athletes can achieve their full potential safely and enjoyably.

References

Alfredson, H., Pietilä, T., Jonsson, P. & Lorentzon, R. (1998) Heavy-load eccentric calf muscle training for the treatment of chronic Achilles tendinosis. American Journal of Sports Medicine 26, 360–366.

Alter, J. (1986) Stretch and Strengthening. Houghton Mifflin, Boston, MA.

Almekinders, L.C. & Gilbert, J.A. (1986) Healing of experimental muscle strains and the effects of non-steroidal anti-inflammatory medication. American Journal of Sports Medicine 14, 303–308.

American Academy of Pediatrics Committee on Sports Medicine (1990) Strength training, weight and power lifting, and body building by children and adolescents. Pediatrics 86, 801–803.

Archambault, J.M., Wiley, J.P. & Bray, R.C. (1995) Exercise loading of tendons and the development of overuse injuries: A review of current literature. Sports Medicine 20, 77–89.

Bahr, R. & Lian, O. (1997) A two-fold reduction in the incidence of acute ankle sprains in volleyball. Scandinavian Journal of Medicine and Science in Sports 7, 172–177.

Baker, K.G., Robertson, V.J. & Duck, F.A. (2001) A review of therapeutic ultrasound: biophysical effects. Physical Therapy 81, 1351–1358.

Bandy, W.D. & Irion, J.M. (1994) The effect of time on static stretch on the flexibility of the hamstring muscles. Physical Therapy 74, 845–850.

Bandy, W.D., Irion, J.M. & Briggler, M. (1998) The effect of static stretch and dynamic range of motion training on the flexibility of the hamstring muscles.

Journal of Orthopaedic and Sports Physical Therapy 27, 295–300.

Beard, G. & Wood, E. (1964) Massage Principles and Techniques. W.B. Saunders, Philadelphia.

Bijur, P.E., Trumble, A., Harel, Y., Overpeck, M.D., Jones, D. & Scheidt, P.C. (1995) Sports and recreation injuries in US children and adolescents. Archives of Pediatrics and Adolescent Medicine 149, 1009–1016.

Bleakley, C., McDonough, S. & MacAuley, D. (2004) The use of ice in the treatment of acute soft-tissue injury: A systemic review of randomized controlled trials. American Journal of Sports Medicine 32, 251–261.

Borsa, P.A., Lephart, S.M., Irrgang, J.J., Safran, M.R. & Fu, F.H. (1997) The effects of joint position and direction of joint motion on proprioceptive sensibility in anterior cruciate ligament-deficient athletes. American Journal of Sports Medicine 25, 336–340.

Canale, S.T., DeLee, J.C. & Drez, D. Jr. (1994) Orthopedic Sports Medicine: Principles and Practice. W.B. Saunders, Philadelphia.

Caraffa, A., Cerulli, G., Projetti, M., Aisa, G. & Rizzo, A. (1996) Prevention of anterior cruciate ligament injuries in soccer. A prospective controlled study of proprioceptive training. Knee Surgery, Sports Traumatology, Arthroscopy 4, 19–21.

Chen, G., Smith, G.A., Deng, S., Hostetler, S.G. & Xiang, H. (2005) Nonfatal injuries among middle-school and high-school students in Guangxi, China. American Journal of Public Health 95, 1989–1995.

Cordova, M.L., Scott, B.D., Ingersoll, C.D. & Leblanc, M.G. (2005) Effects of ankle support on lower extremity functional performance: meta-analysis. Medicine and Science in Sports and Exercise 37, 635–641.

Curkovic, B., Vitulic, V., Babic-Naglic, D. & Durrigl, T. (1993) The influence of heat and cold on the pain threshold in rheumatoid arthritis. Zeitschrift fur Rheumatologie 52, 289–291.

Dahners, L.E. & Mullis, B.H. (2004) Effects of nonsteroidal anti-inflammatory drugs on bone formation and soft-tissue healing. Journal of the American Academy of Orthopaedic Surgeons 12, 139–143.

Decoster, L.C., Vailas, J.C., Lindsay, R.H. & Williams, G.H. (1997) Prevalence and features of joint hypermobility among adolescent athletes. Archives of Pediatrics and Adolescent Medicine 151, 989–992.

Deforest, R.E., Herrick, J.F., Janes, J.M. & Kursen, F.H. (1953) Effects of ultrasound on growing bones: experimental study. Archives of Physical Medicine and Rehabilitation 34, 21–31.

Dialli, O., Dore, E., Duche, P. & Van Praagh, E. (2001) Effects of plyometric training followed by reduced training programme on physical performance in prepubescent soccer players. Journal of Sports Medicine and Physical Fitness 41, 342–348.

Dick, F.W. (2002) Psychological changes in the growing child. In: Sports Training Principles, 4th edn. A & C Black, London: 199–210.

Emery, C.A., Cassidy, J.D., Klassen, T.P., Rosychuk, R.J. & Rowe, B.H. (2005a)

Effectiveness of a home-based balance-training program in reducing sports-related injuries among healthy adolescents: a cluster randomized controlled trial. *Canadian Medical Association Journal* **172**, 749–754.

Emery, C.A., Cassidy, J.D., Klassen, T.P., Rosychuk, R.J. & Rowe, B.H. (2005b) Development of a clinical static and dynamic standing balance measurement tool appropriate for use in adolescents. *Physical Therapy* **85**, 502–514.

Faigenbaum, A.D. & Bradley, D.F. (1998) Strength training in the young athlete. *Orthopedic and Physical Therapy Clinics of North America* **7**, 67–90.

Faigenbaum, A. & Westcott, W. (2004) Strength training guidelines. In: *Youth Strength Training. A Guide for Fitness Professionals from the American Council on Exercise.* Healthy Learning Books & Video, Monterey: 17–26.

Faigenbaum, A.D. & Yap, C.W. (2000) Are plyometrics safe for children? *Journal of Strength and Conditioning Research* **22**, 45–46.

Feldman, D., Shrier, I., Rossignol, M. & Abenhaim, L. (1999) Adolescent growth is not associated with changes in flexibility. *Clinical Journal of Sport Medicine* **9**, 24–29.

Feltz, D.L. & Ewing, M.E. (1987) Psychological characteristics of the elite young athlete. *Medicine and Science in Sports and Exercise* **19**, S98–S105.

Fitzgerald, G.K., Piva, S.R. & Irrgang, J.J. (2003) A modified neuromuscular electrical stimulation protocol for quadriceps strength training following anterior cruciate ligament reconstruction. *Journal of Orthopaedic and Sports Physical Therapy* **33**, 492–501.

Fleck, S.J. & Kramer, W.J. (1997) *Designing Resistance Training Programs*, 2nd edn. Human Kinetics, Champaign, IL: 199–216.

Fotheringham, M.J. & Sawyer, M.G. (1995) Adherence to recommended medical regimens in childhood and adolescence. *Journal of Paediatrics and Child Health* **31**, 72–78.

Frost, H.M. (1989) The biology of fracture healing. An overview for clinicians. Part 1. *Clinical Orthopedics and Related Research* **248**, 283–293.

Gann, N. (1991) Ultrasound: current concepts. *Clinical Management* **11**, 64–69.

Greens, W.B. (1993) *The Clinical Measurement of Joint Motion.* American Academy of Orthopaedic Surgeons, Rosemont, Chigaco.

Heidt, R.S., Sweeterman, L.M., Carlonas, R.L., Traub, J.A. & Tekulve, F.X. (2000) Avoidance of soccer injuries with preseason conditioning. *American Journal of Sports Medicine* **28**, 659–662.

Hewett, T.E., Myer, G.D., Ford, K.R., *et al.* (2005) Biomechanical measures of neuromuscular control and valgus loading of the knee predict anterior cruciate ligament injury risk in female athletes: a prospective study. *American Journal of Sports Medicine* **33**, 492–501.

Hislop, H.J. & Montgomery, J. (1995) *Daniels and Worthingham's Muscle Testing.* W.B. Saunders, Philadelphia.

Hockenberry, M.J., Wilson, D. & Winkelstein, M.L. (2005) *Wong's Essentials of Pediatric Nursing*, 7th edn. Mosby, St. Louis.

Järvinen, M.J. & Lehto, M.U.K. (1993) The effects of early mobilisation and immobilisation on the healing process following muscle injuries. *Sports Medicine* **15**, 78–89.

Józsa, L.G. & Kannus, P. (1997) Effects of activity and inactivity on tendons. In: *Human Tendons, Anatomy, Physiology and Pathology.* Human Kinetics, Champaign, IL: 98–160.

Kahn, J. (1985) *Low Volt Technique.* Syosset, New York.

Kannus, P., Parkkari, J., Järvinen, T.L., Järvinen, T.A. & Järvinen, M. (2003) Basic science and clinical studies coincide: active treatment approach is needed after a sports injury. *Scandinavian Journal of Medicine and Science in Sports* **13**, 150–154.

Kemper, K., Sara, R., Silver-Highfield, E, *et al.* (2000) On pins and needles: pediatric pain patients' experience with acupuncture. *Pediatrics* **105**, 941–947.

Kendall, F.P., McCreary, E.K. & Kendall, E. (1983) *Muscles Testing and Function*, 3rd edn. Williams & Wilkins, Baltimore.

Kendall, H.O. & Kendall, F.P. (1952) *Posture and Pain.* Williams & Wilkins, Baltimore.

Khan, K.M., Cook, J.L., Bonar, F., Harcourt, P. & Åström M. (1999) Histopathology of common tendinopathies: Update and implications for clinical management. *Sports Medicine* **27**, 393–408.

Kibler, W.B. (2000) Closed kinetic chain rehabilitation for sports injuries. *Physical Medicine and Rehabilitation Clinics of North America* **11**, 369–384.

Klemp, P., Steven, J.E. & Isaacs, S. (1984) A hypermobility study in ballet dancers. *Journal of Rheumatology* **11**, 692–696.

Knott, M. & Voss, D. (1956) *Proprioceptive Neuromuscular Facilitation.* Harper and Brother, New York.

Kovacs, E.J., Birmingham, T.B., Forwell, L. & Litchfield, R.B. (2004) Effect of training on postural control in figure skaters: A randomized controlled trial of neuromuscular versus basic off-ice training programs. *Clinical Journal of Sport Medicine* **14**, 215–224.

Lastayo, P.C., Woolf, J.M., Lewek, M.D., *et al.* (2003) Eccentric muscle contraction: Their contribution to injury, prevention, rehabilitation, and sport. *Journal of Orthopaedic and Sports Physical Therapy* **33**, 557–571.

Lephart, S. (1994) Reestablishing proprioception, kinesthesia, joint position sense, and neuromuscular control in rehabilitation. In: *Rehabilitation Techniques in Sports Medicine*, 2nd edn. (Prentice, W.E., ed.) Mosby, St. Louis: 118–137.

Lysens, R., Steverlynck, A. & Van den Auweele, Y. (1984) The predictability of sports injuries. *Sports Medicine* **1**, 6–10.

MacAuley, D. (2001) Ice therapy: How good is the evidence? *International Journal of Sports Medicine* **22**, 379–384.

Mandelbaum, B.R., Silvers, H.J., Watanabe, D.S., *et al.* (2005) Effectiveness of a neuromuscular and proprioceptive training program in preventing anterior cruciate ligament injuries in female athletes: 2 year follow up. *American Journal of Sports Medicine* **33**, 1003–1011.

Maxwell, C. (1978) Sensitivity and accuracy of the visual analogue: A psychophysical classroom experiment. *British Journal of Clinical Pharmacology* **6**, 15–24.

McGuiness, J., Vicenzino, B. & Wright, A. (1997) Influence of a cervical mobilisation technique on respiratory and cardiovascular function. *Manual Therapy* **2**, 216–220.

Micheli, L.J. (1983) Overuse syndrome in children sports: The growth factor. *Orthopaedic Clinics of North America* **14**, 337–360.

Micheli, L.J. (1987) The traction apophysitises. *Clinics in Sports Medicine* **6**, 389–404.

Micheli, L.J. (1995) *The Sports Medicine Bible.* HarperCollins, New York.

Michlovitz, S.L. (1990) *Thermal Agents in Rehabilitation.* F.A. Davis, Philadelphia.

Mishra, D.K., Friden, J., Schmitz, M.C. & Lieber, R.L. (1995) Anti-inflammatory medication after muscle injury. A treatment resulting in short-term improvement but subsequent loss of muscle function. *Journal of Bone and Joint Surgery* **77A**, 1510–1519.

Mukherjee, D., Nissen, S.E. & Topol, E.J. (2001) Risk of cardiovascular events associated with selective COX-2 inhibitors. *Journal of the American Medical Association* **8**, 954–959.

Myklebust, G., Engebretsen, L., Braekken, I.H., Skulberg, A., Olsen, O.E. & Bahr, R. (2003) Prevention of ACL injuries in female handball players: a prospective intervention study over three seasons. *Clinical Journal of Sport Medicine* **13**, 71–78.

Myer, G.D., Ford, K.R., Palumbo, J.B. & Hewett, T.E. (2005) Neuromuscular training imporoves performance in lower extremity biomechanics in female athletes. *Strength Conditioning Research* **19**, 51–60.

Naughton, G., Farpour-Lambert, N.J., Carlson, J., Bradney, M. & Van Praagh, E. (2000) Physiological issues surrounding the performance of adolescent athletes. *Sports Medicine* **30**, 309–325.

Nelson, R. & Currier, D. (1991) *Clinical Electrotherapy*. Appleton & Lange, Norwalk.

Norkin, C. & White, D.J. (1985) *Measurement of Joint Range of Motion A Guide to Goniometry*, 2nd edn. F.A. Davis, Philadelphia.

Noyes, F.R. (1977) Functional properties of knee ligaments and alterations induced by immobilization, *Clinical Orthopaedics and Related Research* **123**, 210–242.

Olsen, O.E., Myklebust, G., Engebretsen, L., Holme, I. & Bahr, R. (2005) Exercises to prevent lower limb injuries in youth sports: cluster randomised controlled trial. *British Medical Journal* **330**, 449–455.

O'Sullivan, P.B., Phyty, G.D., Twomey, L.T. & Allison, G.T. (1997) Evaluation of specific stabilizing exercise in the treatment of chronic low back pain with radiologic diagnosis of spondylolysis or spondylolisthesis. *Spine* **22**, 2959–2967.

Parkkari, J., Kujala, U.M. & Kannus, P. (2001) Is it possible to prevent sports injuries? Review of controlled clinical trials and recommendations for future work. *Sports Medicine* **31**, 985–995.

Passer, M.W. (1988) Psychological issues in determining children's age-readiness for competition. In: *Children in Sport*, 3rd edn. (Smoll, F.L., Magill, R.A. & Ash, M.J., eds.) Human Kinetics, Champaign, IL: 67–78.

Pate, R.R., Trost, S.G., Levin, S., *et al.* (2000) Sports participation and health-related behaviors among US youth. *Archives of Pediatrics and Adolescent Medicine* **154**, 904–911.

Patel, D.R. (2002) Pediatric neurodevelopment and sports participation. When are children ready to play sports? *Pediatric Clinics of North America* **49**, 505–531.

Paxton, E.W., Fithian, D.C., Stone, M.L. & Silva, P. (2003) The reliability and validity of knee-specific and general health instruments in assessing acute patellar dislocation outcomes. *American Journal of Sports Medicine* **31**, 487–492.

Pill, S.G., Flynn, J.M. & Ganley, T.J. (2003) Managing and preventing overuse injuries in young athletes. *Journal of Musculoskeletal Medicine* **20**, 434–442.

Pratt, M. (1989) Strength, flexibility, and maturity in adolescent athletes. *American Journal of Diseases of Children* **143**, 560–563.

Redford, J.B. (1980) *Orthotic Etectera*, 2nd edn. William & Wilkins, Baltimore, MD.

Rennie, G.A. & Michlovitz, S. (1996) Biophysical principles of heat and superficial heating agents. In: *Thermal Agents in Rehabilitation (Contemporary Perspectives in Rehabilitation)*, 3rd edn. (Michlovitz, S., ed.) F.A. Davis, Philadelphia: 107–135.

Robertson, V.J. & Baker, K.G. (2001) A review of therapeutic ultrasound: Effectiveness studies. *Physical Therapy* **8**, 1339–1350.

Robertson, V.J. & Ward, A.R. (2002) Vastus medialis electrical stimulation to improve lower extremity function following a lateral release. *Journal of Orthopaedic and Sports Physical Therapy* **32**, 437–446.

Safran, M.R., Allen, A.A., Lephart, S.M., Borsa, P.A., Fu, F.H. & Harner, C.D. (1999) Proprioception in the posterior cruciate ligament deficient knee. *Knee Surgery, Sports Traumatology, Arthroscopy* **7**, 310–317.

Safran, M.R., Borsa, P.A., Lephart, S.M., Fu, F.H. & Warner, J.J.P. (2001) Shoulder proprioception in baseball pitchers. *Journal of Shoulder and Elbow Surgery* **10**, 438–444.

Safran, M.R., Garrett, W.E. Jr., Seaber, A.V., Glisson, R.R. & Ribbeck, B.M. (1988) The role of warmup in muscular injury prevention. *American Journal of Sports Medicine* **6**, 123–129.

Sales de Gauzy, J., Mansat, C., Darodes, P.H. & Cahuzac, J.P. (1999) Natural course of osteochondritis dissecans in children. *Journal of Pediatric Orthopaedics Part B* **8**, 26–28.

Shrier, I. & Gossal, K. (2000) Myths and truths of stretching: Individualized recommendations for healthy muscles. *The Physician and Sportmedicine* **28**, 57–63.

Simonian, P.T. & Stahlei, L.T. (1995) Periarticular fractures after manipulation for knee contractures in children. *Journal of Pediatric Orthopedics* **15**, 288–291.

Sluijs, E.M., Kok, G.J. & Van der Zee, J. (1993) Correlates of exercise complinace in physical therapy. *Physical Therapy* **73**, 771–782.

Smith, A.D. (1995) Rehabilitation of children following sport- and activity-related injuries. In: *The Encyclopaedia of Sports Medicine: The Young Athlete* (Bar-Or, O., ed.) Blackwell Science, Oxford: 224–239.

Smith, J.L. & Madsen, J.R. (2003) Neurosurgical procedures for the treatment of pain. In: *Pain in Infants, Children and Adolescents* (Schechter, M.L., Berde, C.V. & Yaster, M., eds.) Lippincott Williams & Wilkins, Philadelphia: 329–338.

Sran, M. & Khan, K. (2002) Spinal manipulation versus mobilization. *Canadian Medical Association Journal* **7**, 1–30.

Stamford, B. (1996) Cross-training: Giving yourself a whole-body workout. *The Physician and Sportsmedicine* **24**, 1–4.

Starkey, C. (2004) *Therapeutic Modalities*, 3rd edn. F.A. Davis, Philadelphia.

Sterling, M., Jull, G. & Wright, A. (2001) Cervical mobilisation: concurrent effects on pain, sympathetic nervous system activity and motor activity. *Manual Therapy* **6**, 72–81.

Stricker, P.R. (2002) Sports training issues for the pediatric athlete. *Pediatric Clinics of North America* **49**, 793–802.

Tanner, J.M. (1978) *Foetus into Man*. A. Wheaton, Exeter.

Tippett, S.R. (1997) Lower extremity injuries in the young athlete. *Orthopaedic Physical Therapy Clinics of North America* **6**, 471.

VanDuersen, R.W., Sanchez, M.M., Ulbrecht, J.S. & Cavanagh, P.R. (1998) The role of muscle spindles in ankle movement perception in human subjects with diabetic neuropathy. *Experimental Brain Research* **120**, 1–8.

Verhagen, E.A.L.M., van Mechelen, W. & de Vente, W. (2000) The effect of preventive measures on the incidence of ankle sprains. *Clinical Journal of Sport Medicine* **10**, 291–296.

Vicenzino, B., Collins, D., Benson, H. & Wright, A. (1998) An investigation of the interrelationship between manipulative therapy-induced hypoalgesia and sympathoexcitation. *Journal of Manipulative and Physiological Therapy* **21**, 448–453.

Vickers, A. & Zollman, C. (1999) ABC of complimentary medicine: Acupuncture. *British Medical Journal* **319**, 973–976.

Walsh, M.T. (1996) Hydrotherapy: the use of water as a therapeutic agent. In: *Thermal Agents Rehabilition*, 3rd edn. (Michlovitz, S.L. ed.) F.A. Davis, Philadelphia: 138–168.

Wong, D.L., Hockenberry-Eaton, M., Wilson, D., Winkelstein, M. & Schwartz, P. (2001) *Whaley and Wong's Essentials of Pediatric Nursing*, 5th edn. Mosby, St. Louis: 1301.

Young, M.A., Cook, J.L., Purdam, C.R., Kiss, Z.S. & Alfredson, H. (2005) Eccentric decline squat protocol offers superior results at 12 months compared with traditional eccentric protocol for patellar tendinopathy in volleyball players. *British Journal of Sports Medicine* **39**, 102–105.

Part 4

Non-orthopedic Health Concerns

Chapter 15

The Preparticipation Physical Evaluation

ERIC SMALL

Each year in the USA, 15 million children and adolescents have a sports physical or preparticipation physical evaluation (PPE). Physicians perform these in a variety of ways. Examinations may vary from listening to the heart and lungs to performing a full musculoskeletal examination from head to toe. There are up to 1500 PPE forms available in various states and schools.

One must understand the goals for performing the PPE when certain procedures are adopted or excluded from the process of the PPE. The main goal is to ensure the safety and health of athletes during training and competition. Secondary goals include assessing the risk for sudden death, screening for conditions that may be exacerbated by sports participation, and allowing safe and fun participation amongst athletes.

The PPE is divided into three steps: medical history, physical examination, and clearance. This chapter focuses on the process and highlights the salient features of the three parts.

Evidence base of PPE

There are very few studies systematically assessing the effectiveness of PPE or parts thereof. In other words, the evidence base for the PPE is relatively vague. Wingfield *et al.* (2004) looked at this subject and found that the format of the PPE was not standardized in most settings and did not consistently meet the recommendations of the American Heart Association for cardiovascular screening (medical history and physical examination). However, the majority of the information provided by Wingfield

et al. (2004) is based on type III evidence or expert opinion. A recent article by Corrado *et al.* (2006), who evaluated a preparticipation screening program in young Italian athletes, demonstrated a decreased risk of sudden death from cardiomyopathy.

Timing of the PPE

The PPE should be carried out 4–6 weeks prior to the sports season. This means that any pending medical conditions or musculoskeletal injuries can be addressed and resolved or rehabilitated before the start of the season. For example, if an athlete has infectious mononucleosis, a time period of 4–6 weeks may be necessary before the spleen returns to normal size and the athlete may safely participate in sports. Another example is an athlete who is 5 months post anterior cruciate ligament (ACL) reconstruction. The athlete may be cleared to running and jumping at the time of the PPE but may need another month before he or she can participate in scrimmages, contact activities, and full competition.

Type of examination

There are generally two types of PPEs that can be performed: individual or station. The individual examination is definitely preferred as information from history and physical examination can be integrated with data from medical records to allow for an individual and detailed recommendation. Furthermore, personal health issues, such as eating habits, social habits, possible drug consumption, and family/ school functioning, can be explored more easily in

191

this setting. Ideally, the examination should be carried out by the student's own personal physician who has the relevant records and the rapport and trust of the patient.

The station examination is one in which multiple examiners examine different parts of the body, such as the heart/lung, abdomen, and musculoskeletal systems. There are two variations of the station examination: there may be 6–8 different people examining different body parts, or 6–8 examiners all performing the entire examination. If the station examination is performed it is preferable to have one examiner carry out the entire PPE as more medical information can be gleaned.

General recommendation for the PPE

It is recommended that the physician use the form supplied by the American Academy of Family Physicians, American Academy of Pediatrics, American College of Sports Medicine, American Medical Society for Sports Medicine, American Orthopaedic Society for Sports Medicine, and American Osteopathic Academy of Sports Medicine (2005) (Fig. 15.1).

Table 15.1 summarizes various medical conditions (American Academy of Pediatrics Committee on Sports Medicine and Fitness 2001) that should be specifically sought out during the PPE. For further information on injuries, non-orthopedic health conditions, and psychologic issues, the reader is referred to the respective sections in this volume.

History

Some questions regarding sports participation and past medical history may be asked using standardized questionnaires. However, there are a series of general questions that this author believes must be reviewed with each athlete, even though on the questionnaire it was checked off as a "No" answer. These categories include asthma, allergies (especially history of anaphylaxis, carries adrenaline injector), surgeries, current medication, or recent emergency room visits.

It is important to be cognizant of the sport the athlete will be participating in. For example, if the

youngster is playing football, several questions must be asked as football players are more likely to suffer from heat injury, concussion, and brachial plexus injuries (burners or stingers). In cross-country runners or track athletes, a history of shin pain or stress fractures must be queried. All female athletes, especially those participating in aesthetic sports (dance, gymnastics, figure skating) should be asked about their eating habits, menstrual cycles, and bone health (American Academy of Pediatrics Committee on Sports Medicine and Fitness, 2000b) These are questions that relate to the female athlete triad (disordered eating, amenorrhea, osteopenia; Yeager *et al.* 1993). If a female athlete demonstrates elements of the female athlete triad, referral should be made to a team of professionals including the athlete's primary care physician, a nutritionist, and a psychologist. In baseball players (especially pitchers and catchers), it is important to ask about elbow and shoulder problems.

There are several essential areas on which to focus during the remaining history. These are as follow.

Cardiac disease

SUDDEN DEATH

A student dying on the athletic field is a tragedy for all involved: parents, friends, staff and personnel. Fortunately, these events are rare (perhaps 8–12 deaths per year in the USA). Important questions to screen for individuals at risk for sudden death during the PPE are: Is there a family history of sudden death, a history of Marfan's syndrome, chest pain, or fainting with exercise? If the athlete responds positively to a family history of sudden death, or admits to shortness of breath or chest pain with exercise then clearance should be withheld until further evaluation by a pediatric cardiologist (Maron *et al.* 2003).

HYPERTOPHIC CARDIOMYOPATHY

Hypertrophic cardiomyopathy is the most common cause of sudden death in the athlete under 21 years of age. In a landmark study in 1996 (Maron *et al.* 1996), 36% of deaths in young competitive athletes

Preparticipation Physical Evaluation

DATE OF EXAM _____

Name _____ Sex _____ Age _____ Date of birth _____

Grade _____ School _____ Sport(s) _____

Address _____ Phone _____

Personal physician _____

In case of emergency, contact

Name _____ Relationship _____ Phone (H) _____ (W) _____

Explain "Yes" answers below. Circle questions you don't know the answer to.	Yes	No
1. Has a doctor ever denied or restricted your participation in sports for any reason?	☐	☐
2. Do you have an ongoing medical condition (like diabetes or asthma)?	☐	☐
3. Are you currently taking any prescription or nonprescription (over-the-counter) medicines or pills?	☐	☐
4. Do you have allergies to medicines, pollens, foods, or stinging insects?	☐	☐
5. Have you ever passed out or nearly passed out DURING exercise?	☐	☐
6. Have you ever passed out or nearly passed out AFTER exercise?	☐	☐
7. Have you ever had discomfort, pain, or pressure in your chest during exercise?	☐	☐
8. Does your heart race or skip beats during exercise?	☐	☐

9. Has a doctor ever told you that you have (check all that apply):
☐ High blood pressure ☐ A heart murmur
☐ High cholesterol ☐ A heart infection

	Yes	No
10. Has a doctor ever ordered a test for your heart? (for example, ECG, echocardiogram)	☐	☐
11. Has anyone in your family died for no apparent reason?	☐	☐
12. Does anyone in your family have a heart problem?	☐	☐
13. Has any family member or relative died of heart problems or of sudden death before age 50?	☐	☐
14. Does anyone in your family have Marfan syndrome?	☐	☐
15. Have you ever spent the night in a hospital?	☐	☐
16. Have your ever had surgery?	☐	☐
17. Have you ever had an injury, like a sprain, muscle or ligament tear, or tendinitis, that caused you to miss a practice or game? If yes, circle affected area below.	☐	☐
18. Have you had any broken or fractured bones or dislocated joints? If yes, circle below.	☐	☐
19. Have you had a bone or joint injury that required x-rays, MRI, CT, surgery, injections, rehabilitation, physical, therapy, a brace, a cast, or crutches? If yes, circle below.	☐	☐

Head	Neck	Shoulder	Upper arm	Elbow	Forearm	Hand/ fingers	Chest
Upper back	Lower back	Hip	Thigh	Knee	Calf/shin	Ankle	Foot/toes

	Yes	No
20. Have you ever had a stress fracture?	☐	☐
21. Have you been told that you have or have you had an x-ray for atlantoaxial (neck) instability?	☐	☐
22. Do you regularly use a brace or assistive device?	☐	☐
23. Has a doctor ever told you that you have asthma or allergies?	☐	☐

	Yes	No
24. Do you cough, wheeze, or have difficulty breathing during or after exercise?	☐	☐
25. Is there anyone in your family who has asthma?	☐	☐
26. Have you ever used an inhaler or taken asthma medicine?	☐	☐
27. Were you born without or are you missing a kidney, an eye, a testicle, or any other organ?	☐	☐
28. Have you had infectious mononucleosis (mono) within the last month?	☐	☐
29. Do you have any rashes, pressure sores, or other skin problems?	☐	☐
30. Have you had a herpes skin infection?	☐	☐
31. Have you ever had a head injury or concussion?	☐	☐
32. Have you been hit in the head and been confused or lost your memory?	☐	☐
33. Have you ever had a seizure?	☐	☐
34. Do you have headaches with exercise?	☐	☐
35. Have you ever had numbness, tingling, or weakness in your arms or legs after being hit or falling?	☐	☐
36. Have you ever been unable to move your arms or legs after being hit or falling?	☐	☐
37. When exercising in the heat, do you have severe muscle cramps or become ill?	☐	☐
38. Has a doctor told you that you or someone in your family has sickle cell trait or sickle cell disease?	☐	☐
39. Have you had any problems with your eyes or vision?	☐	☐
40. Do you wear glasses or contact lenses?	☐	☐
41. Do you wear protective eyewear, such as goggles or a face shield?	☐	☐
42. Are you happy with your weight?	☐	☐
43. Are you trying to gain or lose weight?	☐	☐
44. Has anyone recommended you change your weight or eating habits?	☐	☐
45. Do you limit or carefully control what you eat?	☐	☐
46. Do you have any concerns that you would like to discuss with a doctor?	☐	☐

FEMALES ONLY

	Yes	No
47. Have you ever had a menstrual period?	☐	☐

48. How old were you when you had your first menstrual period? ____

49. How many periods have you had in the last 12 months? _____

Explain "Yes" answers here: _____
_____
_____
_____
_____
_____
_____

I hereby state that, to the best of my knowledge, my answers to the above questions are complete and correct.

Signature of athlete _____ Signature of parent/guardian _____ Date _____

Fig. 15.1 History form (a) and physical examination form (b) for the preparticipation examination recommended by the American Academy of Family Physicians, the American Academy of Pediatrics, the American College of Sports Medicine, the American Medical Society for Sports Medicine, the American Orthopaedic Society for Sports Medicine, and the American Osteopathic Academy of Sports Medicine (2005).

Preparticipation Physical Evaluation

PHYSICAL EXAMINATION FORM

Name _____ Date of birth _____

Height _____ Weight _____ % Body fat (optional) _____ Pulse _____ BP ___ /___ (__ /__ , __ /__)

Vision   R 20/ _____ L 20/ _____   Corrected: Y N   Pupils: Equal _____ Unequal _____

Follow-Up Questions on More Sensitive Issues	Yes	No
1. Do you feel stressed out or under a lot of pressure?		
2. Do you ever feel so sad or hopeless that you stop doing some of your usual activities for more than a few days?	☐	☐
3. Do you feel safe?	☐	☐
4. Have you ever tried cigarette smoking, even 1 or 2 puffs? Do you currently smoke?	☐	☐
5. During the past 30 days, did you use chewing tobacco, snuff, or dip?	☐	☐
6. During the past 30 days, have you had at least 1 drink of alcohol?	☐	☐
7. Have you ever taken steroid pills or shots without a doctor's prescription?	☐	☐
8. Have you ever taken any supplements to help you gain or lose weight or improve your performance?	☐	☐
9. Questions from the Youth Risk Behavior Survery (http://www.cdc.gov/HealthyYouth/yrbs/index.htm) on guns, seatbelts, unprotected sex, domestic violence, drugs, etc.	☐	☐

Notes:

	NORMAL	ABNORMAL FINDINGS	INITIALS*
MEDICAL			
Appearance			
Eyes/ears/nose/throat			
Hearing			
Lymph nodes			
Heart			
Murmurs			
Pulses			
Lungs			
Abdomen			
Genitourinary (males only)†			
Skin			
MUSCULOSKELETAL			
Neck			
Back			
Shoulder/arm			
Elbow/forearm			
Wrist/hand/fingers			
Hip/thigh			
Knee			
Leg/ankle			
Foot/toes			

*Multiple-examiner set-up only.
†Having a third party present is recommended for the genitourinary examination.

Notes: _____

Name of physician (print/type) _____ Date _____

Address _____ Phone _____

Signature of physician _____ MD or DO

Fig. 15.1 *(cont'd)*

Table 15.1 Conditions that should be specifically sought out during the preparticipation physical evaluation (PPE).

Sport	Comment	Criteria before return to play	Further information
Concussion			
Football, soccer	Amnesia is the worst prognostic sign	Must do non-contact practice for 1 week without symptoms	
Heat injury			
Football, tennis, cross-country running	Risk factors (obesity, nutritional supplement use, prescription medication)	Athlete must have documented urine specific gravity of 1010 mg/L or lower, returned to baseline weight, and be asymptomatic with exercise	see Chapter 20; American Academy of Pediatrics Committee on Sports Medicine and Fitness (2000a)
Stress fracture of tibia/fibula, metatarsal			
Cross-country running, soccer, basketball	Females need to be worked up for female athlete triad (osteoporosis, amenorrhea, disordered eating)	Practicing, jogging, without pain	see Chapter 12
Low back pain (stress fracture/spondylolysis)			
Gymnastics, figure skating, dance, tennis	Bone scan, CT scan, or MRI generally needed to make the diagnosis	Practice with brace without pain	see Chapter 12
ACL tear			
Basketball/soccer	Decision to perform surgery is based on symptoms (episodes of instability, sport practiced, and whether there is a meniscus tear)	Must have 90% strength and flexibility	see Chapter 14
Nutritional supplements			
Prevalent in strength sports (American football, soccer, wrestling)	Ask if the athlete is taking supplements whether or not they checked the box on the form as a 'No'		see Chapters 16 & 21; American Academy of Pediatrics Committee on Sports Medicine and Fitness (2005)
Obesity		These children do not need to be excluded from sports participation. If there is severe hypertension then some restriction will take place	

ACL, anterior cruciate ligament; CT, computed tomography; MRI, magnetic resonance imaging.

was brought about by hypertrophic obstructive cardiomyopathy, with aortic root dissection being next most common. Other causes of sudden cardiac death under age 18 years include coronary anomalies, myocarditis, and total anomalous pulmonary venous return (Maron *et al.* 1996, 2003; Maron 2003). Hypertophic cardiomyopathy is an autosomal dominant genetic pattern and over 10 genes have been identified. In the majority of cases, there is a negative history and physical exam. A history of chest pain during exercise, fainting or near fainting during exercise, or a family history of sudden death under age 45 years are signs that one should think of hypertophic cardiomyopathy and that further work-up is required.

Musculoskeletal problems (sprains, strains, and overuse injuries)

As part of the history it is important to determine whether the young athlete has ligamentous laxity or is tight in the muscles, by asking such questions as: Have you ever dislocated a joint, are you double jointed, or are you tight in your muscles compared to your peers? As pointed out in other chapters in this book, female athletes are 3–5 times more likely to suffer an ACL tear (Arendt & Dick 1995). Many of these injuries are preventable.

Neurologic issues (concussion, brachial plexus injury)

Concussion, defined as temporary altered mental status with or without altered loss of consciousness, is a serious public health risk that should be questioned during the PPE. There are two types of concussions: simple and complex. In a simple concussion, symptoms resolve within minutes or hours. In a complicated concussion, symptoms persist for 1 day up to weeks or months. With persistent symptoms and/or repeated concussions, neuropsychologic testing is recommended (McCrory *et al.* 2005).

A brachial plexus injury can occur in sports such as American football where there is temporary numbness and/or tingling of one arm. If symptoms persist or bilateral weakness is present, evaluation of cervical disk injury or cervical spine stenosis should be considered.

Bronchial asthma

Bronchial asthma is the most common chronic disease of childhood. It is important to screen for exercise-induced asthma during the history of the PPE by asking such questions as: Do you have difficulty breathing with exercise, chest pain during exercise, or coughing during exercise under extreme conditions (cold, severe physical exertion, or environmental pollutants).

Physical examination

Height, weight, and blood pressure need to be assessed. A body mass index (BMI) should be calculated and assessed using reference centiles to identify athletes who are at risk for eating disorders and those who are overweight.

At a minimum, the heart, lungs, neurologic systems, and musculoskeletal systems should be examined. When there are positives in the written history or the oral history, the respective issues should be expanded on in the physical examination. For example, in an athlete who has a history of multiple concussions, it is indicated to physically stress him or her by performing maximal push-ups or sit-ups in 1 minute or sprinting 100 yards. These physical stressors are performed because they may induce headache or nausea which would mean the athlete is not ready to return to sports. An orthopedic and/or musculoskeletal examination is recommended to check for asymmetry, lack of range of motion, weakness, or muscle atrophy (Figs 15.2–15.13).

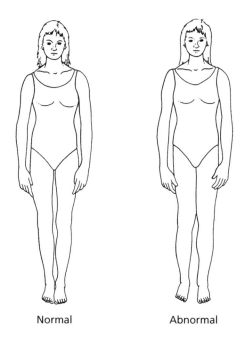

Normal   Abnormal

Fig. 15.2 Stand straight with arms at sides. Check for symmetry of upper and lower extremities and trunk. Common abnormalities: (1) enlarged acromioclavicular joint; (2) enlarged sternoclavicular joint; (3) asymmetrical waist (leg length difference or scoliosis); (4) swollen knee; (5) swollen ankle. Redrawn from Ross Laboratories, Columbus, Ohio.

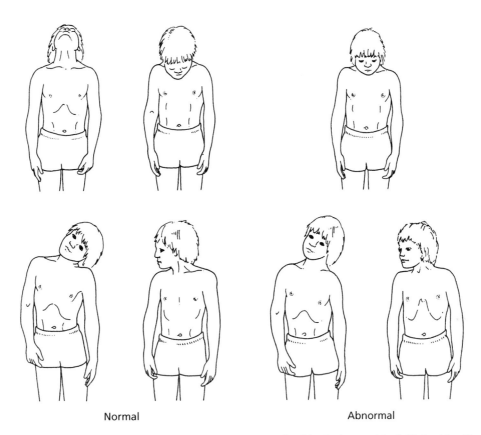

Normal   Abnormal

Fig. 15.3 Look at the ceiling; look at the floor; touch right (left) ear to shoulder; look over right (left) shoulder. The athlete should be able to touch chin to chest, ears to shoulders and look equally over shoulders. Common abnormalities (may indicate previous neck injury). (1) loss of flexion; (2) loss of lateral bending; (3) loss of rotation. Redrawn from Ross Laboratories, Columbus, Ohio.

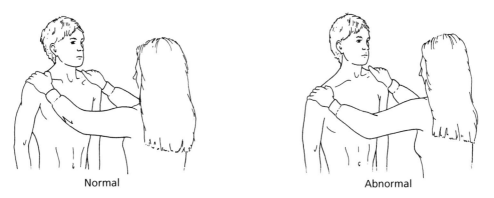

Normal   Abnormal

Fig. 15.4 Shrug shoulders while examiner holds them down. Check that trapezius muscles appear equal; left and right side have equal strength. Common abnormalities (may indicate neck or shoulder problem): (1) loss of strength; (2) loss of muscle bulk. Redrawn from Ross Laboratories, Columbus, Ohio.

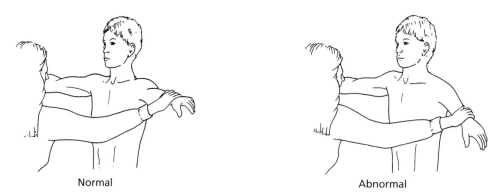

Fig. 15.5 Hold arms out from sides horizontally and lift while examiner holds them down. Strength should be equal and deltoid muscles should be equal in size. Common abnormalities: (1) loss of strength; (2) wasting of deltoid muscle. Redrawn from Ross Laboratories, Columbus, Ohio.

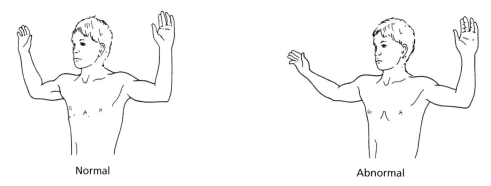

Fig. 15.6 Hold arms out from sides with elbows bent (90°); raise hands back vertically as far as they will go. Check that hands go back equally and at least to upright vertical position. Common abnormality (may indicate shoulder problem or old dislocation) is loss of external rotation. Redrawn from Ross Laboratories, Columbus, Ohio.

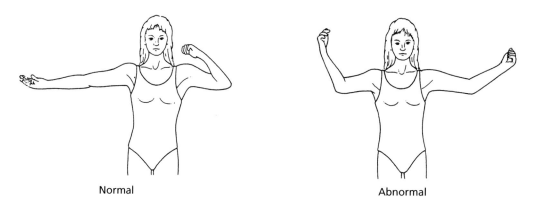

Fig. 15.7 Hold arms out from sides, palms up; straighten elbows completely; bend completely. Check motion is equal left and right sides. Common abnormalities (may indicate old elbow injury, old dislocation, fracture, etc.): (1) loss of extension; (2) loss of flexion. Redrawn from Ross Laboratories, Columbus, Ohio.

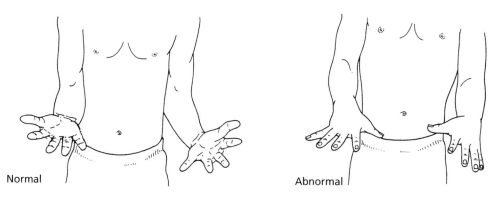

Fig. 15.8 Hold arms down at sides with elbows bent (90°); supinate palms; pronate palms. Palms should go from facing ceiling to facing floor. Common abnormalities (may indicate old forearm, wrist, or elbow injury): (1) lack of full supination; (2) lack of full pronation. Redrawn from Ross Laboratories, Columbus, Ohio.

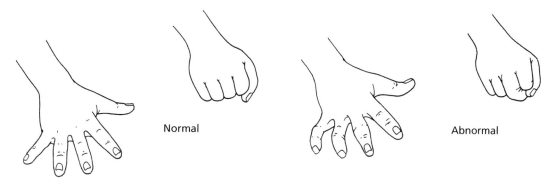

Fig. 15.9 Make a fist; open hand and spread fingers. First should be tight and fingers straight when spread. Common abnormalities (may indicate old finger fractures or sprains): (1) protruding knuckle from fist; (2) swollen and/or crooked finger. Redrawn from Ross Laboratories, Columbus, Ohio.

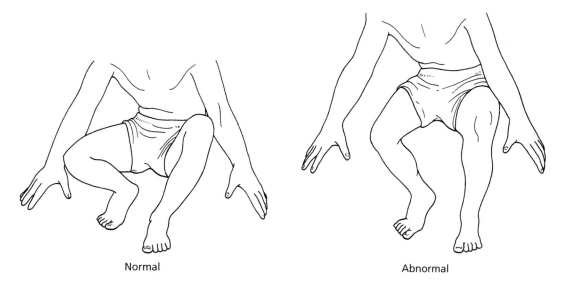

Fig. 15.10 Squat on heels; duck walk four steps and stand up. Check that maneuver is painless; heel to buttock distance is equal left and right; knee flexion is equal during walk; rises straight up. Common abnormalities: (1) inability to fully flex one knee; (2) inability to stand up without twisting or bending to one side. Redrawn from Ross Laboratories, Columbus, Ohio.

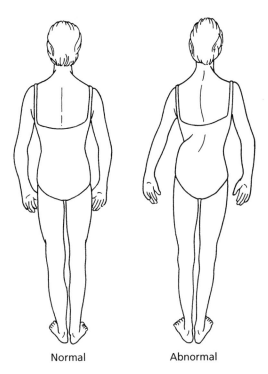

Normal   Abnormal

Fig. 15.11 With back to examiner stand up straight. Check for symmetry of shoulders, waist, thighs, and calves. Common abnormalities: (1) high shoulder (scoliosis) or low shoulder (muscle loss); (2) prominent rib cage (scoliosis); (3) high hip or asymmetrical waist (leg length difference or scoliosis); (4) small calf or thigh (weakness from old injury). Redrawn from Ross Laboratories, Columbus, Ohio.

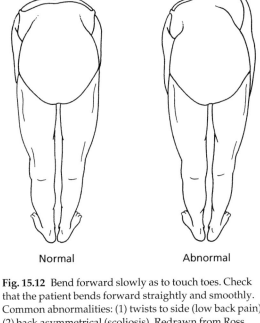

Normal   Abnormal

Fig. 15.12 Bend forward slowly as to touch toes. Check that the patient bends forward straightly and smoothly. Common abnormalities: (1) twists to side (low back pain); (2) back asymmetrical (scoliosis). Redrawn from Ross Laboratories, Columbus, Ohio.

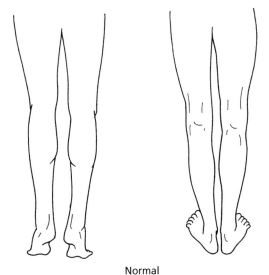

Normal

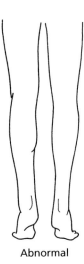

Abnormal

Fig. 15.13 Stand on heels; stand on toes. Check for equal elevation on right and left sides; symmetry of calf muscles. Common abnormality is wasting of calf muscles (Achilles injury or old ankle injury). Redrawn from Ross Laboratories, Columbus, Ohio.

Blood tests and work-up

There are no routine blood tests, urinalysis, or screening electrocardiograms as part of the PPE. Blood tests (hemoglobin and hematocrit) may be performed by the athlete's pediatrician or family doctor. If the PPE is the only contact with the health care system, then a complete blood count (CBC) should be performed in selected individuals. The hemoglobin and hematocrit is analyzed to screen for iron deficiency anemia. A CBC in an endurance female athlete (running, skiing) is likely to be a more cost-effective screening test than a CBC in a male wrestler or a football player. Female athletes are more likely to be anemic than males because of menses and eating patterns.

An electrocardiogram is only recommended if there are any abnormalities suggesting heart disease in the medical history or the physical findings. There is a high percentage of false positives in screening electrocardiograms. At the same time, many young athletes with hypertrophic cardiomyopathy or arrhythmias have negative electrocardiograms.

Clearance

At the conclusion of the PPE, one of three clearance status should be assigned: cleared, not cleared, not cleared pending further evaluation and work-up. In categories two and three, it is extremely critical that there is good communication between everyone (physician, school nurse, athletic director, athlete, athletic trainer). In every school there are different lines of communication. The parent, child, and coach should know why the child was not cleared and what can be done and needs to be done.

Common pitfalls

Having performed a PPE does not guarantee the student athlete will not have an injury, minor or major. In addition, the general public and parents wrongfully assume that without a history of chest pain or fainting with exercise and with a normal cardiac physical examination it is guaranteed there is no underlying heart condition that could result in sudden death. It has been shown from the Italian experience (Corrado *et al.* 2006) that the risk of sudden cardiac death, particularly from cardiomyopathy, can be reduced by the PPE, but not nullified.

General recommendations

Communication and counseling for parents and patients

The PPE can serve as means for reintegrating the child into the health care system. Adolescents are one of the most underserved populations in terms of visits to the health care system. Furthermore, many adolescents—both male and female—are not happy with their weight. Most want to lose weight and some want to gain weight. The PPE is an opportunity to assure these youngsters about their body shape and composition or to initiate referral to appropriate medical specialists, psychologists, and nutritionists. For the overweight child or athlete, suggestions and recommendations can be made for increasing physical activity and improving nutrition.

Conclusions

The majority of young athletes can safely participate in middle and high school sports. It is our goal as a medical community to assist in their safe participation and promote enjoyment. A concerted effort should be made to reintegrate these young athletes into the health care system by encouraging routine visits to their pediatrician or primary health care provider.

Directions for future research

Further evidence-based research needs to be carried out to standardize cardiovascular screening to prevent sudden death and standardize the musculoskeletal history and physical to prevent sports injuries. Furthermore, the effectiveness of each item included in the PPE needs to be assessed.

References

American Academy of Family Physicians, American Academy of Pediatrics, American College of Sports Medicine, American Medical Society for Sports Medicine, American Orthopaedic Society for Sports Medicine, American Osteopathic Academy of Sports Medicine (2005) *The Preparticipation Physical Evaluation*, 3rd edn. McGraw Hill, New York.

American Academy of Pediatrics Committee on Sports Medicine and Fitness (2000a) Climatic heat stress and the exercising child and adolescent. *Pediatrics* **106**, 158–159.

American Academy of Pediatrics Committee on Sports Medicine and Fitness (2000b) Medical concerns in the female athlete. *Pediatrics* **106**, 610–613.

American Academy of Pediatrics Committee on Sports Medicine and Fitness (2001) Medical conditions affecting sports participation. *Pediatrics* **107**, 1205–1209.

American Academy of Pediatrics Committee on Sports Medicine and Fitness (2005) Use of performance enhancing substances. *Pediatrics* **115**, 1103–1106.

Arendt, E. & Dick, R. (1995) Knee injury patterns among men and women in collegiate basketball and soccer. NCAA data and review of literature. *American Journal of Sports Medicine* **23**, 694–701.

Corrado, D., Basso, C., Pavei, A., Michieli, P., Schiavon, M. & Thiene, G. (2006) Trends in sudden cardiovascular death in young competitive athletes after implementation of a preparticipation screening program. *Journal of the American Medical Association* **296**, 1593–1601.

Maron, B.J. (2003) Sudden death in young athletes. *New England Journal of Medicine* **349**, 1064–1075.

Maron, B.J., McKenna, W.J., Danielson, G.K., *et al.*, Task Force on Clinical Expert Consensus Documents, American College of Cardiology; Committee for Practice Guidelines, European Society of Cardiology (2003) American College of Cardiology/European Society of Cardiology clinical expert consensus document on hypertrophic cardiomyopathy: a report of the American College of Cardiology Foundation Task Force on clinical expert consensus documents and the European Society of Cardiology Committee for Practice Guidelines. *Journal of the American College of Cardiology* **42**, 1687–1713.

Maron, B.J., Shirani, J., Poliac, L.C., Mathenge, R., Roberts, W.C. & Mueller, F.O. (1996) Sudden death in young competitive athletes. Clinical, demographic, and pathological profiles. *Journal of the American Medical Association* **276**, 199–204.

McCrory, P., Johnston, K., Meeuwisse, W., *et al.* (2005) Summary and agreement statement of the 2nd International Conference on Concussion in Sport, Prague 2004. *British Journal of Sports Medicine* **39**, 196–204.

Wingfield, K., Matheson, G.O. & Meeuwisse, W.H. (2004) Preparticipation evaluation: an evidence-based review. *Clinical Journal of Sports Medicine* **14**, 109–122.

Yeager, K.K., Agostini, R., Nattiv, A. & Drinkwater, B. (1993) The female athlete triad: disordered eating, amenorrhea, osteoporosis. *Medicine and Science in Sports and Exercise* **25**, 775–777.

Chapter 16

Nutrition for the School Aged Child Athlete

MELVIN H. WILLIAMS

As with adult athletes, the level of performance in any given youth sport is dependent upon two major factors: genetics and training. Young athletes must be genetically endowed with physiologic, psychologic, and biomechanical traits necessary for success in a given sport, and they must optimize these traits through proper physical, mental, and skill training. Beyond genetics and training, the most important factor that may impact sport performance in the young athlete is proper nutrition.

Recent reviews have indicated that for young athletes there is no substitute for a healthy diet consisting of a variety of foods from all food groups with enough energy (calories) to support growth, daily physical activities, and sports activities. Such a diet is critical, not only to their athletic success but, more importantly, to their growth, development, and overall health (American Academy of Pediatrics 2005; Cotunga *et al.* 2005). In essence, the optimal diet for the young athlete is a diet that is optimal for his or her overall health.

Healthful eating for children and adolescents

Dietary recommendations for children and adolescents of school age, approximately 5–18 years, have been developed for all macronutrients and many micronutrients by most countries and some international organizations, such as the World Health Organization (WHO). We will refer to these recommendations for specific nutrients as recommended dietary intakes (RDI). In the past, RDI were developed with the major intention of preventing deficiency diseases. Today, RDI are also designed to optimize health, mainly in attempts to prevent the development of chronic diseases such as obesity, diabetes, heart disease, and cancer.

To promote healthier eating, various dietary guidelines have been developed with the basic premise that the RDI for all nutrients should be obtained from foods commonly available. Dwyer (2006) noted that the immediate goal of dietary guidelines is to promote health by providing healthy consumers science-based advice on food choices and eating patterns. The ultimate goal is to optimize intakes of key nutrients and to change food-related behaviors in desirable directions from the health standpoint.

General dietary guidelines for healthy children

Uauy *et al.* (2006) noted that, from an international perspective, a large variety of foods can be combined in varying amounts to provide a healthy diet. The prevailing view is that a large set of food combinations is compatible with nutritional adequacy and a healthy diet, and food-based dietary guidelines are more closely linked to the diet–health relationships of relevance to a particular country or region of interest. They also noted that the idea of optimal nutrient intake is based on the quest for improved functionality, such as muscle strength, which could be of interest to the athlete.

Heird and Cooper (2006) noted that children have unique nutrient needs for growth and development, but also noted that by 2 years of age, a child's diet should not differ from that of the rest of the family.

All known required nutrients can be supplied by a varied diet selected according to current food guidelines. The following general dietary guidelines for healthy children and adolescents are comparable among various national and international recommendations. Societies can select the foods they prefer and combine them in the way that best suits their tastes and other sensory requirements (Bloch & Shils 2006; Heird & Cooper 2006; Treuth & Griffin 2006; Uauy *et al.* 2006; Willett & Stampfer 2006).

1 Maintain a healthy body weight. Stay lean and active throughout life.
2 Eat a wide variety of natural foods from within and among food groups, such as those in various food guide pyramids.
3 Eat more complex carbohydrates and dietary fiber. Eat simple sugars only in moderation.
4 Choose a diet moderate in unsaturated fats and low in saturated and *trans* fats.
5 Eat a moderate amount of protein, balancing your intake of plant and animal sources.
6 Limit your intake of salt.
7 Drink enough fluids.
Additional details are provided in following sections for specific macronutrients and micronutrients.

Dietary practices and considerations for the school aged athlete

Sports scientists have studied dietary considerations of young athletes in various ways. Surveys have been most common, mainly to determine nutrient intake in various groups of athletes in attempts to determine the nutritional adequacy of their diets. Experimental research evaluating the effect of dietary interventions on performance is more limited.

Dietary practices of school aged athletes

Numerous studies have surveyed the diets of young athletes. Some studies reported that young athletes appear to have better eating patterns than their non-athlete peers. For example, Cavadini *et al.* (2000) reported that athletic adolescents display healthier food habits than non-athletic adolescents. Croll *et al.* (2006) also reported that adolescent athletes

involved in weight-related or power team sports had better eating habits. In general, they found that athletes ate breakfast more frequently and had higher mean protein, calcium, iron, and zinc intakes than non-sport-involved peers.

However, most dietary surveys suggest that many young athletes, particularly elite athletes involved in weight-controlled sports, do not consume adequate or healthful diets. In general, although the findings were mixed among studies, dietary intakes of the athletes were considered deficient in energy, carbohydrate, and various micronutrients, particularly iron, calcium, zinc, and folate, while intake of fats was in excess (Lopez-Varela *et al.* 2000; Beals 2002; Papadopoulou *et al.* 2002; Ziegler *et al.* 2002; Christensen *et al.* 2005; Iglesias-Gutierrez *et al.* 2005; Ruiz *et al.* 2005). Although Ziegler *et al.* (2002) reported that most of the athletes in their study consumed less than 67% of the requirement for several micronutrients, most of the biochemical indexes of nutritional status were within normal limits. This finding, common in dietary surveys of athletes, may be attributed to the fact that elite athletes may underreport energy intakes, which can have a significant impact on reported micronutrient intake (Jonnalagadda *et al.* 2000), or they may consume vitamin and/or mineral dietary supplements (O'Dea 2003) that may compensate for decreased nutrient intake from foods.

Nevertheless, based on the results of their studies, many investigators recommended that well-designed nutrition intervention programs are advisable for optimizing performance and especially for promoting healthy eating habits in young athletes (Greydanus & Patel 2002; Ziegler *et al.* 2002; Iglesias-Gutierrez *et al.* 2005; Ruiz *et al.* 2005).

Dietary considerations for school aged athletes

The goal of nutrition for young athletes, whether a member of a local community sport club or an Olympic champion, is the same as for all athletes—to provide a healthful diet adequate in energy, carbohydrate, fat, protein, vitamins, minerals, and fluids to support the physical and mental demands of their specific training and competition. However, Unnithan and Goulopoulou (2004) indicate that a paucity of literature exists with regard to research on nutrition for the pediatric athlete, and this lack of research makes the development of specific nutritional recommendations for young athletes problematic. Although research regarding specific nutrient needs of young athletes is limited, Bar-Or (2001) counters that nutritional issues are similar for all athletes irrespective of age. Nevertheless, Bar-Or (1995) also notes that children have several physiologic characteristics that distinguish them from adults and require specific nutritional considerations, and such considerations are incorporated in the following discussion.

Energy considerations for school aged athletes

In a review of energy balance in young athletes, Thompson (1998) indicated that the energy intake in certain athletic groups may be marginal or inadequate, which could impair health status and sport performance. On the other hand, excessive energy intake could predispose young athletes to obesity, which also may impair health status and sport performance.

Energy output

Thompson (1998) noted that very little is known about the energy needs of young athletes, as no studies of energy balance in young athletes have been published. However, various formulae have been developed to estimate the energy requirement of children and adolescents, and such formulae have incorporated estimates of energy expenditure through physical activity. Such estimates would be appropriate for young athletes as they calculate energy needs based on basal energy expenditure, activities of daily living, patterns of growth and development, and amount of physical activity. Detailed discussion of energy expenditure is beyond the scope of this chapter. Briefly, however, estimates of energy requirements (EER) for young athletes may be obtained from various governmental health services, such as the MyPyramid food guide (www.MyPyramid.gov) developed by the US Department of Agriculture. The EER is determined from age, weight, height, extra energy for growth and development, and specific amounts of physical activity.

Energy input

Caloric energy is provided by the carbohydrate, fat, and protein content of the foods one eats, and two key concepts are important for athletes of all ages to help attain proper body composition and obtain an adequate supply of micronutrients. The first is the *key nutrient concept*. Eight key nutrients are protein, calcium, iron, vitamin A, vitamin C, thiamin, riboflavin, and niacin. The central theme of the *key nutrient concept* is simply that if these eight key nutrients are adequate in the foods you eat, you will probably receive an ample supply of all nutrients essential to humans. For example, foods rich in iron are usually rich in zinc. The second is the *nutrient density concept*. Per amount of caloric energy, foods with a high nutrient density contain higher concentrations of one or more of the key nutrients. For example, a glass of milk and a can of soda may contain equal calories, but the milk is rich in protein, calcium, vitamin A, and riboflavin. Table 16.1 lists the common food group classifications that are good sources of the listed key nutrients. These food groups serve as the basis for most healthful dietary recommendations, such as MyPyramid.

By eating the recommended amounts of food from each group daily, you can greatly increase your ability to obtain all the nutrients your body needs. MyPyramid (http://www.mypyramid.gov/downloads/MyPyramid_Food_Intake_Patterns.pdf) provides the suggested amounts of food from the

Table 16.1 Common food group classifications rich in selected key nutrients.

Grains	Iron, thiamin, riboflavin, niacin
Vegetables	Vitamin A, vitamin C, iron
Fruits	Vitamin A, vitamin C
Milk, yogurt, and cheese	Calcium, protein, vitamin A, riboflavin
Meat and beans	Protein, thiamin, riboflavin, niacin
Oils	Vitamin A

basic food groups, subgroups, and oils to meet recommended nutrient intakes at 12 different calorie levels. Sample menus are also available.

Healthy weight maintenance or loss for school aged athletes

The American Academy of Pediatrics (2005) notes that weight control is perceived to be advantageous for youths involved in sports such as bodybuilding, cheerleading, dancing, distance running, cross-country skiing, diving, figure skating, gymnastics, martial arts, rowing, swimming, weight-class football, and wrestling, which emphasize thinness, leanness and/or competing at the lowest possible weight for aesthetic appeal or economy of movement. Such athletes may want to maintain or lose body weight, but weight lost should be fat, not muscle.

Use of improper weight-loss methods may predispose young athletes to various health problems and impaired performance. Treuth and Griffin (2006) indicate that adolescence is a time when eating disorders emerge, including anorexia nervosa, bulimia, and a wide range of unhealthy food restriction practices. Such eating disorders may also be prevalent in sports, particularly among young female athletes in weight-control sports, and have been referred to as the female athlete triad which consists of disordered eating, menstrual irregularity, and bone demineralization (Torstveit & Sundgot-Borgen 2005; Nichols et al. 2006; Williams 2007). Increasing caloric intake to offset the high energy demand of intense sport training may be sufficient to reverse menstrual dysfunction and stimulate bone accretion (Warren & Perlroth 2001). This topic is covered in more detail in Chapters 17 and 18.

The American Academy of Pediatrics (2005) has recommended healthy weight maintenance or loss practices for young athletes. Some of its key points for young athletes are to:

1 Start early to permit a gradual weight loss over a realistic time period;
2 Eat enough to cover the energy costs of daily living, growth, building and repairing muscle tissue, and participating in sports;
3 Lose excess fat without reducing lean muscle

mass or causing dehydration, both of which can impair performance;
4 Limit weight loss to a maximum of 1.5% of the total body weight, or 0.5–0.9 kg·week^{-1};
5 Lose excess weight by both diet and extra exercise;
6 Obtain from the diet approximately 55–65% of energy from carbohydrate, 15–20% from protein, and 20–30% from fat;
7 Maintain the desired body weight, once attained, rather than cycling up and down;
8 Discuss any desired weight loss with a health care professional and the family.

Breakfast can be a very important meal for school aged athletes attempting to maintain or lose weight. A breakfast rich in carbohydrate and protein, such as cereal, milk, toast, eggs, and fruit or fruit juice, provides a nutritious start to the day. Children who reported eating breakfast on a consistent basis tended to have superior nutritional profiles than their breakfast-skipping peers. Even though they consumed more daily calories, they were less likely to be overweight (Rampersaud et al. 2005).

Healthy weight gain for school aged athletes

Young athletes in sports such as football, rugby, basketball, and power lifting emphasize gaining weight. However, weight gained should be muscle, not fat. Dietz (2006) indicated that adolescence is a critical period for the onset of overweight, which has been associated with decreased levels of physical activity and a high intake of energy-dense, micronutrient-poor foods (Swinburn et al. 2004; Erlanson-Albertsson & Zetterstrom 2005; Janssen et al. 2005). Juvenile obesity is now a global issue and increasing evidence indicates that adolescents are presenting with what have been traditionally adult-onset diseases, such as hypertension and type 2 diabetes (Silink 2002; Treuth & Griffin 2006).

The American Academy of Pediatrics (2005) has recommended healthy weight gain practices for young athletes. In essence, some of its key points for young athletes are to:

1 Start early to permit a gradual weight gain over a realistic time period;
2 Set a reasonable goal, such as adding 0.45 kg of muscle per week;

3 Consume about 8400–10,500 kJ (2000–2500 kcal) per week more than needed to maintain weight;

4 Consume 1.5–1.75 g protein per kg of body weight plus increased energy intake from healthy carbohydrates and fats;

5 Engage in an appropriate resistance training program.

Dietary considerations for school aged athletes

Carbohydrate

The major dietary energy source for most athletic endeavors is carbohydrate. In the body, dietary carbohydrates are processed into glucose, which can be processed into energy more readily than fats or protein. Moreover, glucose may be stored in the muscle and liver as glycogen, a key energy source for most sports. When blood glucose or muscle glycogen levels fall below a critical level, muscle fatigue occurs and performance suffers (Williams 2007).

Compared with men, research indicates that prepubertal and early pubertal boys oxidize less carbohydrate and more fat during aerobic exercise, such as cycling at 70% peak oxygen uptake (Timmons et al. 2003). Nevertheless, carbohydrate is still the most important fuel for young athletes. Moreover, several studies (Riddell et al. 2000, 2001; Timmons et al. 2003) have shown that boys could use exogenous carbohydrates consumed in sports drinks during exercise very effectively, helping to spare the use of endogenous carbohydrate stores, reduce the rating of perceived exertion during exercise, and enhance performance in prolonged exercise.

Appropriately selected, foods containing natural carbohydrate sources are among the healthiest choices for the school aged athlete, and also the most important for sport performance. For the typical child or adolescent, recommended carbohydrate intake ranges 45–65% of daily energy intake, and the school aged athlete should strive to consume near the upper levels of this recommendation, about 60% or higher. Table 16.2 presents foods rich in carbohydrate content. The following are some general guidelines for consuming healthy, or "good", carbohydrates (Bloch & Shils 2006; Willett & Stampfer 2006).

Table 16.2 Foods rich in carbohydrates (grams of carbohydrate per serving).

Grains (15 g)	Fruits (15 g)	Starchy vegetables (15 g)	Other vegetables (5 g)	Sports drinks/sports bars/ sports gels (14–52 g)
Whole grain	Apples	Black beans	Asparagus	Gatorade
Brown rice	Apricots	Corn	Black beans	Gatorade Energy drink
Bulgar	Bananas	Green peas	Broccoli	PowerAde
Oatmeal	Cantaloupe	Lentils	Carrots	GU
Rye crackers	Dried fruits	Navy beans	Mushrooms	Power gel
Wholewheat cereal	Mangoes	Potatoes	Navy beans	Power Bar
Wholewheat bread	Nectarines	Sweet potatoes	Summer squash	Clif Bar
	Oranges	Winter squash	Tomatoes	
*Enriched**	Peaches		Zucchini	
Bagels	Pears			
Crackers	Pineapple			
Dinner rolls	Plums			
English muffin				
Pasta				
Pancakes				
White bread				
White rice				
Wild rice				

* Some of these products may also be found in wholegrain form.

1 Grains should be consumed primarily in a minimally refined, high-fiber form. Consume 90 g or more (3 or more ounce-equivalents) of wholegrain products per day, with the rest of the recommended grains coming from enriched or wholegrain products. In general, at least half the grains should come from whole grains.

2 Vegetables and fruits should be consumed in abundance. Five servings is minimal and should include green leafy and orange vegetables daily. Choose fiber-rich fruits and vegetables often. Two cups of fruit and 2.5 cups of vegetables per day are recommended for a reference 2000 kcal intake, with higher or lower amounts depending on the calorie level. Choose a variety of fruits and vegetables each day. In particular, select from all five vegetable subgroups (dark green, orange, legumes, starchy vegetables, and other vegetables) several times a week.

3 Refined starches and simple sugars intake should be low, with less than 10% of daily calories coming from simple sugars. Choose and prepare foods and beverages with little added sugars or caloric sweeteners. Practice good oral hygiene to reduce the incidence of dental caries.

Adequate intake of carbohydrate is important before, during, and after exercise; some guidelines are presented later in this chapter.

Fats

In the body, dietary fat is processed into fatty acids, which may be stored in the muscle or in the fat (adipose) cells to provide energy during exercise. Compared with men, research indicates that prepubertal and early pubertal boys oxidize more fat during aerobic exercise, such as cycling at 70% peak oxygen uptake (Timmons *et al.* 2003). However, although fatty acids are an important energy source during exercise, particularly endurance exercise, they are not as efficient as carbohydrate. Moreover, the typical school aged athlete has substantial stores of fatty acids and, contrary to muscle glycogen stores, depletion of fatty acids is not common and has not been documented as a cause of fatigue. Additionally, both acute and chronic high fat diets, as well as various attempts to increase fat metabolism

during exercise, have not been shown to enhance exercise performance in adults and also are not likely to do so in young athletes.

For health reasons, most recommendations for healthful eating recommend consumption of dietary fat in moderation. Although the amount of dietary fat recommended may vary by country, the general range is 15–35% of daily energy intake. However, recommendations also present guidelines for eating healthier fats, such as the following (Bloch & Shils 2006; Willett & Stampfer 2006):

1 Children and adolescents aged 4–18 years should obtain 25–35% of calories from fat. However, this percentage may be slightly lower (20–25%) for young athletes because of the recommended increase in energy from dietary carbohydrates.

2 Most dietary fat should come from sources of monounsaturated and polyunsaturated fatty acids. Limit polyunsaturated fats to 6–10% of daily caloric intake, with about 10–15% from monounsaturated fats.

3 Consume less than 10% of calories from saturated fatty acids and less than 300 mg·day^{-1} cholesterol.

4 Keep *trans* fatty acid consumption as low as possible.

How do these recommendations translate to the actual foods young athletes consume? Here are some guidelines.

1 Check food labels. Select foods with lower levels of daily recommendations for total fat, saturated fat, and *trans* fat. Many healthy food products may be fat-free, but caloric content may still be high because of added sugars.

2 Eat mainly plant-based foods, wholegrain breads and cereals, fruits, and vegetables as discussed in the section on carbohydrates.

3 Drink fat-free or low-fat milk or equivalent milk products.

4 Select leaner cuts of meat and poultry, such as flank steak, eye of round, very lean hamburger, Canadian bacon, and turkey breast. Eat less high-fat meats, such as fried chicken, regular hamburger, bacon, and hot dogs. Avoid highly processed meats, which are high in total and saturated fats.

5 Eat fish several times a week, as fish contains more of the omega-3 fatty acids, a polyunsaturated fat with some health benefits. However, some fish, such as shark, swordfish, and albacore tuna, are high in mercury and should be limited in the diets of younger children.

6 Limit intake of high-fat fried or baked products and desserts, such as French fries, crackers, cakes, and doughnuts, particularly those using partially hydrogenated fats, the main source of *trans* fats in the diet.

7 Limit use of pure fats and oils, such as butter, margarine, and salad oils in food preparation. For cooking oils, use olive or canola oil.

Protein

Protein is a key nutrient for athletes. It is the building block for all tissues in the body, particularly muscle. Protein also provides the basis for the synthesis of enzymes, which control metabolic processes. Finally, protein may also be used as a source of energy during exercise, but not as effectively as carbohydrate or fats.

Compared with adults, children and adolescents need slightly more protein per kilogram body weight. National and international recommendations for young children average about $1.0-1.1$ g·kg body weight^{-1}·day^{-1}, and decline to about $0.80-0.85$ g·kg^{-1}·day^{-1} during late adolescence. Based on percentage of energy intake, national and international recommendations for children and adolescents range $10-30\%$ of total daily calories for children and adolescents $4-18$ years of age.

There is considerable debate as to whether or not adult athletes need more protein than the RDI (Williams 2007). Research with young athletes is limited. Bar-Or (2001) indicated young athletes had a greater need for protein intake to support growth. In support of this viewpoint, Boisseau *et al.* (2002) reported that the growth and development in adolescent soccer players, as well as non-active adolescents, necessitated a higher protein intake than is usually recommended. They observed a positive nitrogen balance with a mean protein intake of 1.57 g·kg body mass^{-1}·day^{-1}. Although this amount is greater than most RDI, it is well within the recommended protein intake based on percentage of daily caloric intake. For example, 1.57 g protein per kilogram body mass for a 70-kg athlete would total

about 110 g protein daily. Consuming 3000 kcal daily, with 15% derived from protein, would provide over 110 g protein. Young athletes do not need exaggerated amount of dietary protein, and may obtain all they need through natural, wholesome foods.

Animal foods provide high-quality protein as they contain a balance of all essential amino acids. Some plant foods are also good sources of protein, but the quality of the protein is somewhat lower as some essential amino acids may be present in limited quantities. Guidelines the young athlete can use to obtain adequate dietary protein are as follow:

1 Consume $170-230$ g ($6-8$ oz) of lean or very lean meat, poultry, or fish daily. Each ounce provides about 7 g high quality protein, or a total of $42-56$ g daily.

2 Drink $3-4$ glasses of skim or low-fat milk daily. Each glass provides about 8 g high quality protein, or a total of $24-32$ g daily.

3 Consume eggs periodically. A large egg contains about 6 g high quality protein. About 3.5 g protein are in the egg white, and the rest in the yolk, which also is high in cholesterol. Liquid egg substitutes made from egg white contain over 7 g protein per _ cup (60 g).

4 Consume plant foods rich in protein, such as nuts and legumes. Nuts such as almonds, cashews, peanuts, and even peanut butter, contain about $5-6$ g protein per 30 g (1 oz), but are high in fat. Legumes such as baked beans, kidney beans, and lentils contain about $7-9$ g protein per 100 g (3.5 oz). Soy beans, or products made from soy, are slightly higher in protein content than other legumes.

5 Other sources of dietary protein include grains such as wholewheat bread and cereals ($2-4$ g per serving) and vegetables (2 g per serving).

6 Some sports drinks, sports bars, and protein powders such as soy and whey are good sources of protein. Check labels for grams of protein.

Vitamins

Vitamins are micronutrients, a class of complex organic compounds found in small amounts in most natural foods. Vitamins are essential for the optimal functioning of many different physiologic processes

Table 16.3 Some essential vitamins and excellent food sources.

Vitamin (other terms)	Major food sources
Vitamin A (retinol; carotenoids)	Liver; whole milk; fortified milk; orange vegetables such as carrots, sweet potatoes; dark, green leafy vegetables; fortified margarine
Vitamin C (ascorbic acid)	Citrus fruits; strawberries; green leafy vegetables; broccoli; peppers; potatoes
Vitamin D (cholecalciferol)	Fortified foods such as dairy products, margarine, and cereals; fish oils
Vitamin E (tocopherol)	Vegetable oils, margarine, green leafy vegetables, wheatgerm, wholegrain products, egg yolks
Thiamin (vitamin B_1)	Lean ham and pork; wholegrain products; enriched breads and cereals; legumes
Riboflavin (vitamin B_2)	Milk and dairy products; lean meat; eggs; whole and enriched grain products; green leafy vegetables; beans
Niacin (nicotinamide; niacinamide)	Lean meats, fish and poultry; wholegrain products; legumes
Vitamin B_6 (pyridoxine; pyridoxal)	High protein foods such as lean meats, fish, poultry, legumes; green leafy vegetables; baked potatoes; bananas
Vitamin B_{12} (cyanocobalamin)	Animal foods only; lean meats, fish, poultry, eggs, milk
Folate (folic acid)	Liver; green leafy vegetables, legumes, nuts, fortified grain products, such as cereals

Note: Some fortified cereals may contain the recommended dietary intakes (RDI) for all vitamins.

in the body. Many vitamins function as coenzymes, facilitating the role of enzymes to regulate a variety of metabolic reactions. Several vitamins function as antioxidants, helping protect body tissues against undesirable effects, such as cellular damage, associated with the formation of free radicals from oxidative reactions in the body. Many of these metabolic and oxidative processes are accelerated during exercise, and an adequate bodily supply of vitamins is essential for these processes to function best.

National and international RDI for most vitamins have been developed for children and adolescents in different age groups. The RDI are usually extrapolated from research with adults, using a metabolic body weight ratio multiplied by a growth factor, and gradually increase through childhood and adolescence. At about age 14–18 years, the vitamin requirements are similar to adults (Shils *et al.* 2006; Treuth and Griffin 2006).

Some dietary surveys of athletes have indicated inadequate dietary intakes of micronutrients, including vitamins, but in many cases biochemical indices of nutritional status were within normal limits. Athletes may consume vitamin supplements (O'Dea 2003), but no research has been uncovered indicating a positive effect on exercise performance. Antioxidant vitamins, mainly C, E, and beta-carotene, do not appear to enhance sport performance and

evidence is equivocal as to whether or not they prevent muscle tissue damage. Most research has been conducted with adults, and no studies have been uncovered regarding antioxidant needs of young athletes (Williams 2007).

Consuming a healthful, nutrient-dense diet with adequate energy content, including a wide variety of foods among and within the various food groups, will provide adequate amounts of all vitamins for young athletes. Some foods, such as breakfast cereals, are fortified with most vitamins. Table 16.3 lists key vitamins along with good food sources. Adequate vitamin D may be provided by safe exposure to sunshine, but in winter months in northern latitudes adequate vitamin D from fortified foods, such as milk, may be required to optimize bone growth and development. As adolescent girls enter puberty, they should increase their folate intake to reduce the risk of neural tube defects in their future children. Many health professionals recommend that for most people, including school aged athletes, taking a daily typical multiple vitamin provides a sensible nutritional safety net (Willett & Stampfer 2006). However, excess vitamin intake, either individual or multiple vitamin preparations, is not recommended as some vitamins, such as A and D, and niacin may cause health problems when consumed in excess.

Minerals

Minerals are micronutrients, inorganic elements found in small amounts in most natural foods. Several minerals serve as building blocks for body tissues, such as bone and teeth. Others, functioning as metalloenzymes to facilitate enzymic activities, are necessary for diverse metabolic processes, including muscle contraction and oxygen transport, both of which are accelerated during exercise and necessitate adequate mineral status to optimize sport performance.

National and international RDI for most minerals have been developed for children and adolescents in different age groups. The amounts recommended vary among different age ranges of childhood and adolescence. During the peak of the adolescent growth spurt, requirements for calcium, iron, and zinc increase (Treuth & Griffin 2006) and at age 14–18 years the mineral RDI vary slightly from those for adults (Shils et al. 2006).

Some dietary surveys (Fogelholm et al. 2000; Croll et al. 2006) indicate that young athletes obtain adequate mineral nutrition, whereas others (Beals 2002; Papadopoulou et al. 2002; Christensen et al. 2005) report that mineral intake is less than recommended. Young athletes in weight-control sports are less likely to obtain adequate mineral nutrition, particularly calcium, iron and zinc, mainly because of suboptimal energy intake. Zinc requirements are relatively high during adolescence as both muscle and bone contains most of the body zinc stores, and these tissues increase rapidly during adolescence. Zinc deficiency is a concern because it may impair growth velocity. However, most concern has focused on implications of inadequate calcium and iron intake for health and sport. The *key nutrient concept* indicates that consuming a healthful natural diet rich in calcium and iron will provide adequate amounts of other essential minerals.

CALCIUM

Calcium is one of the most important minerals in human nutrition. Found in all body cells, it is involved in a variety of physiologic processes. However, 99% of body calcium stores are found in the bones and teeth, and this is the key health issue. Late childhood and adolescence is a key time for optimizing peak bone mass, necessitating a greater need for calcium intake to support bone accretion (Bar-Or 2001; Willett & Stampfer 2006). For some minerals, the requirement can be met both by mobilizing stores and from the diet. However, in the case of calcium, no calcium stores are available that can be used to support bone mineralization, and the adolescent's requirements must be met entirely from dietary sources (Treuth & Griffin 2006). Physical activity, particularly weight-bearing exercise, is also important to optimize bone mass during childhood and adolescence and is discussed in Chapter 9.

The recommended calcium intake for children aged 4–8 years is about 800 mg·day^{-1}, while for those aged 9–18 years it is about 1300 mg·day^{-1}. Dairy products contain the most dietary calcium and, in general, recommendations for children aged 4–8 years are to consume two cups of milk, while those over age 9 should consume three cups of fat-free or low-fat milk or equivalent milk products, such as cheese and yogurt. Some research supports this recommendation. Volek et al. (2003) reported that in boys, aged 13–17 years, three servings per day of fluid milk (1% fat) significantly increased bone mass compared to a group consuming fruit juice over a 12-week period in which they engaged in resistance training. Some guidelines for obtaining dietary calcium are presented in Table 16.4.

IRON

The major function of iron in human metabolism is the formation of compounds, such as hemoglobin and myoglobin, essential for the utilization of oxygen. Inadequate iron intake may lead to iron-deficiency anemia (IDA) or iron deficiency without anemia (IDWA), both of which may impair health and athletic performance (Constantini et al. 2000; Suedekum & Dimeff 2005; Williams 2007).

Dietary iron requirements begin to differ between boys and girls at adolescence, mainly because of the onset of menses. The recommended dietary intake varies somewhat during childhood and adolescence, being about 8–10 mg·day^{-1} for both genders

Table 16.4 Guidelines to increase dietary calcium and iron intake.

Calcium

Consume dairy products. One cup of milk (230 mL; 8 oz) contains about 300 mg calcium. Dairy equivalents include 45 g (1.5 oz) cheese or 1 cup yogurt

Approximate calcium content, per 100 g (3.5 oz), of other foods that are good sources of calcium include almonds (230 mg), baked beans (70 mg), raw collard greens (250 mg), salmon with bones (350 mg), and sardines with bone (350 mg)

Check food labels for foods rich in calcium. Foods that are good sources of calcium contain 10% or more per serving, or approximately 100 mg. Children or adolescents who do not like milk or other dairy products may obtain calcium from fortified products, such as orange juice, bread, and cereals

Calcium supplements may augment food calcium intake to meet requirements

Do not consume calcium in excess

Iron

Consume adequate amounts of meat, fish, shellfish, or poultry, which contain heme iron. Approximate iron content, per 100 g (3.5 oz), includes beef (2.5 mg), pork (1.0 mg), chicken (1.0 mg), fish (1.0 mg) sardines (2.5 mg), shrimp (3.0 mg), pork liver (17.0 mg), and clams (27.0 mg)

Approximate iron content, per 100 g (3.5 oz), of other foods that are good sources of non-heme iron include cooked lentils (3 mg), cooked beans (1.5 mg), cooked greens (1.2 mg), wholegrain products (3 mg); enriched pasta (3 mg); cooked spinach (3 mg); broccoli (0.5 mg), dried apricots and raisins (1.4 mg), and almonds (4 mg)

Consume non-heme iron foods with foods containing vitamin C, which helps iron absorption. Orange juice and toasted wholewheat bread is a good example

Prepare acidic foods, such as tomato sauce for pasta, periodically in iron cookware. Some iron leaches into the food

Check food labels for foods rich in iron. Foods that are good sources of iron contain 10% or more per serving. Some fortified breakfast cereals contain 4–18 mg per serving

Young female athletes may want to consider use of low-dose iron supplements under medical and dietary supervision to prevent a decline in iron status during training

Note: These guidelines are presented to help young athletes obtain adequate dietary calcium and iron. However, excessive intake of either calcium or iron may carry significant health risks. Consuming excessive amounts of fortified food products and/or dietary supplements may exceed the upper limit of recommended amounts. In particular, athletes should consume dietary iron supplements only under the guidance of health professionals.

ages 4–13, and 11 and 15 mg·day^{-1} for boys and girls, respectively, ages 14–18 years.

Adolescence is a particularly common time for the development of iron deficiency anemia. In the USA, approximately 10% of girls aged 12–19 years are anemic, whereas only 1% or less of boys the same age are anemic (Treuth & Griffin 2006). Young athletes may be at particular risk for IDA or IDWA. Studies have shown that endurance training may lead to IDA and/or IDWA in both male and female young athletes (Malczewska *et al.* 2000; Spordaryk 2002). Causes of iron deficiency include poor intake, menstrual losses, gastrointestinal and genitourinary losses resulting from exercise-induced ischemia, foot strike hemolysis, and sweat losses (Suedekum & Dimeff 2005). The prevalence of IDA and IDWA is likely to be higher in athletic populations, particularly younger female athletes, than in healthy sedentary individuals (Beard & Tobin 2000; Suedekum & Dimeff 2005).

Curing IDA with iron supplementation will improve endurance performance; however, results of studies evaluating the effect of iron supplementation on exercise performance in athletes with IDWA are equivocal (Williams 2007), but several studies have shown enhanced performance following such supplementation in young athletes. For example, Friedmann *et al.* (2001) provided either ferrous iron (2 × 100 mg elemental iron) or placebo daily for 12 weeks to young elite male and female athletes with low serum ferritin (<20 µg·L^{-1}) and normal hemoglobin. The iron supplementation increased serum ferritin levels by 20 µg·L^{-1}, but there was no change in red blood cell volume. However, the iron supplementation did increase $\dot{V}O_{2max}$ and oxygen consumption in a test of anaerobic capacity (maximal accumulated oxygen deficit) and these investigators noted an increase in maximal aerobic performance capacity.

Meat, poultry, and fish are the best dietary sources of dietary iron, as they contain heme iron; heme iron is more readily absorbable in the digestive tract compared with non-heme iron, the type found in plant foods. Some guidelines for obtaining dietary iron are presented in Table 16.4.

Water and electrolytes

Proper hydration, particularly when exercising under warm or hot environmental conditions, is critical for athletes of all ages. However, when compared with adults, children possess certain characteristics that may predispose them to dehydration and heat illness (American Academy of Pediatrics 2005). For example, children produce more heat relative to body mass for the same running exercise, have higher thresholds before beginning to sweat, have a lower sweating capacity, have inadequate thirst mechanisms, have decreased thermoregulatory ability during dehydration, and take longer to acclimatize to the heat (American Academy of Pediatrics 2005; Bar-Or 1995).

Adequate hydration is important for the young athlete for both practice and competition, not only to prevent heat illnesses but also to help maintain sport performance. Relative to the latter, recent research has shown that a 2% dehydration will deteriorate basketball skill performance in 12- to 15-year-old players (Dougherty *et al.* 2006). The following guidelines will help ensure adequate hydration during exercise to help optimize performance and prevent heat illnesses.

1 Stay hydrated daily. Drink small amounts more often, not large amounts at one time. Drink about 500 mL fluids 15–30 min prior to practice or competition. Drink about 250 mL fluids every 15–20 min during exercise. Drink fluids after activity to satisfy your thirst.

2 Maintain your body weight. Weigh yourself in the morning before practice; your weight should remain relatively constant. If under your normal weight, you are most likely dehydrated. If you practice or may be involved in competition two or more times a day, weigh yourself periodically to make sure you have adequately rehydrated after the first exercise bout. One-half liter equals 0.5 kg (1 lb).

3 Drink cool water, which is sufficient for most practices and competition that do not last longer than 60 min; this includes most school aged sport events.

4 Consume sports drinks when exercising more than 60 min; sports drinks may be preferable for more prolonged exercise tasks because they contain about 6–8% carbohydrate (Greydanus & Patel 2002). Some research indicates that a sports drink may be more effective than water in minimizing fluid deficits and mean core temperature responses during 120 min of tennis training and other similar training in adolescent athletes (Bergeron *et al.* 2006) and, compared with water rehydration during recovery from dehydration, enhance subsequent performance of various basketball skills during a simulated game (Dougherty *et al.* 2006). Sports drinks may also enhance fluid replacement during recovery as they are more palatable than water. Fruit juices, diluted half with water, may be an alternative.

5 Do not drink excessively. If your body weight exceeds normal, you may be overhydrated. Overhydration may predispose you to hyponatremia (low sodium levels in the body) that may have serious health consequences, including coma and death.

The major electrolyte lost in sweat is sodium. However, young athletes appear to have lower losses of sweat sodium compared to adults (Bar-Or 2001). Nevertheless, young athletes who train in warm environments may need to increase their salt intake somewhat, particularly during the early stages of training and acclimatization to the heat. Simply sprinkling more salt on daily meals should suffice during periods of heavy sweating. Most sports drinks also contain sodium.

For health reasons, salt intake should be moderated. General recommendations for adults suggest sodium intake be limited to less than 2300 mg (approximately 5000 mg salt) per day. Few guidelines are available for children, but healthful recommendations encourage decreased intake of processed high-sodium foods, increased use of salt alternatives in home food preparation, and decreased use of the salt shaker at the dining table. However, as noted above, athletes in training may be advised to add salt to their meals during training.

Salt restriction may benefit some athletes. Milgrom and Taussig (1999) reported that 12% of high school athletes tested positive for exercise-induced asthma (EIA). In their review, Mickleborough and Gotshall (2003) indicated recent research has suggested that salt-restrictive diets can reduce the severity of EIA. Although additional research is merited, young athletes with EIA might experiment with salt-restricted diets, such as the DASH (Dietary Approaches to Stop Hypertension) diet.

Vegetarian diets

Children and adolescents may adopt a vegetarian diet for various reasons, such as health, religion, or love of animals. Many young women, including athletes, opt to become vegetarians for reasons related to body image, body size, and weight, and some may develop eating disorders which they attempt to disguise by adopting a vegetarian lifestyle (Barr & Rideout 2004; Johnston & Sabaté 2006).

There are various classes of vegetarians. Vegans consume only plant foods, whereas other classes may consume dairy products and eggs, and even other classes consume fish or white poultry meat. The American Dietetic Association and Dietitians of Canada (2003) indicate that well-planned vegan and other types of vegetarian diets are appropriate for all stages of the life cycle, including childhood and adolescence. Barr and Rideout (2004) also noted that such well-planned diets, appropriately supplemented, appear to effectively support athletic performance. However, Johnston and Sabaté (2006) noted that intakes of some micronutrients are usually lower than the requirements in adolescent vegetarians. The following recommendations may be appropriate for young vegetarian athletes (Barr & Rideout 2004; Johnston & Sabaté 2006).
1 Consume foods rich in iron. Vegetarians, particularly women, are at increased risk for IDWA, which may limit endurance performance.
2 Consume vitamin and mineral fortified foods. Vitamins B_{12} and D are found only in animal foods, but may be found in fortified foods, such as breakfast cereals. Calcium-fortified products, such as soy milk, are excellent sources for vegetarians who do not consume dairy products.
3 Consider taking a one-a-day multivitamin or mineral supplement with no more than the recommended dietary intake.
4 Possibly take a creatine supplement. As a group, vegetarians have lower mean muscle creatine concentrations than do omnivores, and this may impair supramaximal exercise performance.

Eating before, during, and after competition and hard training

What the young athlete eats and drinks before, during, and after competition and hard training may have an effect on performance and recovery.

Pre-competition

To help optimize muscle glycogen stores, athletes should exercise only lightly or rest and consume a diet rich in carbohydrates for a day or two prior to competition. For young athletes competing in prolonged endurance events, such as running a marathon, tapering of exercise is more prolonged and a carbohydrate-loading protocol may last several days. For some athletes, such as gymnasts, where excess body weight may impair performance, carbohydrate intake may be moderate because muscle glycogen binds water which increases body weight.

An important consideration is the pre-competition meal, which should be designed to:
1 Allow for the stomach to be relatively empty at the start of competition;
2 Help prevent gastrointestinal distress;
3 Help avoid sensations of hunger or fatigue;
4 Provide adequate carbohydrate; and
5 Provide adequate fluids.
The meal should also contain what the athlete enjoys, tolerates well, and usually eats. In general, the pre-competition meal should be eaten about 3–4 h prior to competition. In addition, adequate fluids should be consumed to guard against dehydration. Here are two examples of meals rich in carbohydrate and balanced in other nutrients.

Example 1
Glass of orange juice
Bowl of oatmeal
Two pieces of toast and jam
Sliced peaches with
    skim milk
Fluids as needed

Example 2
Cup of low-fat yogurt
Banana
Toasted bagel
30 g chicken breast
Tomato/lettuce
Half cup of raisins
Fluids as needed

Avoid foods that may cause problems. Young athletes usually learn what foods to avoid prior to competition. Although carbohydrates are recommended, some preparations, such as the "energy" drinks available, may contain concentrated amounts of simple sugars that can cause a reverse osmosis in the gastrointestinal tract, precipitating distress such as diarrhea. Other foods, such as beans, although rich in carbohydrate and protein, can cause intestinal gas and discomfort, and should not be consumed unless well tolerated.

During competition

In general, if pre-competition nutrition is adequate, most school aged athletes need consume nothing except fluids during competition. For prolonged athletic events, those lasting more than an hour or so, sports drinks may be preferable as they provide both fluids and energy in the form of carbohydrate. A 6–8% carbohydrate solution should suffice, consuming 170–230 mL (6–8 oz) every 15–20 min.

Recovery

Following competition or hard training, or during all-day or multiple-day sports competition such as tennis tournaments and swim meets, proper nutrition may facilitate recovery. However, tolerance to eating after hard exercise varies as some can eat while others cannot. In general, athletes are recommended to consume about 1 g carbohydrate for each kilogram of body weight within 2 h after exercise, but the sooner the better. Adding protein, about 1 g protein for every 4 g carbohydrate, may be helpful as it provides nutrients important for muscle recovery. Fluids may be palatable, such as a carbohydrate/protein smoothie based on fruits and high-quality whey or soy protein, but solid foods such as a turkey breast sandwich on wholewheat bread will also provide carbohydrate and protein. Other high carbohydrate, moderate protein snacks may be easily packed. Examples include bagels, fig Newton bars, wholewheat crackers, peanut butter, raisins, bananas, sliced carrots, small containers of fruit juice, dried fruits, almonds, walnuts, liquid meal replacements, sports drinks, and sports bars.

Conclusions

A healthful diet is the basis for feeding the school aged athlete. It should be rich in whole grains, low-fat dairy products, lean meat, fish and poultry, fruits and vegetables in order to provide adequate carbohydrate, protein, calcium, iron, and vitamins, with lower amounts of saturated fats, *trans* fats, cholesterol, and sodium. The diet should be adequate in energy to fit the needs of the athlete's sport and to optimize body weight as recommended. Fluid intake should be adequate to maintain body hydration status for exercise in the heat. A multivitamin and/or mineral supplement may be recommended, particularly for athletes in weight-control sports. Overall, proper nutrition, coupled with proper training, will help the school aged athlete optimize his or her genetic potential for sport.

References

American Academy of Pediatrics (2005) Promotion of healthy weight-control practices in young athletes. Pediatrics **116**, 1557–1564.

American Dietetic Association, Dietitians of Canada (2003) Position of the American Dietetic Association and the Dietitians of Canada: Vegetarian diets.

Journal of the American Dietetic Association **103**, 748–765.

Bar-Or, O. (1995) The young athlete: Some physiological considerations. *Journal of Sports Sciences* **13**, S31–S33.

Bar-Or, O. (2001) Nutritional considerations for the child athlete.

Canadian Journal of Applied Physiology **26**, S186–S191.

Barr, S.I. & Rideout, C.A. (2004) Nutritional considerations for vegetarian athletes. *Nutrition* **20**, 696–703.

Beals, K.A. (2002) Eating behaviors, nutritional status, and menstrual function in elite female adolescent volleyball players. *Journal of the American Dietetic Association* **102**, 1293–1296.

Beard, J. & Tobin, B. (2000) Iron status and exercise. *American Journal of Clinical Nutrition* **72**, 594S–597S.

Bergeron, M.F., Waller, J.L. & Marinik, E.L. (2006) Voluntary fluid intake and core temperature responses in adolescent tennis players: Sports beverage versus water. *British Journal of Sports Medicine* **40**, 406–410.

Bloch, A.S. & Shils, M.E. (2006) Appendices: Section II. National and international recommended dietary reference values. In: *Modern Nutrition in Health and Disease*, 10th edn. (Shils, M.E., et al. eds.) Lippincott Williams & Wilkins, Philadelphia: 1852–1899.

Boisseau, N., Le Creff, C., Loyens, M. & Poortmans, J.R. (2002) Protein intake and nitrogen balance in male non-active adolescents and soccer players. *European Journal of Applied Physiology* **88**, 288–293.

Cavadini, C., Decarli, B., Grin, J., Narring, F. & Michaud, P.A. (2000) Food habits and sport activity during adolescence: Differences between athletic and non-athletic teenagers in Switzerland. *European Journal of Clinical Nutrition* **54**, S16–S20.

Christensen, D.L., Jakobsen, J. & Friis, H. (2005) Vitamin and mineral intake of twelve adolescent male Kalenjin runners in western Kenya. *East African Medical Journal* **82**, 637–642.

Constantini, N.W., Eliakim, A., Zigel, L., Yaaron, M. & Falk, B. (2000) Iron status of highly active adolescents: Evidence of depleted iron stores in gymnasts. *International Journal of Sport Nutrition and Exercise Metabolism* **10**, 62–70.

Cotunga, N., Vickery, C.E. & McBee, S. (2005) Sports nutrition for young athletes. *Journal of School Nursing* **21**, 323–328.

Croll, J.K., Neumark-Sztainer, D., Story, M., Wall, M., Perry, C. & Harnack, L. (2006) Adolescents involved in weight-related and power team sports have better eating patterns and nutrient intakes than non-sport-involved adolescents. *Journal of the American Dietetic Association* **106**, 709–717.

Dietz, W.H. (2006) Childhood obesity. In: *Modern Nutrition in Health and Disease*, 10th edn. (Shils M.E., et al. eds.) Lippincott Williams & Wilkins, Philadelphia: 979–990.

Dougherty, K.A., Baker, L.B., Chow, M. & Kinney, W.L. (2006) Two percent dehydration impairs and six percent carbohydrate drink improves boys basketball skills. *Medicine and Science in Sports and Exercise* **38**, 1650–1658.

Dwyer, J.T. (2006) Dietary guidelines: National perspectives. In: *Modern Nutrition in Health and Disease*, 10th edn. (Shils M.E., et al., eds.) Lippincott Williams & Wilkins, Philadelphia: 1673–1686.

Erlanson-Albertsson, C. & Zetterstrom, R. (2005) The global obesity epidemic: Snacking and obesity may start with free meals during infant feeding. *Acta Paediatrica* **94**, 1523–1531.

Fogelholm, M., Rankinen, T., Isokaanta, M., Kujala, U. & Uusitupa, M. (2000) Growth, dietary intake, and trace element status in pubescent athletes and schoolchildren. *Medicine and Science in Sports and Exercise* **32**, 738–746.

Friedmann, B., Weller, E., Mairbaurl, H. & Bartsch, P. (2001) Effects of iron repletion on blood volume and performance capacity in young athletes. *Medicine and Science in Sports and Exercise* **33**, 741–746.

Greydanus, D.E. & Patel, D.R. (2002) Sports doping in the adolescent athlete: The hope, hype, and hyperbole. *Pediatric Clinics of North America* **49**, 829–855.

Heird, W. & Cooper, A. (2006) Infancy and childhood. In: *Modern Nutrition in Health and Disease*, 10th edn. (Shils M.E., et al. eds.) Lippincott Williams & Wilkins, Philadelphia: 797–817.

Iglesias-Gutierrez, E., Garcia-Roves, P.M., Rodriguez, C., Braga, S., Garcia-Zapico, P. & Patterson, A.M. (2005) Food habits and nutritional status assessment of adolescent soccer players. A necessary and accurate approach. *Canadian Journal of Applied Physiology* **30**, 18–32.

Janssen, I., Katzmarzyk, P.T., Boyce, W.F., et al. (2005) Comparison of overweight and obesity prevalence in school aged youth from 34 countries and their relationships with physical activity and dietary patterns. *Obesity Reviews* **6**, 123–132.

Johnston, P.K. & Sabaté, J. (2006) Nutritional implications of vegetarian diets. In: *Modern Nutrition in Health and Disease*, 10th edn. (Shils M.E., et al. eds.) Lippincott Williams & Wilkins, Philadelphia: 1638–1654.

Jonnalagadda, S.S., Benardot, D. & Dill, M.N. (2000) Assessment of under-reporting of energy intake of elite female gymnasts. *International Journal of Sport Nutrition and Exercise Metabolism* **10**, 315–325.

Lopez-Varela, S., Montero, A., Chandra, R.K. & Marcos, A. (2000) Nutritional status of young female elite gymnasts. *International Journal of Vitamin and Nutrition Research* **70**, 185–190.

Malczewska, J., Raczynski, G. & Stupnicki, R. (2000) Iron status in female endurance athletes and in non-athletes. *International Journal of Sport Nutrition and Exercise Metabolism* **10**, 260–276.

Mickleborough, T. & Gotshall, R. (2003) Dietary components with demonstrated effectiveness in decreasing the severity of exercise-induced asthma. *Sports Medicine* **33**, 671–681.

Milgrom, H. & Taussig, L.M. (1999) Keeping children with exercise-induced asthma active. *Pediatrics* **104**, e38.

Nichols, J.F., Rauh, M.J., Lawson, M.J., Ji, M. & Barkai, H.S. (2006) Prevalence of the female athlete triad syndrome among high school athletes. *Archives of Pediatrics and Adolescent Medicine* **160**, 137–142.

O'Dea, J.A. (2003) Consumption of nutritional supplements among adolescents: Usage and perceived benefits. *Health Education Research* **18**, 98–107.

Papadopoulou, S.K., Papadopoulou, S.D. & Gallos, G.K. (2002) Macro- and micro-nutrient intake of adolescent Greek female volleyball players. *International Journal of Sport Nutrition and Exercise Metabolism* **12**, 73–80.

Rampersaud, G.C., Pereira, M.A., Girard, B.L., Adams, J. & Metzl, J.D. (2005) Breakfast habits, nutritional status, body weight, and academic performance in children and adolescents. *Journal of the American Dietetic Association* **105**, 743–760.

Riddell, M.C., Bar-Or, O., Schwarcz, H.P. & Heigenhauser, G.J. (2000) Substrate utilization in boys during exercise with [13C]-glucose ingestion. *European Journal of Applied Physiology* **83**, 441–448.

Riddell, M.C., Bar-Or, O., Wilk, B., Parolin, M.L. & Heigenhauser, G.J. (2001) Substrate utilization during exercise with glucose and glucose plus fructose ingestion in boys age 10–14 yr. *Journal of Applied Physiology* **90**, 903–911.

Ruiz, F., Irazusta, A., Gil, S., Irazusta, J.U., Casis, L. & Gil, J. (2005) Nutritional intake in soccer players of different ages. *Journal of Sports Sciences* **23**, 235–242.

Shils, M.E., Shike, M., Ross, A.C., Caballero, B. & Cousins, R.J., eds. (2006) *Modern Nutrition in Health and Disease*, 10th edn, Lippincott Williams & Wilkins, Philadelphia.

Silink, M. (2002) Childhood diabetes: A global perspective. *Hormone Research* **57** (Supplement 1), 1–5.

Spodaryk, K. (2002) Iron metabolism in boys involved in intensive physical training. *Physiology and Behavior* **75**, 201–206.

Suedekum, N.A. & Dimeff, R.J. (2005) Iron and the athlete. *Current Sports Medicine Reports* **4**, 199–202.

Swinburn, B.A., Caterson, I., Seidell, J.C. & James, W.P. (2004) Diet, nutrition and the prevention of excess weight gain. *Public Health Nutrition* **7**, 123–146.

Thompson, J.L. (1998) Energy balance in young athletes. *International Journal of Sport Nutrition* **8**, 160–174.

Timmons, B.W., Bar-Or, O. & Riddell, M.C. (2003) Oxidation rate of exogenous carbohydrate during exercise is higher in boys than in men. *Journal of Applied Physiology* **94**, 278–284.

Torstveit, M.K. & Sundgot-Borgen, J. (2005) The female athlete triad: Are elite athletes at increased risk? *Medicine and Science in Sports and Exercise* **37**, 184–193.

Treuth, M.S. & Griffin, I.J. (2006) Adolescence. In: *Modern Nutrition in Health and Disease*, 10th edn. (Shils M.E., *et al.* eds.) Lippincott Williams & Wilkins, Philadelphia: 818–829.

Uauy, R., Hertrampf, E. & Dangour, A. (2006) Food-based dietary guidelines for healthier populations: International considerations. In: *Modern Nutrition in Health and Disease*, 10th edn. (Shils M.E., *et al.* eds.) Lippincott Williams & Wilkins, Philadelphia: 1701–1776.

Unnithan, V.B. & Goulopoulou, S. (2004) Nutrition for the pediatric athlete. *Current Sports Medicine Reports* **14**, 261–266.

Volek, J.S., Gomez, A.L., Scheett, T.P., *et al.* (2003) Increasing fluid milk favorably affects bone mineral density responses to resistance training in adolescent boys. *Journal of the American Dietetic Association* **103**, 1353–1356.

Warren, M.P. & Perlroth, N.E. (2001) The effects of intense exercise on the female reproductive system. *Journal of Endocrinology* **170**, 3–11.

Willett, W.C. & Stampfer, M.J. (2006) Foundations of a healthy diet. In: *Modern Nutrition in Health and Disease*, 10th edn. (Shils M.E., *et al.* eds.) Lippincott Williams & Wilkins, Philadelphia: 1625–1637.

Williams, M.H. (2007) *Nutrition for Health, Fitness & Sport*. McGraw-Hill, Boston.

Ziegler, P., Sharp, R., Hughes, V., Evans, W. & Khoo, C.S. (2002) Nutritional status of teenage female competitive figure skaters. *Journal of the American Dietetic Association* **102**, 374–379.

Chapter 17

Risk for Eating Disorders in the Young Athlete

STEFANIE GILBERT, LAUREN K. SILBERSTEIN, AND J. KEVIN THOMPSON

For many girls and boys, a successful athletic career in ballet, gymnastics, or wrestling begins when they are very young. Typically, the journey of a child athlete can be an extremely competitive one, where excelling at one's sport becomes the primary goal, overshadowing social interactions with one's peers and family and even academic achievement in school. On the positive side, child athletes develop the skill and pride of self-discipline at an early age. They experience the thrill of athletic accomplishment and the excitement of being a star in their chosen field. However, taken to an extreme, the self-discipline, excessive training, and obsessive focus on athletic performance and physical perfection may push at-risk children and adolescents over the edge to adopt disordered eating attitudes and behaviors (Thompson & Smolak 2001).

Because of their emphasis on athletic prowess and a lean body, certain athletic fields, such as ballet, gymnastics, figure skating, and wrestling, have been implicated in the development of eating disorders among children and adolescents (Garner et al. 1998; Walsh et al. 2000). However, research investigating these relationships has produced inconsistent findings. Although some studies indicate that athletics increase the risk of developing an eating disorder (Oppliger et al. 1993; Davis et al. 1994; French et al. 1994; Wiita & Stombaugh 1996) others indicate that athletic participation has no impact on the development of eating disorders (Fulkerson et al. 1999; Hausenblaus & Mack 1999; Rhea 1999; Kirk et al. 2001; Thompson & Digsby 2004), or may even be beneficial in lowering eating disorder risk (Smolak et al. 2000; Pyle et al. 2003). For example, athletic involvement has been associated with increased self-esteem

(Taub & Blind 1992; Pedersen & Seidman 2004) and body satisfaction (Smolak et al. 2000; Hausenblas & McNally 2004) which, in turn, are negatively associated with eating disorder risk (Lindeman 1994).

The suggestion has been made that it is not so much sports participation, per se, that increases a child's risk for developing an eating disorder, but the chosen sport's emphasis on leanness and maintenance of a low body weight. Unfortunately, research addressing this question has only produced more inconsistencies. A number of studies have demonstrated that sports emphasizing leanness or a low body weight place young people at greater risk for developing an eating disorder (Stoutjesdyk & Jevne 1993; Davison et al. 2002; Sherwood et al. 2002), but other studies refute these findings (Benson et al. 1990; Taub & Blinde 1994; Kirk et al. 2001). Likewise, some studies have found sport-by-sport differences (Brooks-Gunn et al. 1988) whereas other studies have not (Taub & Blinde 1992; Kirk et al. 2001; Hausenblaus & McNally 2004).

The cause of these discrepant findings may be, in part, a lack of standardization across studies in assessment measures, the definition of "athlete" used in selecting the study sample, group assignment, diagnostic and risk criteria, mediating variables, and sampling procedures. In other words, studies that appear to be assessing the same phenomenon may produce different results because they are actually analyzing different variables. For example, there is no consensus on how to designate a sport as one that emphasizes leanness, so an activity such as swimming has been alternately categorized as a "lean" sport and "non-lean" sport by different researchers.

Female athlete triad

The female athlete triad is a subclinical syndrome that occurs in physically active girls and women. It was defined in 1993 by the American College of Sports Medicine as the combination of disordered eating, amenorrhea, and osteoporosis. This triad of disorders develops in response to pressure to achieve or maintain an unrealistically low body weight (Otis *et al.* 1997). Thus, involvement in athletics that emphasize a lean physique and low body weight, such as gymnastics and distance runing, may increase the risk of developing the syndrome (Hobart & Smucker 2000). Alone or in any combination, the three conditions of the female athlete triad can decrease athletic performance and result in morbidity and mortality (Otis *et al.* 1997).

The disordered eating component of the triad refers to a range of pathologic eating behaviors like those found in anorexia nervosa and bulimia nervosa, including dietary restriction, purging, and body image problems (Thompson & Smolak 2001; Thompson 2004). Osteoporosis is the second component of the triad. A disease characterized by fragile bones and low bone density, osteoporosis places the young athlete at risk for stress fractures and more severe fractures of the hips or vertebral column (Hobart & Smucker 2000). Furthermore, it is significantly associated with morbidity and can result in permanent bone loss (Hobart & Smucker 2000).

Contrary to popular belief, the third component of the triad, amenorrhea, is not a normal or benign consequence of athletic training. In reality, it can result in both infertility and osteoporosis (Lo *et al.* 2003). In fact, half of all athletes with amenorrhea have bone densities at least one standard deviation below the mean (Walsh *et al.* 2000). Risk of bone loss increases with the duration of amenorrhea, and after 3 years of amenorrhea, irreplaceable bone loss can occur (Hobart & Smucker 2000). Adolescents with the female athlete triad may have primary or secondary amenorrhea. Primary amenorrhea occurs if there is a lack of spontaneous menstruation either by age 14 years without the development of secondary sex characteristics or by age 16 years with normal development of secondary sex characteristics. Secondary amenorrhea is the abnormal cessation of menstruation in a woman who previously has had menstrual cycles. Although 6 months without menses is a common standard, there is disagreement concerning the point at which oligomenorrhea (menses occurring at intervals more than 35 days) becomes secondary amenorrhea. Nevertheless, any irregularity in the menstrual cycle should be assessed immediately as a possible sign of illness. Physicians can make the first step in diagnosing the athlete triad in its early stages by taking a menstrual history (Hobart & Smucker 2000).

Research supporting the athletics–eating disorder connection

A substantial subset of children and adolescents who are hospitalized for eating disorders were competitive athletes before the onset of their disorder, with steady increases in physical activity and steady decreases in food intake and weight typically preceding their hospital admissions (Davis *et al.* 1994; French *et al.* 1994). In a study of 5461 adolescent girls (Loud *et al.* 2005), mothers reported their daughters' weight and height, menarchal status, physical activity, dietary intake, and disordered eating behaviors on annual surveys. According to their mothers' reports, approximately 16% of the girls participated in 16 or more hours per week of moderate to vigorous activity, 3% engaged in disordered eating, using fasting, vomiting, diet pills, or laxatives to control their weight, and 2.7% had a history of stress fracture. Independent of age and body mass index (BMI), girls who participated in at least 16 hours per week of activity were more likely to have a history of stress fracture and to engage in disordered eating than were girls who participated in fewer than 4 hours per week of activity. Independent of age and BMI, risk of stress fracture significantly increased with each hour per week of high impact physical activity. Running, cheerleading, and gymnastics were independently associated with greater odds of stress fracture.

Other studies provide additional support for the athletics–eating disorder connection. In a large-scale study of 7th to 12th grade female athletes participating in school-sponsored sports, Roberts *et al.* (2003) found that 19 of the 226 participants (8.4%)

scored above 20 on the Eating Attitudes Test-26 (EAT), which is indicative of an eating disorder. Of the 139 athletes who were at least 1 year postmenarchal and had not taken contraceptives during the past year, 3.5% reported secondary amenorrhea (three or fewer menstrual periods during the past year or no periods in the past 3 months), and 13.7% reported oligomenorrhea (4–6 periods during the past year).

Running

Although most studies addressing this issue have been retrospective, preventing conclusions about causation from being drawn, data from one longitudinal study supports the athletics–eating disorder connection. Wiita and Stombaugh (1996) assessed changes in the nutritional knowledge, eating practices, and health of female adolescent runners. After 3 years of competitive running, fewer athletes responded correctly to statements about healthy fluid intake and the dangers of skipping meals. In addition, they significantly decreased their mean energy intake and mean protein, calcium, potassium, and sodium intake. Importantly, the incidence of eating disorders and stress fractures increased, and menstrual irregularities continued to be high.

Wrestling

The deaths of three collegiate wrestlers in 1997 brought widespread attention to disordered eating among male athletes. Wrestlers commonly utilize extreme weight-loss strategies, such as fasting, purging, and induced dehydration, in order to meet required weights for competition. Close to 2% of wrestlers meet diagnostic criteria for bulimia nervosa, but almost half engage in dangerous weight-loss practices such as restricting fluids, fasting 20 hours prior to being weighed, using rubber suits while exercising, and vomiting after eating (Oppliger et al. 1993).

It has been argued that weight preoccupation and body dissatisfaction that can accompany athletic participation may be misidentified as psychopathology rather than as a means to athletic excellence (Skowron & Friedlander 1994). In support of this premise, Dale and Landers (1999) reported no significant differences in risk for bulimia nervosa between junior high and high school in-season wrestlers and non-wrestlers. However, significantly more in-season wrestlers than non-wrestlers and significantly more in-season than off-season wrestlers scored in the at-risk range in levels of drive for thinness (an indicator of restrictive eating and body dissatisfaction). Interviews with the in-season athletes indicated that their weight concerns were caused solely by the demands of their sport and did not meet the criteria for an eating disorder diagnosis. The researchers concluded that wrestlers' weight consciousness was transient, a result of their sport participation rather than pathologic feelings and attitudes.

Competitive weight-lifting

In a study of the psychiatric effects of anabolic steroids on male bodybuilders, Pope et al. (1993) found athletes to be suffering from both anorexia nervosa and muscle dysmorphia (discussed later in this chapter). Approximately 3% of the athletes reported a history of anorexia nervosa, a rate significantly higher than expected among men.

Football

A self-report study (Depalma et al. 1993) of male college lightweight football players (n = 131) revealed that 42% of the athletes had a pattern of dysfunctional eating, and 9.9% engaged in a degree of binge–purge behavior that could warrant an eating disorder diagnosis. Furthermore, 66% of the players had fasted, almost 4% had used laxatives, and approximately 2% had used diet pills, diuretics, or enemas to control their weight during the month prior to administration of the survey.

Research negating the athletics–eating disorder connection

Some research suggests that participation in sports is without risk or can even be protective against the development of eating disorders. A recent study (Thompson & Digsby 2004) found no significant difference in the occurrence of eating disorders between female high school cheerleaders, often cited as a high-risk group for eating disorders, and other adolescent girls. Even more surprising, a meta-analysis (Smolak *et al.* 2000) showed that female gymnasts, another group considered to be at high risk for eating disorders, were slightly *less* likely than non-athletes to exhibit signs of eating problems.

A study of male and female high school athletes demonstrated an association between competitive sports participation and mental health (Pyle *et al.* 2003). Compared with students who were less active, those involved in competitive sports exhibited fewer mental health problems as well as fewer eating and dietary problems. More recently, Pedersen and Seidman (2004) found that girls' team sports achievement experiences in early adolescence were positively associated with self-esteem in middle adolescence.

Fulkerson *et al.* (1997) compared high school athletes from 14 sports, including soccer, basketball, swimming, and long-distance running, Nordic skiing, slalom skiing, volleyball, tennis, football, wrestling, hockey, danceline, cheerleading, and gymnastics, with students who were not involved in organized sports. The researchers found no significant differences between the athletes and non-athletes on most indices of eating disordered behaviors and attitudes. In the few cases where significant differences were found, the athletes reported more positive attitudes and behaviors than did the non-athletes. Female athletes demonstrated greater self-efficacy than did female non-athletes, and both male and female athletes reported fewer negative views of life than did their non-athletic counterparts.

Ethnic differences

Surprisingly few studies have examined whether ethnicity might moderate the relationship between sports participation and eating disorder risk. The majority of studies have either neglected to report the ethnic make-up of their sample or have focused exclusively on Caucasian samples. This lack of attention to ethnicity may stem from the common

misconception that eating disorders are exclusive to affluent, Caucasian women and girls. However, to date, no study has demonstrated an absence of eating disorder symptoms in ethnic minorities (Gordon *et al.* 2002). Furthermore, evidence suggests that eating disorders are becoming increasingly prevalent among diverse ethnic and socio-economic groups (National Eating Disorders Association 2002), indicating the critical need for research that addresses ethnic differences in eating disorder risk, manifestation, and effective treatments.

Rhea (1995, 1997, 1999) is one of the few researchers who has focused on eating disorders among adolescent athletes from diverse ethnic backgrounds. In her study of female athlete (*n* = 604) and non-athlete (*n* = 463) high school students from urban areas with ethnically diverse populations, Rhea (1995) found that as many as 11% of the sample met diagnostic criteria for an eating disorder. However, there was no difference in eating disorder risk between athletes and non-athletes or any distinctions based on type of sport. Examining ethnic group differences, Rhea found that Caucasian and Hispanic students reported significantly greater eating pathology than did black and Asian students.

In two subsequent studies, Rhea (1997, 1999) evaluated Caucasian, African-American, and Hispanic urban and suburban female athletes in a southern, metropolitan city. In both of these studies, Rhea found that Caucasian and Hispanic athletes scored significantly higher than African-American athletes on measures of eating pathology. Interestingly, Rhea (1999) found that athletes and non-athletes had an equal risk for developing an eating disorder. These results suggest that the risk for eating pathology among female high school athletes is greater among those who are Hispanic and Caucasian and that body dissatisfaction may not be the primary correlate of eating disturbance for these groups of women. Similarly, in Thompson and Digsby's (2004) recent study of female, high school cheerleaders, significantly more white athletes (73.5%) than black athletes (50%) reported body dissatisfaction, one well-documented risk factor for eating disorders.

In sum, the limited number of studies that have examined ethnic differences in eating disorder risk among athletes indicates that Hispanic and

Caucasian athletes have a greater risk than African-American or Asian athletes for developing an eating disorder. However, caution is warranted in interpreting these findings until this research is replicated with other samples and localities. Because no studies to date have examined ethnic differences across a variety of sports, it is unclear whether ethnic group differences in risk for eating disorders are moderated by the type of sport in which individuals participate.

Male athletes

The majority of research on eating disorders among athletic youth has not included male samples. This omission is unfortunate because it perpetuates the misconception that men and boys are exempt from eating disorders. Although eating disorders in the general population are more prevalent among women than men, the manifestation of eating disorders in athletes is similar for both sexes (French et al. 1994; Muise et al. 2003). Furthermore, the reported prevalence rates for eating disorders among male athletes may be conservative because of underreporting by those who are afraid of being characterized as having a woman's disorder and underidentification by parents, sports personnel, and athletes themselves, all of whom may be influenced by the stereotype that eating disorders affect only women and girls (Sherman & Thompson 2001).

A relatively new concern has emerged about male athletes developing "muscle dysmorphia," a body image disorder in which individuals inaccurately believe they look small and weak. Also known as "reverse anorexia" and "bigorexia," muscle dymorphia is not exclusive to male athletes. However, it is thought to predominate among men because of the Western cultural ideals that define female beauty as petite and extremely thin and masculine beauty as large and muscular (Anorexia Nervosa and Related Eating Disorders [ANRED] 2004). The actual prevalence of the disorder is unknown. Eating disorder specialists consider it to be a subtype of body dysmorphic disorder, which is a variant of obsessive–compulsive disorder (ANRED 2004). Patients persistently worry, or obsess, about their body size and feel compelled to exercise to reduce these

worries. They also display two primary criteria for anorexia nervosa and bulimia nervosa: harmful body-shaping behaviors and disturbance in perception of body shape and weight (Cafri et al. 2005).

In their drive to achieve a lean, muscular figure, individuals with muscle dysmorphia may use steroids and ephedrine, exercise compulsively, and engage in strict dieting (Cafri et al. 2005). They are preoccupied with eating the right foods and attribute greater importance to the acquisition of muscle mass than to anything else in their lives (Eating Disorder Recovery Center [EDRC] 2004). While they spend countless hours exercising, their social, emotional, educational, and occupational lives suffer. The experience of missing just a single session at the gym can be fraught with severe anxiety and stress. In extreme causes, the overexercising typical of individuals with muscle dysmorphia can result in permanent muscle damage (EDRC 2004).

Pope et al. (1993) conducted structured interviews with 55 bodybuilders who used anabolic steroids and 53 non-users. Nine participants (8.3%) reported symptoms consistent with muscle dysmorphia (and nearly 3% reported a history of anorexia nervosa), believing they appeared small and weak when they were actually large and muscular. These men reported that they turned down social invitations, refused to go to the beach, and wore heavy clothing during the summer because they feared appearing too small. All nine men with muscle dysmorphia were steroid users, four of whom reported that their muscle dysmorphia contributed to their decision to use steroids. The researchers concluded that anorexia nervosa and muscle dysmorphia may occur frequently among male bodybuilders and that muscle dysmorphia may precipitate or perpetuate the use of anabolic steroids.

Prevention efforts for coaches and parents

Although the prevalence of eating disorders among athletic youth is unclear (Ricciardelli & McCabe 2004), it is evident that participation in sports can increase some children's and adolescents' risk for developing an eating disorder. For this reason, nutrition and eating disorder education is warranted for athletics coaches, who have considerable influence on their athletes' eating behaviors, weight concern, and body image (Depalma *et al.* 1993; Biesecker & Martz 1999). Although not explicitly encouraging harmful weight-loss practices, coaches who stress the importance of maintaining a low body weight or who make critical remarks about an athlete's body may unwittingly promote restrictive dieting practices that may later develop into full-blown eating disorders. The power of a single comment from an influential person was demonstrated when elite gymnast Christy Henrich died in 1994 of complications from anorexia and bulimia nervosa. Henrich believed her pathologic eating was triggered in 1988 when a US judge at a gymnastics meet in Budapest told her she was fat and needed to lose weight in order to qualify for the Olympic team.

Many coaches believe excessive training and restrictive diet regimens are necessary to achieve athletic success (Thompson & Sherman 2005). Thus, education programs should cover the health risks associated with eating disorders and their potential negative impact on athletic performance. Coaches can be encouraged to shift their focus from the athlete's performance to his or her overall health. In addition, they can be trained to recognize signs of eating disorders and to provide help for those affected. This includes confronting and supporting the athlete, informing the athlete's parents about the problem, and insuring that the athlete receives proper psychologic and medical care. A physician should monitor the athlete's health and evaluate physical limitations on sports participation. With parental and patient consent, the coach and physician can work together to monitor the athlete's recovery.

Athletic personnel may realize the importance of their positions but may feel ill-equipped to deal with eating disorders. In a recent survey of 171 athletic trainers in the National Collegiate Athletic Association Division 1A and 1AA schools (Vaughan *et al.* 2004), almost all respondents (91%) reported that they had dealt with a female athlete who had an eating disorder, yet only 27% felt confident to identify a female athlete with an eating disorder, and only 38% felt confident to ask an athlete if she had an eating disorder. The vast majority felt that eating

disorder prevention for female athletes needs more attention and that, as athletic trainers, they have a responsibility to identify and help athletes with eating disorders. One-quarter of the respondents worked at institutions that lacked a policy regarding eating disorders. Trainers at schools that had such policies reported greater confidence in their ability to identify and assist athletes with eating disorders.

Despite research evidence supporting a connection between dieting and the development of an eating disorder, some coaches may continue to promote, condone, or fail to detect unhealthy weight-loss practices among their athletes regardless of institutional policies or the amount of eating disorder education they receive. Consequently, parents need to become informed about eating disorders and their child's athletic life. Parents can observe training sessions and interview their children's coaches to determine if weight standards are extreme or if harmful weight-loss practices are being encouraged. In such cases, parents can voice their concerns to their child's coach or seek the help of an athletic director or school principal. Ultimately, if these efforts fail, parents may have to remove their child from the team.

Parents must also be careful not to communicate harmful messages about food, weight, and athletic performance because their comments may increase their children's vulnerability to developing an eating disorder. One study (Keel *et al.* 1997) showed that girls were most likely to diet if their mothers described them as overweight and made comments about their weight. Similarly, girls were more likely to report weight dissatisfaction if their fathers were dissatisfied with their own weight or commented negatively about their daughters' weight.

Prevention programs for athletes

Given the significant risk posed by rigid weight and exercise requirements inherent in various sports, child and adolescent athletes would benefit from health and eating disorder education. Several trials of such programs have yielded major reductions in eating disorder risk among athletes. In a recent controlled study (Elliot *et al.* 2004), a peer-led prevention program, Athletes Targeting Healthy Exercise and Nutrition Alternative (ATHENA), was implemented to evaluate its impact on eating and body-shaping drug use among female, high school athletes. The program consisted of 8 weekly, 45-min sessions addressing issues that included media images of women, depression prevention, healthy sports nutrition, effective exercise training, drug use, and the effects of other unhealthy behaviors on athletic performance. A confidential questionnaire was administered to athletes before and after their sports season. ATHENA athletes reported significantly less ongoing and new use of diet pills than at baseline and significantly less new use of amphetamines, anabolic steroids, and sports supplements. They also reported significant decreases in their intent to use tobacco, muscle-building supplements, and diet pills, and to vomit to lose weight. Finally, participants reported significantly better strength-training self-efficacy and healthy eating behaviors.

A similar program consisting of sports training and health education was tested with 322 girls aged 8–12 years (DeBate & Thompson 2005). Following the running and wellness program, girls showed significant improvement on measures of self-esteem, body-size satisfaction, and eating attitudes and behaviors.

Other prevention programs have targeted specific populations of athletes. An eating disorder prevention program was tested on ballet students aged 10–18 years (Piran 1999), a group considered to be at high-risk for developing eating disorders. Participants included three cohorts of male and female students who attended a renowned, residential ballet school. Based on the health promoting schools paradigm developed by the World Health Organization, the program consisted of systematic changes and direct interventions with students. School-wide surveys incorporating the EAT, the Diagnostic Survey for Eating Disorders, and the Eating Disorder Inventory were administered in 1987, for a baseline measure, 1991, and 1996. Compared to the baseline cohort, the second and third cohorts showed significant reductions in disordered eating behaviors and attitudes and significant increases in healthy eating practices.

Another prevention program implemented in recent years was designed to prevent extreme weight-loss practices among adolescent wrestlers (Oppliger et al. 1998). Wisconsin high school wrestlers were surveyed 1 year before and 2 years after the program was implemented. Following the intervention, most weight lost, weight lost to certify for competition, weekly weight fluctuations, longest fast, frequency of cutting weight (i.e., rapid weight reduction), and weight-loss methods decreased significantly. Furthermore, wrestlers reporting more than one of the DSM, 3rd edition, revised criteria for bulimia nervosa significantly decreased by 11%, whereas those reporting all five remained the same. The researchers concluded that a minimal weight limit combined with nutritional education could reduce deleterious weight-loss practices among high school wrestlers.

Directions for future research

There is a clear need for standardization across studies assessing eating disorders in young athletes. Currently, there are no criteria for differentiating between athletes and non-athletes, sports emphasizing leanness and those that do not, and levels of competition. Until a consensus is made on such issues, researchers must provide more thorough explanations of their categorical variables so that proper comparisons among studies can be made. This effort may be the key to understanding the discrepant findings in the literature.

Nevertheless, comparisons of athletes engaged in sports that require the maintenance of low body weights with those engaged in "non-lean" sports are important. These can be accompanied by comparisons with age-comparable non-athletes who engage in non-competitive exercise as well as those who engage in little or no exercise. These methodologies can help to isolate the specific variables that increase eating disorder risk, whether they are the increased time spent in exercise, the competitive aspect of the exercise, or the increased emphasis on achieving and maintaining a low body weight.

Large-scale longitudinal studies assessing risk for eating disorders by sport are sorely needed. Such studies should include equal numbers of male and female athletes as well as ethnically diverse samples that allow for statistical analyses of ethnic group differences. Standardized instruments should be utilized that have appropriate reliability and validity for these subgroups. Ideally, measurements should be taken at several regular intervals beginning at prepuberty to assess whether the onset of puberty affects the relationship between sports participation and eating disorder risk. Furthermore, groups of athletes should be compared with same-age nonathletes to examine the specific effect of athletic participation on eating disorder risk that cannot be attributed to simple maturation.

As noted earlier, a few researchers have begun to evaluate treatment and prevention programs for athletes with eating disordered problems or related behaviors (steroid use among males); however, much more work needs to be carried out in this area. It will be important to adapt effective strategies that have been previously found to work for female and male adolescents, with the hopes of preventing or addressing early signs of disturbance before the symptoms develop into an intractable eating disorder (Thompson 2004; Thompson & Cafri, 2007).

References

Anorexia Nervosa and Related Eating Disorders, Inc. (2004) Muscle dysmorphic disorder (bigorexia). http://www.anred.com. Accessed September 2005.

Benson, J.E., Allemann, Y., Theintz, G.E. & Howald, H. (1990) Eating problems and calorie intake levels in Swiss adolescent athletes. *International Journal of Sports Medicine* 11, 249–252.

Biesecker, A.C. & Martz, D.M. (1999) Impact of coaching style on vulnerability for eating disorders: An analog study. Eating Disorders. *Journal of Treatment and Prevention* 7, 235–244.

Brooks-Gunn, J., Burrow, C. & Warren, M.P. (1988) Attitudes toward eating and body weight in different groups of female adolescent athletes. *International Journal of Eating Disorders* 7, 749–757.

Cafri, G., Thompson, J.K., Ricciardelli, L., McCabe, M., Smolak, L. & Yesalis, C. (2005) Pursuit of the muscular ideal: Physical and psychological consequences and putative risk factors. *Clinical Psychology Review* 25, 215–239.

Dale, K.S. & Landers, D.M. (1999) Weight control in wrestling: Eating disorders or disordered eating? *Medicine and Science in Sports and Exercise* 31, 1382–1389.

Davis, C., Kennedy, S.H., Ravelski, E. & Dionne, M. (1994) The role of physical activity in the development and maintenance of eating disorders. *Psychological Medicine* 24, 957–967.

Davison, K.K., Earnest, M.B. & Birch, L.L. (2002) Participation in aesthetic sports and girls' weight concerns at ages 5 and 7 years. *International Journal of Eating Disorders* 31, 312–317.

Debate, R.D. & Thompson, S.H. (2005) Girls on the run: Improvements in self-esteem, body size satisfaction and eating attitudes/behaviors. *Eating and Weight Disorders Studies on Anorexia, Bulimia and Obesity* 10, 25–32.

Depalma, M.T., Koszewski, W.M., Case, J.G., *et al.* (1993) Weight control practices of lightweight football players. *Medicine and Science in Sports and Exercise* 25, 694–701.

Eating Disorder Recovery Center (Addictions & More) (2004) Muscle dysmorphia. http://www.addictions.net Accessed September 2005.

Elliot, D.L., Goldberg, L., Moe, E.L., DeFrancesco, C.A., Durham, M.B. & Hix-Small, H. (2004) Preventing substance use and disordered eating: Initial outcomes of the ATHENA (Athletes Targeting Healthy Exercise and Nutrition Alternatives) program. *Archives of Pediatrics and Adolescent Medicine* 158, 1043–1049.

French, S.A., Perry, C.L., Leon, G.R. & Fulkerson, J.A. (1994) Food preferences, eating patterns, and physical activity among adolescents: Correlates of eating disorders symptoms. *Journal of Adolescent Health* 15, 286–294.

Fulkerson, J.A., Keel, P.K., Leon, G.R. & Dorr, T. (1999) Eating-disordered behaviors and personality characteristics of high school athletes and nonathletes. *International Journal of Eating Disorders* 26, 73–79.

Garner, D.M., Rosen, L.W. & Barry, D. (1998) Eating disorders among athletes. Research and recommendations. *Child and Adolescent Psychiatric Clinics of North America* 7, 839–857.

Gordon, K.H., Perez, M. & Joiner, T.E. (2002) The impact of racial stereotypes on eating disorder recognition. *International Journal of Eating Disorders* 32, 219–224.

Hausenblas, H.A. & Mack, D.E. (1999) Social physique anxiety and eating disorder correlates among female athletic and nonathletic populations. *Journal of Sport Behavior* 22, 502–513.

Hausenblas, H.A. & McNally, K.D. (2004) Eating disorder prevalence and symptoms for track and field athletes and nonathletes. *Journal of Applied Sport Psychology* 16, 274–286.

Hobart J.A. & Smucker, D.R. (2000) The female athlete triad. *American Family Physician* 61, 3357–3364.

Keel, P.K., Heatherton, T.F., Harnden, J.L. & Hornig, C.D. (1997) Mothers, fathers, and daughters: Dieting and disordered eating. *Eating Disorders: Journal of Treatment and Prevention* 5, 216–228.

Kirk, G., Singh, K. & Getz, H. (2001) Risk of eating disorders among female college athletes and nonathletes. *Journal of College Counseling* 4, 122–132.

Lindeman, A.K. (1994) Self-esteem: Its application to eating disorders and athletes. *International Journal of Sports Nutrition* 4, 237–252.

Lo, B.P., Hebert, C. & McClean, A. (2003) The Female Athlete Triad no pain, no gain. *Clinical Pediatrics* **42**, 573–580.

Loud, K.J., Gordon, C.M., Micheli, L.J. & Field, A.E. (2005) Correlates of stress fractures among preadolescent and adolescent girls. *Pediatrics* **11**, e399–406.

Muise, A.M., Stein, D.G. & Arbess, G. (2003) Eating disorders in adolescent boys: A review of the adolescent young adult literature. *Journal of Adolescent Health* **33**, 427–435.

National Eating Disorders Association (2002) Eating disorders in women of color: Explanations and implications. http://www.nationaleatingdisorders.org. Accessed September 2005.

Oppliger, R.A., Landry, G.L., Foster, S.W. & Lambrecht, A.C. (1993) Bulimic behaviors among interscholastic wrestlers: A statewide survey. *Pediatrics* **91**, 826–831.

Oppliger, R.A., Landry, G.L., Foster, S.W. & Lambrecht, A.C. (1998) Wisconsin minimum weight program reduces weight-cutting practices of high school wrestlers. *Clinical Journal of Sports Medicine* **8**, 26–31.

Otis, C.L., Drinkwater, B., Johnson, M., Loucks, A. & Wilmore, J. (1997) The female athlete triad. *Medicine and Science in Sports and Exercise* **29**, i–ix.

Pedersen, S. & Seidman, E. (2004) Team sports achievement and self-esteem development among urban adolescent girls. *Psychology of Women Quarterly* **28**, 412–422.

Piran, N. (1999) Eating disorders: A trial of prevention in a high risk school setting. *Journal of Primary Prevention* **20**, 75–90.

Pope, H.G., Katz, D.L. & Hudson, J.L. (1993) Anorexia nervosa and "reverse anorexia" among 108 male bodybuilders. *Comprehensive Psychiatry* **34**, 406–409.

Pyle, R.P., McQuivey, R.W., Brassington, G.S. & Steiner, H. (2003) High school student athletes: Associations between intensity of participation and health

factors. *Clinical Pediatrics* **42**, 697–701.

Rhea, D.J. (1995) Risk factors for the development of eating disorders in ethnically diverse high school athlete and non-athlete populations. *Dissertations International* **56**, 1670A. (UMI No. 4194209)

Rhea, D.J. (1997) Eating disorders: Ethnic differences of volleyball players. *USA Volleyball Journal* **10**, 18–19.

Rhea, D.J. (1999) Eating disorder behaviors of ethnically diverse urban female adolescent athletes and non-athletes. *Journal of Adolescence* **22**, 379–388.

Ricciardelli, L.A. & McCabe, M.P. (2004) A biopsychosocial model of disordered eating and the pursuit of muscularity in adolescent boys. *Psychological Bulletin* **130**, 179–205.

Roberts, T.A., Glen, J. & Kreipe, R.E. (2003) Disordered eating and menstrual dysfunction in adolescent female athletes participating in school-sponsored sports. *Clinical Pediatrics* **42**, 561–564.

Sherman, R.T. & Thompson, R.A. (2001) Athletes and disordered eating: Four major issues for the professional psychologist. *Professional Psychology: Research and Practice* **32**, 27–33.

Sherwood, N.E., Neumark-Sztainer, D., Story, M., Beuhring, T. & Resnick, M.D. (2002) Weight-related sports involvement in girls: Who is at risk for disordered eating? *American Journal of Health Promotion* **16**, 341–344.

Skowron, E.A. & Friedlander, M.L. (1994) Psychological separation, self-control, and weight preoccupation among elite women athletes. *Journal of Counseling and Development* **72**, 310–315.

Smolak, L., Murnen, S.K. & Ruble, A.E. (2000) Female athletes and eating problems: A meta-analysis. *International Journal of Eating Disorders* **27**, 371–380.

Stoutjesdyk, D. & Jevne, R. (1993) Eating disorders among high performance athletes. *Journal of Youth and Adolescence* **22**, 271–282.

Taub, D.E. & Blinde, E.M. (1992) Eating disorders among adolescent female athletes: Influence of athletic participation and sport team membership. *Adolescence* **27**, 833–848.

Taub, D.E. & Blinde, E.M. (1994) Disordered eating and weight control among adolescent female athletes and performance squad members. *Journal of Adolescent Research* **9**, 483–497.

Thompson, J.K. & Smolak, L., eds. (2001) *Body Image, Eating Disorders, and Obesity in Youth: Assessment, Treatment and Prevention*. Washington, DC: American Psychological Association.

Thompson, J.K., ed. (2004) *Handbook of Eating Disorders and Obesity*. New York: Wiley.

Thompson, J.K. & Cafri, G. (2007) *The Muscular Ideal*. Washington, DC: American Psychological Association.

Thompson, R.A. & Sherman, R.T. (2005) The last word: Athletes, eating disorders, and the four-minute mile. *Eating Disorders: The Journal of Treatment and Prevention* **13**, 321–324.

Thompson, S.H. & Digsby, S. (2004) A preliminary survey of dieting, body dissatisfaction, and eating problems among high school cheerleaders. *Journal of School Health* **74**, 85–90.

Vaughan, J.L., King, K.A. & Cottrell, R.R. (2004) Collegiate athletic trainers' confidence in helping female athletes with eating disorders. *Journal of Athletic Training* **39**, 71–76.

Walsh, J.M.E., Wheat, M.E. & Freund, K. (2000) Detection, evaluation, and treatment of eating disorders: The role of the primary care physician. *Journal of General Internal Medicine* **15**, 577–590.

Wiita, B.G. & Stombaugh, I.A. (1996) Nutrition knowledge, eating practices, and health of adolescent female runners: A 3-year longitudinal study. *International Journal of Sport Nutrition* **6**, 414–425.

Chapter 18

Delayed Puberty in Girls and Primary and Secondary Amenorrhea

ALAN D. ROGOL

The purpose of this chapter is to describe the pubertal process in girls, its variation in timing and *tempo*, and the effects of pathophysiologic processes on its onset, progression, and completion. Because the emphasis of this volume is on the athlete, the effects of athletic training are considered in greater depth.

Because breast budding is considered the first sign of pubertal development in girls, those beyond 13.3 years (+2 standard deviations [SD] from a mean of 11.2 years) are considered to have delayed puberty. This is a statistical definition. One should be concerned, certainly, by age 14 years and an evaluation by a subspecialist is indicated. If the girl is an athlete and quite thin, one might consider her activity to be causative; however, that would be quite improper, because athletic amenorrhea (and delayed puberty caused by excessive energy expenditure in relationship to inadequate energy intake) is a diagnosis of exclusion.

Amenorrhea may be primary—a girl of 15 years or older who has never had a menstrual period—or secondary, meaning that the adolescent has had at least one period, but now has had ceased menses for at least 6 months. Excessive energy expenditure relative to caloric intake is only one of a long list of causes of secondary amenorrhea which, for example, includes hyperandrogenism, hyperprolactinemia, and pregnancy.

The link between athletic activity and operation of the hypothalamic–pituitary–gonadal axis has been reported by Loucks (2004) and Redmond and Loucks (2005), who have noted a very significant threshold relationship between luteinizing hormone (LH) pulsatility, reflecting the hypothalamic gonadotrophin-releasing hormone (GnRH) pulse generator and net energy intake. When the net intake (total intake minus energy expenditure) dips below $30 \text{ kcal·kg}^{-1}\text{·day}^{-1}$, then the hypothalamic GnRH pulse generator slows, and the gonadotropic signal to the steroid-secreting cells of the ovary is inadequate to signal for enough estradiol production.

Normal pubertal development

Growth and sexual maturation in both boys and girls is a complex process involving the dynamic

Table 18.1 Pubic hair development in the female.

Stage	Characteristics	Age (years) mean and 95% confidence limits
I	Prepubertal, no sexual hair	
II	Sparse growth of long, slightly pigmented hair over mons veneris or labia majora	11.7 (9.2–14.1)
III	Further darkening and coarsening of hair with spread over the symphysis pubis	12.4 (10.2–14.6)
IV	Hair is adult in character but not in distribution, has not spread to medial surface of the thighs	13 (10.8–15.1)
V	Hair is adult with extension to the medial thighs	14.4 (12.2–16.7)

interplay of genetic constitution, nutrition, and a number of hormones. Ultimate height, the biologic timing of pubertal development, and the tempo and degree of that development are encoded in the genome. However, the process of pubertal development can be significantly modified by alterations in nutritional intake, psychologic state, physical exercise, and hormonal activity.

Female adolescent development has been extensively reviewed by Tanner and colleagues (Marshall & Tanner 1969). They have developed a staging system that defines the normal progression of adolescent sexual development as well as defining some of the variations (particularly in onset) that are considered to represent the range of normal. Their method simply relies on a careful physical examination of the child or adolescent and does not require any endocrine laboratory or radiologic studies. Female sexual maturation is characterized by pubic hair development as well as by changes in breast size and contour (see Chapter 31).

Although puberty progresses in an orderly process, there is much variability in its onset and completion. Once entrained, however, the variability between stages (tempo), although present, is much less. Given this basic premise, one can describe how adolescent females mature and have a firm basis for accurately pinpointing alterations and aberrations of this developmental process. Pubic hair and breast development are divided into five stages of maturation, which are shown in Tables 18.1 and 18.2. The greatest variation is in the age of onset of pubertal development; this is usually heralded by breast budding, although in 10–20% of girls pubic hair development will precede breast enlargement (Tables 18.1–18.3). These two events may be considerably disparate; for example, among girls in breast stage III, all stages of pubic hair (PH) development may be noted as 25% may have none (Tanner PH stage I) and 10% will have reached full adult status (Tanner PH stage V) (Tanner 1990). For details about the methods for assessing the Tanner stages, see Chapter 31.

The uterus begins to enlarge early in puberty, attaining a threefold increase by Tanner breast stage III and virtually a fivefold increase at full maturity. The ovaries may begin to increase in size well before

Table 18.2 Breast development.

Stage	Characteristics	Age (years) mean and 95% confidence limits
I	Prepubertal	
II	Breast budding, widening of areola with elevation of the breast and papilla as a small mound	11.1 (9.0–13.3)
III	Continued enlargement of both breast and areola but without separation of their contours	12.2 (10.0–14.3)
IV	Formation of the areola and papilla as a secondary mound projecting above the contour of the breast	13.1 (10.8–15.3)
V	Adult, project of the papilla only with the areola recessed to the contour of the breast. Not all girls pass through stage V; others may maintain stage IV development	15.3 (11.9–18.8)

Table 18.3 Typical age ranges for normal female pubertal development.

Characteristic	Age (years) mean and 95% confidence limits
First breast budding	11.2 (9.0–13.3)
First pubic and axillary hair (adrenarche)	11.7 (9.3–14.1)
Menarche	12.8 (10.8–14.8)

external signs of puberty become apparent, as many small primordial follicles mature to a stage in which follicle-stimulating hormone (FSH) bound to its receptor induces the aromatase enzyme system and the production of estrogen. Most girls will experience menarche between 2 and 2.5 years later. In the USA, the average age at menarche is 12.8 ± 1.2 (SD) years. The sequence of these events is shown in Fig. 18.1.

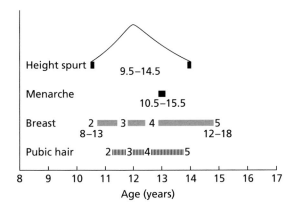

Fig. 18.1 Diagram of sequence of events at puberty. An average girl is represented in relation to the scale of ages: the range of ages within which some of the changes occur is indicated by the figures below them. Redrawn from Marshall & Tanner 1969.

At menarche there is a considerable range of breast development. Most girls are in breast stage IV (projection of the nipple and areola above the level of the rest of the breast; see Table 18.2). However, some 25% are in breast stage III, with a small percentage in stage II. Similarly, most girls at menarche are in PH stages III or IV, but some are in stage V, and a very few have yet to have pubarche (stage I).

Menarche does not necessarily mark the end of sexual development or mean that the adolescent has attained full reproductive capacity, because ovulation does not occur with each cycle. Young women have great variability in their menstrual cycles (Vollman 1977) and appear particularly susceptible to stressors (e.g., psychologic and athletic) that may alter the function of the brain–hypothalamic–pituitary–ovarian axis, especially within the first 2 years after menarche (see below). In addition, at menarche adolescent females have not reached their adult body composition.

Growth at adolescence occurs relatively early in girls—in some, peak height velocity is reached soon after breast buds appear. When menarche occurs, the height velocity is declining. On average girls will continue to grow 6 cm after menarche (95% confidence interval [CI], 0–12 cm) (Tanner 1990). The adolescent growth spurt is also accompanied by alterations in body shape and size. In fact, the greatest alterations in the sexually dimorphic char-

acteristics occur during adolescent development. Nearly all skeletal and muscular dimensions (length, breadth, and girth) are altered during pubertal maturation, although not necessarily in a proportional manner (Malina *et al.* 2004). The greatest sexual dimorphism occurs at the shoulders and hips. Girls have a very large adolescent increase in bi-iliac diameter, but a much smaller one (compared to boys) in the bi-acromial diameter. Other skeletal changes at puberty include widening of the pelvic inlet.

The *tempo* of the pubertal growth spurt refers to the rate at which the child passes through these developmental stages. Although the timing of the onset of puberty may be quite variable, parameters of pubertal development have considerably less dispersion with biologic age than with chronologic age. For example, the variation (95% CI) for the age at menarche is 11–15 years in terms of chronologic age, but only 12–14 years in terms of skeletal (bone) age (Tanner 1990). In part, the tempo of pubertal development is determined genetically as is the adult height and body habitus, although all may be affected by undernutrition, physical activity, or hormonal deficiencies.

The adolescent growth spurt in female gymnasts was considered to be abnormal in that it had been suggested that high level gymnastics *training* leads to disproportionate short stature with virtually all of the deficit in the lower segment (below the pubic ramus; Theintz *et al.* 1993). This seemed at odds with the very large number of (short) adult, formerly elite gymnasts, who seemed proportionate in their adult stature. Thoms *et al.* (2005) tracked the growth of 15 Belgian gymnasts and showed that each athlete had a clearly defined adolescent growth spurt (height) as well as sitting height and leg length, although the athletes were below average in height and had their spurts late by contemporary standards. They concluded that the pattern of adolescent growth and maturation is *similar* to that of other athletes, short normal late-maturing girls, and late-maturing girls with short parents (Thoms *et al.* 2005). It should be noted that the training for nationally competitive gymnasts is about as tough as it gets. Thus, it seems that if there is an alteration in adolescent growth, it is no different than that noted as a "physiologic" variant.

Body composition and the relative proportions of fat and fat-free mass (and its subdivisions into water, bone, and muscle) also change predictably during puberty. Fat-free mass, bone mass, and percent body fat are nearly equal in prepubertal boys and girls; by full maturity women have almost twice the percent body fat but only two-thirds the fat-free body mass and skeletal mass of men. Children are chemically as well as biologically immature when compared with adults (who have a diminished amount of total body water compared to less mature individuals). Excess subcutaneous fat can be stored at several sites. The health implications can be (and increasing evidence shows that they are) vastly different (Bouchard et al. 1993; Despres et al. 2001; Ardern et al. 2003, 2004). Traditional measures of anthropometry have been expanded to take into account these concepts of regional distribution of fat, because there is growing evidence that abdominal fat and upper body truncal fat are more closely related to health risk than any other fat depots (Bouchard et al. 1993; Despres et al. 2001; Ardern et al. 2003, 2004).

Considerable recent evidence suggests that body fat content and its regional distribution, especially to the abdominal area, are related to increased estrogen levels and lower androgen : estrogen ratios in plasma (de Ridder et al. 1990). The earlier maturing girl has an abdominal accumulation of fat (Frisancho & Flegel 1982). Whether the tempo of puberty contributes to body composition and fat patterning has not been adequately evaluated.

Hormonal control of puberty in the female

Gonadal steroid hormones are important for the growth process because they are responsible in large part for the augmented growth hormone (GH) secretion characteristic of the adolescent growth spurt of maturing girls (Rose et al. 1991). The increase in mean GH level is most evident at night and occurs, as it does in boys (Mauras et al. 1987; Martha et al. 1989), by an increase in the amplitude of the GH pulse rather than in the frequency of release. In both girls and boys the amount of GH released is inversely correlated to the body mass index [BMI = body mass (kg) × length^{-2} (m)]

(Rose et al. 1991; Martha et al. 1992; Roemmich et al. 1998).

Gonadotropins

Pulsatile release of LH is found at all stages of pubertal development because there are now immunoassays that faithfully track biologically active hormone. Truly pulsatile LH (and FSH) release can be detected in prepubertal (stage I) as well as early pubertal children. Such secretion can be distinguished from that in children with permanent hypogonadotropic hypogonadism (Haavisto et al. 1990). From early puberty onward the data are consistent (although not quantitatively) with those from many previous studies using less sensitive assays. They show augmented, pulsatile release of LH—at first, only at night—followed by a period of unbalanced secretion with the great majority at night, and finally to the adult pattern of intermittent pulsatile release with a frequency of one pulse approximately every 90 min in the early follicular phase of the menstrual cycle. The ovary is stimulated to produce increasing quantities of estradiol by the increasing concentrations of biologically active gonadotropins.

Primary amenorrhea without sexual development

Constitutional (normal) variations of growth and puberty are less common in girls than in boys. The normal ranges for growth (and sexual development) are often defined as the 95% confidence intervals for children at a specific chronologic age. Individuals outside of this statistically defined range may be uncommon, but not necessarily abnormal; they may represent constitutional (i.e., physiologic) variants. Adult height (target height) depends also on the adult heights of the parents. On average, the adult height of a girl will be the average of her mother's height and that of her father minus 6.5 cm, with one SD of approximately 5 cm:

Adult target height (mid-parental target height)
= [maternal height + (paternal height − 13 cm)]/2

The 13 cm difference is to put the father on the same height percentile on the chart for females that he has on the chart for males. Children with constitutionally delayed growth and pubertal development usually have normal birth weight and length. The growth rate is normal for the first 6–12 months, but then decreases significantly over the next 1–2 years until the child has a steady, although low normal growth velocity at approximately 2.5–3 years. This slow but steady rate continues for the major portion of the next decade. However, the normal early pubertal deceleration (pre-adolescent "dip") in growth velocity is often prolonged and accentuated in magnitude.

Constitutional variants are often characterized by a familial occurrence and a normal relationship between the timing of the onset of puberty and skeletal maturation. However, constitutional delayed growth and puberty may be diagnosed only following careful evaluation that excludes other causes of delay and longitudinal follow-up that shows *normal* sexual development. The further below the third percentile (approximately −2 SD) the young girl finds herself, the less likely that constitutional explanations are correct.

Management

Most girls will require only reassurance. If therapy is needed, it is usually with gonadal steroid hormones, often 0.15–0.3 mg·day^{-1} conjugated equine estrogens, ethinyl estradiol, 5–20 µg·day^{-1} or one of the low-dose estrogen patches (cutaneous therapy) for several months. If prolonged therapy is required, the addition of medroxyprogesterone acetate 5–10 mg·day^{-1} for 10–14 days of each month to induce menstrual flow is prudent. The latter is rarely necessary for girls with constitutional delay of puberty, but is required for those with permanent hypogonadotropic hypogonadism (see below).

Pathologic variations in growth and adolescent development

Hypogonadotropic hypogonadism

Hypogonadotropic hypogonadism defines the status of diminished or absent gonadotropin secretion; but it is not in itself a pathologic diagnosis. There are both familial and sporadic causes and the

Table 18.4 Hypogonadotropic hypogonadism in childhood and adolescence.

Isolated gonadotropin deficiency

Syndromes
Kallmann
Prader–Labhardt–Willi
Laurence–Moon–Bardet–Biedl
Many more

Multiple pituitary hormone deficiencies
Congenital
    Transcription factor deficiencies (HESX1, LHX3, PROP1)
    Midline defects
    Orphan nuclear receptor deficiencies (DAX1, SF1)
    Leptin or leptin receptor deficiency
    G-protein related receptor (GP54R) deficiency
Acquired
    Hypothalamic-pituitary tumors
    Langerhans cell histiocytosis
    Thalassemia major
    Pituitary stalk section (traumatic)
    Cranial irradiation
    Psychogenic/stress
    Large volume of exercise at low energy intake

Chronic illness (many)

---

differential diagnosis is broad (Table 18.4). Isolated gonadotropin deficiency as noted in a number of sporadic conditions or familial clustering is usually hypothalamic in origin; that is, it is one of a number of disorders of the GnRH pulse generator rather than a failure of the pituitary to produce gonadotropins. After a period of priming of the gonadotrophs with GnRH, they can begin to secrete gonadotropins in synchrony with the rhythmic (pulsatile) administration of exogenous GnRH. This form of treatment can produce normal puberty in permanently hypogonadotropic individuals and induce normal, fertile menstrual cycles. The various syndromes noted have GnRH deficiency in common, but differ in their other characteristics. Kallmann's syndrome is accompanied by anosmia, brought about by defective development of the olfactory bulbs; the Prader–Labhardt–Willi sy drome by obesity, short stature, hypogonadism, small hands and feet (acromicria), mental retardation, and infantile hypotonia; the Laurence–Moon–Bardet–Biedl syndrome by retinitis pigmentosa, postaxial polydactyly, obesity, and hypogonadism. Multiple pituitary hormone deficiencies may be congenital (usually hypothalamic in origin) and either part of an inherited constellation of findings or sporadic (Parks *et al.* 1999; Silveira *et al.* 2002). If GH or thyroid-stimulating hormone (TSH) concentrations are also subnormal, growth as well as adolescent development will be delayed. These, of course, should permit an earlier diagnosis than if gonadotropin deficiency is isolated. Many are secondary to deficiencies in one of multiple pituitary transcription factors (Parks *et al.* 1999; Silveira *et al.* 2002). Gonadotropin deficiency (along with other deficiencies) may occur in association with midline cranial defects, such as septo-optic dysplasia (underdevelopment of the optic disks or nerves and usually an absent septum pellucidum; Dattani *et al.* 2000; Dattani & Preece 2004).

A long list of tumors of the hypothalamic and pituitary regions can cause a hypogonadotropic state. These are relatively uncommon in children, except for craniopharyngioma. This tumor is usually suprasellar and may be asymptomatic well into the second decade (and beyond) when patients may present with headache, visual disturbances, short stature and/or growth failure, delayed puberty, or diabetes insipidus. Visual field deficits (including bilateral temporal hemianopsia), optic atrophy, or papilledema may be noted on physical examination. Laboratory evaluation often confirms the deficits in pituitary hormone concentrations; however, the circulating concentration of prolactin may be increased because of the interruption of hypothalamic dopamine inhibition of tonic prolactin release. Radiographically, the tumor may be solid or cystic with evidence of calcification. Other central nervous system (CNS) disorders that may lead to delayed puberty include infiltrative diseases such as Langerhans' cell histiocytosis; particularly the type formerly known as Hand–Schüller–Christian disease (Nezelof & Basset 1998). Diabetes insipidus is the most common endocrinopathy (caused by infiltration of the supraoptic hypothalamic nucleus), although growth failure (GH deficiency) and delayed puberty (gonadotropin deficiency) are relatively common. The pathogenesis is apparently infiltration of the hypothalamic nuclei producing the specific releasing hormones.

Radiation therapy to the CNS for leukemia or for other tumors may result in hypothalamic dysfunction. Although GH deficiency is most common, a small minority of patients will have partial or complete gonadotropin (releasing hormone) deficiency (Richards *et al.* 1976; Rappoport & Brauner 1989) or even precocious puberty, especially if irradiated at a young age.

Severe, chronic systemic disorders, often with attendant malnutrition, may cause slow growth and delayed adolescent development. Weight loss of virtually any cause to less than 80–85% of ideal body weight will often produce hypothalamic GnRH deficiency. When the weight is regained, puberty can commence or continue. If adequate nutrition and body weight are maintained in conditions such as Crohn's disease or in chronic pulmonary or renal disease, sufficient gonadotropin release usually occurs to initiate and maintain pubertal development. Anorexia nervosa is a special condition (see below) in which weight loss and significant psychologic dysfunction occur simultaneously. Weight gain is often enough to permit these mainly young women to obtain pubertal development; however, severe psychologic distress may continue the hypogonadotropic state.

Hyperprolactinemia resulting from a pituitary tumor is uncommon in adolescent girls. However, if present it may inhibit the hypothalamic control of gonadotropin release. A common cause of mild hyperprolactinemia is therapy with antidopaminergic agents such as chlorpromazine. In most cases, however, these adolescents will show some pubertal development, although they may not attain menarche or may have secondary amenorrhea. Both Cushing's disease and hypothyroidism are listed as causes of delayed adolescence without sexual development. More often they merely delay sexual development or prolong the time before menarche.

Hypergonadotropic hypogonadism (gonadal failure)

The list of definable causes of hypergonadotropic hypogonadism without sexual development is relatively small. The overwhelming majority of these females have Turner's syndrome (45,X gonadal dysgenesis) or one of its many variants (Sybert 2004; Stratakis & Rennert 2005; for the adult consequences see El Sheikh *et al.* 2002). Girls with this condition grow slowly beginning at birth; they may have many of the associated stigmata: lymphedema at birth, webbed neck, multiple pigmented naevi, disorders of the heart (left-sided), kidneys (horseshoe) and great vessels (e.g., coarctation of the aorta), and small hyperconvex fingernails. As they get older there is significant short stature, growth failure, and absence of adolescent development, often in the presence of either pubic or axillary hair. The latter is because of an appropriate adrenarche with failure of gonadarche. Although less severe, short stature and even some adolescent development may occur with chromosomal mosaicism; the dictum that any short, poorly growing, sexually infantile girl has Turner's syndrome until proven otherwise is useful because this condition is so prevalent (approximately 1 in 2500 newborn phenotypic females).

The term pure gonadal dysgenesis refers to 46,XX phenotypic females who have streak ovaries; this condition may be inherited as an autosomal recessive trait. Affected girls are of average height, have none of the stigmata of Turner's syndrome, but have elevated (to the menopausal range) circulating levels of gonadotropins, especially FSH, because the streak ovaries produce neither steroid hormones nor inhibin.

The availability of recombinant human GH has made mandatory early diagnosis of Turner's syndrome (i.e., much earlier than the subsequent delayed puberty), because treatment with GH is not only efficacious in increasing the growth rate, but will add 8–10 cm to the average adult height of approximately 146 cm for untreated females with Turner's syndrome. Low dose replacement therapy with 0.15–0.3 mg conjugated estrogens, or estradiol itself, should be administered to the girl at the usual age of puberty, if the height deficit has been lessened with GH therapy. For those with a late diagnosis of Turner's syndrome or with a large height deficit, one should begin estrogen therapy later, but in almost all cases before age 15 or 16 years to permit maximal accrual of bone mineral. After 6–12

months medroxyprogesterone acetate (5–10 mg) is added on days 12–25 of the month to induce menstrual cycles. Subsequently, the estrogen dose is increased to 0.3–0.6 mg on days 1–25 of the month (see above for equivalent doses of ethinyl estradiol and the estrogen patch).

For completeness, galactosemia is mentioned. Pre- or postnatal ovarian failure is caused, perhaps, by an abnormal metabolite of galactose, and is later manifested by delayed puberty. This condition should be detected at birth by the mandated screening procedure or by symptoms in the perinatal period. Gonadal steroid hormone treatment is the same as noted for young women with Turner's syndrome.

Primary amenorrhea with sexual development

The disorders described here assume some form of ovarian function—at least enough to permit the ovary to produce some estrogen to feminize the adolescent, but not necessarily enough to induce menarche. This is a heterogeneous group of disorders, consisting mainly of anomalies of the distal reproductive tract.

Disorders of the outflow tract and uterus

The simplest single disorder is that of the imperforate hymen, which does not permit the outward passage of uterine mucous and endometrial blood. These accumulate in the vagina (hydrocolpos) or uterus (hydrometrocolpos) and produce a bulging hymen, and/or one may elicit a vague history of abdominal pain that may have monthly exacerbations.

Mullerian agenesis or hypoplasia leads to disorders of the upper portion of the vagina and uterus. These disorders produce a very short vagina ending in a blind pouch and primary amenorrhea; however, the differential diagnosis includes imperforate hymen, other disorders of the vagina, and the androgen insensitivity syndromes (see below).

Disorders of the ovary

The common disorders of the ovary, Turner's syndrome and XX "pure" gonadal dysgenesis usually present as primary amenorrhea without sexual development and are discussed above. A small percentage of girls with Turner's syndrome—especially those with mosaic variants—may have sexual development including menarche. Those with advanced stages of development may be as short as the typical young woman with classic 45,X gonadal dysgenesis (approximately 146 cm), but are usually taller.

Premature menopause may occur at any age or stage of sexual development, even in the rare girl with Turner's syndrome who advances to menarche. Although this presents mainly as secondary amenorrhea (see below), occasionally primary amenorrhea may be the presenting complaint. The pathogenesis may include circulating antiovarian antibodies, either as a rare singular entity or more commonly as part of an expanded syndrome of antiendocrine tissue autoimmune syndrome (Betterle et al. 2002).

Malignancies and radiation therapy or chemotherapy

Malignancies can directly cause premature ovarian failure. Furthermore, the nitroso compounds 1,3-bis(2-chloroethyl)-1-nitrosourea (BCNU) and 1-(-2-chloroethyl)-3-cyclohexyl-1-nitrosourea (CCNU) or procarbazine used for the chemotherapy of malignancies can produce ovarian failure, but amenorrhea is usually secondary.

Androgen insensitivity syndromes and other disorders of androgen action

Complete androgen insensitivity (testicular feminization)

This syndrome (with some incomplete varieties) is the most common form of male pseudohermaphroditism. There is no genital ambiguity, and these 46,XY individuals have the external appearance of normal females. At puberty they have a growth spurt and feminize completely, except that they have no pubic or axillary hair. The circulating levels of androgens are high, and significant quantities of estrogen are produced by the aromatization process. The estrogen receptors are intact, permitting development along female lines, but there is a defect in the androgen receptor that does not permit the production of androgen-dependent proteins. Because the chromosomal complement is XY, there are no internal female genital structures that derive from the Mullerian ducts, the uterus and fallopian tubes. The vagina is short and ends in a blind pouch, because the upper portion is derived from the Mullerian duct system. Incomplete forms of androgen insensitivity occur, but they may present with ambiguous genitalia (partial male differentiation).

Disorders of androgen action

This group also includes the syndromes associated with deficiency of 5α-reductase, the enzyme that reduces testosterone to dihydrotestosterone. A series of reports concerning patients in the Dominican Republic have described families with a 46,XY chromosomal complement raised as females, who underwent a striking degree of virilization at puberty. The genitalia had a female appearance at birth and throughout childhood, with a single perineal opening and a short vaginal pouch. As expected there are no Mullerian derivatives.

Secondary amenorrhea

In adolescents, the most common single cause of secondary amenorrhea is pregnancy. Hypergonadotropic amenorrhea is most often brought about by variants of Turner's syndrome (mosaicism) and less commonly to the other causes noted above, including surgical removal of the ovaries and uterus. However, chronic anovulation of central (hypothalamic and suprahypothalamic) origin is very common in the adolescent and includes polycystic ovary syndrome and partial forms of isolated gonadotropin deficiency described earlier. Secondary amenorrhea is the presenting symptom for a large array of conditions whose final pathway usually includes disruption of the GnRH signal to the pituitary gonadotrophs (Table 18.4). These conditions are represented schematically in Fig. 18.2. The diagram shows the interrelationships among the various purported factors that may lead to secondary amenorrhea.

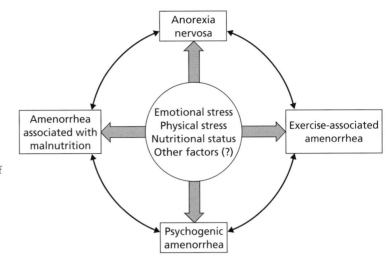

Fig. 18.2 Schematic representation of postulated associations among various forms of hypothalamic chronic anovulation and commonly linked factors. These disorders appear to be closely interrelated. From Rebar 1983.

Weight loss and related conditions

Simple weight loss is a very common cause of secondary amenorrhea, especially when social pressure is placed on adolescents to be thin. These adolescent women do not fulfill the strict psychiatric criteria for anorexia nervosa, although this latter condition is a well-described antecedent to secondary amenorrhea (Chapter 17). A useful differential point for diagnosis is that amenorrhea uniformly follows weight loss in the former condition, but often precedes weight loss in young women with anorexia nervosa. Its extreme form is noted in the desert-dwelling hunter-gatherers of the

Kalahari desert. Poor nutrition during the months of drought with increased energy expenditure to gather food and wood leads to low body weight and suppression of ovulation. During the rainy season, when food is more abundant and the work to gather food and fuel is less intense, the women regain cyclic ovulatory function and exhibit a peak time of giving birth exactly 9 months after attainment of maximal weight (van der Walt *et al.* 1978).

The important clinical features of anorexia are listed in Table 18.5. Malnutrition is often extreme and may far outstrip that of simple weight loss. The psychoneuroendocrine aspects may be secondary to

Table 18.5 DSM IV diagnostic criteria for anorexia nervosa (American Psychiatric Association 2000).

1 Refusal to maintain body weight at or above a minimally normal weight for age and height (e.g., weight loss leading to maintenance of body weight less than 85% of that expected; or failure to make expected weight gain during period of growth, leading to body weight less than 85% of that expected)

2 Intense fear of gaining weight or becoming fat, even though underweight

3 Disturbance in the way in which one's body weight or shape is experienced, undue influence of body weight or shape on self-evaluation, or denial of the seriousness of the current low body weight

4 In postmenarcheal females, amenorrhea (i.e., the absence of at least three consecutive menstrual cycles). A woman is considered to have amenorrhea if her periods occur only following hormone (e.g., estrogen, administration).

5 Two specific types:

(a) Restricting type: during the current episode of anorexia nervosa, the person has not regularly engaged in binge-eating or purging behavior (i.e., self-induced vomiting or the misuse of laxatives, diuretics, or enemas)

(b) Binge-eating/purging type: during the current episode of anorexia nervosa, the person has regularly engaged in binge-eating or purging behavior (i.e., self-induced vomiting or the misuse of laxatives, diuretics, or enemas) the central inhibition of the GnRH pulse generator resulting from metabolic signals from the inadequately nourished peripheral organs and/or may be a result of primary psychogenic causes. In either case there is inadequate GnRH stimulation to the gonadotrophs; this may be considered a protective mechanism to prevent the caloric drain of the menstrual cycle and pregnancy. Other neuroendocrine correlates include disorders of the circadian pattern of cortisol release indicative of significant activation ("stress"), but with suppression of adrenal androgen release. In a similar manner the hypothalamic–pituitary–thyroid axis is affected with a proportionately more profound decrease in tri-iodothyronine (T_3) than in thyroxine (T_4)—and an increase in reverse T_3 (rT_3). Teleologically, this pattern may serve as a protective mechanism to decrease the caloric expenditure (fuel savings), as manifest by significant and often severe abnormalities of thermoregulation.

Hyperprolactinemia

Hyperprolactinemia is a common cause of secondary amenorrhea in women of reproductive age; however, it is relatively uncommon in adolescents. Microadenomas and therapy with dopamine-antagonist drugs are the more common etiologies of hyperprolactinemia. Therapy of the former with dopamine agonists (e.g., bromocriptine or cabergoline) restores cyclic ovarian cycles and reduces the size of the tumor.

Psychogenic hypothalamic amenorrhea

Secondary amenorrhea may occur in women with depressive illness and in those with a history of other significant psychologic stresses. The stressors usually lead to hypogonadotropism based on inadequate suprahypothalamic stimulation of the hypothalamic GnRH pulse generator (Lachelen & Yen 1978). The mechanism may be related to inadequate positive feedback by estrogen or prolonged estrogen negative feedback (Santen *et al.* 1978).

Exercise-associated conditions

Delayed menarche, luteal phase dysfunction, and secondary amenorrhea have been associated with chronic endurance training, such as long-distance running and ballet dancing (Cumming & Rebar 1983; Keizer & Rogol 1990). Although reproductive system alterations are relatively common in chronically exercising women, no single etiology has been proven. This is not surprising given the multiplicity of factors involved: dietary changes, the hormonal effects of acute bouts of exercise performed chronically, probable alterations in steroid hormone metabolism and of altered body composition, and the psychologic and physical stress of the exercise itself (Fig. 18.3) (Rebar 1984).

Interpretation of the available epidemiologic and cross-sectional data does not provide a clear depiction of the pathogenetic mechanism(s) responsible for the reported alterations. A wide range for the

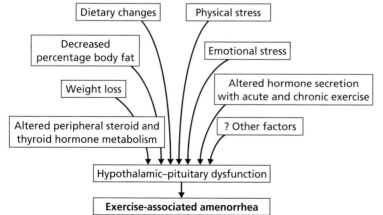

Fig. 18.3 Some factors apparently involved in the pathophysiology of exercise-associated amenorrhea. From Rebar 1984.

prevalence of "athletic amenorrhea" has been reported: 1–43% compared to 2.5% in the general population (for reviews see Bonen & Keizer 1984; Loucks & Horvath 1985; Keizer & Rogol 1990). This range is a result, to a large degree, of methodologic limitations, including the definition of amenorrhea which varies from 4 to 12 months, and wide variations that are included in the reports regarding chronologic age, gynecologic age, prior menstrual status, coincident health problems, and training duration and intensities. Younger competitive athletes appear to have a much higher incidence than older recreational joggers. Collectively, available cross-sectional studies indicate that the incidence of amenorrhea is considerably higher in young, intensively training, competitive athletes than in the general population. However, it must be recognized that alterations in cycle length may occur that do not produce amenorrhea. For example, three alterations —the short luteal phase, luteal phase insufficiency, and anovulation—can easily be missed when only menstrual data are obtained (DeSouza 2003). The highest incidence (5–7%) of anovulatory cycles is found in the early post-menarcheal years (Vollman 1977). The shortened luteal phase (Strott et al. 1970) may be regarded as a sequel to aberrant folliculogenesis (Sherman & Korenman 1974; DiZerega et al. 1981). However, a luteal phase of less than 10 days is also characteristic of the early post-menarcheal years, with a reported incidence of approximately 55% at a gynecologic age of less than 5 years (Vollman 1977). The available data indicate that strict standardization of gynecologic age, type of training, and training volume and intensity according to the subject's capabilities (standardized on lactate threshold or maximal oxygen uptake) is needed to compare data that might link exercise and athletic menstrual disorders.

Cross-sectional studies in intensively training adolescents have revealed that menstrual cycle lengths are not different from controls, whereas luteal phase insufficiency, short luteal phase, and anovulation are much more common in young athletes. There is an indication (Marx et al. 1986) that different types of activity evoke different hormonal responses, although selection criteria cannot be excluded. Estradiol, progesterone, and FSH levels have been consistently lower in intensively training adolescents or young women, whereas LH levels are either not different or higher than in controls. In more mature women, who began to train at a later gynecologic age, the prevalence of secondary amenorrhea is much lower than in younger individuals.

There are very few longitudinal studies available in which the lengths of the phases of the menstrual cycle were determined before and after training. Most involve few subjects, few hormone determinations, or a relatively short training period. Bullen et al. (1984) showed that modest training at 70% of $\dot{V}o_{2max}$ caused subtle changes in urinary hormone excretion. This study and that of Bonen and Keizer (1984) might be biased by the relatively short training period and the more moderate exercise intensity. The follow-up study by Bullen et al. (1985) carefully showed marked alterations in reproductive system function (e.g., lack of mid-cycle LH surge despite few indications of menstrual cycle disorders). However, the very marked vigorous training schedule over 2 months may have confounded the results because some of the women may have been overreached or overtrained (Keizer & Rogol 1990). Thus, a sudden increase in training volume and/or intensity may alter reproductive system function. Boyden et al. (1984) investigated 19 eumenorrheic (mean age 29.3 years) moderately trained women preparing for a marathon during 14–15 months of training (48–80 km·week^{-1}). Although menstrual cyclicity remained unaltered, subtle reproductive changes occurred including decreased LH and estradiol (single samples) and a decreased GnRH responsivity (in contrast to highly trained competitive runners, Veldhuis et al. 1985).

Our own prospective studies in older, previously sedentary women (average age 31.4 ± 1.4 years, 17.8 ± 0.9 years beyond menarche) produced remarkably little alteration in clinical reproductive status (e.g., menstrual cyclicity) in eumenorrheic, previously non-training women, despite running almost 1300 km in the first year (Rogol et al. 1992). Minimal changes were noted in the pulsatile release of LH, indicating little if any alteration in the hypothalamic GnRH pulse generator. We conclude that a progressive exercise program of moderate distance and intensity does not significantly alter the robust reproductive system of gynecologically mature eumenorrheic women who are likely in energy balance. Thus, the so-called "athletic amenorrhea" reported in cross-sectional studies may result from associated, or prior, non-exercise-dependent variables (especially younger gynecologic age and diminished energy intake compared to energy expenditure) that alone or in the aggregate affect the activity of the hypothalamic–pituitary–ovarian axis.

Although many possible mechanisms of altered brain–hypothalamic–pituitary–gonadal function in endurance training women have been proposed (Keizer & Rogol 1990), none has been unequivocally proven. The mechanism of stress-altered GnRH and gonadotropin release in runners has been suggested to include mediation by corticotropin-releasing hormone (CRH) and central endorphin pathways (Loucks & Horvath 1985; Villaneuva et al. 1986; Ding et al. 1988; Loucks et al. 1989). These mechanisms may be involved in many forms of hypothalamic (central) amenorrhea (Biller et al. 1990). Thus, in both eumenorrheic and amenorrheic runners, these mechanisms, along with others, may conspire to alter reproductive function. Although there are relatively direct effects of the endorphins and CRH on the adrenocorticotropic hormone (ACTH) rhythm and on the brain–GnRH–gonadotropin–gonadal axis, there are a host of other indirect actions at multiple hierarchical levels.

Exercise activates the hypothalamic–pituitary–adrenal axis acutely to varying degrees depending upon the intensity and duration of exercise (Farrell et al. 1983) and probably diminishes the firing rate of the GnRH pulse generator by increasing local levels of pro-opiomelanocortin-related peptides.

Others have suggested an interaction between the brain–hypothalamic–pituitary–adrenal and gonadal axes. Loucks et al. (1989) reported a blunted ACTH response to CRH and very mild hypercortisolism despite normal ACTH levels. Gambacciani et al. (1986) speculate from data in rats that a loss of negative feedback of cortisol at the level of the hippocampus may lead to increased CRH levels in the hypothalamus, which subsequently inhibits GnRH release. Taken together these data point to a central (brain or hypothalamic) mediation of altered gonadotropin release with a major input of the brain–

hypothalamic portion of the adrenal axis. Similar results (caused by "stress"?) have been reported in non-exercising women with hypothalamic amenorrhea (Biller et al. 1990). In addition to a certain poorly defined predisposition of certain women to menstrual cycle disorders, there is apparently a relationship between physical training and reproductive system alterations in endurance training women. However, evidence suggests that training must exceed a certain duration and/or intensity to inhibit pulsatile GnRH release. One may hypothesize that "overreaching" or "overtraining" (for definitions see Kuipers & Keizer 1988) may have an important role in altering the reproductive system. According to this thesis, a certain amount of training and/or a sudden increase in the amount or intensity of training is required to become "overreached." In this case, inappropriate or incomplete adaptation has occurred (Selye 1939).

Leptin is an adipose tissue-derived hormone (messenger) that signals the energy balance to the brain to regulate a number of metabolic processes, including reproduction (Moschos et al. 2002). Leptin affects GnRH neurons and GnRH pulsatility through a number of neuropeptides, including cocaine and amphetamine-regulated transcript peptide (CART), galanin-like peptide, and/or melanocortin-concentrating hormone (MCH) (Moschos et al. 2002). It may very well have a role in exercise-induced amenorrhea and other forms of functional hypothalamic amenorrhea (FHA). Short-term leptin administration studies (3 months) in women with FHA showed remarkable recovery of cyclic pituitary and ovarian function, including ovulation (Welt et al. 2004). Whether there is a role for leptin in exercise-associated hypothalamic amenorrhea, including those younger women with markedly delayed pubertal development, will await further studies. However, this new avenue for research holds more promise than almost anything else that has transpired in the past 20 years in this area of scientific inquiry.

Over the last decade the seemingly inconsistent data have been synthesized into the syndrome of the "female athlete triad" (Birch 2005). This syndrome is comprised of a constellation of signs and symptoms in three broad categories: disordered eating, menstrual dysfunction, and decreased bone mineral density. The American College of Sports Medicine Position Stand on the Female Athlete Triad (Otis *et al.* 1997) states that the triad "is a morbid condition comprising some degree of inadequate eating (in the extreme, a diagnostic eating disorder), some form of menstrual disorder (in the extreme, amenorrhea), and some degree of skeletal demineralization (in the extreme, osteoporosis)." I would add that for the adolescent athlete, amenorrhea could be primary or secondary and the skeletal disturbance could be failure to accrue an adequate peak bone mass. The complete syndrome, especially in adolescent athletes, is not only a risk at present —stress fractures, but also in the long term as osteoporosis becomes more and more likely if the accrued peak bone mass is well below the ideal.

If one considers not only the end points of the triad continuum—*clinical* eating disorders, amenorrhea, and osteoporosis—but to go beyond these three features and consider disordered eating, signs of menstrual dysfunction (e.g., luteal phase disturbances), and stress fractures, the number of young women who should have medical surveillance and consideration for treatment increases markedly (Torstveit & Sundgot-Borgen 2005). Treatment modalities such as increased food intake and decreased volume (and perhaps intensity) of exercise show low adherence especially in those athletes whose sports require the lean silhouette. There is now compelling evidence that restricting energy availability rather than an overly lean body composition (or stress) is the most likely factor in the etiology of reproductive system dysfunction in athletes (Loucks 2003). It seems merely a reflection of energy balance:

Energy retention = (energy intake − energy output)

where energy output includes resting metabolic rate, activity energy expenditure, and the thermal effect of feeding (digestion). Imbalance can come from either side of the equation.

A clinical example may put these thoughts into perspective. A 15.5-year-old female presents because of primary amenorrhea. She has had breast development for 1.5 years, but is growing slowly and her weight remains virtually constant. Her appetite, while not robust, is not much different than her not so seriously training sisters. She has no significant complaints of headache, nausea, vomiting, abdominal pain, or discomfort; but she has had one fibular stress fracture and multiple musculoskeletal injuries especially of the wrists and ankles. She is a competitive gymnast with approximately 20 h of training a week. Her mother had menarche at 14 years, but her two sisters who do not train seriously had menarche at 12.5 years.

She is an excellent student, but does not have much time for activities other than school and training. The height is 150 cm and the weight 40 kg. Her heart rate is 56 beats·min^{-1} and her blood pressure 103/66 mmHg. Her appearance is that of a much younger child. The general physical examination is normal and she has 12-year molars in all quadrants. The optical fundi are normal. The thyroid is not palpably enlarged. She has axillary hair and PH Tanner stage III. The breasts are early Tanner stage III with very little development of the areolae and nipples.

The bone age is 12.5 years, the biochemical profile is normal as is the complete blood count. Endocrine laboratory data: LH 0.6 IU/L, FSH 2.1 IU/L, estradiol <10 pg/mL, prolactin 4.4 ng·mL^{-1}, IGF-I 140 ng·mL^{-1}, free T$_4$ 1.2 ng·dL^{-1}, and TSH 1.1 μ IU·mL^{-1}. The interpretation of the data is that she has short stature, delayed pubertal development, and no obvious endocrine abnormality (hypothyroidism, hyperprolactinemia, or growth hormone deficiency). The gonadotropin and estradiol levels are consistent with hypogonadotropic hypogonadism, but most likely merely denote that the transition from the prepubertal hiatus to puberty has not occurred; that is, it is physiologic and not pathologic.

In summary, the history, including that of her diet, exercise, and medical are consistent with "athletic amenorrhea," but no test is diagnostic. The important point is that she will be at risk for osteoporosis later in life if she remains hypoestrogenemic. She clearly loads her skeleton to a sufficient degree to sufficiently mineralize bone.

Treatment may be difficult. The most straightforward approach would be to prescribe a larger caloric intake. That would likely surpass the "energy" deficiency and the hypothalamic–pituitary–gonadal axis would awaken from its prepubertal hiatus. That is a difficult treatment plan for a highly competitive gymnast. The drug of choice would be medroxyprogesterone acetate, a progestational agent to attempt to induce menses. If successful that would suggest adequate estrogenization and would medically induce sloughing of the endometrium. That outcome is unlikely given the lack of outward signs or biochemical evidence for pubertal development. What likely will be efficacious as well as acceptable would be a 12.5–25 μg dose of estradiol, transcutaneously, by patch twice weekly; that is, change patches every 3.5 days. Medroxyprogesterone may be added after about a year (escalating doses of estradiol) if spontaneous uterine bleeding has not started.

The American Academy of Pediatrics Committee of Sports Medicine and Fitness, 1999–2000 has presented a series of recommendations (2000). Those key to the female athlete triad include:
- Dietary practices; exercise intensity, duration, and frequency; and menstrual history should be reviewed during evaluations that precede participation in sports.
- Amenorrhea should not be considered a normal response to exercise.
- Disordered eating should be considered in adolescents with amenorrhea.
- Education and counseling should be provided to athletes, parents, and coaches regarding disordered eating, menstrual dysfunction, decreased bone mineralization, and adequate energy and nutrient intake to meet energy expenditure and maintain normal growth and development.

- An adolescent with menstrual dysfunction attributed to exercise should be encouraged to increase energy intake and modify excessive exercise activity to get back into energy balance.
- Estrogen–progesterone supplementation may be considered in mature amenorrheic (late adolescent) athletes.
- Measurement of bone mineral density should be considered a tool to help make treatment decision. Remember the adolescent athlete has not reached her peak bone mass; therefore, comparison of bone density should be made on age-appropriate z- (*not* t-) scores.

Challenges for future research

- To determine the role of leptin and other metabolic and neuropeptides in the genesis and maintenance of functional hypothalamic amenorrhea.
- To determine the influence of the CRH–pituitary–adrenal axis on the GnRH–pituitary–gonadal axis and its modulation by exercise.
- To determine the genetic, nutritional, hormonal, and neuropeptide mechanisms that subserve alterations in body composition and the regional distribution of fat in girls at adolescence. This is to determine: (i) the influence on menarche itself; and (ii) the mechanisms by which endurance exercise alters these relationships.
- To determine the nutritional, stress, and hormonal mechanisms for secondary amenorrhea in athletes and their non-exercising cohort.

References

American Academy of Pediatrics: Committee on Sports Medicine and Fitness (2000) Medical concerns in the female athlete. *Pediatrics* 106, 610–613.

American Psychiatric Association (2000) *Diagnostic and Statistical Manual of Mental Disorders*, 4th edn. Text revision. American Psychiatric Association, Washington DC.

Ardern, C.I., Janssen, I., Ross, R. & Katzmarzyk, P.T. (2004) Development of health-related waist circumference thresholds within BMI categories. *Obesity Research* 12, 1094–1103.

Ardern, C.I., Katzmarzyk, P.T., Janssen, I. & Ross, R. (2003) Discrimination of

health risk by combined body mass index and waist circumference. *Obesity Research* 11, 135–142.

Betterle, C., Dal Pra, C., Mantero, F. & Zanchetta, R. (2002) Autoimmune adrenal insufficiency and autoimmune polyendocrine syndromes: autoantibodies, autoantigens, and the applicability in diagnosis and disease prediction. *Endocrine Reviews* 23, 327–364.

Biller, B., Federoff, H. & Koenig, J. (1990) Abnormal cortisol secretion and responses to corticotropin releasing hormone in women with hypothalamic amenorrhea. *Journal of Clinical*

Endocrinology and Metabolism 70, 311–317.

Birch, K. (2005) Female athlete trial. *British Medical Journal* 330, 244–246.

Bonen, A. & Keizer, H. (1984) Athletic menstrual cycle irregularity: endocrine response to exercise and training. *The Physician and Sportsmedicine* 12, 78–94.

Bouchard, C., Depres, J.-P. & Mauriege, P. (1993) Genetic and nongenetic determinants of regional fat distribution. *Endocrine Reviews* 14, 72–93.

Boyden, T.W., Pamenter, R.W., Stanforth, P., Rotkis, T. & Wilmore, J. (1984)

Impaired gonadotropin responses to gonadotropin-releasing hormone stimulation in 20 endurance-trained women. *Fertility and Sterility* **41**, 359–363.

Bullen, B., Skrinar, G., Beitins, L., *et al.* (1984) Endurance training effects on plasma hormonal responsiveness and sex hormone excretion. *Journal of Applied Physiology: Respiratory, Environmental and Exercise Physiology* **56**, 1453–1463.

Bullen, B., Skrinar, G., Beitins, I., VonMering G., Twinbull, B. & McArthur, J. (1985) Induction of menstrual cycle disorders by strenuous exercise in untrained women. *New England Journal of Medicine* **312**, 1349–1353.

Cumming, D. & Rebar, R. (1983) Exercise and reproductive function in women: a review. *American Journal of Industrial Medicine* **4**, 113–125.

Dattani, M., Martinez-Barbera, J., Thomas, P.Q., *et al.* (2000) Molecular genetics of septo-optic dysplasia. *Hormone Research* **53** (Supplement 1), 26–33.

Dattani, M. & Preece, M. (2004) Growth hormone deficiency and related disorders: insights into causation, diagnosis, and treatment. *Lancet* **363**, 1977–1987.

de Ridder, C., Bruning, P., Zonderland, M., *et al.* (1990) Body fat mass, body fat distribution and plasma hormones in early puberty in females. *Journal of Clinical Endocrinology and Metabolism* **70**, 888–893.

DeSouza, M.J. (2003) Menstrual disturbance in athletes: a focus on luteal phase defects. *Medicine and Science in Sports and Exercise* **35**, 1553–1563.

Després, J.P., Lemieux, I. & Prud'homme, D. (2001) Treatment of obesity: need to focus on high risk abdominally obese patients. *British Medical Journal* **322**, 716–720.

Ding, J.-H., Sheckter, C., Drinkwater, B., Soules, M. & Bremner, W. (1988) High serum cortisol levels in exercise-associated amenorrhea. *Annals of Internal Medicine* **108**, 530–534.

DiZerega, G., Turner, C., Stouffer, R., Anderson, L., Charming, C. & Hodgen, G. (1981) Suppression of follicle stimulating hormone-dependent folliculogenesis during the primate ovarian cycle. *Journal of Clinical Endocrinology and Metabolism* **52**, 451–456.

ElSheikh, M., Dunger, D.B., Conway, G.S. & Wass, J.A.H. (2002) Turner's syndrome in adulthood. *Endocrine Reviews* **23**, 120–140.

Farrell, P., Garthwaite, T. & Gustafson, A. (1983) Plasma adrenocorticotropin and cortisol responses to submaximal and exhaustive exercise. *Journal of Applied Physiology: Respiratory, Environmental and Exercise Physiology* **55**, 1441–1444.

Frisancho, A. & Flegel, P. (1982) Advanced maturation with centripetal fat pattern. *Human Biology* **54**, 717–727.

Gambacciani, M., Yen, S. & Rasmussen, D. (1986) GnRH release from the mediobasal hypothalamus: *in vitro* inhibition by corticotropin-releasing factor. *Neuroendoerinology* **43**, 533–536.

Haavisto, A.-M., Dunkel, L., Petterson, K. & Huhtaniemi, I. (1990) LH measurements by *in vitro* bioassay and a highly sensitive immunofluorometric assay improve the distinction between boys with constitutional delay of puberty and hypogonadotropie hypogonadism. *Pediatric Research* **27**, 211–214.

Keizer, H. & Rogol, A. (1990) Physical exercise and menstrual cycle alterations: what are the mechanisms? *Sports Medicine* **10**, 218–235.

Kuipers, H. & Keizer, H. (1988) Overtraining in elite athletes. *Sports Medicine* **6**, 79–92.

Lachelin, G. & Yen, S. (1978) Hypothalamic chronic anovulation. *American Journal of Obstetrics and Gynecology* **130**, 825–831.

Loucks, A. (2004) Energy balance and body composition in sports and exercise. *Journal of Sports Medicine* **22**, 1–14.

Loucks, A. & Horvath, S. (1985) Athletic amenorrhea: a review. *Medicine and Science in Sports and Exercise* **17**, 56–72.

Loucks, A.B. (2003) Introduction to menstrual disturbances in athletes. *Medicine and Science in Sports and Exercise* **35**, 1551–1552.

Loucks, A.B., Laughlin, G.A., Mortola, J.F., Girton, L., Nelson, J.C. & Yen, S.S.C. (1989) Alterations in the hypothalamic-pituitary-ovarian and the hypothalamic-pituitary-adrenal axes in athletic women. *Journal of Clinical Endocrinology and Metabolism* **75**, 514–518.

Malina, R.M., Bouchard, C. & Bar-Or, O. (2004) *Growth, Maturation, and Physical Activity*. Human Kinetics Press, Champaign, IL.

Marshall, W.A. & Tanner, J. (1969) Variations in pattern of pubertal changes in girls. *Archives of Disease in Childhood* **44**, 291–303.

Martha, P. Jr., Gorman, K., Blizzard, R., Rogol, A. & Veldhuis, J. (1992) Endogenous growth hormone secretion and clearance rates in normal boys as determined by deconvolution analysis: relationship to age, pubertal status and body mass index. *Journal of Clinical Endocrinology and Metabolism* **74**, 336–344.

Martha, P. Jr., Rogol, A., Veldhuis, J., Kerrigan, J., Goodman, D. & Blizzard, R. (1989) Alterations in the pulsatile properties of circulating growth hormone concentrations during puberty in boys. *Journal of Clinical Endocrinology and Metabolism* **69**, 563–570.

Marx, K., Kische, B., Lenz, H. & Hoffmann, P. (1986) Die Gonadotropin and Sexualsteroide wdhrend des Menstruationszyklus bei jungen sporttreibenden Frauen. *Medizin und Sport* **26**, 51–54.

Mauras, N., Blizzard, R., Link, K., Johnson, M., Rogol, A. & Veldhuis, J. (1987) Augmentation of growth hormone secretion during puberty: evidence for a pulse amplitude-modulated phenomenon. *Journal of Clinical Endocrinology and Metabolism* **64**, 596–601.

Moschos, S., Chan, J.L. & Mantzoros, C.S. (2002) Leptin and reproduction: a review. *Fertility and Sterility* **77**, 433–444.

Nezelof, C. & Basset, F. (1998) Langerhans cell histiocytosis research: past, present, and future. *Hematology Oncology Clinics of North America* **12**, 385–406.

Otis, C.L., Drinkwater, B.L., Johnson, M., Loucks, A.B. & Wilmore, J.H. (1997) ACSM Position Stand on the female athlete triad. *Medicine and Science in Sports and Exercise* **29**, i–ix.

Parks, J.S., Brown, M.R., Hurley, D.L., Phelps, C.J. & Wajnrajch, M.P. (1999) Heritable disorders of pituitary development. *Journal of Clinical Endocrinology and Metabolism* **84**, 4362–4370.

Rappoport, R. & Brauner, R. (1989) Growth and endocrine disorders secondary to cranial irradiation. *Pediatric Research* **25**, 561–567.

Rebar, R.W. (1983) The reproductive age: chronic anovulation. In: *The Ovary* (Serra, G.B., ed.) Raven Press, New York: 217–240.

Rebar, R.W. (1984) Effect of exercise on reproductive function in females. In: *The Hypothalamus in Health and Disease* (Givens, J.R., ed.) Year Book, Chicago: 245.

Redmond, L.M. & Loucks, A.B. (2005) Menstrual disorders in athletes. *Sports Medicine* **35**, 747–755.

Richards, G., Wara, W., Grumbach, M., Kaplan, S., Sheline, G. & Conte, F. (1976) Delayed onset of hypopituitarism: sequelae of therapeutic irradiation of central nervous system, eye and middle ear tumors. *Journal of Pediatrics* **89**, 533–539.

Roemmich, J.N., Clark, P.A., Mai, V., *et al.* (1998) Alterations in growth and body composition during puberty, III. Influence of maturation, gender, body composition, body fat distribution, aerobic fitness and total energy expenditure on nocturnal growth hormone release during puberty. *Journal of Clinical Endocrinology and Metabolism* **83**, 1440–1447.

Rogol, A., Weltman, A., Weltman, J. et al. (1992) Durability of the reproductive axis in eumenorrheic women during 1 year of endurance training. *Journal of Applied Physiology* **72**, 1571–1580.

Rose, S., Municchi, G., Barnes, K., *et al.* (1991) Spontaneous growth hormone secretion increases during puberty in normal girls and boys. *Journal of Clinical Endocrinology and Metabolism* **73**, 428–435.

Santen, R., Friend, J., Trejanowski, D., Davis, B., Samojlike, E. & Barden, C. (1978) Prolonged negative feedback suppression after estradiol administration: proposed mechanism

of eugonadal secondary amenorrhea. *Journal of Clinical Endocrinology and Metabolism* **47**, 1220–1229.

Selye, H. (1939) The effect of adaptations to various damaging agents on the female sex organs in the rat. *Endocrinology* **25**, 615–624.

Sherman, B. & Korenman, S. (1974) Measurement of plasma LH FSH, estradiol and progesterone in disorders of the human menstrual cycle: the short luteal phase. *Journal of Clinical Endocrinology and Metabolism* **38**, 89–93.

Silveira, L.F.G., MacColl, G.S. & Bouloux, P.M.G. (2002) Hypogonadotropic hypogonadism. *Seminars in Reproductive Medicine* **20**, 327–338.

Stratakis, C.A. & Rennert, O.M. (2005) Turner syndrome: an update. *The Endocrinolgist* **15**, 27–36.

Strott, C., Cargille, C., Ross, G. & Lipsett, M. (1970) The short luteal phase. *Journal of Clinical Endocrinology and Metabolism* **30**, 246–251.

Sybert, V.P. (2004) Turner's syndrome. *New England Journal of Medicine* **351**, 1227–1238.

Tanner, J. (199) *Foetus into Man: Physical Growth from Conception to Maturity.* Harvard University Press, Cambridge, MA: 1–103.

Theintz, G.E., Howals, H., Weiss, U. & Sizonenko, P.C. (1993) Evidence for a reduction of growth potential in adolescent female gymnasts. *Journal of Pediatrics* **122**, 306–313.

Thoms, M., Claessens, A.L., LeFevre, J., Philippaerts, R., Beunen, G.P. & Malina, R.M. (2005) Adolescent growth spurt in female gymnasts. *Journal of Pediatrics* **146**, 239–244.

Torstveit, M.K. & Sundgot-Borgen, J. The female athlete triad: Are elite athletes at increased risk? *Medicine and Science in Sports and Exercise* **37**, 184–193.

van der Walt, L., Wilmsen, E. & Jenkins, T. (1978) Unusual sex hormone patterns among desert dwelling hunter-gatherers. *Journal of Clinical Endocrinology and Metabolism* **46**, 658–663.

Veldhuis, J., Evans, W., Demers, L., Thorner, M., Wakat, D. & Rogol, A. (1985) Altered neuroendocrine regulation of gonadotropin secretion in women distance runners. *Journal of Clinical Endocrinology and Metabolism* **61**, 557–563.

Villaneuva, A., Schlosser, C., Hopper, B., Liu, J., Hoffmah, D. & Rebar, R. (1986) Increased cortisol production in women runners. *Journal of Clinical Endocrinology and Metabolism* **63**, 133–136.

Vollman, R. (1977) *The Menstrual Cycle.* W.B. Saunders, Philadelphia.

Welt, C.K., Chan, J.L., Bullem, J., *et al.* (2004) Recombinant human leptin in women with hypothalamic amenorrhea. *New England Journal of Medicine* **351**, 987–997.

Chapter 19

Cardiovascular Concerns in the Young Athlete

THOMAS W. ROWLAND

Ironically, the same cardiovascular responses to exercise that provide the physical and psychosocial benefits of sports play may—albeit rarely—impose serious risk. Fortunately, the number of individuals in jeopardy is very small, and current evidence suggests that risk is incurred only by those with underlying abnormalities of the cardiovascular system. Certain issues notwithstanding (see "Cardiac fatigue" below), young athletes with a normal cardiovascular system do not appear to be vulnerable to cardiac damage or sudden death during sports training or competition. In this chapter we address the forms of heart disease that pose danger for sports play in youth, the mechanisms and clinical expressions of that risk, and the means by which adverse or tragic outcomes might be avoided.

Cardiac fatigue

Exercise places heavy work demands on myocardial function. During even moderate intensity endurance exercise, myocardial oxygen uptake may increase three- to fivefold compared to resting values (Heiss *et al.* 1976). During resistance exercise, which places less demand on blood circulation, elevations in blood pressure cause a significant rise in myocardial wall stress. Moreover, in comparison to skeletal muscle, the myocardium is not permitted time to stop and recover during physical activities—that is, for the heart muscle there are no time outs, water stops, or coasting downhill. The heart is metabolically an obligatory aerobic organ so, because periods of oxygen starvation are not permitted, no opportunity can be provided to build up an oxygen debt.

Given these high demands, it will come as no surprise that the stresses of sustained high levels of exercise may result in fatigue and microdamage of cardiac muscle. Such effects have been clearly identified in skeletal muscle, but the extent that exercise stress can diminish contractile force and disrupt integrity of cell membranes in cardiac muscle has not been clearly demonstrated. Moreover, the clinical consequences of any such effects as well as their potential influence on exercise performance are not clear.

Studies in adults

Several echocardiographic studies in adult athletes competing in events such as ultramarathons or 24-h runs have indicated a transient pre-race to post-race decline in left ventricular contractility as indicated by a fall in shortening fraction (for review see Dawson *et al.* 2003). For example, Niemela *et al.* (1984) reported a 16% decline in left ventricular shortening fraction and 9% fall in mean velocity of circumferential fiber shortening in 13 adult male runners after a 24-h race. In many of these studies, however, the influences of modifying factors on shortening fraction, particularly decreased ventricular filling volume from dehydration, were not clearly assessed. Shortening fraction values typically normalize by 24–48 h post-race, without evidence of sequelae.

In reviewing these studies, Dawson *et al.* (2003) concluded that the major factor in the development of diminished contractility was duration of the event. A fall in shortening fraction in adult athletes has not been reported during competitions less prolonged than a half triathlon.

Evidence of cellular disruption following intense or prolonged exercise by a rise in serum enzymes associated with myocardial ischemia or necrosis has been equally ambivalent. Some early studies revealed a small rise following marathon running in the muscle–brain isoenzyme of creatine kinase (CK-MB), which typically increases in adults with ischemic heart events from atherosclerotic coronary artery disease (Apple *et al.* 1984). However, as no other markers of myocardial ischemia were evident, this finding may instead reflect the release of CK-MB found in trained skeletal rather than cardiac muscle.

More recent exercise studies have indicated small increases in blood levels of cardiac troponin I and T, more specific markers of myocardial damage, such that "it is tempting to speculate that stressful, prolonged intense exercise may result in minor, reversible myocyte degeneration in humans" (Koller 2003). On the other hand, other reports have failed to demonstrate troponin changes with exercise, a confusion that may reflect differences in factors such as imprecision in different types of troponin assays and timing of procuring blood specimens (Dawson *et al.* 2003).

In summary, whether intense exercise can truly cause myocardial fatigue and injury is not well documented. Current information in adult athletes suggests that if such damage does occur, it only follows extreme bouts of exercise, is transient, and has no obvious detrimental effect. This question may bear particular significance, however, for young endurance athletes, whose myocardial stresses during competition and training occur in a *developing* myocardium. That is, recurrent exercise-induced myocardial injury might have no significance for the mature heart, but could theoretically have detrimental effects on growing cardiac tissue.

Studies in youths

The very limited available information on this issue in child athletes is reassuring. When Rost (1987) studied young swimmers with serial echocardiograms over a 10-year period, "there was no evidence to suggest that the early start of high-performance training had any bearing on the development of cardiac damage." Rowland *et al.* (1997) performed echocardiograms before and immediately after a 4-km road race in nine trained boys aged 9–14 years. Mean values of left ventricular shortening fraction did not change, while body weight and ventricular end-diastolic dimension declined, presumably as a result of dehydration. These returned to pre-race values on a follow-up test 24 h afterwards.

Importantly, there have been no clinical reports of cardiac complications as an increasing number of immature endurance athletes have become involved in highly intensive training regimens. This informal mass "experiment" is further indication that intense athletic training in the growing years does not create risk of stress-induced injury to the growing heart. Continued scrutiny of cardiac findings in elite level child athletes will be important, however, in verifying this conclusion.

The question of cardiac fatigue with exercise becomes more pertinent in youths with heart disease who wish to participate in sports. Intuitively, those who demonstrate evidence of depressed myocardial function at rest (i.e., patients with dilated cardiomyopathy, postoperative cyanotic heart disease) might incur further damage from augmented heart work demands, and participation in high intensity sports is therefore not advised (Graham *et al.* 1994).

Defining the potential impact of sports training on myocardial function in youth with milder forms of heart disease becomes more problematic. For example, what recommendations should be made to an adolescent cross-country runner with mild to moderate aortic valve insufficiency who has minimal left ventricular enlargement, normal shortening fraction, and no dysrhythmias? The concern in this athlete is that:

1 Long-standing volume overload on the left ventricle from valvular regurgitation might eventuate in myocardial dysfunction; and

2 The cardiac responses to endurance exercise create additive myocardial stress and could potentially hasten this process.

On the other hand, cardiac responses to endurance training that improve myocardial efficiency might prove beneficial.

At the present time there is no research information by which this dilemma might easily be resolved.

Generally, athletes in this category who are clinically stable have been permitted full sports participation with serial exercise testing and echocardiography (Cheitlin *et al.* 1994). Any evidence of progression (enlarging left ventricular size, fall in shortening fraction, diminished exercise capacity) would signal a need to restrict at least some forms of sports play.

Sudden death with heart disease

Sudden death from heart disease, with or without exercise, is fortunately a rare event in the pediatric population. Unlike adults with coronary artery disease, the common forms of cardiac abnormalities in children (congenital heart anomalies) are not typically associated with mechanisms for sudden death. In a small minority, however, the potential exists for fatal events from myocardial ischemia, ventricular dysrhythmias, or elevations in pulmonary blood pressure. As these mechanisms are potentiated by the myocardial demands of physical activity, patients with severe aortic outflow obstruction, cyanotic heart disease, ventricular tachyarrhythmias, and primary or secondary pulmonary hypertension are usually restricted from intense sports play (Graham *et al.* 1994).

The larger difficulty for clinicians—and the fear of parents and coaches—is the grim tragedy of sudden unexpected cardiac death in young athletes who have occult, unrecognized cardiovascular abnormalities. The high public visibility of these shocking events has generated a great deal of anxiety regarding this risk as well as considerations of how such tragedies might be prevented. The good news is that sudden cardiac death of an apparently healthy young athlete during participation in sports is exceedingly rare. The incidence of such an event is considered to be about 1 in every 250,000 athletes (Maron *et al.* 1996). The unfortunate news is that in many cases the current approach to preparticipation screening may fail to detect would-be athletes who are at risk.

The forms of covert cardiovascular abnormalities that predispose the young athlete for sudden death during sports play have been well defined (Table 19.1). In general, it is the lack of premonitory symptoms and clinical findings that permit the

Table 19.1 Etiology of sudden cardiac death in young athletes in 134 cases reported by Maron *et al.* (1996).

Cardiovascular abnormality	Cases (%)
Hypertrophic cardiomyopathy	36.0
Aberrant coronary arteries	13.0
Other coronary abnormalities	10.0
Unexplained increased cardiac mass	10.0
Ruptured aortic aneurysm	5.0
Valvular aortic stenosis	4.0
Myocarditis	3.0
Dilated cardiomyopathy	3.0
Arrhythmogenic right ventricle	3.0
Other	10.0
Unexplained	2.0

more common, such as hypertrophic cardiomyopathy and congenital coronary artery anomalies, to head this list.

Hypertrophic cardiomyopathy

Hypertrophic cardiomyopathy is an autosomal dominant inherited condition characterized by dramatic myocardial thickening, particularly of the ventricular septum (thus, the alternative name, asymmetric septal hypertrophy). In some cases, more commonly in adults, muscular hypertrophy causes obstruction to aortic outflow (consequently yet another name, idiopathic hypertrophic subaortic stenosis). The cause of sudden death in patients with hypertrophic cardiomyopathy is not certain but presumably occurs as a consequence of coronary insufficiency and ischemia within the thickened ventricular wall.

Vigorous physical activity increases risk of sudden death with hypertrophic cardiomyopathy, and individuals with this condition are therefore restricted from competitive athletic play. The reason it ranks as the most common cause of sudden unexpected cardiac death in young athletes reflects the notorious difficulty in detecting hypertrophic cardiomyopathy by physical examination. Hence, would-be athletes with this condition frequently go undetected during the preparticipation sports evaluation (Maron *et al.* 1982).

A family history of individuals with hypertrophic cardiomyoapthy can typically only be obtained in approximately 20% of cases. Previous symptoms of chest pain, dizziness, or syncope can be indicators of the presence of this disease but are usually absent. A heart murmur, if present, may sound functional. Abnormalities in pulses, changes in murmur with body position, and the presence of a murmur of mitral insufficiency are usually observed in adult but not adolescent patients.

The electrocardiogram is almost always abnormal, demonstrating deep Q waves over the left precordial leads, left ventricular hypertrophy, and/or ischemic ST-T wave changes. The echocardiogram provides the definitive diagnosis, with a ventricular septum usually measuring over 15–16 mm, over twice the normal measurement. Consequently, it has been suggested that the echocardiogram should become a standard component of the preparticipation evaluation. Such an approach, although intuitively attractive, is rendered difficult not only by the expense but also by the large number of false positive cases that would be identified of mild ventricular thickening, particularly in a group of trained athletes. The same prohibitive problem would occur with use of the electrocardiogram as a routine screening tool.

Coronary artery anomalies

Atherosclerotic coronary artery disease does not pose a risk for athletes in the growing years. However, rare cases of congenital anomalous origin of coronary blood vessels may compromise flow to heart muscle with physical activity and cause sudden death during sports play. The most common is an origin of the left main coronary artery from the right sinus of Valsalva, which may limit coronary flow either by its compression between the aorta and main pulmonary artery or by functional obstruction at its os. Many other variations have been observed, including right coronary artery arising from the left sinus and the left coronary originating from the pulmonary artery. Also included in this list of anomalies that restrict coronary flow with exercise are congenital hypoplasia or stenosis of coronary vessels and coronary arteries buried in heart muscle.

Although life-threatening congenital anomalies of the coronary arteries are exceedingly rare, they typically rank second among causes of sudden unexpected cardiac death in young athletes. Even more so than hypertrophic cardiomyopathy, they are usually clinically silent, without symptoms or abnormalities on cardiac examination. Indeed, often the first sign of this condition is the sudden collapse of an apparently healthy young athlete during sports play (Basso *et al.* 2000).

Marfan's syndrome

Marfan's syndrome is a hereditary disease of exaggerated laxity of connective tissue. In its most serious manifestation, the base of the ascending aorta widens, with progressive aneurysmal dilatation, rupture, and sudden death. Because conditions of high cardiac output might accelerate this progression, and sudden blows to the chest might trigger aneurysm rupture, individuals with Marfan's syndrome are often restricted from sports play (Braverman 1998).

The diagnosis is suspected by the multiple phenotypic findings that constitute the syndrome: tall stature with long arms, arachnodactyly, and hyperextensible joints; scoliosis, pectus excavatum deformity, and flat feet; ocular findings of dislocated lens and myopia; and evidence of mitral valve prolapse, mitral regurgitation, and aortic insufficiency on cardiac auscultation. Typically, only portions of the syndrome are evident in a given patient, and because at present there is no "test" for this disease, the diagnosis of Marfan's syndrome is sometimes problematic. Echocardiographic findings of aortic root dilatation and mitral valve prolapse confirm cardiac manifestations of Marfan's syndrome and may signal a need for sports restriction.

Recognition of the physical findings of Marfan's syndrome on preparticipation sports screening, particularly if there is a family history of individuals with this disorder, should prompt referral to a cardiologist. Besides sports restriction, prescription of beta-blocker medication is often warranted to diminish progression of aortic root dilatation, and surgical intervention can be offered when the aortic root diameter reaches a concerning size (about 55 mm).

Long QT syndrome

Conduction abnormalities may also pose a risk to the young athlete. In patients with long QT syndrome, myocardial electrical recovery is delayed, a condition that creates a risk for life-threatening ventricular tachyarrhythmias. The diagnosis is made by identifying an overly long QT interval, a marker of ventricular repolarization, on the electrocardiogram. The normal QT interval, corrected for heart rate, is 0.36–0.44 s, while in those with long QT syndrome corrected values are typically at least 0.50 s. Long QT syndrome can be inherited in both an autosomal dominant and recessive pattern, but in one-third of cases there is no family history (Vincent 2000).

Sudden death in individuals with long QT syndrome is frequently associated with hyperadrenergic situations such as sports play and times of anger, fear, or fright. Interestingly, swimming appears to place these patients at particular risk (Schwartz et al. 1991). The contribution of such events to the frequency of sudden death during sports play is not certain. In autopsy series of these deaths there always remains a few percent that are "unexplained." It has been surmised that long QT syndrome may have been responsible for these cases.

It is important, then, to identify young would-be athletes with long QT syndrome and restrict them from competitive sports play. Detection may come from a screening electrocardiogram performed in a child with a family history of unexplained sudden death. Alternatively, ventricular tachyarrhythmias from long QT syndrome is in the differential diagnosis of patients who experience syncope or seizures, with or without sports play. An electrocardiogram is an essential part of the evaluation of these youngsters to assess QT interval duration.

Sudden death without structural heart disease

It has generally been considered that children and adolescents without underlying structural or electrical heart disease are not at risk for cardiac catastrophes during sports play. There are, however, certain conditions that afflict the healthy heart and may be responsible for sudden collapse and death during athletic training and/or competition.

Commotio cordis

It has long been recognized that sudden death may be precipitated by a non-penetrating blow to the chest in the region overlying the heart (commotio cordis, or concussion of the heart). Such tragedies have occurred in youths who have been struck with a variety of sports equipment (baseballs, hockey pucks, lacrosse balls, hockey sticks) as well as body parts (knees, fists, feet, elbows). Sudden death appears to occur by ventricular fibrillation, although cases of cardiac asystole have been reported. Fibrillation is triggered in these cases by the blow occurring at a vulnerable period in the cardiac cycle (near the peak of the T wave, at 60–90% of the QT interval) (Geddes & Roeder 2005).

The risk of these unfortunate incidents is very small but seems to be largely confined to children and young adolescents. The average age of reported cases is 11–12 years, with an age range of 3–19 years. Inexplicably, almost all cases have involved males (Maron et al. 1995).

Myocarditis

Instances of sudden death during exercise have been reported in young athletes as well as military recruits in the midst of viral respiratory infections, with histologic evidence of subclinical myocarditis at autopsy (Lynch 1980). Death in these cases is presumably secondary to ventricular dysrhythmias in inflamed conduction tissue. Given the ubiquitous nature of viral infections in the pediatric population, the risk of such an event would seem extraordinarily small. Still, concern has been raised regarding the risks of intense sports play during viral infections. However, as McCaffrey et al. (1991) have noted, "to restrict participation on he basis of a low-grade fever, or to recommend evaluation of such non-cardiac symptoms by a cardiologist is both impractical and unrealistic." Some have suggested restricting athletes from play who do not "feel well" or have muscle aching (as a marker of muscle involvement) as part of their viral syndrome.

Drugs

Although not expected in young athletes, older adolescents may suffer sudden death from cocaine use, and other drugs, particularly adrenergic stimulants, have been suspected. Cocaine causes constriction of the coronary arteries, with resulting myocardial ischemia and ventricular tachyarrhythmias. Sudden death can occur regardless of dose (Isner *et al.* 1986).

Conclusions

There exists an exceedingly small but finite risk for sudden death or heart injury during sports play in young athletes. The chance of these occurrences may be reduced by identification of at-risk athletes during the preparticipation evaluation. To achieve this, a careful cardiac examination and medical history (with particular attention to previous chest pain or syncope with exercise, as well as a family history of unexpected early cardiac death) remain the most appropriate screening diagnostic tools. It should be recognized, however, that some risk of adverse cardiac events must be accepted as an inevitable aspect of sports participation.

Challenges for future research

More information is needed regarding the possibility of myocardial fatigue during prolonged exercise in young athletes. Defining this risk could influence limitations on immature competitors in events such as marathon running.

Genetic markers for hereditary cardiac abnormalities such as hypertrophic cardiomyopathy, long QT syndrome, and Marfan's syndrome need to be refined and made clinically available. Such testing would greatly improve the chance of detecting would-be athletes at risk for sudden death during sports play.

The balance of salutary and injurious effects on the myocardium during sports training in children with heart disease needs to be lineated.

References

Apple, F.S., Rogers, M.A. & Sherman, W.M. (1984) Profile of creatine kinase isoenzymes in skeletal muscle of marathon runners. *Clinical Chemistry* **30**, 413–416.

Basso, C., Maron, B.J., Corrado, D. & Thiene, G. (2000) Clinical profile of congenital coronary artery anomalies with origin from the wrong aortic sinus leading to sudden death in young competitive athletes. *Journal of the American College of Cardiology* **35**, 1493–1501.

Braverman, A.C. (1998) Exercise and the Marfan syndrome. *Medicine and Science in Sports and Exercise* **30** (Supplement), S387–S395.

Cheitlin, M.D., Douglas, P.S. & Parmley, W.W. (1994) Acquired valvular heart disease. *Circulation* **26** (Supplement), S254–S260.

Dawson, E., George, K., Shave, R., Whyte, G. & Ball, D. (2003) Does the human heart fatigue subsequent to prolonged exercise? *Sports Medicine* **33**, 365–380.

Geddes, L.A. & Roeder, R.A. (2005) Evolution of our knowledge of sudden death due to commotio cordis. *American Journal of Emergency Medicine* **23**, 67–65.

Graham, T.P., Bricker, J.T., James, F.W. & Strong, W.B. (1994) Congenital heart disease. *Medicine and Science in Sports and Exercise* **26** (Supplement), S246–S253.

Heiss, H.W., Barmeyer, J., Wink, K., Cerny, F.J., Keul, J. & Reindell, H. (1976) Studies on the regulation of myocardial blood flow in man. *Basic Research in Cardiology* **71**, 658–675.

Isner, J.M., Estes, M. & Thompson, P.D. (1986) Acute cardiac events temporally related to cocaine abuse. *New England Journal of Medicine* **315**, 1438–1443.

Koller, A. (2003) Exercise-induced increases in cardiac troponins and prothrombotic markers. *Medicine and Science in Sports and Exercise* **35**, 444–448.

Lynch, P. (1980) Soldiers, sport, and sudden death. *Lancet* **1**, 1235–1237.

Maron, B.J., Poliac, L.C., Kaplan, J.A. & Mueller, F.O. (1995) Blunt impact to the chest leading to sudden death from cardiac arrest during sports activities. *New England Journal of Medicine* **333**, 337–342.

Maron, B.J., Roberts, W.C. & Epstein, S.E. (1982) Sudden death in hypertrophic cardiomyopathy: a profile of 78 patients. *Circulation* **65**, 1388–1394.

Maron, B.J., Shirani, J., Poliac, L.C., Mathenge, R., Roberts, W.O. & Mueller, F.O. (1996) Sudden death in young competitive athletes. *Journal of the American Medical Association* **276**, 199–204.

McCaffrey, F.M., Braden, D.S. & Strong, W.B. (1991) Sudden cardiac death in young athletes. A review. *American Journal of Diseases of Children* **145**, 177–182.

Niemala, K.O., Palatski, I.J. & Ikaheimo, M.J. (1984) Evidence of impaired left ventricular performance after an uninterrupted competitive 24-hour run. *Circulation* **70**, 350–356.

Rost, R. (1987) *Athletics and the Heart.* Year Book Medical, Chicago.

Rowland, T.W., Goff, D., DeLuca, P. & Popowski, B. (1997) Cardiac effects of a competitive road race in trained runners. *Pediatrics* **100**, E2.

Schwartz, P.J., Zaza, A., Locati, E. & Moss, A.J. (1991) Stress and sudden death. The case of the long QT syndrome. *Circulation* **83** (Supplement 2), 71–80.

Vincent, G.M. (2000) The long QT syndrome. *Cardiology Clinics* **18**, 309–320.

Chapter 20

Physiologic and Health Aspects of Exercise in Hot and Cold Environments

BAREKET FALK AND RAFFY DOTAN

In the realm of pediatric exercise physiology, as in other fields, children cannot be regarded as being small adults. This is also certainly true in the area of thermoregulation. However, careful scrutiny of the available literature suggests that much—surely not all—of what has traditionally been regarded as maturational differences between children and adults may actually be because of size and proportional differences. We try to highlight this change in interpretation in this chapter.

Body temperature (T_{body}) may be regulated by behavioral and physiologic means. Behavioral means involve the conscious selection of a microenvironment or the adjustment of exertion level. Physiologic temperature regulation involves the control of metabolic heat production, peripheral blood flow, and sweating.

During exercise, metabolic heat produced by the working muscles may be as high as 15–20 times that produced during rest. The heat is convected from the body core to the periphery and is subsequently dissipated through evaporation, convection, conduction, or radiation from the body's surface to the environment. Thermoregulation may be affected by the environmental conditions, as well as by the physical and physiologic state of the body. Physical factors affecting thermoregulation include body size and composition. More specifically, and quite considerably in the case of children, higher ratio of surface (skin) area : body mass has a prime role in thermoregulation. For any given environmental condition and physical characteristic, the physiologic response to exercise in the heat may be affected by factors such as the individual's level of acclimat-

ization, aerobic fitness, and hydration state. It is not clear how or to what extent these factors affect the thermoregulatory response to cold exposure. Furthermore, it is unclear whether these factors influence thermoregulation to the same extent in children as in adults.

This chapter outlines the differences in thermoregulation between children and adults and the changes that take place during growth and maturation in the physiologic response to exercise in the heat and in the cold. Some of the observed differences may simply be a result of body size and proportional differences, while others are likely the result of age-determined physiologic differences. The distinction between these two is not always clear-cut. Thus, this chapter emphasizes relevant recent findings in the area of thermoregulation in children and tries to provide alternative interpretations to some of the available data. The early signs and symptoms of various heat and cold disorders are described to facilitate their early identification. Finally, the adverse effects of hyperthermia and hypothermia and their prevention are discussed.

Thermoregulation: children, adolescents, and adults

The effectiveness of thermoregulation is reflected by heat and cold tolerance, and by the stability of core temperature (T_{re}) and the circulatory system, while performing various tasks in the heat and cold. This section outlines reported physical and physiologic characteristics that can affect heat or cold tolerance, and the different thermoregulatory strategies of children and adults.

Heat tolerance

Heat tolerance is mainly dependent on maintaining T_{re}, blood pressure, and circulatory sufficiency within physiologic limits. From a methodologic standpoint, the criteria used for defining heat tolerance and prematurely terminating a given subject's exposure are problematic. For example, the subjective exhaustion criterion does not take into account known age-dependent differences in the subjective rating of perceived exertion and possibly motivation. Moreover, using a uniform T_{re} cut-off value does not take into account possible age- or maturity-related differences in core temperature tolerance and could considerably affect heat storage comparisons. This should be borne in mind when considering the results and conclusions of the studies below.

When ambient temperature (T_{amb}) is lower than skin temperature (T_{sk}), thermoregulation in general, and exercise tolerance in particular, are apparently similar in children and adults (Drinkwater et al. 1977; Davies 1981; Delamarche et al. 1990). Nevertheless, children may use their thermoregulatory means differently to adults. Specifically, they appear to rely more on their relatively higher cutaneous surface area and blood flow and sweat less (Shibasaki et al. 1997b). That is, children's higher relative skin area allows them to utilize relatively more radiative, convective and conductive heat transfer, and less evaporative heat dissipation (see "Physical and physiological characteristics related to thermoregulation" below for further detail).

In warmer environments, when T_{amb} is similar to, or slightly higher than T_{sk}, children have been shown to tolerate at least 1 h of moderate exercise (Haymes et al. 1974, 1975; Drinkwater et al. 1977; Docherty et al. 1986; Delamarche et al. 1990; Shibasaki et al. 1997a,b). Inbar et al. (2004) suggested that this may be because of children's greater efficiency of evaporating smaller amounts of sweat (see also "Sweating rate") and, in fact, reflects their better thermoregulation. When compared with adults, however, children's T_{body} and heat storage are often found to be higher (Sohar & Shapiro 1965; Haymes et al. 1975; Drinkwater et al. 1977). If this is

true, possible differences between children and adults in warm environments may become apparent only after prolonged exposures. However, there are reservations concerning the suitability of current T_{body} and heat storage formulae for children and, therefore, the validity of the findings. In most studies where T_{body} is calculated, a weighted average of T_{re} and T_{sk} is used (e.g., $0.8T_{re} + 0.2T_{sk}$), based on estimated adult proportions of core vs. periphery. Such a formula, even if not accurate, is satisfactory in dimensionally uniform populations. However, children's larger relative skin area should entail a higher periphery : core volume ratio and consequently a higher T_{sk} proportion in the T_{body} and heat storage formulae. The current indiscriminate use of the existing formulae most likely overestimate children's T_{body} and heat content under most conditions.

In very high heat loads, as T_{amb} rises above 40°C, children's tolerance to a given exercise task appears lower than that of adults (Haymes et al. 1974; Drinkwater et al. 1977) vs. (Bar-Or et al. 1968; Wagner et al. 1972). Their T_{body} (Sohar & Shapiro 1965; Wagner et al. 1972; Leppaluoto 1988) and relative heat storage (Haymes et al. 1974; Drinkwater et al. 1977) were found higher. It has been suggested that children's lower observed heat tolerance is caused, at least in part, by size-related cardiovascular insufficiency (Jokinen et al. 1990; Falk et al. 1992c; see "Body dimensions" and "Circulatory characteristics" below). Children's reduced heat tolerance has also been attributed to lower sweating rates (Sohar & Shapiro 1965; Wagner et al. 1972; Haymes et al. 1974; Meyer et al. 1992), and a consequently compromised evaporative cooling. In a recent paper, on the other hand, Inbar et al. (2004) found prepubertal boys, exercising in 41°C heat to be more efficient sweaters and better thermoregulators than their adult counterparts.

While children do sweat less than adults, it has not been established whether this is a limitation or rather a manifestation of a different thermoregulatory strategy (see "Sweating rate" below).

Cold tolerance

There are only three reported studies in which cold stress was severe enough to result in decreased

T_{body} in exercising children and adolescents (Sloan & Keatinge 1973; Falk *et al.* 1997; Klentrou *et al.* 2004). In one study, 11- to 12-year-old boys were exposed to variable conditions (7–22°C), resting for 110 min, with a light 10-min exercise bout midway through that period (Falk *et al.* 1997). Although the children were dressed in sweat suits throughout the exposure, T_{re} decreased during the 7°C exposure. More importantly, even after 30 min of "rewarming recovery" in a thermoneutral environment, T_{re} continued to decrease. Klentrou *et al.* (2004) and Sloan and Keatinge (1973) demonstrated a greater drop in T_{re} and oral temperature, respectively, in younger, less mature children compared with older children, while cycling in the cold (5°C) or swimming in cool water (20°C). In both studies, the greater surface area : body mass ratio was related to the greater drop in temperature, demonstrating the importance of body dimensions and composition, rather than age per se, for thermoregulation in the cold.

Smolander *et al.* (1992) reported that in spite of obvious differences in body dimensions, pre- and early pubescent boys were able to maintain T_{re} as effectively as adults while exercising at 30% $\dot{V}o_{2max}$ in 5°C. The children's strategy was to increase their metabolic rate while vasoconstricting peripheral vessels to a greater degree than did the adults. The age-related difference in strategy was also apparent in two boys and two adults of similar surface area : mass ratio, suggesting a maturational influence on the selection of coping strategy. Similar differences were observed during rest in moderately cool air (16–20°C) (Wagner *et al.* 1974; Araki *et al.* 1980) and water (28°C) (Anderson & Mekjavic 1996).

Thus, in summary, children's thermoregulation, although achieved by a different strategy, appears as effective as that of adults in moderate conditions but may be lacking in extreme environments (Fig. 20.1).

Physical and physiologic characteristics related to thermoregulation

The apparent difference in thermoregulatory effectiveness between children and adults in extreme environments may be attributed to several physical and physiologic differences that diminish with

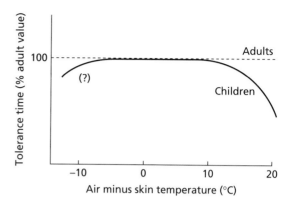

Fig. 20.1 Schematic representation of heat and cold tolerance in children (solid line) compared with adults (dashed line) in relation to the skin–air temperature gradient. After Bar-Or (1989).

pubertal growth and maturation. Table 20.1 relates size and maturation to different thermoregulatory responses to heat and cold exposures.

Body dimensions

In mild or warm environments, children's larger relative skin area allows them to rely more heavily on convective and radiative heat transfer and depend less on evaporative cooling (Gullestad 1975; Davies 1981; Delamarche *et al.* 1990; Shibasaki *et al.* 1997b). However, in more extreme hot or cold environments, the larger relative area becomes a liability. In extreme heat, the body absorbs heat from the environment and evaporative heat dissipation may not be sufficient for adequate cooling. In the cold, a small body dissipates relatively more heat to the environment compared with a larger one, and may not be able to compensate by elevating metabolic heat production, or additional vasoconstriction.

Metabolic characteristics

The oxygen cost of locomotion per unit mass is higher in children than in adults (Robinson 1938; Astrand 1952), resulting in a higher relative heat production. This places an added strain on the thermoregulatory system during exercise in the heat. During relatively short exposures to cold, the elevated metabolic heat production in prepubertal boys may be advantageous (Smolander *et al.* 1992;

Thermoregulatory response difference (children vs. adults)	Size-related	Maturation-related
Heat		
Higher dry heat exchange	+	?
Higher skin blood flow	+	?
Lower sweating rate per gland	+	+
Lower sweating "sensitivity"*	?	?
Higher heat-activated-sweat-gland density	+	−
Lower electrolyte concentration of sweat	−	+
Lower cardiac output	+	?
Lower tolerance to extreme heat	+	+
Higher T_{re} response to dehydration[†]	?	?
Slower initial rate of acclimation	?	+
Cold		
Higher dry heat loss	+	?
Greater vasoconstriction	+	?
Higher metabolic heat production	?	+
Higher shivering threshold[‡]	+	?

Table 20.1 Child–adult differences in thermoregulatory responses and their relationship to size and maturation.

−, Unrelated; ?, possibly related; +, clearly related.
* Sweating sensitivity is defined as the change in sweating rate relative to the change in rectal temperature ($\Delta SR/\Delta T_{re}$).
[†] Rectal temperature response to dehydration is defined as the change in T_{re} relative to the change in percent body mass ($\Delta T_{re}/\Delta BW$ loss).
[‡] Shivering threshold is defined as the core temperature at which shivering begins.

Anderson & Mekjavic 1996). However, during prolonged exercise in the cold, children's higher metabolic rate may leave them with lower energy reserves (Smolander *et al.* 1992). The problem is amplified by children's lower proportion of muscle mass where most of the glycogen is stored.

In premenarcheal adolescent girls, on the other hand, under similar environmental conditions to those of Smolander *et al.* (1992), the higher heat production was insufficient to compensate for the apparently larger convective and radiative heat losses from the skin and T_{re} did decrease (Klentrou *et al.* 2004). It is unclear whether the boys' and girls' different T_{re} response (Smolander *et al.* 1992 vs. Klentrou *et al.* 2004) is a result of gender, age, maturation, or body size differences.

Circulatory characteristics

Compared with adults, children have a considerably smaller blood volume relative to their skin area

(Astrand 1952). This fact, combined with children's greater reliance on cutaneous blood flow, implies that under thermal load a much larger proportion of their cardiac output must be diverted to the periphery for cooling. This is especially so in more extreme conditions, when the heat dissipating system is considerably stressed (Drinkwater *et al.* 1977). A direct result is a compromised venous return, leading to a greater reduction in stroke volume (Jokinen *et al.* 1990). Regardless of whether this is a result of dimensional or maturational differences, under high environmental heat loads, the result is a compromised heat convection from the body's core to the skin and the environment. This readily translates into children's lower exercise capacity under these conditions.

Cutaneous blood flow has been reported to be higher in children than in adults (Wagner *et al.* 1972; Drinkwater *et al.* 1977; Shibasaki *et al.* 1997b), and in pre- and mid-pubertal boys compared with post-pubertal ones (Falk *et al.* 1992c), during or immediately following exercise in the heat. A similar pattern was seen in pre-, mid-, and late-pubertal girls (Brien *et al.* 2000). This may explain the higher T_{sk} often observed in children (Wagner *et al.* 1972; Drinkwater *et al.* 1977; Araki *et al.* 1980; Delamarche *et al.* 1990; Tochihara *et al.* 1995). Furthermore, Shibasaki *et al.* (1997b) reported that exercising in the heat, boys had a greater increase of cutaneous blood flow for a given increase in T_{re} than men. These differences were even more evident when cutaneous vascular resistance was calculated (dividing skin blood flow by mean arterial pressure). Examining the relationship between local sweating rate and skin blood flow, Shibasaki *et al.* (1999) concluded that the boys' higher cutaneous blood flow was because of a greater initial withdrawal of vasoconstrictor tone, and a greater subsequent vasodilatation.

Children's circulatory response to cold stress is not well documented. Several studies reported that, in the cold, children's T_{sk} was lower at rest (Wagner *et al.* 1974; Araki *et al.* 1980; Smolander *et al.* 1992) as well as during exercise (Smolander *et al.* 1992). The lower T_{sk} reflects a greater reduction in skin blood flow to minimize heat loss.

Sweating rate

Tsuzuki-Hoyakaw *et al.* (1995) reported a higher sweating rate (SR) in children aged 9 months to 4.5 years than in their mothers while resting in a warm, humid environment (35°C, 70% relative humidity, RH). Thus, child–adult SR differences may not exist at a very young age.

In older children, however, any given environmental or metabolic thermoregulatory load will induce a lower SR than in adults (for reviews see Bar-Or 1980, 1989, 1996; Falk 1998; Inoue *et al.* 2004) and increases during puberty (Araki *et al.* 1979; Falk *et al.* 1992b). Children exhibit lower SR relative to whole body or regional surface area, as well as per sweat gland. Sweating response is also lower relative to a given rise in T_{body} or T_{re} (Anderson & Mekjavic 1996; Inbar *et al.* 2004). This child–adult difference becomes more evident as exercise intensity or heat stress increase (Inoue *et al.* 2004).

Maximal SRs of both children and adults remain unknown. Therefore, it could not have been established whether SRs indeed are limiting factors in thermoregulation. Rivera-Brown *et al.* (1999) reported considerably high SRs (>500 mL·h^{-1}) in 13-year-old trained and heat-acclimated boys exercising in the heat. Previous studies reported ~200–300 mL·h^{-1} in untrained unacclimatized boys (Bar-Or *et al.* 1980; Falk *et al.* 1992c).

In reviewing previous studies, it is difficult to explain why sweat production has typically not been related to body mass or metabolic load and its attendant heat production. Indeed, re-examination of reported group data in this manner reveals comparable SRs in children and adults (Falk & Dotan, unpublished; Falk 1991). Re-analysis of individual data of past studies and normalizing SRs for whole body, lean body, or muscle mass in future ones, may elucidate the question of whether children's metabolic load-relative SR is indeed different from adults' and—if so—how.

If such normalized SRs are comparable between children and adults, then what characterizes children's thermoregulation is not deficient sweating but rather a larger relative skin area. That is, a larger surface area is available for heat exchange and for evaporating smaller amounts of sweat. This, in turn, could explain why adults are more prone to excess sweating (i.e., dripping) and why children may be regarded as more efficient sweaters (Inbar *et al.* 2004).

Falk *et al.* (1992b) attempted to refine the investigation of the observed child–adult differences in SR by comparing pre-, mid-, and late pubertal boys, exercising at 50% $\dot{V}o_{2max}$ in 42°C, 20% RH. SR per body surface area and per gland increased with physical maturity (Fig. 20.2). Inoue *et al.* (2004) suggested that sweat gland function starts changing with the *onset* of puberty. This was based on a report by Araki *et al.* (1979), who showed SR to increase with age in 7- to 16-year-old boys, but most significantly so around 12–13 years of age, corresponding to the onset of puberty. Because of the linkage between onset of puberty and accelerated changes in bodily dimensions and hormonal function, it is yet to be determined whether the maturation-related SR change (Falk *et al.* 1992b) is primarily brought about by the hormonal or the dimensional changes of the pubertal growth spurt.

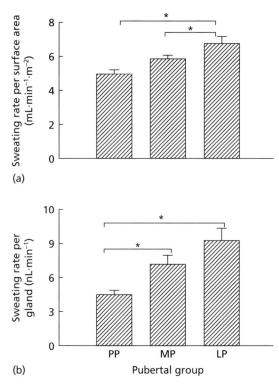

Fig. 20.2 Sweating rate: (a) per skin surface area; and (b) per gland among pre-, mid-, and late pubertal boys (PP, MP, LP, respectively), exercising in the heat (50% $\dot{V}O_{2max}$; 42°C, 20% relative humidity). After Falk *et al.* (1992a,b).

SWEAT GLAND SIZE AND POPULATION DENSITY

The changes in sweating response from childhood to adulthood may be explained by changes in sweat gland size and by modifications in sweat gland function. During childhood, sweat gland size is directly related to age (r = 0.77) and to height (r = 0.81) (Landing *et al.* 1968). Sato and Sato (1983) also reported that large glands (biopsied from adults) exhibited enhanced SR compared with small ones. In view of the relationship between sweat gland function and size, it is tempting to suggest that the difference in glandular size between children and adults (Landing *et al.* 1968; Wolfe *et al.* 1970) is directly related to the observed differences in SR.

The total number of sweat glands is believed to be determined by the age of 2–3 years (Kuno 1956) and does not change thereafter. Therefore, as skin surface area increases with age, sweat gland density decreases (Bar-Or 1980; Falk *et al.* 1992a).

When the response of heat-activated sweat glands to exercise in the heat was compared among pre-, mid-, and late pubertal boys (Falk *et al.* 1992a), the sweat gland population density was found to decrease while sweat bead size increased with maturity. However, the percentage of skin area covered by sweat beads did not differ among groups. Therefore, it may be speculated that although sweat gland output and distribution pattern differ among age groups, the resultant evaporative cooling capacity per unit surface area may be similar (Falk *et al.* 1992a), or possibly even more efficient in the younger boys (Inbar *et al.* 2004).

Reviewing the sweating efficiency issue more critically, it could be suggested that sweat bead size and distribution density are of little importance because sweat normally wets the entire skin area shortly after sweating onset. A more pertinent question is how much sweat actually evaporates off and cools the skin, as opposed to how much sweat drips off. As water is a vital commodity, its efficient use becomes a crucial issue in prolonged heat exposure, particularly in children whose body composition and possibly other factors render them more susceptible to the effects of dehydration (Bar-Or *et al.* 1980). The question, then, is how much of the excreted sweat drips onto or is absorbed by the environment rather than how much of it evaporates off the skin and cools it. Although not specifically documented, it appears that excessive sweating is more prevalent in adults and especially in men. It is not known what, if any, could be the advantage of excessive profuse sweating, or whether it merely is a symptom of an imperfect thermoregulatory system.

Relevant to this issue is the distinction between thermoregulatory sweating with its cholinergic neural control (Randall 1953) and stress-induced sweating, which is adrenergic in nature and probably greater in adults. The question here is whether stress-related sweating is a significant component of the sweating response to exercising in the heat. If so, to what extent can it account for the excessive sweating in adults. This needs to be experimentally addressed.

Several studies reported a greater increase in T_{sk} in children compared with adults at a given heat load (Wagner *et al.* 1972; Drinkwater *et al.* 1977; Araki *et al.* 1979; Delamarche *et al.* 1990). This may be explained by increased cutaneous vasodilatation, by a delay in the onset of sweating in children (Araki *et al.* 1979), or by a lower sweating response to a given change in T_{re} (Inbar *et al.* 2004). Some evidence suggests that concurrent with sweat gland growth during puberty, there is an increased sensitivity to both cholinergic (Sato & Sato 1983) and adrenergic (Wada 1950) stimuli, contributing to an elevated SR. Children's lower response has often been referred to as lower sweating "sensitivity." In light of the interpretations presented in this review, the use of this term appears rather misleading. That is, in view of children's greater reliance on radiative and convective heat dissipation via their larger relative skin area, it does not appear to be an issue of lower sensitivity but rather a lesser need for utilizing the sweating mechanism, conserving precious fluids in the process.

The SR increase, observed from childhood to adulthood, may also be explained by a maturation-related increase in the sweat gland's own metabolic capacity. Lactate is a product of anaerobic glycolysis at the sweat gland and the rate of lactate excretion is used as an index of sweat gland metabolism (Wolfe *et al.* 1970; Fellmann *et al.* 1985; Falk *et al.* 1991b). In pubertal boys, SR was shown to be directly related to the glandular lactate excretion rate (Fig. 20.3) and both were shown to increase with physical maturity (Falk *et al.* 1992a).

Sweat is excreted from gland to skin in a pulsatile fashion. The SR response relative to the pulsing frequency has been shown to be lower in boys than men (Shibasaki *et al.* 1997a). Such age-related difference could not be shown for gland pulsing frequency in relation to T_{body}. The authors' interpretation was that the boys' lower SR was the result of an immature peripheral mechanism (e.g., sweat

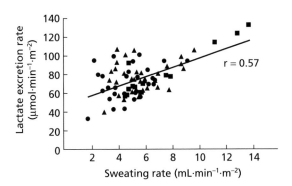

Fig. 20.3 The relationship between lactate excretion rate per gland and sweating rate per gland in pre- (solid circle), mid- (solid triangle), and late pubertal (solid square) boys exercising in the heat (50% $\dot{V}o_{2max}$; 42°C, 20% relative humidity). After Falk *et al.* (1991b).

gland metabolism and output) rather than a central sudomotor mechanism.

Hormonal status

Of the hormones associated with pubertal changes, two have been implicated in thermoregulation: testosterone and prolactin. Kawahata (1960) showed a sudorific effect of testosterone in adults although Rees and Shuster (1981) could not confirm this. Prolactin has been implicated in affecting sweat electrolyte composition in adults (Robertson *et al.* 1986; Kaufman *et al.* 1988; Kulczycki & Robertson 1988; Robertson 1989) and in adolescents (Falk *et al.* 1991a). However, the thermoregulatory roles of both testosterone and prolactin during childhood and adolescence remain unclear.

The endocrine response to exercise in the heat has been studied extensively in adults, mainly in relation to hormones associated with fluid and electrolyte balance (for reviews see Francesconi 1988; Radomski *et al.* 1998), but has scarcely been studied in children. Increases in aldosterone and other stress-related hormones, similar to those observed in adults, were reported in children (Jokinen *et al.* 1991) and adolescents (Falk *et al.* 1991a) during both rest and exercise in the heat, respectively. Nevertheless, it is still unclear how particular hormones may modify the thermoregulatory response during growth and maturation.

The endocrine response to cold stress has been studied in adults (e.g., Leduc 1961; Golstein-Golaire *et al*. 1970) but not in children. It is therefore unknown whether this response is different in childhood, or whether differences in the thermoregulatory response to cold can be attributed to maturation-related hormonal differences.

Heat disorders

Athletes exercising in the heat can experience various heat-related disorders ranging in intensity and severity from hypotension and headache to a potentially fatal heat stroke. Often, the victims of hyperthermia are young, healthy, and highly motivated individuals who are unaware of the early symptoms of heat illness. In fact, because hyperthermia is not associated with any painful sensation, motivated athletes may even increase exercise intensity during the last stages of competition, when hyperthermia is likely to occur.

Heat disorders have frequently been divided into three syndromes: (i) heat cramps; (ii) heat exhaustion; and (iii) heat stroke, often referred to as exertional heatstroke when associated with exercise. The three syndromes are not always distinct and an overlap exists in the signs and symptoms of each condition (Table 20.2). In fact, some argue that the various heat-related illnesses may be a continuum rather than separate distinct pathophysiologic

Table 20.2 Symptoms and signs of heat disorders. From Shibolet *et al.* 1962, 1976; Knochel 1974; Callaham 1979; Bar-Or 1983; Hubbard & Armstrong 1988; Shapiro & Seidman 1990; American College of Sports Medicine 1996.

Symptom or sign	Heat cramps	Heat exhaustion	Heat stroke
Pain	+	+*	
Headache	+*	+	+
Nausea	+*	+	+
Vomiting		+*	
Diarrhea			+*
Thirst		+*	
Fatigue, weakness	+	+	+
Loss of skin turgor	+	+	+
Dry skin			+*
Apathy	+	+	
Coma			+*
Confusion, agitation, seizures, convulsions			+
Hypotension			+
Tachycardia	+	+	+
Flattened or inverted T waves			+*
High rectal temp.		+ (<40°C)	+ (>40°C)
Pupillary changes			+*
Hyperventilation	+*	+*	+
Oliguria and anuria			+*
Hypernatremia		+†	
Hyponatremia	+	+‡	
Hypochloremia	+		
Low urine sodium	+	+‡	
High urinary nitrogen, CPK, creatinine, inorganic phosphate	+*		
Acute renal failure			+*
Clotting dysfunction			+*

CPK, creatine phosphokinase.
* Sometimes.
† When caused by water deprivation.
‡ When caused by salt depletion.

entities (Shibolet *et al.* 1967; Costrini *et al.* 1979; Hubbard & Armstrong 1988; Bytomski & Squire 2003).

Heat disorders may occur in athletes as well as in spectators in seemingly harmless environmental conditions (e.g., a warm day with a moderate breeze) (Bar-Or 1983; Coris *et al.* 2004), or they may develop over several days (Hubbard & Armstrong 1988). Squire (1990) reported that in a national junior Olympic track-and-field meet held during the last 3 days of July, 1983, in southeastern USA, cumulative fluid losses resulted in an increased incidence of heat disorders. Most distance events were held on the first day of competition and the remainder took place on the second day. However, the highest incidence of heat illness was observed on the third day of the meet.

Treatment of all heat disorders should focus on reduction of T_{body} and rehydration. Lowering of T_{body} may be attained by simply stopping activity, or by moving to a shaded area. Spraying the body with water and using a fan can enhance evaporative cooling (Chesney 2003). In the case of more severe symptoms, cool (Shapiro & Seidman 1990) or ice-cold (Costrini 1990) water immersion have been recommended. Rehydration may be achieved by oral ingestion or, in more severe cases, by intravenous fluid administration (for detailed treatment procedures see Costrini 1990; Shapiro & Seidman 1990).

Prevention of heat disorders

It is notable that heat disorders are the only conditions (other than trauma) that are potentially fatal in healthy individuals. Yet, they are all preventable. With adequate preparation, involving sound hydration practices, proper conditioning and acclimatization, and the identification of individuals at risk, all heat disorders may be averted (for reviews of prevention and treatment procedures see American College of Sports Medicine 1996; Chesney 2003).

Drug abuse, although not common in children, is becoming troublesome in adolescents (Hindmarsh & Opheim 1990). Drug abuse may physiologically or behaviorally alter thermoregulatory capacity. Drugs such as amphetamines, ephedrine, alkaloids, and other stimulants may increase exertional drive, heat production, and T_{re}, while lowering perceived stress (Gill *et al.* 2000). Diuretics (e.g., caffeine, alcohol, or pharmaceutical diuretics) could predispose to hypohydration and electrolyte imbalance, while atropine and beta-blockers can adversely affect the cardiovascular system and the sweating response (Gordon *et al.* 1984; Kolka *et al.* 1987). It is unknown how anabolic steroids may affect the thermoregulatory response to exercise in the heat. Drugs suggested to affect thermoregulation are listed in Table 20.3.

This section focuses on the way in which hydration status, conditioning, and acclimatization can affect heat disorders.

HYDRATION

SR is elevated during exercise, especially in the heat. If not accompanied by sufficient fluid replacement, sweating will result in a net fluid loss and lead to a state of hypohydration. When water is available ad libitum, children (Bar-Or *et al.* 1980, 1992),

Table 20.3 Drugs that may affect thermoregulation.

Drug	Effect on thermoregulation
Beta-blockers	Increase sweating and may lead to dehydration
Amphetamines, LSD	Increase metabolic rate and thus, heat production
Anticholinergics	Decrease sweating and thus, decrease evaporative cooling
Antihistamines	Decrease sweating and thus, decrease evaporative cooling
Diuretics	Predispose to hypohydration. Alter electrolyte balance
Ephedrine alkaloids	Increase metabolic rate and thus, heat production
Thyroid hormone	Increases metabolic rate and thus, heat production
Vasodilators	Increase skin blood flow and thus, increase heat gain in a hot environment and increase heat loss in cold environment

adolescents (Iuliano *et al.* 1998), and adults (Pugh *et al.* 1967; White & Ford 1983) fail to drink sufficiently to counteract fluid loss. Although water may be readily available, children will drink more if the beverage is flavored (Meyer *et al.* 1994; Wilk & Bar-Or 1996; Rivera-Brown *et al.* 1999). Another way to enhance thirst is to add carbohydrates (CHO, ~8%) and NaCl (15–20 mmol·L^{-1}) to the flavored beverage (as in commercial sports drinks). This has been shown to increase voluntary fluid consumption and retention by as much as 90% in children exercising in the heat (Bar-Or & Wilk 1996; Wilk & Bar-Or 1996; Hall *et al.* 2005). Indeed, several reports indicate that adding CHO and NaCl to their beverages consistently prevented dehydration in 9- to 12-year-old boys exercising in the heat (Wilk & Bar-Or 1996; Wilk *et al.* 1998; Rivera-Brown *et al.* 1999). Attempting to increase osmolality and fluid retention, via use of salt tablets, should be avoided because of their typically unbalanced electrolyte content and the intestinal cramps or other disorders that often follow.

Interestingly, a recent preliminary report (Wilk *et al.* 2005) demonstrated that, contrary to previous findings, a CHO-NaCl beverage was not sufficient to prevent dehydration in 12- to 15-year-old athletes exercising in the heat. This might have partially been because of the higher exercise intensity than in previous studies (65 vs. 50–60% $\dot{V}o_{2max}$). More important, however, were the much shorter rest intervals (5 vs. 25 min) that likely prevented adequate hydration even by the more informed and willing subjects. These findings emphasize the need to adjust training and competition protocols to allow for proper hydration.

Hypohydration compromises thermoregulation by reducing both skin blood flow and SR (Fortney *et al.* 1984). This has been demonstrated in adults but has not been confirmed in children. Nevertheless, in view of the lower SR in children and their greater reliance on skin blood flow for radiative and convective cooling, it is highly likely that hypohydration imposes a higher risk for children than for adults. In fact, Bar-Or *et al.* (1980) demonstrated that for any given percentage of body mass, lost by sweating, T_{re} increased more in children than it did in adults (Fig. 20.4).

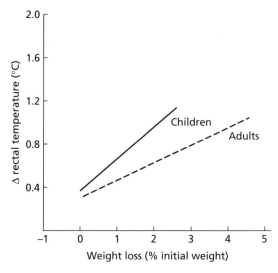

Fig. 20.4 Comparison of the relationship between the level of hypohydration, expressed as percentage change in initial body weight, and the rise in rectal temperature in children (solid line) and adults (dashed line). After Bar-Or *et al.* (1980).

In spite of the widely reported decrements in physical performance in adults as a result of dehydration, "voluntary" dehydration is still practiced by many athletes (Webster *et al.* 1990; Shirreffs 2005). In adults, Walsh *et al.* (1994) reported mild dehydration (2% body mass) to result in performance decrement. In children, a single preliminary report suggested that even a 1% decrease in body mass could decrease endurance performance (Wilk *et al.* 2002). Further studies are required to determine the level of dehydration critical to exercise capacity and heat tolerance in children and adolescents. It is noteworthy that, while CHO-NaCl beverages have been demonstrated to improve performance in adults exercising in the heat (Carter *et al.* 2005; for review see Maughan 2001), a similar effect in children has not been shown (Meyer *et al.* 1995a,b).

Many child and adolescent athletes arrive at practice sessions already with a fluid deficit, which is exaggerated during the ensuing workout (Casa *et al.* 2005; De Felix-Davila *et al.* 2005; Yeargin *et al.* 2005). Moreover, before competition wrestlers, boxers, judoka, and body builders commonly lose 3–5% of

Table 20.4 Modification in athletic activity using the wet bulb globe temperature (WBGT)* index. After Bar-Or 1983; American College of Sports Medicine 1987, 1996; Squire 1990.

WBGT (°C)	Risk of thermal disorders	Modification of activity
>28	Extreme	Stop all athletic activities
23–28	High	Stop activities of individuals at risk, such as the unacclimated, unfit, obese, and those with a history of heat disorders Increase rest periods of all other participants Reduce exercise intensity Increase fluid intake
18–23	Moderate	Increase rest periods and fluid intake Be alert for signs and/or symptoms of heat disorders.
10–18	Low	All activities are allowed
<10	Low	All activities are allowed but beware of signs of hypothermia

* WBGT $= 0.7T_{wb} + 0.2T_g + 0.1T_{db}$, where T_{wb}, wet bulb temperature; T_g, black globe temperature; T_{db}, dry bulb temperature.

their body mass for "making weight" (Tipton *et al.* 1976). In fact, some wrestlers, mostly in the lightweight categories, lose as much as 10% or more of their body mass before competition (Tipton & Tcheng 1970). Although the American National Collegiate Athletic Association has adopted weight-control rules, intended to eliminate such rapid weight loss procedures (Oppliger *et al.* 2003), these practices continue. Sansone and Sawyer (2005) recently reported a 5-year-old boy who was pressured to lose weight in order to wrestle at a lower weight category.

Once hypohydration sets in, it is seldom possible to correct during exercise of any significant intensity. Therefore, an adequate hydration level must be ascertained before participation in physical activity, especially in the heat. This can be achieved with 7–8 mL fluids per kilogram of body mass (e.g., 300–360 mL for a 45-kg child) 20–30 min before warm-up. Although more fluid is emptied from the stomach and enters the blood stream faster with larger ingested volumes (Costill & Saltin 1974), it could be very uncomfortable and adversely affect performance. Therefore, it is recommended that during activity, small volumes (2–3 mL per kilogram body mass, or 90–135 mL for a 45-kg child) be ingested at 15–20-min intervals (American College of Sports Medicine 1987, 1996). In running events, hydration stations should be positioned accordingly.

In sports such as soccer, rugby, or field hockey, it is suggested that when environmental conditions are stressful (Table 20.4), the games be divided into quarters rather than halves, in order to provide an additional rehydration breaks (Squire 1990).

The fluid selected should stimulate further drinking and athletes should be encouraged to drink beyond thirst quenching (Greenleaf 1992). The beverage should be cool (not too cold), non-carbonated, lightly sweetened, and flavored (Bar-Or & Wilk 1996; Horswill *et al.* 2005). Children's taste preferences may differ (Meyer *et al.* 1995b), although Meyer *et al.* (1994) demonstrated that on average, fluid consumption was highest with grape or orange flavoring. Although sports beverages may not be necessary at most sporting events in terms of energy replenishment, their main prophylactic advantages are the facilitation of enhanced water absorption, and retention (Johnson *et al.* 1988).

ACCLIMATIZATION AND ACCLIMATION

Heat acclimatization and acclimation are the processes by which the body adapts to heat stress —naturally or via planned repeated exposures, respectively. The associated physiologic adaptations lead to improved thermoregulation, higher exercise capacity in the heat, and enhanced thermal comfort.

Children and adolescents are capable of heat acclimation similar to adults. The main difference is in the initial rate of acclimation, as demonstrated by Inbar (1978), during a 2-week acclimation program (Inbar 1978; Bar-Or 1983). Wagner et al. (1972) demonstrated a lower level of acclimation in adolescent boys compared to men following an 8-day protocol. Additionally, Inbar et al. (1981) reported increased heat-activated sweat gland density, following acclimation in 8- to 10-year-old boys, with no associated rise in SR. This may reflect a better distribution of sweat, as suggested by Shvartz et al. (1979). It should also be noted that in children, heat acclimation can be attained by conditioning without exposure to a hot environment (Inbar et al. 1981; see "Conditioning" below).

Conversely, the perceived difficulty of a given exercise-in-the-heat stress was shown to decrease faster during acclimation in boys compared to men (Bar-Or & Inbar 1977). Although this may appear advantageous, it is also potentially dangerous because children may not recognize the imminence of a potentially dangerous exposure and consequently fail to stop or modify their activity during exercise in the heat.

Proper acclimation is especially important during the transitory and unpredictable spring season, particularly for athletes for whom this is the early training or competitive season. There are several reports of heat stroke in high school and college football players during the first practices of the season (Fox et al. 1966; Redfearn & Murphy 1969; Barcenas et al. 1976; Savdie et al. 1991) which could have been prevented by suitable acclimation. Proper acclimation is also essential for those athletes traveling to warmer geographic regions.

In adults, reasonable acclimation may be attained following 4–7 exposures to exercise (>50% $\dot{V}O_{2max}$) in the heat, while 8–14 exposures may suffice for maximal acclimation (Armstrong & Maresh 1991). In children, less stringent protocols may be adequate. For example, exercise in a mild environment or rest in the heat have been shown as effective in acclimating prepubertal children as exercise in the heat, or nearly so (Inbar et al. 1981). It is also important to remember that because acclimation increases SR, it also increases fluid loss. Therefore, sound hydration practices, as described above, should be emphasized.

Loss of acclimation can be fairly rapid. In adults, Williams et al. (1967) demonstrated more than 50% of the T_{re} acclimation effect to have been lost within 3 weeks of no heat exposure, while over 50% of SR adaptation disappeared within a week. It is unknown whether acclimation loss is similar in children and adolescents but the advantages of acclimation in these populations should not be taken for granted beyond a few days (Armstrong & Maresh 1991).

CONDITIONING

It is widely accepted that physical training in a mildly warm environment improves physiologic responses to heat stress (for reviews see Armstrong & Pandolf 1988; McLellan 2001). High maximal aerobic power may be very effective in enhancing exercise-in-heat tolerance in adults, probably because of the higher blood volume associated with both innate and acquired high $\dot{V}O_{2max}$ (Noakes 2005).

Delmarche et al. (1990) did not observe any relationship between $\dot{V}O_{2max}$ (43–65 mL·min^{-1}·kg^{-1}) and the thermoregulatory response to passive heat in prepubertal boys. Likewise, Araki et al. (1980) reported no difference in T_{body} in response to a passive heat load in prepubertal boys prior to and following training. The common denominator in those passive exposures was likely the low required cardiac output, which probably did not strain the circulatory system. Conversely, the same authors (Matsushita & Araki 1980) observed higher SRs at any given T_{re}, in trained vs. untrained boys. Additionally, skin blood flow during heat stress was correlated with $\dot{V}O_{2max}$ in children (Inoue et al. 2004). Similarly, Inbar et al. (1981) reported that in 8- to 10-year-old boys, heat acclimation could be attained either by mere rest in the heat or by physical conditioning with no additional heat load (training at 65% $\dot{V}O_{2max}$). That is, when high skin blood flow and cardiac output are required (exercise in the heat), prior conditioning or high aerobic power facilitate effective thermoregulation. Therefore, as is the case in adults, the fit child and adolescent will better tolerate exercise stress in the heat than the unfit.

ENVIRONMENTAL CONDITIONS

Radiative and convective heat dissipation is diminished, or even reversed, at high T_{amb}, and thermoregulatory reliance must be shifted to evaporative cooling. High humidity further stresses the thermoregulatory system by inhibiting sweat evaporation and limiting evaporative cooling. Exposure to solar radiation can considerably add to the accumulated heat that must be dissipated. Relative air movement, on the other hand, such as that caused by wind, fan, or riding a bicycle outdoors, can greatly improve heat dissipation by enhancing convection and evaporation, depending on ambient conditions.

The most commonly applied heat stress index is the wet bulb globe temperature (WBGT) (American College of Sports Medicine 1987, 1996; American Academy of Pediatrics 2000) which takes into account temperature, humidity, and radiation. Modifications for outdoor activities (e.g., longer and more frequent rest periods), according to the WBGT index, are outlined in Table 20.4. A possible means of increasing rest periods is frequent substitution of players and/or having more time-outs available to coaches. In addition, it is recommended that in summer, activities be planned for the early morning or later evening hours. The worst scenario is a hot, humid day, with solar radiation and little or no wind. The associated risks are considerably amplified in spring, and particularly early spring, when participants have not had a chance to heat acclimatize.

Clothing should be suitable for the environmental conditions. Loose, light-colored, lightweight or net-like material, is appropriate for hot humid days, and provided solar radiation is not excessive, skin should be exposed to allow for sweat evaporation. Sweat-saturated clothing should be replaced. It should be noted that most sunscreen lotions are lipid-based and may therefore hinder heat transfer, uniform skin wetting, and, consequently, compromise evaporative cooling. Special gear such as football helmets and protective equipment, long-sleeved heavy rugby jerseys, or fashionable track suits will impede heat dissipation and impair thermoregulation.

Cold injuries

Cold injuries involve peripheral frostbite or systemic hypothermia. The early symptoms of frostbite include local pain and skin redness which may turn white with increased severity. It is interesting to point out that frostbite may occur even under elevated T_{re} conditions. This may well be another symptom of thermoregulatory imperfection.

To the authors' knowledge, there are no reports of hypothermia ($T_{re} < 35°C$) in children during exercise in the cold. This is because of the significantly elevated metabolic rate, associated with most athletic activities, that compensates for heat lost to the environment. However, exercise does not render immunity against hypothermia. It is certainly conceivable that extreme cold or exercise that is too light will eventually lead to hypothermia. Smolander et al. (1992) reported prepubertal boys exercising in 5°C while maintaining T_{re} as effectively as adults (Fig. 20.5). To accomplish this, they increased metabolic heat production more than did the adults, leading to greater energy expenditure. Hence, the authors argue that in physical activities of extended durations, children may experience earlier exhaustion. During locomotive activities, especially weight-bearing ones, children's lower economy (Robinson

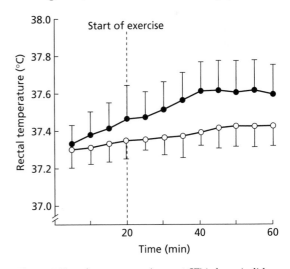

Fig. 20.5 Rectal temperature (mean ± SE) in boys (solid circle) and in men (open circle) during rest and exercise (30% $\dot{V}o_{2max}$) in 5°C. Redrawn from Smolander et al. (1992).

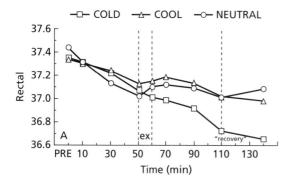

Fig. 20.6 Rectal temperature pre-entry, during, and following exposure to 22°C (open circle, neutral), 13°C (open triangle, cool), and 7°C (open square, cold). Temperature decreased significantly with time and a significant condition–time interaction was observed. Redrawn from Falk *et al.* (1997).

1938; Astrand 1952) and resultant higher relative heat production may fully or partially provide the added metabolic heat needed to prevent net heat loss to the environment.

During a 110-min rest and exercise exposure to 7°C, 11- to 12-year-old boys exhibited a progressive drop in T_{re} (Falk *et al.* 1997). T_{re} lowering persisted even during the subsequent 30-min recovery in a thermoneutral environment (22°C) (Fig. 20.6), likely because of the vasodilatory pooling of core blood with the cold peripheral blood in the warmer environment. As a result of their relatively larger skin area and likely larger periphery : core volume ratio, children are expected to exhibit this phenomenon more markedly than adults. Likewise, discontinuous or sporadic exercise (high intensity exertion followed by low intensity or rest) may increase the risk of cold injury resulting from the increased peripheral blood flow and sweat excretion during exercise followed by high convective, radiative, and evaporative heat loss during recovery. Children may be especially susceptible as they are often characterized by intermittent type of exercise (Bailey *et al.* 1995).

During exercise in the cold outdoors, one must consider the wind-chill factor. For example, when air temperature is 0°C, a 24 km·h^{-1} air velocity will result in a perceived and effective air temperature

equivalent to −10.5°C. A 40 km·h^{-1} air velocity will bring the effective temperature down to −16°C. The wind-chill factor is important not only in winter sports but may also be significant during running or cycling, where the relative air velocity may result in cold injury to exposed skin, or even hypothermia in severe conditions. This applies both to children and adults. However, children's larger relative surface area predisposes them to greater exposure risks than adults.

Heat conduction of water is ~25 times greater than that of air. Body movements, especially in water, greatly increase convective heat loss. Thus, compared with dry land, aquatic activities can result in a much greater rate of heat loss. Children's greater relative skin area is thus a distinct disadvantage in such activities and could result in a dangerously large heat loss (Sloan & Keatinge 1973). With the current popularity of triathlon, and the increasingly higher number of young competitors in that sport, these issues deserve more attention.

In contrast to heat acclimation, there appears to be little adaptation to cold (Young 1988). It is mainly characterized by elevated skin blood flow to frequently exposed extremities (Krog *et al.* 1960; Daanen 2003). This adaptation, which may help to prevent frostbite, has been demonstrated in adults but not studied in children.

A higher fitness level may facilitate maintenance of a higher level of physical activity and heat production. Reliance on elevated metabolism does, however, require greater energy expenditure and may shorten potential exposure duration. Moreover, well-trained individuals are often leaner than others, a fact that can more than counteract the said fitness advantage, making them more cold-intolerant and susceptible to cold injuries.

Finally, prevention of hypothermia is primarily dependent on proper clothing. Clothing material should allow for some insulation, yet permit sweat evaporation (i.e., wicking and breathing materials). Additionally, layering of clothing is advantageous over a single heavy garment because it provides a better insulation : weight ratio and allows adjustments to changing conditions. In very cold conditions, hat and gloves are recommended, or even essential, for frostbite avoidance as well as the prevention of excessive heat loss via the exposed hands and particularly the head. The head loses disproportionately more heat than other body parts because of its limited degree of effective vasoconstriction.

During aquatic activity in cool water (≤23°C), it is recommended to allow children frequent (every 10–15 min) exits for rewarming, and/or have them use neoprene vests or other specialized cold water clothing.

Challenges for future research

The physiologic effects and health-related aspects of exercise in the heat or in the cold have been extensively investigated in adults but scarcely in children. There is a particular lack of information regarding cold exposure. Numerous topics merit further research.

1 The definition of heat tolerance is central to comparing thermoregulatory capacity of children and adults. At this point, several pertinent questions remain:
- Is the critical upper limit of T_{re} different in children than in adults and, if so, how does it change from infancy to adulthood?
- How should circulatory insufficiency (e.g., blood pressure drop) be objectively defined for proper comparison?
- Could children and possibly adults be coaxed into continuing heat exposures beyond subjective exhaustion when objective physiologic limits have not been reached (e.g., as is typically the case in testing of maximal aerobic capacity)?

2 There remain several questions as to the relationships between SR and age, maturation, and body size:
- How much is SR dependent on the absolute metabolic and total heat load?
- Relative to adults, in extreme heat, are children limited by their maximal SR or by the heat they absorb from the environment?
- Do sweat gland size and SR go hand in hand during growth and maturation? How are they related to the pubertal growth spurt and other growth landmarks? To what extent and how are they related to pubertal hormonal or neurologic changes?
- In view of children's lower SR yet higher relative skin area, under what conditions (exercise intensity, T_{amb}, RH), if at all, is evaporative cooling in children more efficient than in adults?

3 Involuntary hypohydration has been documented in children and in adults. The thermoregulatory consequences of hypohydration on exercise performance are likely more severe in children. Unknown at present is children's critical degree of detrimental dehydration.

4 Children respond to cold exposure with a greater increase in metabolic rate. Also, indirect evidence suggests enhanced peripheral vasoconstriction in children. Further study is needed to clarify the circulatory and hormonal responses to cold exposure in children, and the extent to which it is determined by maturation or dimensional growth per se.

5 No protocols or efficacy estimates are available for acclimating or habituating children and adolescents to the cold. Nor is it known whether, in children, enhanced physical fitness provides any advantage during prolonged cold exposure above and beyond the greater exercise capacity and endurance.

6 Most studies have investigated responses to heat or cold in young or adolescent boys. There is relatively little information on girls and on possible gender-related thermoregulatory and heat or cold tolerance differences.

7 Many studies have investigated children's physiologic responses to heat or cold stress yet only a few have attempted to determine children's cognitive or behavioral responses.

8 Because of their larger relative skin area, children are likely more susceptible to heat- or cold-induced disorders in extreme environments. There are some experimental data to support this statement. Epidemiologic data, however, while demonstrating increased susceptibility in the elderly, fail to do so in children. Additional reliable epidemiologic information is particularly important in view of children's increasing participation in outdoor sports.

References

American Academy of Pediatrics. Committee on Sports Medicine and Fitness (2000) Climatic heat stress and the exercising child and adolescent. *Pediatrics* **106**, 158–159.

American College of Sports Medicine (1987) Position statement on the prevention of thermal injuries during distance running. *Medicine and Science in Sports and Exercise* **19**, 529–533.

American College of Sports Medicine (1996) Position stand on heat and cold illnesses during distance running. *Medicine and Science in Sports and Exercise* **28**, i–x.

Anderson, G.S. & Mekjavic, I.B. (1996) Thermoregulatory responses of circumpubertal children. *European Journal of Applied Physiology and Occupational Physiology* **74**, 404–410.

Araki, T., Toda, Y., Matsushita, K. & Tsujino, A. (1979) Age differences in sweating during muscular exercise. *Japanese Journal of Fitness and Sports Medicine* **28**, 239–248.

Araki, T., Tsujita, J., Matsushita, K. & Hori, S. (1980) Thermoregulatroy responses of prepubertal boys to heat and cold in relation to physical training. *Human Ergonomics* **9**, 69–80.

Armstrong, L.E. & Maresh, C.M. (1991) The induction and decay of heat acclimatisation in trained athletes. *Sports Medicine* **12**, 302–312.

Armstrong, L.E. & Pandolf, K.B. (1988) Physical training, cardiorespiratory physical fitness and exercise-heat tolerance. In: *Human Performance Physiology and Environmental Medicine at Terrestrial Extremes* (Pandolf, K.B., Sawka, M.N. & Gonzalez, R.R., eds.) Benchmark Press, Indianapolis, IN: 199–226.

Astrand, P.O. (1952) *Experimental Studies of Physical Work Capacity in Relation to Sex and Age*. Mundsgaard, Copenhagen.

Bailey, R.C., Olson, J., Pepper, S.L., Porszasz, J., Barstow, T.J. & Cooper, D.M. (1995) The level and tempo of children's physical activities: an observational study. *Medicine and Science in Sports and Exercise* **27**, 1033–1041.

Bar-Or, O. (1980) Climate and the exercising child: a review. *International Journal of Sports Medicine* **1**, 53–65.

Bar-Or, O. (1983) *Pediatric Sports Medicine for the Practitioner*. Springer-Verlag, New York.

Bar-Or, O. (1989) Temperature regulation during exercise in children and adolescents. In: *Youth, Exercise and Sports* (Gisolfi, C.V. & Lamb, D.R., eds.), Benchmark Press, Indianapolis: 335–362.

Bar-Or, O. (1996) Thermoregulation in females from a life span perspective. In: *Exercise and the Female: A Life Span Approach* (Bar-Or, O., Lamb, D.R. & Clarkson, P.M., eds.) Cooper Publishing Group, IN.

Bar-Or, O., Blimkie, C.J., Hay, J.A., MacDougall, J.D., Ward, D.S. & Wilson, W.M. (1992) Voluntary dehydration and heat intolerance in cystic fibrosis, *Lancet* **339**, 696–699.

Bar-Or, O., Dotan, R., Inbar, O., Rotshtein, A. & Zonder, H. (1980) Voluntary hypohydration in 10- to 12-year-old boys. *Journal of Applied Physiology* **48**, 104–108.

Bar-Or, O. & Inbar, O. (1977) Relationship between perceptual and physiological changes during heat acclimatization in 8–10-year-old boys. In: *Frontiers of Activity and Child Health* (Lavalee, H. & Shephard, R.J., eds.) Pelican Press, Quebec: 205–214.

Bar-Or, O., Magnusson, L.I. & Buskirk, E.R. (1968) Distribution of heat-activated sweat glands in obese and lean men and women. *Human Biology* **40**, 235–248.

Bar-Or, O. & Wilk, B. (1996) Water and electrolyte replenishment in the exercising child. *International Journal of Sport Nutrition* **6**, 93–99.

Barcenas, C., Hoeffler, H.P. & Lie, J.T. (1976) Obesity, football, dog days and siriasis: a deadly combination. *American Heart Journal* **92**, 237–244.

Brien, E.K., Wilk, B., Iwata, M. & Bar-Or, O. (2000) Forearm blood flow in pre/early-, mid, and late-pubertal girls exercising in the heat. *Medicine and Science in Sports and Exercise* **32**, S157.

Bytomski, J.R. & Squire, D.L. (2003) Heat illness in children. *Current Sports Medicine Reports* **2**, 320–324.

Callaham, M.L. (1979) Emergency management of heat illness. In: *Emergency Physician Series*, Abbott Laboratories, North Chicago, IL: 1–23.

Carter, J., Jeukendrup, A.E. & Jones, D.A. (2005) The effect of sweetness on the efficacy of carbohydrate supplementation during exercise in the heat. *Canadian Journal of Applied Physiology* **30**, 379–391.

Casa, D.J., Yeargin, S.W., Decher, N.R., McCaffrey, M. & James, C.T. (2005) Incidence and degree of dehydration and attitudes regarding hydration in adolescents at summer football camp. *Medicine and Science in Sports and Exercise* **37**, S463.

Chesney, M.L. (2003) Pediatric exertional heatstroke. *Air Medical Journal* **22**, 6–8.

Coris, E.E., Ramirez, A.M. & Van Durme, D.J. (2004) Heat illness in athletes: the dangerous combination of heat, humidity and exercise. *Sports Medicine* **34**, 9–16.

Costill, D.L. & Saltin, B. (1974) Factors limiting gastric emptying during rest and exercise. *Journal of Applied Physiology* **37**, 679–683.

Costrini, A. (1990) Emergency treatment of exertional heatstroke and comparison of whole body cooling techniques. *Medicine and Science in Sports and Exercise* **22**, 15–18.

Costrini, A.M., Pitt, H.A., Gustafson, A.B. & Uddin, D.E. (1979) Cardiovascular and metabolic manifestations of heat stroke and severe heat exhaustion. *American Journal of Medicine* **66**, 296–302.

Daanen, H.A. (2003) Finger cold-induced vasodilation: a review. *European Journal of Applied Physiology* **89**, 411–426.

Davies, C.T. (1981) Thermal responses to exercise in children. *Ergonomics* **24**, 55–61.

De Felix-Davila, R.A., Rivera-Brown, A.M. & Lebron, L.E. (2005) Hydration status and sweat electrolyte loss in adolescent judokas training in hot and humid conditions. *Medicine and Science in Sports and Exercise* **37**, S167–168.

Delamarche, P., Bittel, J., Lacour, J.R. & Flandrois, R. (1990) Thermoregulation at rest and during exercise in prepubertal boys. *European Journal of Applied Physiology and Occupational Physiology* **60**, 436–440.

Docherty, D., Eckerson, J.D. & Hayward, J.S. (1986) Physique and thermoregulation in prepubertal males during exercise in a warm, humid environment. *American Journal of Physical Anthropology* **70**, 19–23.

Drinkwater, B.L., Kupprat, I.C., Denton, J.E., Crist, J.L. & Horvath, S.M. (1977) Response of prepubertal girls and college women to work in the heat. *Journal of Applied Physiology* **43**, 1046–1053.

Falk, B. (1991) *The Thermoregulatory Response of Pre-, Mid- and Late-pubertal Boys Exercisign in the Heat*. McMaster University, Hamilton, ON.

Falk, B. (1998) Effects of thermal stress during rest and exercise in the paediatric population. *Sports Medicine* **25**, 221–240.

Falk, B., Bar-Eli, M., Dotan, R., *et al.* (1997) Physiological and cognitive responses to cold exposure in 11–12 year-old boys. *American Journal of Human Biology* **9**, 39–49.

Falk, B., Bar-Or, O., Calvert, R. & MacDougall, J.D. (1992a) Sweat gland response to exercise in the heat among pre-, mid-, and late-pubertal boys. *Medicine and Science in Sports and Exercise* **24**, 313–319.

Falk, B., Bar-Or, O., MacDougall, D., Goldsmith, C. & McGillis, L. (1992b) A longitudinal analysis of the sweating response of pre-, mid- and late-pubertal boys during exercise in the heat. *American Journal of Human Biology* **4**, 527–535.

Falk, B., Bar-Or, O. & MacDougall, J.D. (1991a) Aldosterone and prolactin response to exercise in the heat in circumpubertal boys. *Journal of Applied Physiology* **71**, 1741–1745.

Falk, B., Bar-Or, O. & MacDougall, J.D. (1992c) Thermoregulatory responses of pre-, mid-, and late-pubertal boys to exercise in dry heat. *Medicine and Science in Sports and Exercise* **24**, 688–694.

Falk, B., Bar-Or, O., MacDougall, J.D., McGillis, L., Calvert, R. & Meyer, F. (1991b) Sweat lactate in exercising children and adolescents of varying physical maturity. *Journal of Applied Physiology* **71**, 1735–1740.

Fellmann, N., Labbe, A., Gachon, A.M. & Coudert, J. (1985) Thermal sweat lactate in cystic fibrosis and in normal children. *European Journal of Applied Physiology and Occupational Physiology* **54**, 511–516.

Fortney, S.M., Wenger, C.B., Bove, J.R. & Nadel, E.R. (1984) Effect of hyperosmolality on control of blood flow and sweating. *Journal of Applied Physiology* **57**, 1688–1695.

Fox, E.L., Mathews, D.K., Kaufman, W.S. & Bowers, R.W. (1966) Effects of football equipment on thermal balance and energy cost during exercise. *Research Quarterly* **37**, 332–329.

Francesconi, R.P. (1988) Endocrinological responses to exercise in stressful environments. *Exercise and Sport Sciences Reviews* **16**, 255–284.

Gill, N.D., Shield, A., Blazevich, A.J., Zhou, S. & Weatherby, R.P. (2000) Muscular and cardiorespiratory effects of pseudoephedrine in human athletes. *British Journal of Clinical Pharmacology* **50**, 205–213.

Golstein-Golaire, J., Vanhaelst, L., Bruno, O.D., Leclercq, R. & Copinschi, G. (1970) Acute effects of cold on blood levels of growth hormone, cortisol, and thyrotropin in man. *Journal of Applied Physiology* **29**, 622–626.

Gordon, N.F., Kruger, P.E., van Rensburg, J.P., van der Linde, A., Kielbloack, A.J. & Cilliers, J.F. (1984) Effect of beta-adrenoreceptor blockade on thermoregulation during prolonged exercise in the heat. *Medicine and Science in Sports and Exercise* **16**, S138.

Greenleaf, J.E. (1992) Problem: thirst, drinking behavior, and involuntary dehydration. *Medicine and Science in Sports and Exercise* **24**, 645–656.

Gullestad, R. (1975) Temperature regulation in children during exercise. *Acta Paediatrica Scandinavica* **64**, 257–263.

Hall, E.L., Bergeron, M.F., Brenner, J.S., Wang, X. & Ludwig, D.A. (2005) Voluntary fluid intake and core temperature responses in children during exercise in the heat. *Medicine and Science in Sports and Exercise* **37**, S28.

Haymes, E.M., Buskirk, E.R., Hodgson, J.L., Lundegren, H.M. & Nicholas, W.C. (1974) Heat tolerance of exercising lean and heavy prepubertal girls. *Journal of Applied Physiology* **36**, 566–571.

Haymes, E.M., McCormick, R.J. & Buskirk, E.R. (1975) Heat tolerance of exercising lean and obese prepubertal boys. *Journal of Applied Physiology* **39**, 457–461.

Hindmarsh, K.W. & Opheim, E.E. (1990) Drug abuse prevalence in western Canada and the North West Territories: a survey of students in grades 6–12. *International Journal of the Addictions* **25**, 301–305.

Horswill, C.A., Passe, D.H., Stofan, J.R., Horn, M.K. & Murray, R. (2005) Adequacy of fluid ingestion in adolescents and adults during moderate-intensity exercise. *Pediatric Exercise Science* **17**, 41–50.

Hubbard, R.W. & Armstrong, L.E. (1988) The heat illnesses: biochemical, ultrastructural and fluid-electrolyte considerations. In: *Human Performance Physiology and Environmental Medicine at Terrestrial Extremes*. (Pandolf, K.B., Sawka, M.N. & Gonzalez, R.R., eds.) Benchmark Press, Indianapolis: 305–360.

Inbar, O. (1978) Acclimatization to dry and hot environments in young adults and children 8–10 years old. Doctoral thesis. Columbia University, New York.

Inbar, O., Bar-Or, O., Dotan, R. & Gutin, B. (1981) Conditioning versus exercise in heat as methods for acclimatizing 8- to 10-yr-old boys to dry heat. *Journal of Applied Physiology* **50**, 406–411.

Inbar, O., Morris, N., Epstein, Y. & Gass, G. (2004) Comparison of thermoregulatory responses to exercise in dry heat among prepubertal boys, young adults and older males. *Experimental Physiology* **89**, 691–700.

Inoue, Y., Kuwahara, T. & Araki, T. (2004) Maturation- and aging-related changes in heat loss effector function. *Journal of Physiological Anthropology and Applied Human Science* **23**, 289–294.

Iuliano, S., Naughton, G., Collier, G. & Carlson, J. (1998) Examination of the self-selected fluid intake practices by junior athletes during a simulated duathlon event. *International Journal of Sport Nutrition* **8**, 10–23.

Johnson, H.L., Nelson, R.A. & Consolazio, C.F. (1988) Effects of electrolyte and nutrient solutions on performance and metabolic balance. *Medicine and Science in Sports and Exercise* **20**, 26–33.

Jokinen, E., Valimaki, I., Antila, K., Seppanen, A. & Tuominen, J. (1990) Children in sauna: cardiovascular adjustment. *Pediatrics* **86**, 282–288.

Jokinen, E., Valimaki, I., Marniemi, J., Seppanen, A., Irjala, K. & Simell, O. (1991) Children in sauna: hormonal adjustments to intensive short thermal stress. *Acta Physiologica Scandinavica* **142**, 437–442.

Kaufman, F.L., Mills, D.E., Hughson, R.L. & Peake, G.T. (1988) Effects of bromocriptine on sweat gland function during heat acclimatization. *Hormone Research* **29**, 31–38.

Kawahata, A. (1960) Sex differences in sweating. In: *Essential Problems in Climate Physiology* (Yoshimura, H., Ogata, K. & Itoh, S., eds.) Nankodo, Kyoto: 169–184.

Klentrou, P., Cunliffe, M., Slack, J., *et al.* (2004) Temperature regulation during rest and exercise in the cold in premenarcheal and menarcheal girls. *Journal of Applied Physiology* **96**, 1393–1398.

Knochel, J.P. (1974) Environmental heat illness. An eclectic review. *Archives of Internal Medicine* **133**, 841–864.

Kolka, M.A., Stephenson, L.A., Bruttig, S.P., Cadarette, B.S. & Gonzalez, R.R. (1987) Human thermoregulation after atropine and/or pralidoxime administration. *Aviation, Space, and Environmental Medicine* **58**, 545–549.

Krog, J., Folkow, B., Fox, R.H. & Andersen, K.L. (1960) Hand circulation in the cold of Lapps and North Norwegian fisherman. *Journal of Applied Physiology* **15**, 654–658.

Kulczycki, L.L. & Robertson, M.T. (1988) The sweat chloride concentration and prolactin activity in cystic fibrosis. *Scandinavian Journal of Gastroenterology Supplement* **143**, 28–30.

Kuno, Y. (1956) *Human Perspiration.* C.C. Thomas, Springfield, IL.

Landing, B.H., Wells, T.R. & Williamson, M.L. (1968) Studies on growth of eccrine sweat glands. In: *Human Growth: Body Composition, Cell Growth, Energy and Intelligence* (Cheek, D.B., ed.) Lea & Febiger, Philadelphia, PA: 382–394.

Leduc, J. (1961) Catecholamine production and release in exposure and acclimation to cold. *Acta Physiologica Scandinavica Supplement* **183**, 1–101.

Leppaluoto, J. (1988) Human thermoregulation in sauna. *Annals of Clinical Research* **20**, 240–243.

Matsushita, K. & Araki, T. (1980) The effect of physical training on thermoregulatory responses of pre-adolescent boys to heat and cold. *Japanese Journal of Fitness and Sports Medicine* **29**, 69–74.

Maughan, R.J. (2001) Food and fluid intake during exercise. *Canadian Journal of Applied Physiology* **26**, S71–78.

McCormick, R.J. & Buskirk, E.R. (1974) Heat tolerance of exercising lean and obese middle-aged men. *Federation Proceedings* **33**, 441.

McLellan, T.M. (2001) The importance of aerobic fitness in determining tolerance to uncompensable heat stress. *Comparative Biochemistry and Physiology Part A Molecular Integrative Physiology* **128**, 691–700.

Meyer, F., Bar-Or, O., MacDougall, D. & Heigenhauser, G.J. (1992) Sweat electrolyte loss during exercise in the heat: effects of gender and maturation. *Medicine and Science in Sports and Exercise* **24**, 776–781.

Meyer, F., Bar-Or, O., MacDougall, D. & Heigenhauser, G.J. (1995a) Drink composition and the electrolyte balance of children exercising in the heat. *Medicine and Science in Sports and Exercise* **27**, 882–887.

Meyer, F., Bar-Or, O., Salsberg, A. & Passe, D. (1994) Hypohydration during exercise in children: effect on thirst, drink preferences, and rehydration. *International Journal of Sport Nutrition* **4**, 22–35.

Meyer, F., Bar-Or, O. & Wilk, B. (1995b) Children's perceptual responses to ingesting drinks of different compositions during and following exercise in the heat. *International Journal of Sport Nutrition* **5**, 13–24.

Noakes, T.D. (2005) High $\dot{V}o_{2max}$ with no history of training is due to high blood volume: an alternative explanation. *British Journal of Sports Medicine* **39**, 578.

Oppliger, R.A., Steen, S.A. & Scott, J.R. (2003) Weight loss practices of college wrestlers. *International Journal of Sport Nutrition and Exercise Metabolism* **13**, 29–46.

Pugh, L.G., Corbett, J.L. & Johnson, R.H. (1967) Rectal temperatures, weight losses, and sweat rates in marathon running. *Journal of Applied Physiology* **23**, 347–352.

Radomski, M.W., Cross, M. & Buguet, A. (1998) Exercise-induced hyperthermia and hormonal responses to exercise. *Canadian Journal of Physiology and Pharmacology* **76**, 547–552.

Randall, W.C. (1953) The physiology of sweating. *American Journal of Physical Medicine* **32**, 292–318.

Redfearn, J.A. Jr. & Murphy, R.J. (1969) History of heat stroke in a football trainee. *Journal of the American Medical Association* **208**, 699–700.

Rees, J. & Shuster, S. (1981) Pubertal induction of sweat gland activity. *Clinical Science (London)* **60**, 689–692.

Rivera-Brown, A.M., Gutierrez, R., Gutierrez, J.C., Frontera, W.R. & Bar-Or, O. (1999) Drink composition, voluntary drinking, and fluid balance in exercising, trained, heat-acclimatized boys. *Journal of Applied Physiology* **86**, 78–84.

Robertson, M.T. (1989) Prolactin, human nutrition and evolution, and the relation to cystic fibrosis. *Medical Hypotheses* **29**, 87–99.

Robertson, M.T., Boyajian, M.J., Patterson, K. & Robertson, W.V. (1986) Modulation of the chloride concentration of human sweat by prolactin. *Endocrinology* **119**, 2439–2444.

Robinson, S. (1938) Experimental studies of physical fitness in relation to age. *Internationale Zeitschrift fur angewandte Physiologie, einschliesslich Arbeitsphysiologie* **10**, 251–323.

Sansone, R.A. & Sawyer, R. (2005) Weight loss pressure on a 5 year old wrestler. *British Journal of Sports Medicine* **39**, e2.

Sato, K. & Sato, F. (1983) Individual variations in structure and function of human eccrine sweat gland. *American Journal of Physiology* **245**, R203–R208.

Savdie, E., Prevedoros, H., Irish, A., *et al.* (1991) Heat stroke following Rugby League football. *Medical Journal of Australia* **155**, 636–639.

Shapiro, Y. & Seidman, D.S. (1990) Field and clinical observations of exertional heat stroke patients. *Medicine and Science in Sports and Exercise* **22**, 6–14.

Shibasaki, M., Inoue, Y. & Kondo, N. (1997a) Mechanisms of underdeveloped sweating responses in prepubertal boys. *European Journal of Applied Physiology and Occupational Physiology* **76**, 340–345.

Shibasaki, M., Inoue, Y., Kondo, N., Aoki, K. & Hirata, K. (1999) Relationship between skin blood flow and sweating rate in prepubertal boys and young men. *Acta Physiologica Scandinavica* **167**, 105–110.

Shibasaki, M., Inoue, Y., Kondo, N. & Iwata, A. (1997b) Thermoregulatory responses of prepubertal boys and young men during moderate exercise. *European Journal of Applied Physiology and Occupational Physiology* **75**, 212–218.

Shibolet, S., Coll, R., Gilat, T. & Sohar, E. (1967) Heatstroke: its clinical picture and mechanism in 36 cases. *Quarterly Journal of Medicine* **36**, 525–548.

Shibolet, S., Fisher, S., Gilat, T., Bank, H. & Heller, H. (1962) Fibrinolysis and hemorrhages in fatal heatstroke. *New England Journal of Medicine* **266**, 169–173.

Shibolet, S., Lancaster, M.C. & Danon, Y. (1976) Heat stroke: a review. *Aviation, Space, and Environmental Medicine* **47**, 280–301.

Shirreffs, S.M. (2005) The importance of good hydration for work and exercise performance. *Nutrition Reviews* **63**, S14–S21.

Shvartz, E., Bhattacharya, A., Sperinde, S.J., Brock, P.J., Sciaraffa, D. & Van Beaumont, W. (1979) Sweating responses during heat acclimation and moderate conditioning. *Journal of Applied Physiology* **46**, 675–680.

Sloan, R.E. & Keatinge, W.R. (1973) Cooling rates of young people swimming in cold water. *Journal of Applied Physiology* **35**, 371–375.

Smolander, J., Bar-Or, O., Korhonen, O. & Ilmarinen, J. (1992) Thermoregulation during rest and exercise in the cold in pre- and early pubescent boys and in young men. *Journal of Applied Physiology* **72**, 1589–1594.

Sohar, E. & Shapiro, Y. (1965) The physiological reactions of women and children marching during heat. In: *Israel Physiology and Pharmacology Society* 50.

Squire, D.L. (1990) Heat illness. Fluid and electrolyte issues for pediatric and adolescent athletes. *Pediatric Clinics of North America* 37, 1085–1109.

Tipton, C.M. & Tcheng, T.K. (1970) Iowa wrestling study. Weight loss in high school students. *Journal of the American Medical Association* 214, 1269–1274.

Tipton, C.M., Tcheng, T.K. & Zambraski, E.J. (1976) Iowa wrestling study: weight classification systems. *Medicine and Science in Sports* 8, 101–104.

Tochihara, Y., Ohnaka, T. & Nagai, Y. (1995) Thermal responses of 6- to 8-year-old children during immersion of their legs in a hot water bath. *Applied Human Science* 14, 23–28.

Tsuzuki-Hayakawa, K., Tochihara, Y. & Ohnaka, T. (1995) Thermoregulation during heat exposure of young children compared to their mothers. *European Journal of Applied Physiology and Occupational Physiology* 72, 12–17.

Wada, M. (1950) Sudorific action of adrenalin on the human sweat glands and determination of their excitability. *Science* 111, 376–377.

Wagner, J.A., Robinson, S. & Marino, R.P. (1974) Age and temperature regulation of humans in neutral and cold

environments. *Journal of Applied Physiology* 37, 562–565.

Wagner, J.A., Robinson, S., Tzankoff, S.P. & Marino, R.P. (1972) Heat tolerance and acclimatization to work in the heat in relation to age. *Journal of Applied Physiology* 33, 616–622.

Walsh, R.M., Noakes, T.D., Hawley, J.A. & Dennis, S.C. (1994) Impaired high-intensity cycling performance time at low levels of dehydration. *International Journal of Sports Medicine* 15, 392–398.

Webster, S., Rutt, R. & Weltman, A. (1990) Physiological effects of a weight loss regimen practiced by college wrestlers. *Medicine and Science in Sports and Exercise* 22, 229–234.

White, J. & Ford, M.A. (1983) The hydration and electrolyte maintenance properties of an experimental sports drink. *British Journal of Sports Medicine* 17, 51–58.

Wilk, B. & Bar-Or, O. (1996) Effect of drink flavor and NaCL on voluntary drinking and hydration in boys exercising in the heat. *Journal of Applied Physiology* 80, 1112–1117.

Wilk, B., Jae-Hyun, L. & Bar-Or, O. (2005) Drink composition, voluntary drinking and aerobic performance in heat-acclimated adolescent male athletes. *Medicine and Science in Sports and Exercise* 37, S464.

Wilk, B., Kriemler, S., Keller, H. & Bar-Or, O. (1998) Consistency in preventing voluntary dehydration in boys who drink a flavored carbohydrate-NaCl beverage during exercise in the heat. *International Journal of Sport Nutrition* 8, 1–9.

Wilk, B., Yuxiu, H. & Bar-Or, O. (2002) Effect of hypohydration on aerobic performance of boys who exercise in the heat. *Medicine and Science in Sports and Exercise* 34, S48.

Williams, C.G., Wyndham, C.H. & Morrison, J.F. (1967) Rate of loss of acclimatization in summer and winter. *Journal of Applied Physiology* 22, 21–26.

Wolfe, S., Cage, G., Epstein, M., Tice, L., Miller, H. & Gordon, R.S. Jr. (1970) Metabolic studies of isolated human eccrine sweat glands. *Journal of Clinical Investigation* 49, 1880–1884.

Yeargin, S.W., Casa, D.J., Decher, N.R. & O'Connor, C.B. (2005) Incidence and degree of dehydration and attitutdes regarding hydration in children at summer football camp. *Medicine and Science in Sports and Exercise* 37, S463.

Young, A.J. (1988) Human adaptation to cold. In: *Human Performance Physiology and Environmental Medicine at Terrestial Extremes* (Pandolf, K.B., Sawka, M.N. & Gonzalez, R.R., eds.) Benchmark Press, Indianapolis: 401–434.

Chapter 21

Doping in Children and Adolescents

ERIC S. RAWSON AND ADAM M. PERSKY

At the age of 8 years, Richard Sandrak could bench press twice his body weight. Called "The Little Hercules," he received notoriety not only because of his physical prowess but also because his father was giving him powdered food supplements with vitamin and minerals as concoctions to promote strength and muscle mass. There was outcry by many parents that this was tantamount to child abuse, but Richard continued to earn money through appearances and endorsement deals. At the age of 13 years, Freddy Adu was offered $750,000 by Inter Milan to oversee his development as a soccer player. His mother refused the money, as well as dozens of other offers, claiming that Freddy was too young to play professionally. Subsequently, Freddy became an American citizen and joined the US Major League Soccer Under 17 team, where he was the highest paid player in the league ($500,000/year) at the age of 14 years. Additionally, he received a $1 million endorsement deal with Nike. Few people expected LeBron James to attend college following high school and play collegiate basketball. James was so skilled at basketball as a high school student, that National Basketball Association (NBA) coach John Lucas ignored NBA rules and invited the 17-year-old James to work out with the Cleveland Cavaliers. Lucas was fined $150,000 and suspended for two games, but believed it was worth it to watch James play in person. LeBron James entered the NBA Draft after high school, and began his professional basketball career with a $90 million Nike contract, and a 3-year $10.8 million dollar salary. While such child prodigies are rare, eager parents, coaches, and trainers of talented young athletes often have

been cited as promoting a "winning-at-all-costs" attitude.

The pressure to succeed in athletics, and the potential financial benefits of such success, can be overwhelming for children and adolescents. Weight gain, weight loss, increased energy levels, and improved sports performance are goals that are not exclusive to adults. Not coincidentally, the use of performance-enhancing substances, which may aid in the accomplishment of these goals, is also not exclusive to adults. Numerous substances are used by children and adolescents to gain an edge, but few of these compounds have been specifically studied and proven to be safe, enhance performance, or modulate body composition in youth. The most common substances used by children and adolescents are the nutritional supplement creatine, the herbal central nervous stimulant ephedra and its synthetic counterpart ephedrine, the drug caffeine, and anabolic-androgenic steroids and their precursor hormones. Each of these substances should be considered candidates for use and/or abuse by young individuals.

Creatine

Creatine became popular as a nutritional supplement in the early 1990s when Olympic Gold Medal winners Linford Christie and Sally Gunnell were reported to have used creatine (Hawes 1998). In addition to anecdotal reports of creatine's effectiveness as an ergogenic aid, scientific publications reported that dietary creatine supplementation could increase muscle creatine stores (Harris *et al.*

1992) and improve the performance of brief, high-power exercise (Greenhaff *et al.* 1993). We have previously reviewed the function of creatine and efficacy of creatine supplementation as an ergogenic aid (Rawson & Clarkson 2003) and summarize part of that review in the next few paragraphs. Although much research has been conducted on creatine, these studies have been in adults. We know little about the potential benefits or harm of creatine supplementation in children and adolescent athletes.

Creatine is a non-essential compound that can be obtained in the diet or synthesized by the liver, pancreas, and kidneys (Walker 1979). Approximately 95% of the body's creatine is stored in skeletal muscle, where its primary function is as an energy buffer. During times of increased energy demand, phosphocreatine (PCr) donates its phosphate to adenosine diphosphate (ADP) to produce adenosine triphosphate (ATP). Exercise tasks such as sprinting and weight lifting that involve brief, intense efforts rely heavily on the ATP-PCr energy system, which is the only fuel system in the muscles that can produce energy at sufficiently high rates to accomplish these tasks. Because the ATP-PCr energy system can provide ATP at maximal rates for only seconds before PCr stores are depleted, it has been theorized that increased PCr stores would provide an energy reserve available to support short-term, high-intensity activity.

Creatine is typically ingested as a loading dose of about 20 g·day^{-1} for 5 days and then a maintenance dose of 2–5 g·day^{-1}. The loading dose has been shown to increase muscle creatine stores and may also increase phosphocreatine resynthesis (Greenhaff *et al.* 1994; Yquel *et al.* 2002), although this has not been shown in every case (Vandenberghe *et al.* 1999). Following the creatine loading phase, muscle creatine levels increase approximately 25% to what appears to be a maximum of about 160 mmol·kg^{-1} dry muscle, although individual responses vary considerably (Harris *et al.* 1992; Hultman *et al.* 1996). It is worth noting that this high variability in response may explain why creatine supplementation appears to be ineffective as an ergogenic aid in some individuals and some studies.

Creatine supplementation and exercise performance

Several hundred studies have examined the effects of creatine supplementation on exercise performance and have been summarized and reviewed elsewhere (Lemon 2002; Kreider 2003; Rawson & Clarkson 2003; Rawson & Volek 2003). In controlled laboratory tests (e.g., cycling), creatine supplementation appears to improve performance of short-term (<30 s), high-intensity exercise, particularly when there are repeated bouts (Kreider 2003). Creatine supplementation is effective in improving performance during sprinting episodes within and at the end of certain prolonged events such as cycling races (Engelhardt *et al.* 1998; Vandebuerie *et al.* 1998). Field tests have also confirmed benefits of creatine supplementation. For example, in track events, Skare *et al.* (2001) reported increased velocity in the 100-m sprint and reduced total time of six intermittent 60-m sprints in subjects ingesting creatine compared with no changes in the placebo-supplemented subjects. The finding of improved sports performance resulting from creatine supplementation, however, is not consistent. As one of many examples, Op't Eijnde *et al.* (2001) found no effect of creatine supplementation on either power or precision of first and second services, baseline strokes, volleys, and shuttle run time in trained tennis players. However, the position of the American College of Sports Medicine (ACSM) is that "exercise performance involving short periods of extremely powerful activity can be enhanced, especially during repeated bouts" by creatine supplementation (Terjung *et al.* 2000).

Rawson and Volek (2003) reviewed 22 studies of the effects of creatine ingestion during resistance training. Sixteen of the studies reported a greater improvement in muscle strength and/or weight-lifting performance (maximal repetitions at a given percentage of maximal strength) in subjects ingesting creatine compared with placebo, one brief investigation (7 days) reported gains in the creatine group and no change in the placebo group, and five studies found no difference between creatine and placebo groups. Two meta-analyses concluded that body composition and performance of strength tests were improved with creatine supplementation (Branch 2003; Nissen & Sharp 2003). The ACSM consensus statement on creatine supplementation reached a similar conclusion regarding the combined effects of creatine ingestion and resistance training and states that "creatine supplementation is associated with enhanced accrual of strength in strength-training programs" (Terjung *et al*. 2000).

The safety of creatine supplements has been questioned but, despite a few case reports of adverse events with creatine use (Lawrence & Kirby 2002), other studies have not found problems (Greenwood *et al*. 2003; Kreider *et al*. 2003). However, it is important to note that all studies to assess the safety of creatine were carried out in adults. We do not know the long-term consequences of creatine supplementation in developing children.

Prevalence of creatine use

Given the proven benefits of creatine supplementation and lack of evidence that it is unsafe, it is no wonder that creatine is the most popular nutritional supplement with athletes. Use of creatine by younger athletes, as might be expected, lagged behind use by adult athletes. Massad *et al*. (1995) published a paper that examined the use of nutritional supplements in high school athletes. Twenty-two supplements were listed in the report including standards such as vitamins, minerals, protein and amino acids, and fluid replacement drinks as well as the more esoteric supplements such as ginseng, royal jelly, and bee pollen. Creatine is not mentioned in the report. It appears that creatine was not considered to be used by young athletes in 1995, but over the course of the next 10 years, it has become one of the most popular ergogenic aids in youth sports. In 1998, the popularity of creatine supplements led clinicians at the Mayo Clinic Sports Medicine Center to suspect that high school athletes were taking creatine supplements (Smith & Dahm 2000). They provided the first evidence of prevalence of creatine use in high school athletes by surveying athletes during a preparticipation examination, and found that the profile of a typical creatine user was a 16-year-old male involved in several sports with football as the primary sport (Smith & Dahm 2000).

Athletes as young as grade 6 were documented to be using creatine supplements, with a prevalence of 2.9% (2 of 69 athletes surveyed) (Metzl *et al*. 2001). Three studies reported that creatine use in high school athletes was greatest for grade 12 with prevalence rates of 44% (Metzl *et al*. 2001), 24.6% (McGuine *et al*. 2002), and 22% (Ray *et al*. 2001). It was noted that specifically for football players, the highest use was in grade 12 with a prevalence rate of 50.5% (McGuine *et al*. 2001). Other studies combining all grades of high school football players or college freshman football players found prevalence rates of 27.7% (Swirzinski 2000) and 36% (Jonnalagadda *et al*. 2001). From these studies, it appears that about 20–50% of high school athletes, especially seniors and football players, are taking creatine supplements. However, two studies reported lower rates of creatine use in high school athletes of 8.2% (and 21% for just football players) (Smith & Dahm 2000) and 6% (Mason *et al*. 2001), but it should be noted that the former study collected surveys in a preparticipation physical and the latter study had students return the surveys to the coaches. Students may have been reluctant, despite assurance of anonymity, to provide this information to a physician who must clear them to participate in the sport or the coach who controls whether they get to play. In other studies mentioned above, the surveys were administered by the study investigators, the athletic trainer, or the teacher (McGuine *et al*. 2001, 2002; Reeder 2003).

Most of the studies of high school athletes reported that creatine was used to improve performance (Smith & Dahm 2000; Mason *et al*. 2001; Metzl *et al*. 2001), improve strength (McGuine *et al*. 2002; Reeder 2003), enhance recovery (McGuine *et al*. 2001) or increase body weight and build muscle (Swirzinski 2000). Friends and teammates were the most common source of information about creatine (Smith & Dahm 2000; Swirzinski 2000; McGuine *et al*. 2001, 2002; Ray *et al*. 2001; Reeder 2003). One study reported that 26% of the high school athletes experienced side effects of muscle cramps, increased thirst, and stomach cramps (Ray *et al*. 2001). Forty percent of high school athletes who used creatine took an incorrect dose, and 70% took excessive amounts for the maintenance dose (Ray *et al*. 2001).

Creatine supplementation in young athletes

Two studies were identified that examined the effect of creatine supplementation on swimming performance of young athletes (Dawson *et al.* 2002; Theodorou *et al.* 2005). Dawson *et al.* (2002) tested 20 junior swimmers (mean age 16.4 years) before and after creatine (20 g·day^{-1} for 5 days followed by 5 g·day^{-1} for 22 days) or placebo ingestion. The supplementation did not affect single sprint performance in the pool or body composition. However, the supplement did improve total work scores in a 30-s Biokinetic Swim Bench test compared with the placebo. Theodorou *et al.* (2005) compared the effects of creatine (25 g·day^{-1} for 4 days) and creatine plus 400 g carbohydrate supplementation on repeated bouts of maximal swimming in swimmers from the British National Team (mean age 17.8 years). Both creatine and creatine plus carbohydrate supplementation improved swim velocity by a similar amount ($\approx$0.03 m·s^{-1}) over 8–10 repeated intervals, with no difference between the two treatments. Although these studies did find some benefit of creatine supplementation, it is still too preliminary to state that creatine is effective or safe in growing children.

Central nervous system stimulants

The use of central nervous systems stimulants, which may aid in weight loss, increase energy levels, or improve sports performance, is becoming increasingly common. Two drugs that have been studied extensively in adults, and are being used more frequently by younger persons, are ephedrine and caffeine. Both drugs can be ingested in the form of herbal dietary supplements or synthetic drugs or when added to food supplements such as energy drinks. Although a great deal is known about ephedrine and caffeine ingestion in adults, we currently know little about the possible beneficial or harmful effects of ephedrine or caffeine in children and adolescent athletes.

Ephedrine

The most controversial dietary supplements, and the ones that may be most likely to be abused by young people, are those that contain ephedrine. Ephedrine is a sympathomimetic drug and central nervous system stimulant (Hoffman & Lefkowitz 1996), which can be purchased as synthetic ephedrine or in herbal supplements that naturally contain ephedra (Ma Huang, Ephedra Sinica). Ephedra is a herb that contains a combination of alkaloids including ephedrine, pseudoephedrine, norephedrine, and methylephedrine (Gurley *et al.* 1998, 2000). According to the 2005 World Anti-Doping Agency 2005 list, ephedrine and methylephedrine are banned when urine concentrations exceed 10 μg·mL^{-1}, but related compounds such as phenylpropanolamine, synephrine, and pseudoephedrine are not prohibited. Ephedrine has been studied as a weight loss aid (Astrup *et al.* 1992a) because it has both thermogenic and anorectic properties (Dulloo & Miller 1986; Astrup & Toubro 1993). More recently, the effect of ephedrine on exercise performance has been studied because it is a central nervous system stimulant (Bell *et al.* 1998, 2000, 2001, 2002; Bell & Jacobs 1999; Jacobs *et al.* 2003).

ADVERSE EFFECTS OF EPHEDRINE

The highly publicized deaths of several athletes and several thousand reports of adverse events associated with ephedrine have made its ingestion controversial. Haller and Benowitz (2000) reviewed 140 case reports and determined that 31% of adverse events were considered to be definitely or probably related to the use of ephedra alkaloid containing supplements, and 31% were judged to be possibly related. Of the adverse events considered related to ephedra use, there were 10 deaths, 13 events that produced permanent disability, 17 reports of hypertension, 13 reports of palpitations, tachycardia, or both, 10 cases of stroke, and 7 cases of seizures. In a similar analysis, of 926 cases of ephedra toxicity, Samenuk *et al.* (2002) concluded that:

1 Ephedra use is temporally related to stroke, myocardial infarction, and sudden death;

2 Underlying heart or vascular disease is not a prerequisite for ephedra-related adverse events; and

3 The cardiovascular toxic effects associated with ephedra were not limited to massive doses.

Points 2 and 3 are important messages to relay to young athletes, and their trainers, coaches, or parents, who may mistakenly believe that only persons with pre-existing disease or those taking higher than recommended doses of ephedrine are at risk. Shekelle *et al.* (2003) evaluated safety data from 50 ephedrine/ephedra studies and reported a 2.2- to 3.6-fold increase in odds of psychiatric, autonomic or gastrointestinal symptoms, and heart palpitations. The authors concluded that they had adequate statistical power to detect adverse events that occur at a frequency of 1 per 1000 or higher, and observed no serious adverse events in any of the trials ($n = 1706$). However, the data were insufficient to draw conclusions about adverse events that occur at a rate less than 1 per 1000.

PREVALENCE OF EPHEDRINE USE

A study of more than 14,000 National Collegiate Athletic Association (NCAA) student athletes at 991 institutions reported that 3.5% ingest ephedrine (Green *et al.* 2001). However, because ephedrine is banned by the NCAA it is likely that the true prevalence of ephedrine use was underreported. In physically active adults exercising in commercial fitness centers, 25% of men and 13% of women reported ephedrine use (Kanayama *et al.* 2001). If the sample size in this study were extrapolated to approximate the number of adults currently exercising at commercial fitness centers in the USA, it could be estimated that nearly 3 million exercising adults are ingesting ephedrine. The widely divergent results of these two studies reveal the difficulty in obtaining an accurate portrayal of ephedrine use among physically active adults. In a study of 752 adults, Harnack *et al.* (2001) reported that 12% used ephedra (52% for boosting energy and 46% for weight loss) while Blanck *et al.* (2001) reported a 1% prevalence of ephedra use in 14,679 adults in the Behavioral Risk Factor Surveillance System Survey, demonstrating the difficulty in obtaining data on ephedrine use in the general population.

Even less is known about ephedrine use in children and adolescents, as studies of dietary supplement behaviors in younger persons often do not specifically address ephedrine ingestion, but instead collapse multiple "energy boosters" into one cate-

gory. In many countries, ephedrine is a prescription drug used for weight loss, but in the USA ephedrine/ephedra containing supplements can be purchased without a prescription. Subsequent to the high profile deaths of several professional athletes and numerous reports of adverse events (Haller & Benowitz 2000; Rawson & Clarkson 2002; Samenuk *et al.* 2002; Bent *et al.* 2003; Shekelle *et al.* 2003), the US Food and Drug Administration (FDA) banned the sale of the ephedrine-containing herb ephedra on April 12, 2004. Although herbal ephedra became unavailable in stores, synthetic ephedrine was still readily available. Additionally, dietary supplements containing synephrine (contained in citrus aurantium, bitter orange, sour orange, Seville orange), which has little information available regarding safety and efficacy, were heavily marketed for weight loss. Only 1 year after ephedra was banned, a US District Court in Utah determined that the FDA did not prove by a preponderance of evidence that a dose of 10 mg or less of ephedra alkaloids presents a "significant or unreasonable risk of injury." Thus, it may be legal to sell ephedra supplements with a recommended daily dose of less than 10 mg. Despite the fact that ephedrine is a banned substance by many professional and amateur sports organizations, and despite the risk of adverse events, athletes continue to use ephedrine.

EPHEDRINE AND WEIGHT LOSS

The effects of ephedrine on weight loss and exercise performance in adults have been previously reviewed (Rawson & Clarkson 2002; Shekelle *et al.* 2003). Ephedrine is both an α and β agonist and it causes the release of norepinephrine from sympathetic neurons (Hoffman & Lefkowitz 1996). Although ephedrine is marketed primarily as a "thermogenic" supplement that induces weight loss through increased metabolic rate, it is estimated that 75% of weight loss from ephedrine/caffeine combinations is brought about by appetite suppression (Dulloo & Miller 1986; Astrup & Toubro 1993). Ephedrine slows down the rate at which food exits the stomach, which could affect satiety (Jonderko & Kucio 1991). When combined with caffeine and aspirin (acetylsalicylic acid), ephedrine becomes a more effective weight loss drug by acting on the prejunctional inhibitors of norepinephrine, adenosine, and prostaglandins (Dulloo 1993; Dulloo *et al.* 1994). To capitalize on this, many ephedra products contain herbal sources of caffeine (e.g., guarana, kola nut) and salicylic acid (e.g., white willow bark). Adenosine, which is stimulated by norepinephrine, negatively modulates norepinephrine levels. Caffeine blunts the effects of adenosine, thus disrupting the feedback system that regulates norepinephrine release. Similarly, prostaglandins are stimulated by norepinephrine, which also regulate norepinephrine release. Acetylsalicylic acid inhibits the production of prostaglandins, increasing norepinephrine release (Dulloo 1993).

In a recent meta-analysis, Shekelle *et al.* (2003) reported that ephedrine, ephedrine plus caffeine, ephedra, and ephedra plus caffeine (from herbal sources) promote weight loss, but these effects are modest when compared with placebo (0.9 kg per month > placebo). For instance, Astrup *et al.* (1992a) reported the effects of a 24-week diet plus either an ephedrine/caffeine combination (20 mg/200 mg), ephedrine (20 mg), caffeine (200 mg), or placebo. The ephedrine/caffeine group lost significantly more weight than the placebo group (ephedrine/caffeine 16.6 kg vs. placebo 13.2 kg), but Astrup *et al.* (1992a,b) described the additional weight loss attributed to ephedrine (1.7 kg) as "clinically irrelevant" compared with the weight loss achieved through diet, nutritional education, frequent monitoring, and behavior therapy (13 kg). Finally, it is doubtful yet unknown whether the weight-reducing effects of ephedrine/caffeine combinations are sustained once the use of these drugs is discontinued.

EPHEDRINE AND PERFORMANCE

Several studies of the effects of ephedrine on exercise performance in adults have been conducted by the Canadian military (Bell *et al.* 1998, 2000, 2001, 2002; Bell & Jacobs 1999; Jacobs *et al.* 2003). Bell *et al.* (1998) first reported ≈5 min increase in time to exhaustion (17.5 vs. 12.6 min) on a cycle ergometer following ephedrine plus caffeine ingestion (1 mg·kg body mass^{-1} ephedrine; 5 mg·kg body mass^{-1} caffeine). In a field study, Bell and Jacobs (1999) reported ≈1.5 min performance improvement of the

Canadian Forces Warrior Test (a 3.2-km run wearing 11 kg of military gear) following the combined ingestion of ephedrine (75 mg) and caffeine (375 mg). Because the combined effects of high-dose ephedrine and caffeine made about 25% of the subjects vomit or nauseous, Bell *et al.* (2000) investigated whether reduced levels of ephedrine (0.8 vs. 1.0 mg·kg body mass^{-1}) plus caffeine (4 vs. 5 mg·kg body mass^{-1}) would preserve the ergogenic effect with fewer adverse events. Time to exhaustion on a cycle ergometer at 85% $\dot{V}o_{2peak}$ was improved (≈10 min) compared to the placebo condition regardless of the dose of ephedrine or caffeine. There were no incidents of nausea or vomiting with the lowest doses of ephedrine and caffeine. In a demonstration that ephedrine can improve performance during short-term sprint exercise, Bell *et al.* (2001) reported increased power output during the first 10 s of a 30-s Wingate test following ephedrine ingestion (1 mg·kg body mass^{-1}). Subsequently, Bell *et al.* (2002) examined the impact of ephedrine (0.8 mg·kg body mass^{-1}) or ephedrine plus caffeine (4 mg·kg body mass^{-1}) on endurance performance, and showed a 48 s (≈2%) decrease in 10-km run time. Thus, ephedrine, especially when combined with caffeine, can improve exercise performance during tasks lasting from 30 s to 45 min.

Jacobs *et al.* (2003) studied the effects of ephedrine ingestion (0.8 mg·kg body weight^{-1}) and ephedrine plus caffeine ingestion (4 mg·kg body weight^{-1}) on resistance training performance. The treatments resulted in a 4 (ephedrine) and 6 (ephedrine plus caffeine) repetition increase during the first of five sets of leg presses at 80% of 1 RM, and a 1 (ephedrine) and 2 (ephedrine plus caffeine) increase in bench press repetitions at 70% of 1 RM during the first of five sets of bench presses. The finding that ephedrine can improve performance of weight-lifting tasks may not be surprising to athletes, as ephedrine has long been marketed and consumed chronically by athletes as a training aid before resistance training workouts.

EPHEDRINE INGESTION IN YOUNG PERSONS

One study was identified that specifically examined the effects of ephedrine plus caffeine on weight loss in obese adolescents (Molnar *et al.* 2000). Molnar *et al.* (2000) supplemented 32 obese adolescents (Tanner stage III–IV; >140% body mass for height; mean age 16 years) with 10–30 mg ephedrine and 100–300 mg caffeine for 30 weeks. Participants were advised how to reduce daily energy intake by 500 kcal·day^{-1} and were encouraged to be physically active. Weight loss in the treatment group was markedly greater than the placebo group (7.9 vs. 0.5 kg), no serious adverse reactions were noted, and the total number of mild and moderate adverse effects (e.g., nausea, insomnia, tremor) was not different between groups, indicating that ephedrine plus caffeine is an effective weight loss therapy in obese adolescents enrolled in a medically supervised weight loss program. No studies have examined the effects of ephedrine ingestion on exercise performance in young persons.

Caffeine

Caffeine occurs naturally in more than 60 plant species (e.g., coffee, tea, kola nuts, bissy nuts, guarana, cocoa) and is often added to beverages, dietary supplements, and medications. The effects of caffeine on muscular work have been studied for 100 years (Rivers & Webber 1907), and research on caffeine has been extensively reviewed (Spriet & Howlett 2000; Graham 2001; Spriet 2002; Magkos & Kavouras 2004). Spriet (2002) and Graham (2001) have referred to caffeine as the "most widely abused" and "most commonly consumed" drug in the world. Caffeine use by athletes is common and socially acceptable, and this laissez-faire attitude may encourage caffeine abuse in children and adolescents.

The mechanisms responsible for the improved exercise performance associated with caffeine ingestion are difficult to determine conclusively, but there are three theories (Spriet & Howlett 2000; Spriet 2002). In the metabolic theory, caffeine may stimulate lipolysis by increasing circulating epinephrine levels, thus sparing muscle glycogen. Additional metabolic effects of caffeine include inhibition of glycogen phosphorylase, antagonism of adenosine receptors, and inhibition of phosphodiesterase. A second possibility is that caffeine may directly affect skeletal muscle through ion handling by stimulating Na^+-K^+ ATPase activity and altering calcium kinetics. Specifically, caffeine may increase the release of calcium from the sarcoplasmic reticulum, increase troponin and myosin calcium sensitivity, and decrease reuptake of calcium by the sarcoplasmic reticulum. Finally, caffeine may directly affect the central nervous system by stimulating the release of neurotransmitters or altering motor unit recruitment, causing decreased perceived exertion (Spriet & Howlett 2000; Spriet 2002).

PREVALENCE OF CAFFEINE USE

Over the past two decades, caffeine consumption has increased in all age groups (Frary *et al.* 2005). The Continuing Surveys of Food Intakes by Individuals (CSFII) provides the largest database to identify caffeine intake in persons aged 2 and older ($n = 15,716$ caffeine consumers) (Frary *et al.* 2005). Overall, 87% of the population consumes caffeine (mean: 193 mg·day^{-1}; 1.2 mg·kg^{-1}·day^{-1}), and 76% of persons younger than 18 years of age consume caffeine (Frary *et al.* 2005). When stratified by age groups, it can be seen that 76% of those aged 2–5 years (16 mg·day^{-1}), 86% of those aged 6–11 years (26 mg·day^{-1}), and ≈90% of those aged 12–17 years (70 mg·day^{-1}) consume caffeine (Frary *et al.* 2005). A significant percentage of caffeine intake in younger persons comes from soft drink consumption, which has increased from 11 to 47 gallons·year^{-1} over the last five decades (USDA 2004). Although coffee intake has decreased by nearly 50% during this time period (USDA 2004), the introduction of specialty coffee beverages has attracted younger persons to coffee houses, and caffeine intake in young persons may be increasing via consumption of these drinks. Caffeine was recently removed (January 2004) from the International Olympic Committee (IOC) banned substance list. Previously, a 12 μg·mL^{-1} urinary concentration limit was set by the IOC, although caffeine doses of 3 mg·kg body weight^{-1} are ergogenic and up to 9 mg·kg body weight^{-1} taken 1 h before exercise is unlikely to cause a positive drug test (Graham 2001). It is unknown if the decision to remove caffeine from the IOC banned substance list will increase caffeine consumption among young athletes, because caffeine ingestion was already widely accepted and health risks are perceived to be minimal. For instance, in 1996, 27% of high school athletes in Canada reported purposefully ingesting caffeine to improve sports performance (Melia *et al.* 1996).

CAFFEINE AND EXERCISE PERFORMANCE

It is generally accepted that caffeine can improve endurance exercise performance (40–80 min) in adults. For instance, in running or cycling trials at 80–90% of $\dot{V}_{O_{2max}}$, elite and recreationally trained athletes show a 20–50% improvement in performance following caffeine ingestion. More recently, the effect of caffeine on shorter-term exercise performance (30 s to 35 min) has been studied. Although the data are somewhat discrepant, caffeine appears to improve performance during exercise lasting 20–35 min at 85–95% $\dot{V}_{O_{2max}}$ and during exercise lasting 4–8 min at 95–110% $\dot{V}_{O_{2max}}$, but not during sprint exercise lasting 30–90 s (Spriet & Howlett 2000; Graham 2001; Spriet 2002).

CAFFEINE INGESTION IN YOUNG PERSONS

Little is known about the effects of caffeine in exercising children. Sasaki *et al.* (1987) reported that caffeine ingestion (384 mg), sucrose ingestion (81 g), or caffeine plus sucrose (396 mg caffeine; 72 g sucrose) equally improved endurance running performance at 80% of $\dot{V}_{O_{2max}}$ in five high school distance runners (mean age 15.6 years). Additionally, fat utilization was highest in the caffeine only treatment. In a preliminary study, Turley *et al.* (2004) reported no changes in oxygen consumption or respiratory exchange ratio in six 7- to 9-year-old children ingesting caffeine (5 mg·kg body weight^{-1}) or placebo prior to a submaximal ergometer test at 25 and 50 W. However, heart rate was lower and systolic and diastolic blood pressures were higher during the caffeine condition. In a second preliminary study, DeSisso *et al.* (2005) reported that caffeine (5 mg·kg^{-1} body weight) decreased exercise heart rate and increased exercise blood pressure in boys (7–9 years) but not men (18–25 years). Although it is possible that caffeine has similar ergogenic effects in children and adolescents, few data are available.

Anabolic-androgenic steroids

Testosterone was isolated in 1935 and, based on its known physiologic actions, was suggested as a performance enhancer as early as 1939 (Boje 1939). Much of the athletic community appeared to take little notice of the potential performance-enhancing effects of testosterone until 1954, when Dr. John Ziegler, a team physician for the US weight lifting team, learned from a Soviet physician that Soviet weight lifters were using testosterone (Bahrke & Yesalis 2002). Dr. Ziegler returned to the USA and along with several weight lifters at the York Barbell Club, experimented with testosterone. It was known by this time that testosterone had both anabolic properties (i.e., the ability to increase muscle size and strength) and androgenic properties (i.e., the ability to increase virilization and aggression), and Dr. Ziegler was concerned about the androgenic effects of testosterone. Dr. Ziegler worked with Ciba Pharmaceutical Company to develop an anabolic drug, with reduced androgenic effects. Together, Dr. Ziegler and Ciba Pharmaceuticals developed the anabolic-androgenic steroid (AAS) Dianabol®. AASs are synthetic testosterone derivatives and mimic some degree of the anabolic and androgenic effects of testosterone (Rahwan 1988; Clarkson & Persky 2002). Reports of the effectiveness of steroids on increasing muscle size and strength spread through the athletic community. More recently, prohormones have been marketed as dietary supplements; these prohormones are precursors to testosterone and include androstenedione and dehydroepiandrosterone (DHEA).

The effects of AASs on skeletal muscle are the primary interest to athletes, despite their effects on other tissues, including reproductive tissue (Feinberg *et al.* 1997), bone (Katznelson *et al.* 1996), adipose tissue (Hislop *et al.* 1999), brain (Rubinow & Schmidt 1996), prostate (Jin *et al.* 1996), liver (Boada *et al.* 1999), and kidney (Martorana *et al.* 1999). The classic theory for steroid action is modulation of gene transcription through direct interaction with the androgen receptor. The androgen receptor is part of the steroid hormone receptor superfamily which also includes receptors for glucocorticoids, estradiol, retinoids, thyroid hormone, progesterone, and mineralcorticoids (Brinkmann *et al.* 1999). Androgens, like other endogenous steroids, can have nongenomic effects (Heinlein & Chang 2002; Estrada *et al.* 2003); additionally AAS act indirectly on skeletal muscle to control muscle mass (Sheffield-Moore 2000).

Effects of testosterone and anabolic-androgenic steroids

The main effect testosterone and AAS have on the body is to alter body composition by increasing muscle mass. As early as the 1970s, several studies showed increases in body mass with AAS use including stanozolol (Winstrol®) (Casner *et al.* 1971) and methandrostenlone (Dianabol®) (Ward 1973). More recently, Ferrando *et al.* (1998) administered intramuscular testosterone (200 mg·day^{-1} testosterone enanthate) for 5 days to assess protein synthesis in males using fractional synthetic rate across the leg. The investigators found no change in protein breakdown but a twofold increase in protein synthetic rate with testosterone administration. This group used the same technique again in males to examine the effects of the oral AAS, oxandrolone (Anavar®) 15 mg·day^{-1} for 5 days (Sheffield-Moore *et al.* 1999). Like testosterone, there was no change in protein catabolic rates but there was a 44% increase in fractional synthetic rate. Other studies have also found testosterone administration increases protein synthesis (Griggs *et al.* 1989; Urban *et al.* 1995; Brodsky *et al.* 1996).

Prevalence of anabolic-androgenic steroid and testosterone use

The application of surveys to determine the AAS use in athletes may underestimate the actual prevalence, because AAS are banned by many national and international governing bodies in sports including the IOC, the NCAA, and almost all professional sports organizations. As such, athletes are unlikely to report using banned substances for fear of being discovered and disqualified. Alternatively, positive drug tests could be used to determine prevalence; however, many athletes know how to administer AAS so they do not test positive. Prevalence of use

by those in the general public, including adolescents and children, is also difficult to assess because these drugs are illegal. Thus, the data provided are probably an underestimation of actual use.

The pharmacoepidemiology of AAS use has been recently reviewed (Bahrke & Yesalis 2002; Thiblin & Petersson 2005). Thiblin and Petersson (2005) reviewed the prevalence of AAS use among exercisers, and prevalence of use in athletes ranged between 6.2 and 38.4%. However, these data should be treated with some caution as response rate to the surveys was at best 66%. Prevalence rates from nonathletes typically range from 0.4% to 6.7% in males (Thiblin & Petersson 2005). Most of the data in these surveys included children, adolescents, and young adults, with ages ranging from 8 years old (Tanner *et al.* 1995) up to the early 20s. The survey results not only characterize the prevalence in the USA, but also in South Africa (Schwellnus *et al.* 1992; Lambert *et al.* 1998), Sweden (Nilsson *et al.* 2001a,b), Canada (Melia *et al.* 1996), the UK (Korkia 1996), and Europe as a whole (Thiblin & Petersson 2005). Table 21.1 is a partial list of studies on the prevalence of AAS use in adolescents.

Effectiveness of testosterone and anabolic-androgenic steroids

Since the first use of testosterone for performance enhancement in the 1950s, there has been equivocal evidence that AAS are ergogenic (for reviews see Haupt & Rovere 1984; Lamb 1984; Clarkson & Thompson 1997; Sturmi & Diorio 1998; Blue & Lombardo 1999; Bahrke & Yesalis 2002; Hartgens & Kuipers 2004) until a definitive study in 1996. Bhasin *et al.* (1996) examined the cumulative impact of resistance exercise and testosterone administration in healthy males aged 19–40 years. Testosterone enanthate (600 mg·week^{-1} i.m.) was administered for 10 weeks in a parallel, 4-arm, placebo controlled study. Subjects administered testosterone had a 3.2 kg increase in fat-free mass and subjects receiving testosterone who exercised had a 6.1 kg increase in fat-free mass; the placebo + exercise control group had a 1.9 kg increase in fat-free mass. The groups receiving testosterone also had significant increases in muscle cross-sectional areas for both the triceps

Table 21.1 Prevalence of anabolic-androgenic steroid and testosterone use in young individuals.

Region	Age group	n	Gender	Prevalence of use (%)
Canada (Melia et al. 1996)	11–18	16119	M and F combined	2.8
Europe (Thiblin & Petersson 2005)	15–16	10000	M/F	2.0/1.0
Norway (Wichstrom & Pedersen 2001)	15–22	8508	M and F combined	0.8
South Africa (Lambert et al. 1998)	16–18	2547	M/F	2.8/1.5
Sweden (Thiblin & Petersson 2005)	15–16	5349	M	1
Sweden (Thiblin & Petersson 2005)	18	36085	M	0.8
Sweden (Nilsson 1995)	14–19	688/695	M/F	5.8/1.0
Sweden (Nilsson et al. 2001b)	16–17	2785	M/F	3.0/0
Sweden (Kindlundh et al. 1998)	16–17	1353/1364	M/F	2.7/0.4
USA (Windsor & Dumitru 1989)	17 (average)	1010	M/F	5.0/1.4
USA (Buckley et al. 1988)	16–18	3403	M	6.6
USA (Komoroski & Rickert 1992)	16–17	672/806	M/F	7.6/1.5
USA (Radakovich et al. 1993)	12–13	1624	M/F	4.7/3.2
USA (Tanner et al. 1995)	8–17	3438/3492	M/F	4.0/1.3
USA (DuRant et al. 1995)	15–19	6253/6000	M/F	4.08/1.2
USA (Scott et al. 1996)	13–19	2136/2522	M/F	4.5/0.8
USA (Stilger & Yesalis 1999)	14–18	873	M	6.3
USA (Irving et al. 2002)	14–18	4746	M/F	5.4/2.9
USA (Elliot et al. 2004)	15.4	668	M/F	0.1
USA (Faigenbaum et al. 1998)	9–13	466/499	M/F	2.6/2.8

(~12% from baseline for testosterone alone; and ~14% from baseline for testosterone + exercise) and quadriceps (~6% from baseline for testosterone alone; and ~14% from baseline for testosterone + exercise); muscle strength also increased as assessed by the bench press (~9% from baseline for testosterone alone; and ~23% from baseline for testosterone + exercise), and the squat (~11% from baseline for testosterone alone; and ~37% from baseline for testosterone + exercise). Thus, testosterone, even in the absence of exercise, can improve muscular performance. Although the results from this study confirm that AAS can improve muscle size and strength, these increases may be underestimated, because AASs are commonly used in conjunction with other AASs or other anabolic/anti-catabolic agents (e.g., growth hormone), human chorionic gonadotropin, anti-estrogens, and clenbuterol.

Effectiveness of prohormones

Whereas testosterone and its synthetic derivatives have been studied as ergogenic aids since the 1950s, dietary supplements purported to increase endogenous testosterone have only been recently studied, beginning with the 1996 marketing of androstenedione. Studies of these prohormones have been reviewed (Kraemer et al. 2002; Ziegenfuss et al. 2002). While some studies have shown increases in testosterone after androstenedione (Uralets & Gillette 1999; Leder et al. 2000; Brown et al. 2001, 2002) or DHEA administration (Barnhart et al. 1999; Genazzani et al. 2003), others have shown no increase in testosterone after androstenedione (Ballantyne et al. 2000; Rasmussen et al. 2000; Colker et al. 2001) or DHEA administration (Bosy et al. 1998). Despite the possible changes in testosterone, most studies fail to show performance enhancement. In an 8-week placebo controlled trial, healthy men (age 19–29 years, $n = 20$) were randomized to resistance exercise plus 300 mg·day^{-1} androstenedione or placebo. An additional 10 men were used for pharmacokinetic analysis. Free and total testosterone did not change but serum estradiol increased after 2, 5, and 8 weeks of supplementation. Strength gains were similar between the active arm and placebo control. Wallace et al. (1999) found that both androstenedione (100 mg·day^{-1} for 12 weeks) and DHEA (100 mg·day^{-1} for 12 weeks) failed to improve strength compared to placebo. These results were confirmed by Broeder *et al.* (2000) who found that androstenedione (200 mg·day^{-1} for 12 weeks) or androstenediol (200 mg·day^{-1} for 12 weeks) failed to improve muscle performance. The lack of performance-enhancing effects in these studies is supported by a more mechanistic study investigating the fractional synthetic rate after administration of androstenedione (100 mg·day^{-1} for 5 days); androstenedione failed to increase fractional synthetic rate or reduce muscle degradation rates.

Like anabolic-steroid use in the 1970s, prohormone use at the turn of the century came under scrutiny. The quality of androstenedione supplements came under suspicion when the University of California, Los Angles Olympic Analytical Laboratory tested the content of various prohormone supplements and found no androstenedione in one product, 10 mg testosterone in another, and four products that contained 90% or less of the amount claimed on the label (Catlin *et al.* 2000). In an androstenedione supplementation study, 20 of 24 of the treated subjects exceeded the cut-off for urinary 19-norandrosterone, the marker for the AAS nandrolone. Thus, athletes could potentially fail a drug test for the AAS nandrolone by taking the dietary supplement androstenedione. As of 2005, most sporting organizations have banned the use of prohormones. In 2004, the US FDA called for the removal of prohormones from the market, until safety issues had been addressed. In early 2005, prohormones, with the exception of DHEA, were removed from the US market.

Testosterone and anabolic androgenic steroids in children and adolescents

For ethical reasons it is difficult to study AAS in children and adolescents. The initial information stems from the secret doping programs of the German Democratic Republic (GDR). The GDR is one of the largest pharmacologic experiments in history spanning nearly three decades (1960s–1990s) (Franke & Berendonk 1997). During this period, adolescent girls and boys were given AAS to improve athletic performance. The GDR scientists noted numerous side effects in their adolescent population including muscle tightness and cramps, acne and hirsutism, alterations in libido, liver damage, amenorrhea, and even death (see Table 21.2 for a summary on potential side effects of AAS). These results do not include the various pathologies these adults now face because of their AAS use as adolescents. Under the GDR system, athletes experienced a dramatic increase in performance. For example, a 5–10 s decrease in running time for the women's 800 m, a 10–12 m increase in men's discus throw, and an 11–20 m increase in women's discus throw (Franke & Berendonk 1997). In the Montreal Olympics in 1976, 11 out of the 13 female swimming events were won by GDR athletes (Franke & Berendonk 1997).

The most recent studies of AAS and children are in burns patients, although this is not directly linked to performance enhancement. Children with major burns (>40% of body surface) are in a catabolic state with respect to muscle and bone for up to 1 year after injury; this catabolic state impairs their normal growth pattern (Murphy *et al.* 2004). Anabolic agents such as AAS and growth hormone are used to enhance the muscle and bone growth to aid normal developmental patterns. In one study (Murphy *et al.* 2004), a total of 84 children aged 1.1–18.8 years (mean 8.5 years in the active group, 8.2 years in placebo group) who had burns on >40% of their total body surface area were enrolled. The active arm ($n = 42$) received oxandrolone orally (0.1 mg·kg^{-1} b.i.d.) for up to 1 year. Children in the placebo group lost nearly 5% more additional lean body mass over the first 6 months, whereas the active arm did not lose lean body mass over the first 6 months after discharge. Twelve months after discharge the active arm increased lean body mass by 13.5% and the placebo arm by 2.6%. When examining changes in bone mass, patients in the active arm had 12.5% increase in bone mineral density at 12 months post-discharge compared to 4% in the placebo controlled group. There were no notable side effects in the oxandrolone treated patients except two female patients sustained some degree of "clitoromegaly" at which time the drug was stopped but was deemed more likely caused by post-burn edema than drug-related. Markers of hepatoxicity such as alanine aminotransaminase (ALT) and aspartate aminotransaminase (AST), bilirubin and gamma-glutaryltransferase remained

Table 21.2 Selected adverse events from AAS use.

Reproductive (male)	*Cardiovascular*
↓ Reproductive hormones	↑ Total cholesterol
Testicular atrophy	↓ HDL*
Impotence	↑ Triglycerides
Prostate hypertrophy/carcinoma	Hypertension
Priapism	Thrombosis
Gyncomastia	↑ Left ventricular mass
↑ Estrogen*	
Reproductive (female)	*Musculoskeletal*
Menstrual irregularities	Early epiphyseal
Clitoral hypertrophy	(growth plate) closure in children
Atrophy of uterine and breast tissue	↑ Risk of muscle strains/tears
Viriliztion	
Liver[†]	*Endocrine (not reproductive)*
Cholestasis and associated	↓ Glucose tolerance
hepatocellular damage	
Tumor (adenoma/carcinoma)	
Other	*Psychologic*
Acne	Mood swings
Allopecia	Aggression
Hirsutism	Depression
Edema	Addiction
	Psychosis

HDL, high density lipoprotein.
* Also noted with androstenedione use (King *et al.* 1999).
[†] Most histologic changes in the liver are associated with oral steroids (Yesalis & Bahrke 2002).

within the normal range. Serum alkaline phosphatase was less in the oxandrolone group at discharge, but was significantly greater in treated patients by 6, 9, and 12 months. These data are consistent with improvements in bone mineral density but not consistent with other liver function variables, thus indicating that the increased alkaline phosphatase is likely to be produced by new bone deposition (Murphy *et al.* 2004). The data for the improvements in muscle mass have been confirmed by monitoring changes in protein synthesis rates (Wolf *et al.* 2003) and mRNA expression (Barrow *et al.* 2003; Wolf *et al.* 2003).

Conclusions

The prevalence of creatine use by high school athletes, particularly football players, in grade 12 is high, with prevalence rates generally greater than 20%. Younger athletes are also taking creatine although the prevalence rates are lower at about 3–10% (McGuine *et al.* 2001, 2002; Metzl *et al.* 2001; Ray *et al.* 2001). We know little about possible side effects or negative consequences of long-term creatine use because there have been no controlled clinical trials in young athletes. Furthermore, we do not know if creatine will benefit performance in this young population because, with two exceptions, controlled studies of creatine supplementation on exercise performance have not been carried out. The National Federation of State High School Associations reports that there are 17,346 member high schools, and approximately 10 million young people are involved in high school activity programs (www.nfhs.org). Considering a very conservative prevalence rate for use of creatine by high school athletes of 10% means that about 1 million high school athletes are taking creatine supplements in the USA alone.

Ephedrine and caffeine ingestion by young athletes may be increasing. While the use of caffeine is socially acceptable, and it is not a banned substance, the use of ephedrine is banned by many sports organizations. The prevalence of ephedrine use in adults ranges from 1% to 25% depending on the segment of the population surveyed (e.g., collegiate athletes, physically active adults, general population) (Blanck et al. 2001; Green et al. 2001; Harnack et al. 2001; Kanayama et al. 2001), while the prevalence of ephedrine use in children and adolescents is unknown. Although the weight-reducing effects of ephedrine are small, sales of dietary supplements containing ephedrine/ephedra exceeded $1 billion in 2002. Ephedrine, especially when combined with caffeine, appears to improve sports performance across a wide range of exercise intensities and durations, but ephedrine remains a banned substance and is associated with both type A (common) and type B (rare/severe) adverse events. Ingesting caffeine with the intent of increasing energy levels or improving sports performance is both socially acceptable by athletes and legal. Seventy-six percent of persons under 18 years of age consume caffeine, and caffeine consumption is increasing in young persons, primarily from soft drink consumption (Frary et al. 2005). Additionally, there are many caffeine-containing energy drinks marketed towards children and adolescents. Although caffeine appears to be relatively safe in healthy adults and capable of producing an ergogenic effect under a variety of different exercise intensities and durations, little is known about the effects of caffeine on exercise performance in children and adolescents.

Data on anabolic androgenic steroids use by young persons are perhaps more difficult to obtain accurately than other performance-enhancing substances. These drugs are illegal to possess and use unless prescribed by a physician, and they are banned by most sports organizations. The available data show that up to 7.6% of adolescents have used AAS (Buckley et al. 1988). While data clearly show that AAS and testosterone increase muscle mass, strength, and protein synthesis in exercising adults, prohormones appear to be ineffective. The consequences of AAS use in children and adolescents can be devastating, because AAS affects numerous tissues in addition to skeletal muscle (e.g., reproductive tissue, bone, adipose, brain, prostate, liver, and kidney).

Doping in children can be controlled through educational and rigorous drug testing programs. However, society places a strong emphasis on success in sports, and winning athletes can receive tremendous financial rewards for their achievements. Athletes will always be interested in gaining an edge, and sometimes this involves doping. Unfortunately, as long as adult athletes are seen as role models, some children will consider using performance-enhancing substances.

Acknowledgment

The authors thank Priscilla M. Clarkson, PhD, for her insightful review of and her guidance in the preparation of this chapter.

References

Astrup, A., Breum, L., Toubro, S., Hein, P. & Quaade, F. (1992a) The effect and safety of an ephedrine/caffeine compound compared to ephedrine, caffeine and placebo in obese subjects on an energy restricted diet. A double blind trial. *International Journal of Obesity and Related Metabolic Disorders* **16**, 269–277.

Astrup, A., Breum, L., Toubro, S., Hein, P. & Quaade, F. (1992b) Ephedrine and weight loss. *International Journal of*
Obesity and Related Metabolic Disorders **16**, 715.

Astrup, A. & Toubro, S. (1993) Thermogenic, metabolic, and cardiovascular responses to ephedrine and caffeine in man. *International Journal of Obesity and Related Metabolic Disorders* **17** (Supplement 1), S41–S43.

Bahrke, M.S. & Yesalis, C.E. (2002) Anabolic-androgenic steroids. In: *Performance-Enhancing Substances in Sport and Exercise* (Bahrke, M.S. &
Yesalis, C.E., eds.) Human Kinetics, Champaign, IL: 33–46.

Ballantyne, C.S., Phillips, S.M., MacDonald, J.R., Tarnopolsky, M.A. & MacDougall, J.D. (2000) The acute effects of androstenedione supplementation in healthy young males. *Canadian Journal of Applied Physiology* **25**, 68–78.

Barnhart, K.T., Freeman, E., Grisso, J.A., et al. (1999) The effect of dehydroepiandrosterone supplementation to symptomatic perimenopausal women on serum endocrine profiles, lipid parameters, and health-related quality of life. *Journal of Clinical Endocrinology and Metabolism* **84**, 3896–3902.

Barrow, R.E., Dasu, M.R., Ferrando, A.A., *et al.* (2003) Gene expression patterns in skeletal muscle of thermally injured children treated with oxandrolone. *Annals of Surgery* **237**, 422–428.

Bell, D.G. & Jacobs, I. (1999) Combined caffeine and ephedrine ingestion improves run times of Canadian Forces Warrior Test. *Aviation, Space, and Environmental Medicine* **70**, 325–329.

Bell, D.G., Jacobs, I. & Ellerington, K. (2001) Effect of caffeine and ephedrine ingestion on anaerobic exercise performance. *Medicine and Science in Sports and Exercise* **33**, 1399–1403.

Bell, D.G., Jacobs, I., McLellan, T.M. & Zamecnik, J. (2000) Reducing the dose of combined caffeine and ephedrine preserves the ergogenic effect. *Aviation, Space, and Environmental Medicine* **71**, 415–419.

Bell, D.G., Jacobs, I. & Zamecnik, J. (1998) Effects of caffeine, ephedrine and their combination on time to exhaustion during high-intensity exercise [see comments]. *European Journal of Applied Physiology* **77**, 427–433.

Bell, D.G., McLellan, T.M. & Sabiston, C.M. (2002) Effect of ingesting caffeine and ephedrine on 10-km run performance. *Medicine and Science in Sports and Exercise* **34**, 344–349.

Bent, S., Tiedt, T.N., Odden, M.C. & Shlipak, M.G. (2003) The relative safety of ephedra compared with other herbal products. *Annals of Internal Medicine* **138**, 468–471.

Bhasin, S., Storer, T.W., Berman, N., *et al.* (1996) The effects of supraphysiologic doses of testosterone on muscle size and strength in normal men. *New England Journal of Medicine* **335**, 1–7.

Blanck, H.M., Khan, L.K. & Serdula, M.K. (2001) Use of nonprescription weight loss products: results from a multistate survey. *Journal of the American Medical Association* **286**, 930–935.

Blue, J.G. & Lombardo, J.A. (1999) Steroids and steroid-like compounds. *Clinics in Sports Medicine* **18**, 667–689, ix.

Boada, L.D., Zumbado, M., Torres, S., *et al.* (1999) Evaluation of acute and chronic hepatotoxic effects exerted by anabolic-androgenic steroid stanozolol in adult male rats. *Archives of Toxicology* **73**, 465–472.

Boje, O. (1939) Doping. *Bulletin of the Health Organization of the League of Nations* **8**, 439–469.

Bosy, T.Z., Moore, K.A. & Poklis, A. (1998) The effect of oral dehydroepiandrosterone (DHEA) on the urine testosterone/epitestosterone (T/E) ratio in human male volunteers. *Journal of Analytical Toxicology* **22**, 455–459.

Branch, J.D. (2003) Effect of creatine supplementation on body composition and performance: a meta-analysis. *International Journal of Sport Nutrition and Exercise Metabolism* **13**, 198–226.

Brinkmann, A.O., Blok, L.J., de Ruiter, P.E., *et al.* (1999) Mechanisms of androgen receptor activation and function. *Journal of Steroid Biochemistry and Molecular Biology* **69**, 307–313.

Brodsky, I.G., Balagopal, P. & Nair, K.S. (1996) Effects of testosterone replacement on muscle mass and muscle protein synthesis in hypogonadal men: a clinical research center study. *Journal of Clinical Endocrinology and Metabolism* **81**, 3469–3475.

Broeder, C.E., Quindry, J., Brittingham, K., *et al.* (2000) The Andro Project: physiological and hormonal influences of androstenedione supplementation in men 35 to 65 years old participating in a high-intensity resistance training program. *Archives of Internal Medicine* **160**, 3093–3104.

Brown, G.A., Martini, E.R., Roberts, B.S., Vukovich, M.D. & King, D.S. (2002) Acute hormonal response to sublingual androstenediol intake in young men. *Journal of Applied Physiology* **92**, 142–146.

Brown, G.A., Vukovich, M.D., Martini, E.R., *et al.* (2001) Effects of androstenedione-herbal supplementation on serum sex hormone concentrations in 30- to 59-year-old men. *International Journal for Vitamin and Nutrition Research* **71**, 293–301.

Buckley, W.E., Yesalis, C.E. 3rd, Friedl, K.E., Anderson, W.A., Streit, A.L. & Wright, J.E. (1988) Estimated prevalence of anabolic steroid use among male high school seniors. *Journal of the American Medical Association* **260**, 3441–3445.

Casner, S.W. Jr., Early, R.G. & Carlson, B.R. (1971) Anabolic steroid effects on body composition in normal young men. *Journal of Sports Medicine and Physical Fitness* **11**, 98–103.

Catlin, D.H., Leder, B.Z., Ahrens, B., *et al.* (2000) Trace contamination of over-the-counter androstenedione and positive urine test results for a nandrolone

metabolite. *Journal of the American Medical Association* **284**, 2618–2621.

Clarkson, P.M. & Persky, A.M. (2002) Steroid misuse in athletes: effects on skeletal muscle. In: *Skeletal Muscle: Pathology, Diagnosis and Management of Disease* (Preedy, V.R. & Peters, T.J., eds.) Greenwich Medical Media, San Francisco: 97–108.

Clarkson, P.M. & Thompson, H.S. (1997) Drugs and sport. Research findings and limitations. *Sports Medicine* **24**, 366–384.

Colker, C.M., Antonio, J. & Kalman, D. (2001) The metabolism of orally ingested 19-nor-4-androstene-3,17-dione and 19-nor-4-androstene-3,17-diol in healthy, resistance-trained men. *Journal of Strength and Conditioning Research* **15**, 144–147.

Dawson, B., Vladich, T. & Blanksby, B.A. (2002) Effects of 4 weeks of creatine supplementation in junior swimmers on freestyle sprint and swim bench performance. *Journal of Strength and Conditioning Research* **16**, 485–490.

DeSisso, T.D., Gerst, J.W., Carnathan, P.D., *et al.* (2005) Effects of caffeine on metabolic and cardiovascular responses to submaximal exercise: Boys versus men. *Medicine and Science in Sports and Exercise* **37**, S465.

Dulloo, A.G. (1993) Ephedrine, xanthines and prostaglandin-inhibitors: actions and interactions in the stimulation of thermogenesis. *International Journal of Obesity and Related Metabolic Disorders* **17** (Supplement 1), S35–S40.

Dulloo, A.G. & Miller, D.S. (1986) The thermogenic properties of ephedrine/methylxanthine mixtures: human studies. *International Journal of Obesity* **10**, 467–481.

Dulloo, A.G., Seydoux, J. & Girardier, L. (1994) Paraxanthine (metabolite of caffeine) mimics caffeine's interaction with sympathetic control of thermogenesis. *American Journal of Physiology* **267**, E801–804.

DuRant, R.H., Escobedo, L.G. & Heath, G.W. (1995) Anabolic-steroid use, strength training, and multiple drug use among adolescents in the United States. *Pediatrics* **96**, 23–28.

Elliot, D.L., Goldberg, L., Moe, E.L., Defrancesco, C.A., Durham, M.B. & Hix-Small, H. (2004) Preventing substance use and disordered eating: initial outcomes of the ATHENA (athletes targeting healthy exercise and nutrition alternatives) program. *Archives of Pediatrics and Adolescent Medicine* **158**, 1043–1049.

Engelhardt, M., Neumann, G., Berbalk, A. & Reuter, I. (1998) Creatine supplementation in endurance sports. *Medicine and Science in Sports and Exercise* **30**, 1123–1129.

Estrada, M., Espinosa, A., Muller, M. & Jaimovich, E. (2003) Testosterone stimulates intracellular calcium release and mitogen-activated protein kinases via a G protein-coupled receptor in skeletal muscle cells. *Endocrinology* **144**, 3586–3597.

Faigenbaum, A.D., Zaichkowsky, L.D., Gardner, D.E. & Micheli, L.J. (1998) Anabolic steroid use by male and female middle school students. *Pediatrics* **101**, E6.

Feinberg, M.J., Lumia, A.R. & McGinnis, M.Y. (1997) The effect of anabolic-androgenic steroids on sexual behavior and reproductive tissues in male rats. *Physiology & Behavior* **62**, 23–30.

Ferrando, A.A., Tipton, K.D., Doyle, D., Phillips, S.M., Cortiella, J. & Wolfe, R.R. (1998) Testosterone injection stimulates net protein synthesis but not tissue amino acid transport. *American Journal of Physiology* **275**, E864–E871.

Franke, W.W. & Berendonk, B. (1997) Hormonal doping and androgenization of athletes: a secret program of the German Democratic Republic government. *Clinical Chemistry* **43**, 1262–1279.

Frary, C.D., Johnson, R.K. & Wang, M.Q. (2005) Food sources and intakes of caffeine in the diets of persons in the United States. *Journal of the American Diet Association* **105**, 110–113.

Genazzani, A.D., Stomati, M., Bernardi, F., Pieri, M., Rovati, L. & Genazzani, A.R. (2003) Long-term low-dose dehydroepiandrosterone oral supplementation in early and late postmenopausal women modulates endocrine parameters and synthesis of neuroactive steroids. *Fertility and Sterility* **80**, 1495–1501.

Graham, T.E. (2001) Caffeine and exercise: metabolism, endurance and performance. *Sports Medicine* **31**, 785–807.

Green, G.A., Uryasz, F.D., Petr, T.A. & Bray, C.D. (2001) NCAA study of substance use and abuse habits of college student-athletes. *Clinical Journal of Sport Medicine* **11**, 51–56.

Greenhaff, P.L., Bodin, K., Söderlund, K. & Hultman, E. (1994) Effect of oral creatine supplementation on skeletal muscle phosphocreatine resynthesis. *American Journal of Physiology* **266**, E725–E730.

Greenhaff, P.L., Casey, A., Short, A.H., Harris, R., Söderlund, K. & Hultman, E. (1993) Influence of oral creatine supplementation of muscle torque during repeated bouts of maximal voluntary exercise in man. *Clinical Science (London)* **84**, 565–571.

Greenwood, M., Kreider, R.B., Greenwood, L. & Byars, A. (2003) Cramping and injury incidence in collegiate football players are reduced by creatine supplementation. *Journal of Athletic Training* **38**, 216–219.

Griggs, R.C., Kingston, W., Jozefowicz, R.F., Herr, B.E., Forbes, G. & Halliday, D. (1989) Effect of testosterone on muscle mass and muscle protein synthesis. *Journal of Applied Physiology* **66**, 498–503.

Gurley, B.J., Gardner, S.F. & Hubbard, M.A. (2000) Content versus label claims in ephedra-containing dietary supplements. *American Journal of Health-System Pharmacy* **57**, 963–969.

Gurley, B.J., Wang, P. & Gardner, S.F. (1998) Ephedrine-type alkaloid content of nutritional supplements containing Ephedra sinica (Ma-huang) as determined by high performance liquid chromatography. *Journal of Pharmaceutical Science* **87**, 1547–1553.

Haller, C.A. & Benowitz, N.L. (2000) Adverse cardiovascular and central nervous system events associated with dietary supplements containing ephedra alkaloids. *New England Journal of Medicine* **343**, 1833–1838.

Harnack, L.J., Rydell, S.A. & Stang, J. (2001) Prevalence of use of herbal products by adults in the Minneapolis/St Paul, Minn, metropolitan area. *Mayo Clinic Proceedings* **76**, 688–694.

Harris, R.C., Söderlund, K. & Hultman, E. (1992) Elevation of creatine in resting and exercised muscle of normal subjects by creatine supplementation. *Clinical Science (London)* **83**, 367–374.

Hartgens, F. & Kuipers, H. (2004) Effects of androgenic-anabolic steroids in athletes. *Sports Medicine* **34**, 513–554.

Haupt, H.A. & Rovere, G.D. (1984) Anabolic steroids: a review of the literature. *American Journal of Sports Medicine* **12**, 469–484.

Hawes, K. (1998) Creatine boom creates administrative challenges. http://www.ncaa.org/news/1998/19980914/active/3532n03.html. Accessed September 2003.

Heinlein, C.A. & Chang, C. (2002) The roles of androgen receptors and androgen-binding proteins in nongenomic androgen actions. *Molecular Endocrinology* **16**, 2181–2187.

Hislop, M.S., Ratanjee, B.D., Soule, S.G. & Marais, A.D. (1999) Effects of anabolic-androgenic steroid use or gonadal testosterone suppression on serum leptin concentration in men. *European Journal of Endocrinology* **141**, 40–46.

Hoffman, B.B. & Lefkowitz, R.J. (1996) Catecholamines, sympathomimetic drugs, and adrenergic receptor antagonists. In: *Goodman & Gilman's The Pharmacological Basis of Therapeutics*, 9th edn. (Hardman, J.G., Limbird, L.E., Molinoff, P.B., Ruddon, R.W. & Gilman, A.G., eds.) McGraw-Hill, New York: 199–248.

Hultman, E., Söderlund, K., Timmons, J.A., Cederblad, G. & Greenhaff, P.L. (1996) Muscle creatine loading in men. *Journal of Applied Physiology* **81**, 232–237.

Irving, L.M., Wall, M., Neumark-Sztainer, D. & Story, M. (2002) Steroid use among adolescents: findings from Project EAT. *Journal of Adolescent Health* **30**, 243–252.

Jacobs, I., Pasternak, H. & Bell, D.G. (2003) Effects of ephedrine, caffeine, and their combination on muscular endurance. *Medicine and Science in Sports and Exercise* **35**, 987–994.

Jin, B., Turner, L., Walters, W.A. & Handelsman, D.J. (1996) The effects of chronic high dose androgen or estrogen treatment on the human prostate [corrected]. *Journal of Clinical Endocrinology and Metabolism* **81**, 4290–4295.

Jonderko, K. & Kucio, C. (1991) Effect of anti-obesity drugs promoting energy expenditure, yohimbine and ephedrine, on gastric emptying in obese patients. *Alimentary Pharmacology & Therapeutics* **5**, 413–418.

Jonnalagadda, S.S., Rosenbloom, C.A. & Skinner, R. (2001) Dietary practices, attitudes, and physiological status of collegiate freshman football players. *Journal of Strength and Conditioning Research* **15**, 507–513.

Kanayama, G., Gruber, A.J., Pope, H.G. Jr., Borowiecki, J.J. & Hudson, J.I. (2001) Over-the-counter drug use in gymnasiums: an underrecognized substance abuse problem? *Psychotherapy and Psychosomatics* **70**, 137–140.

Katznelson, L., Finkelstein, J.S., Schoenfeld, D.A., Rosenthal, D.I., Anderson, E.J. & Klibanski, A. (1996) Increase in bone density and lean body mass during testosterone administration in men with acquired hypogonadism.

Journal of Clinical Endocrinology and Metabolism 81, 4358–4365.

Kindlundh, A.M., Isacson, D.G., Berglund, L. & Nyberg, F. (1998) Doping among high school students in Uppsala, Sweden: A presentation of the attitudes, distribution, side effects, and extent of use. *Scandinavian Journal of the Social Medicine* 26, 71–74.

King, D.S., Sharp, R.L., Vukovich, M.D., *et al.* (1999) Effect of oral androstenedione on serum testosterone and adaptations to resistance training in young men: a randomized controlled trial. *Journal of the American Medical Association* 281, 2020–2028.

Komoroski, E.M. & Rickert, V.I. (1992) Adolescent body image and attitudes to anabolic steroid use. *American Journal of Diseases of Children* 146, 823–828.

Korkia, P. (1996) Use of anabolic steroids has been reported by 9% of men attending gymnasiums. *British Medical Journal* 313, 1009.

Kraemer, W.J., Rubin, M.R., French, D.N. & McGuigan, M.R. (2002) Physiological effects of testosterone precursors. In: *Performance-Enhancing Substances in Sport and Exercise* (Bahrke, M.S. & Yesalis, C.E., eds.) Human Kinetics, Champaign, IL: 79–88.

Kreider, R.B. (2003) Effects of creatine supplementation on performance and training adaptations. *Molecular and Cellular Biochemistry* 244, 89–94.

Kreider, R.B., Melton, C., Rasmussen, C.J., *et al.* (2003) Long-term creatine supplementation does not significantly affect clinical markers of health in athletes. *Molecular and Cellular Biochemistry* 244, 95–104.

Lamb, D.R. (1984) Anabolic steroids in athletics: how well do they work and how dangerous are they? *American Journal of Sports Medicine* 12, 31–38.

Lambert, M.I., Titlestad, S.D. & Schwellnus, M.P. (1998) Prevalence of androgenic-anabolic steroid use in adolescents in two regions of South Africa. *South African Medical Journal* 88, 876–880.

Lawrence, M.E. & Kirby, D.F. (2002) Nutrition and sports supplements: fact or fiction. *Journal of Clinical Gastroenterology* 35, 299–306.

Leder, B.Z., Longcope, C., Catlin, D.H., Ahrens, B., Schoenfeld, D.A. & Finkelstein, J.S. (2000) Oral androstenedione administration and serum testosterone concentrations in young men. *Journal of the American Medical Association* 283, 779–782.

Lemon, P.W. (2002) Dietary creatine supplementation and exercise performance: why inconsistent results? *Canadian Journal of Applied Physiology* 27, 663–681.

Magkos, F. & Kavouras, S.A. (2004) Caffeine and ephedrine: physiological, metabolic and performance-enhancing effects. *Sports Medicine* 34, 871–889.

Martorana, G., Concetti, S., Manferrari, F. & Creti, S. (1999) Anabolic steroid abuse and renal cell carcinoma. *Journal of Urology* 162, 2089.

Mason, M.A., Giza, M., Clayton, L., Lonning, J. & Wilkerson, R.D. (2001) Use of nutritional supplements by high school football and volleyball players. *Iowa Orthopaedic Journal* 21, 43–48.

Massad, S.J., Shier, N.W., Koceja, D.M. & Ellis, N.T. (1995) High school athletes and nutritional supplements: a study of knowledge and use. *International Journal of Sport Nutrition* 5, 232–245.

McGuine, T.A., Sullivan, J.C. & Bernhardt, D.A. (2002) Creatine supplementation in Wisconsin high school athletes. *WMJ* 101, 25–30.

McGuine, T.A., Sullivan, J.C. & Bernhardt, D.T. (2001) Creatine supplementation in high school football players. *Clinical Journal of Sport Medicine* 11, 247–253.

Melia, P., Pipe, A. & Greenberg, L. (1996) The use of anabolic-androgenic steroids by Canadian students. *Clinical Journal of Sport Medicine* 6, 9–14.

Metzl, J.D., Small, E., Levine, S.R. & Gershel, J.C. (2001) Creatine use among young athletes. *Pediatrics* 108, 421–425.

Molnar, D., Torok, K., Erhardt, E. & Jeges, S. (2000) Safety and efficacy of treatment with an ephedrine/caffeine mixture. The first double-blind placebo-controlled pilot study in adolescents. *International Journal of Obesity and Related Metabolic Disorders* 24, 1573–1578.

Murphy, K.D., Thomas, S., Mlcak, R.P., Chinkes, D.L., Klein, G.L. & Herndon, D.N. (2004) Effects of long-term oxandrolone administration in severely burned children. *Surgery* 136, 219–224.

Nilsson, S. (1995) Androgenic anabolic steroid use among male adolescents in Falkenberg. *European Journal of Clinical Pharmacology* 48, 9–11.

Nilsson, S., Baigi, A., Marklund, B. & Fridlund, B. (2001a) The prevalence of the use of androgenic anabolic steroids by adolescents in a county of Sweden. *European Journal of Public Health* 11, 195–197.

Nilsson, S., Baigi, A., Marklund, B. & Fridlund, B. (2001b) Trends in the

misuse of androgenic anabolic steroids among boys 16–17 years old in a primary health care area in Sweden. *Scandinavian Journal of Primary Health Care* 19, 181–182.

Nissen, S.L. & Sharp, R.L. (2003) Effect of dietary supplements on lean mass and strength gains with resistance exercise: a meta-analysis. *Journal of Applied Physiology* 94, 651–659.

Op't Eijnde, B., Vergauwen, L. & Hespel, P. (2001) Creatine loading does not impact on stroke performance in tennis. *International Journal of Sports Medicine* 22, 76–80.

Radakovich, J., Broderick, P. & Pickell, G. (1993) Rate of anabolic-androgenic steroid use among students in junior high school. *Journal of the American Board of Family Practice* 6, 341–345.

Rahwan, R.G. (1988) The pharmacology of androgens and anabolic steroids. *American Journal of Pharmaceutical Education* 52, 167–177.

Rasmussen, B.B., Volpi, E., Gore, D.C. & Wolfe, R.R. (2000) Androstenedione does not stimulate muscle protein anabolism in young healthy men. *Journal of Clinical Endocrinology and Metabolism* 85, 55–59.

Rawson, E.S. & Clarkson, P.M. (2002) Ephedrine as an ergogenic aid. In: *Performance-Enhancing Substances in Sport and Exercise* (Bahrke, M.S. & Yesalis, C.E., eds.) Human Kinetics, Champaign, IL: 289–298.

Rawson, E.S. & Clarkson, P.M. (2003) Scientifically debatable: Is creatine worth its weight. *Sports Science Exchange* 16, 1–6.

Rawson, E.S. & Volek, J.S. (2003) Effects of creatine supplementation and resistance training on muscle strength and weightlifting performance. *Journal of Strength and Conditioning Research* 17, 822–831.

Ray, T.R., Eck, J.C., Covington, L.A., Murphy, R.B., Williams, R. & Knudtson, J. (2001) Use of oral creatine as an ergogenic aid for increased sports performance: perceptions of adolescent athletes. *South Medical Journal* 94, 608–612.

Reeder, B. (2003) Nutritional supplement use by high school students: a survey of two high-schools in the united states. *International Pediatrics* 18, 170–177.

Rivers, W.H.R. & Webber, H.N. (1907) The action of caffeine on the capacity for muscular work. *Journal of Physiology* 36, 33–47.

Rubinow, D.R. & Schmidt, P.J. (1996) Androgens, brain, and behavior. *American Journal of Psychiatry* **153**, 974–984.

Samenuk, D., Link, M.S., Homoud, M.K., *et al.* (2002) Adverse cardiovascular events temporally associated with ma huang, an herbal source of ephedrine. *Mayo Clinic Proceedings* **77**, 12–16.

Sasaki, H., Maeda, J., Usui, S. & Ishiko, T. (1987) Effect of sucrose and caffeine ingestion on performance of prolonged strenuous running. *International Journal of Sports Medicine* **8**, 261–265.

Schwellnus, M.P., Lambert, M.I., Todd, M.P. & Juritz, J.M. (1992) Androgenic anabolic steroid use in matric pupils. A survey of prevalence of use in the western Cape. *South African Medical Journal* **82**, 154–158.

Scott, D.M., Wagner, J.C. & Barlow, T.W. (1996) Anabolic steroid use among adolescents in Nebraska schools. *American Journal of Health-System Pharmacy* **53**, 2068–2072.

Sheffield-Moore, M. (2000) Androgens and the control of skeletal muscle protein synthesis. *Annals of Medicine* **32**, 181–186.

Sheffield-Moore, M., Urban, R.J., Wolf, S.E., *et al.* (1999) Short-term oxandrolone administration stimulates net muscle protein synthesis in young men. *Journal of Clinical Endocrinology and Metabolism* **84**, 2705–2711.

Shekelle, P.G., Hardy, M.L., Morton, S.C., *et al.* (2003) Efficacy and safety of ephedra and ephedrine for weight loss and athletic performance: a meta-analysis. *Journal of the American Medical Association* **289**, 1537–1545.

Skare, O.C., Skadberg, Ø. & Wisnes, A.R. (2001) Creatine supplementation improves sprint performance in male sprinters. *Scandinavian Journal of Medicine and Science in Sports* **11**, 96–102.

Smith, J. & Dahm, D.L. (2000) Creatine use among a select population of high school athletes. *Mayo Clinic Proceedings* **75**, 1257–1263.

Spriet, L.L. (2002) Caffeine. In: *Performance-Enhancing Substances in Sport and Exercise* (Bahrke, M.S. & Yesalis, C.E., eds.) Human Kinetics, Champaign, IL: 267–278.

Spriet, L.L. & Howlett, R.A. (2000) Caffeine. In: *Nutrition in Sport. The Encyclopedia of Sports Medicine. An IOC Medical Commission Publication in Collaboration with the International Federation of Sports Medicine* (Maughan

R.J., ed.) Blackwell Science, Oxford: 379–392.

Stilger, V.G. & Yesalis, C.E. (1999) Anabolic-androgenic steroid use among high school football players. *Jounral of Community Health* **24**, 131–145.

Sturmi, J.E. & Diorio, D.J. (1998) Anabolic agents. *Clinics in Sports Medicine* **17**, 261–282.

Swirzinski, L. (2000) A survey of sport nutrition supplements in high school football players. *Journal of Strength and Conditioning Research* **14**, 464–469.

Tanner, S.M., Miller, D.W. & Alongi, C. (1995) Anabolic steroid use by adolescents: prevalence, motives, and knowledge of risks. *Clinical Journal of Sport Medicine* **5**, 108–115.

Terjung, R.L., Clarkson, P., Eichner, E.R., *et al.* (2000) American College of Sports Medicine roundtable. The physiological and health effects of oral creatine supplementation. *Medicine and Science in Sports and Exercise* **32**, 706–717.

Theodorou, A.S., Haventidis, K., Zanker, C.L., *et al.* (2005) Effects of acute creatine loading with or without carbohydrate on repeated bouts of maximal swimming in high-performance swimmers. *Journal of Strength and Conditioning Research* **19**, 265–269.

Thiblin, I. & Petersson, A. (2005) Pharmacoepidemiology of anabolic androgenic steroids: a review. *Fundamental and Clinical Pharmacology* **19**, 27–44.

Turley, K.R., Gerst, J.W. & Kukta, L.C. (2004) Effects of caffeine on submaximal responses to exercise in children. *Medicine and Science in Sports and Exercise* **36**, S18.

Uralets, V.P. & Gillette, P.A. (1999) Over-the-counter anabolic steroids 4-androsten-3,17-dione; 4-androsten-3beta,17beta-diol; and 19-nor-4-androsten-3,17-dione: excretion studies in men. *Journal of Analytical Toxicology* **23**, 357–366.

Urban, R.J., Bodenburg, Y.H., Gilkison, C., *et al.* (1995) Testosterone administration to elderly men increases skeletal muscle strength and protein synthesis. *American Journal of Physiology* **269**, E820–E826.

United States Department of Agriculture Economic Research Service (USDA) (2004) Food Consumption (per capita) Data System. http://www.ers.usda.gov/data/foodconsumption/. Accessed August 2005.

Vandebuerie, F., Vanden Eynde, B., Vandenberghe, K. & Hespel, P. (1998) Effect of creatine loading on endurance capacity and sprint power in cyclists. *International Journal of Sports Medicine* **19**, 490–495.

Vandenberghe, K., Van Hecke, P., Van Leemputte, M., Vanstapel, F. & Hespel, P. (1999) Phosphocreatine resynthesis is not affected by creatine loading. *Medicine and Science in Sports and Exercise* **31**, 236–242.

Walker, J.B. (1979) Creatine: biosynthesis, regulation, and function. *Advances in Enzymology and Related Areas of Molecular Biology* **50**, 177–242.

Wallace, M.B., Lim, J., Cutler, A. & Bucci, L. (1999) Effects of dehydroepiandrosterone vs androstenedione supplementation in men. *Medicine and Science in Sports and Exercise* **31**, 1788–1792.

Ward, P. (1973) The effect of an anabolic steroid on strength and lean body mass. *Medicine and Science in Sports and Exercise* **5**, 277–282.

Wichstrom, L. & Pedersen, W. (2001) Use of anabolic-androgenic steroids in adolescence: winning, looking good or being bad? *Journal of Studies on Alcohol* **62**, 5–13.

Windsor, R. & Dumitru, D. (1989) Prevalence of anabolic steroid use by male and female adolescents. *Medicine and Science in Sports and Exercise* **21**, 494–497.

Wolf, S.E., Thomas, S.J., Dasu, M.R., *et al.* (2003) Improved net protein balance, lean mass, and gene expression changes with oxandrolone treatment in the severely burned. *Annals of Surgery* **237**, 801–810; discussion 810–811.

Yesalis, C.E. & Bahrke, M.S. (2002) Anabolic-androgenic steroids and related substances. *Current Sports Medicine Reports* **1**, 246–252.

Yquel, R.J., Arsac, L.M., Thiaudiere, E., Canioni, P. & Manier, G. (2002) Effect of creatine supplementation on phosphocreatine resynthesis, inorganic phosphate accumulation and pH during intermittent maximal exercise. *Journal of Sports Science* **20**, 427–437.

Ziegenfuss, T.N., Berardi, J.M. & Lowery, L.M. (2002) Effects of prohormone supplementation in humans: a review. *Canadian Journal of Applied Physiology* **27**, 628–646.

Part 5

Psychosocial Issues

Chapter 22

Personal Development through Sport

DANIEL GOULD AND SARAH CARSON

"For each individual, sport is a possible source for inner improvement."

"Olympism seeks to create a way of life based on the joy found in effort, the educational value of a good example and respect for universal fundamental ethical principles."

"The most important thing in the Olympic Games is not winning but taking part; the essential thing in life is not conquering but fighting well."

(www.brainyquote.com/quotes/authors/p/
pierre_de_coubertin.html)

As the above quotes clearly show, Barron Pierre de Coubertin, the founder of the modern Olympic Games, had a strong belief that sport could and should be used for the personal development of young people. After visits to British and US universities, de Coubertin was motivated to improve the education and personal development of young people through sports participation. In fact, he used personal psychosocial development through sport as a key component of the justification to initiate the modern games.

The importance of sport as a vehicle for personal development is an idea consistent with one of the central objectives of contemporary sport psychology—to understand how participation in sport and physical activity influences the psychologic development of the participant (Weinberg & Gould 2007). In fact, in recent years there has been increased interest in using sport as an arena for developing life skills in youth (Danish *et al.* 2004), with life skills being viewed as those internal personal assets, characteristics, and skills such as goal setting, emotional control, self-esteem, and hard work ethic that can be facilitated or developed in sport and potentially transferred for use in non-sport settings.

In the year 2000, for example, a special issue of the journal *Community Youth Development* was devoted to an examination of extracurricular activities, especially sport, and their potential to contribute to youth and community development (Terry 2000). Similarly, in 1997 the exercise and sport science journal *Quest* devoted a special issue to teaching life skills through sport.

Given the contemporary interest in this area, a need exists to review the scientific literature on the topic. This chapter is designed to critique and review the literature on personal psychosocial development through sport and to outline practical implications as well as critical issues and future research directions.

Psychologic development through sport

Personal development through sport is a broad area including an array of specific topics ranging from perceived competence to delinquency. However, many of these specific topics can be classified into two general themes:

1 General psychological development through sport; and

2 Development of "specific" personal and psychologic qualities through sport.

The research in each of these two general categories are summarized.

General development through sport

The psychosocial development of children through sport and other extracurricular activities has taken on increased importance in the general field of youth development in recent years (Larson 2000; Dworkin *et al.* 2003). For example, Larson (2000) has suggested that extracurricular and community-based after-school activities are often pastimes in which adolescents are highly motivated and involve intense concentration. Hence, they may be particularly useful in allowing adolescents to develop positive skills such as initiative and the ability to set and achieve goals.

This assertion was supported in a recent study of 55 high school adolescents involved in extracurricular and community-based activities (72% were involved in sport) in which Dworkin *et al.* (2003) conducted 10 focus groups to explore adolescents' accounts of their developmental growth experiences. These young people reported that sport and other extracurricular activities were important personal growth experience arenas where psychologic skills such as goal setting, time management, and emotional control were learned. These researchers also reported that new peer relationships were acquired, that participants developed valuable connections to adults, learned how to take responsibility, and learned how to function as a team. Finally, these young people described themselves as agents, or active producers, of their own development.

In a second, more comprehensive investigation, Hansen *et al.* (2003) studied high school students who reported the developmental gains they associated with involvement in a variety of extracurricular activities, including sports. Specifically, 450 high school students completed the Youth Experiences Survey (YES). This self-report measure was used to assess the personal development of the youth relative to participation in:

1 Structured youth activities,
2 Hanging out with friends, and
3 Math and/or English class.

Results revealed that participants reported greater rates of learning experiences (e.g., identity development, initiative, physical skills, teamwork/social skills, interpersonal relationships, adult networks) in extracurricular activities versus comparison activities (academic classes and socializing with friends).

Sport participation was associated with higher rates for some learning experiences such as self-knowledge (e.g., learned what I am good at), emotional regulation (e.g., control temper or stress), and physical skills development. However, students involved in sports also indicated higher rates of negative peer interactions (e.g., felt peer pressure to do something they did not want to) and inappropriate adult behavior (e.g., adults encouraged them to do something they believed morally wrong). Thus, sports were found to be a frequent context for identity work and emotional development. However, participation in sports was also associated with negative experiences such as peer pressure and inappropriate adult behaviors.

In a similar but independent line of research, Eccles and Barber (1999) and Eccles *et al.* (2003) examined risks and benefits associated with participation in several types of extracurricular activities (pro-social organizations such as church, school involvement, the performing arts, academic clubs, and team sports). Longitudinal survey data were collected on 1259 male and female adolescent high school students relative to risk behaviors (e.g., drinking, skipping school, using drugs); academic achievement (e.g., liking of school, academic performance); and family characteristics. Results revealed that involvement in pro-social activities in general were linked to positive educational trajectories and lower rates of involvement in risky behaviors. Team sports in particular were linked to positive educational trajectories (e.g., better liking of school, higher grade point average, college attendance) and high rates of involvement in one risky behavior, drinking alcohol. Thus, sport participation was found to be associated with both positive and negative personal development experiences.

Finally, Steen *et al.* (2003) found that adolescents reported characteristics such as leadership, wisdom, and social intelligence were acquired through life experiences like those fostered in extracurricular activities. And, in a slightly different line of research, young people who had natural mentors such as relatives, coaches, counselors, and teachers felt that those mentors had a pivotal role in the lives

(Zimmerman *et al.* 2002). Specifically, in a sample of 770 urban youth it was found that having a mentor in one's life was associated with less alcohol use, marijuana use, and violent delinquency. The process by which mentors influence youth is relatively unknown, however, and literature on the process of how coaches in particular influence youth development is badly needed.

One recent study specifically focused on how coaches developed life skills in their athletes. Gould *et al.* (2007) studied the characteristics of high school coaches who were recognized for developing character and positive personal characteristics in their players. Specifically, the researchers examined the process of how outstanding high school football coaches developed life skills and desirable personality characteristics in their players. In-depth phone interviews were conducted with 10 finalists for the National Football League Charities "Coach of the Year Program", a national award given for positively influencing players' lives. Coaches averaged 31 years of coaching experience and were highly successful, winning an average of 161 games (76.6%) over their careers. Results revealed that while highly motivated to win, these coaches made the personal development of their players a top priority. The coaches were also found to have well thought-out philosophies which were characterized by clear expectations relative to rules, player behavior, and team expectations. Several coaches emphasized what they called tough love in that they "demanded" maximum effort and discipline, but always made it clear that they cared about their players as people. While results reveal general patterns in coaching behaviors and strategies, the qualitative findings also showed that each coach was unique.

In some of the most important and methodologically sound youth sports research conducted to date, Smith *et al.* (1979) and Smoll *et al.* (1993) examined the relationship between the behaviors characterizing youth coaches and the psychosocial development of children. In this line of research the investigators examined how the feedback and behaviors exhibited by a coach influences athletes' self-esteem, motivation, and sense of satisfaction with the coach, season, and teammates. More specifically, it was found that youth coaches who under-

went Coach Effectiveness Training (CET) to learn techniques for encouragement, effective skill instruction, and avoiding punishment were perceived in a different way than those coaches who did not undergo the training. Coaches trained in "positive coaching" techniques were better liked by their athletes, and these athletes had more satisfaction with their teammates and the competitive season. Athletes of CET trained coaches also exhibited higher levels of motivation. Further, those children who started the season with lower self-esteem and played for a CET trained coach showed a greater increase in self-esteem over the season than those with lower self-esteem playing for non-trained coaches. An interesting note on this line of research is that the win–loss records of the team seemed not to impact athletes' perceptions of satisfaction with coach and season. Thus, this research has shown that training coaches to be more positive and encouraging has led to a number of positive psychosocial consequences.

Coaching style training such as CET has also been found to affect attrition rates in youth sports. In a follow-up investigation, it was found that those athletes who played for untrained coaches reported an attrition rate of 26% (typical rate in youth sports); whereas those athletes playing for a CET trained coach reported rates of only 5% (Barnett *et al.* 1992). Players who had played for these positively oriented coaches also exhibited lower anxiety levels (Smith *et al.* 1995). These findings clearly substantiate the powerful effects of positive coaching behaviors on both keeping young people active in sports and ensuring positive psychosocial consequences such as enhanced esteem and lower anxiety.

Development of specific personal qualities and psychologic characteristics

Past literature has identified a long list of academic, social, and psychologic outcomes that sport participation can foster including goal setting, effective communication, responsibility, problem solving, dealing with conflict, risk taking, managing emotions, providing and receiving feedback, accepting interdependence, appreciating differences, managing time and stress, persistence, courage, and self-control (Kleiber & Roberts 1981; Holland & Andre

1987; Kleiber & Kirshnit 1991; Marsh 1993; Danish *et al.* 2003). While the space allotted for this chapter does not allow for a thorough discussion of all outcomes mentioned above, several key life skills and their relationship with sport participation have been introduced and outlined below.

SELF-ESTEEM

A child's self-esteem and feelings of competence have a remarkable effect on the daily choices they make and the avenues they choose to pursue throughout life. More specifically, how we see ourselves directs our behaviors and our perceptions of what we can achieve and what we should try to accomplish in the future. Sports have been proposed as a means of helping children build a sense of competence that could transfer to positive beliefs about self-worth and ability inside and outside of athletics.

When reviewing the literature on the effectiveness of sport and exercise in affecting individuals' self-esteem, Fox (2000) found that 78% of the studies (conducted from 1970 to 1999) reviewed suggested sport and exercise influenced positive changes in certain aspects of physical self-perceptions. The importance of this finding extends beyond the effects these changes may have on sport motivation and participation because increases in physical self-worth have also been linked to increases in global (general) self-esteem and various positive mental health indicators. Thus, the consequences of these changes in self-perceptions appear to transfer outside of the physical realm. The analysis also indicated that about half of the studies reviewed suggested direct changes to global self-esteem occurred in conjunction with sport and exercise participation.

Because young athletes are not always completely accurate in their self-assessments and because they often rely on feedback from significant others to help develop the perceptions of their abilities, much research has focused on the role coaches have in helping young athletes develop a positive sense of self in sport (Ewing *et al.* 2000). By testing the effectiveness of the previously discussed coaching program designed to develop a more positive approach to coaching, recall that Smith *et al.* (1979) discovered that coaches who had received the training had athletes with greater levels of self-esteem than coaches who had not received the training. Furthermore, those athletes who initially had the lowest levels of self-esteem were those to have the largest gains in self-esteem related to changes in their coaches' practices. This study was later replicated and its results were confirmed with additional positive findings. Trained coaches were found to not only have athletes who had greater perceptions of the self at the time of the study, but also had athletes who were more likely to continue with the sport a year later compared to a group of athletes of coaches who had not received CET training (Barnett *et al.* 1992).

More recently, Paterson (1999) investigated the relationship between 222 youth cricketers' self-perceptions and their views of the strategies used by their coaches. Players' self-esteem, self-perceptions, affective outcomes of participation, and their motivation orientation were measured pre- and post-season, and player observations of their coaches' instructional strategies were collected post-season. Results were mixed, but indicated that players who viewed their coaches as significant others were more likely to have positive perceptions of their own competence and success in cricket. Also, most athletes (excluding the 14 and under, low-skilled group) who had a coach who used strategies such as encouraging self-discipline and involving athletes in the decision-making process had higher global self-worth scores. Coaching internal control in one's athletes was also found to be significantly and positively related to constructs such as global self-worth, general athletic and cricket-specific competence and success perceptions, and plans to continue cricket participation. Thus, while differences between age groups and skill ability needs further investigation, it appears that several aspects of coaching instruction have significant implications for athletes' beliefs about themselves (as athletes and as people outside of sport) and motivation to continue sport participation in the future.

LEADERSHIP

Sport, and those who have a central role in shaping the sport experience (e.g., coaches, parents, and peers), have the capability of providing youth with a unique opportunity to develop the skills essential for leaders in today's society. When provided with an appropriate sporting environment, individual athletes can develop competence in skills such as using and encouraging in others effective communication, taking part in planning and discipline decisions, and acting as a role model for other players (Mosher & Roberts 1981). However, it does not appear that all athletes have equal opportunity to adopt leadership roles, and thus develop the skills of an effective leader.

It has been suggested that those players who are in positions that involve high levels of interaction with other players and who are more frequently involved in team-related decision making and coordinating are the individuals who are more likely to gain leadership positions and develop the skills in sport that will transfer to the adoption of leadership roles outside of sport (Grusky 1963; Loy & Sage 1970; Gill & Perry 1979; Melnick & Loy 1996). This explanation supports the tendency for players such as baseball pitchers, volleyball setters, and football quarterbacks to assume leadership positions on a team.

An opposing view of leadership opportunities has suggested that it is not the centrality of a player's role on a team that leads to leadership development. Instead, these researchers have posited that the level of independence and relative importance of the tasks performed by an athlete are what determines the likelihood that he or she will adopt a leadership role (Tropp & Landers 1979). For example, while a field hockey goalie's position is not one that demands a great deal of constant interaction with other players, it is a position that often carries a lot of responsibility and places the athlete in a position in which the team as a whole and its individual members depend highly on his or her actions.

In a recent study, Wright and Côté (2003) conducted interviews with six male athletes who were classified as members of and leaders within a Canadian Intercollegiate Athletic Union to determine what factors had a role in the development of their leadership skills. It was concluded that the aspects of the sporting environment that aided in the leadership development of these individuals were a focus on skill development, encouragement of a strong work ethic, opportunity to be engaged in the cognitive side of sport and cognitive sport knowledge, and the fostering of positive relationships with others. These athletes were surrounded by inspiring and motivating coaches who were engaged and interested in the athletes' lives, helped the young boys develop both the physical and cognitive (e.g., strategy and tactics) skills of their game, provided opportunities for leaders to emerge on their teams, and engaged the athletes in team-related decision making and problem solving. The parents of these athletes encouraged participation in a variety of organized sports and provided moral support, mentoring, and encouragement for the young individuals. Additionally, these athletes were involved with older peers at an early age, which may have helped develop high level physical, emotional, and cognitive skills. Finally, the young leaders were placed in a sporting environment that was nonthreatening and that provided increasingly challenging competitive opportunities over time. While the athletes in this study came from similar backgrounds, which may have provided unique influences on their leadership development, many of the components mentioned above are most likely common elements in the development of leadership skills in general.

In summary, it appears that sport can develop leadership in participants who play certain positions or have parents and coaches who purposefully teach leadership behaviors. However, the effectiveness of such training, the degree to which it occurs, and the transferability of leadership skills developed in sport to other life situations awaits further research.

ACADEMIC SUCCESS

Various factors associated with academic success also have been of great interest to those studying outcomes of youth sport participation. With school-aged children engaging in athletics both within and outside the school environment, it has been questioned whether or not sport participation has a facilitative or debilitative effect for individuals during the years that are thought to build the foundation for general success in life.

Much research has supported the notion that sport participation is, in fact, related to many positive academic outcomes. More specifically, youth athletes, when compared with their peers not participating in sport, are found to have better school attendance, tend to take more demanding coursework, spend more time on homework, are more likely to report academic aspirations both during and after secondary school, more often pursue higher education, have reduced rates of dropout, and receive fewer discipline referrals (Marsh 1993; McNeal 1995; Mahoney & Cairns 1997; Eccles & Barber 1999; Whitley 1999).

At first, these positive results were questioned because the samples studied were not controlled for pre-existing individual differences such as previous academic success or background variables such as social economic status (Marsh & Kleitman 2003). However, recent studies have addressed and responded to these past limitations and have still found correlations between sport engagement and academic success. Eccles and Barber (1999) controlled for social class, gender, and intellectual aptitude (e.g., grade 9 verbal and numerical ability subscores on the Differential Aptitude Test) in their sample who were studied across grades 6, 7, 10, and 12 and when participants were approximately 21–22 years of age and about 25–26 years old. When interviewed during these periods, it was discovered that student-athletes were more likely than their non-sport engaged peers to report a greater liking of school at grades 10 and 12, were more likely to attend a college or university and to have graduated by 25–26 years of age, reported a greater liking of school at grade 12 than at grade 10, attained higher than expected grade 12 point averages, and accumulate more total years of graduate education by age 25–26. Furthermore, at age 24 years, sport participants were more likely to have a job that provided a sense of autonomy than their non-athlete counterparts.

Similarly, Marsh and Kleitman (2003) conducted a longitudinal study with students across the USA from grade 8 to grade 12. These researchers also accounted for background and pre-existing variables, such as past assessment scores, socioeconomic status, school type (private vs. public), gender,

ethnicity, previous grades, etc. Participation in sports (e.g., baseball, basketball, football, soccer, swimming, hockey, and volleyball) was found to be associated with positive academic outcome variables such as better school grades, more challenging coursework selection, greater homework records, greater number of university applications, and greater college/university enrollment in the grade 12 year. Interestingly, these results were more significant among students who participated in extramural vs. intramural and team vs. individual sports.

Along with Marsh and Kleitman (2003), several researchers have posited that a mediator for the sport participation–academic outcome relationship is the sense of identification with and commitment to one's school and academic values that sport participation often fosters (Snyder & Spreitzer 1990; Eccles & Barber 1999; Barber *et al.* 2001; Marsh & Kleitman 2003). The process of defending one's school in competition, having reinforcement from coaches through "no pass, no play" policies, and developing a social network with one's teammates who also value school and plan on attending college are just a few ways in which sport may impact young athletes' participation and engagement in their academic careers.

Finally, in a recent intervention study, Petitpas *et al.* (2004) evaluated the implementation of the "Play it Smart Program," a national intervention that uses sport as a vehicle to facilitate academic achievement and life skill development in underserved urban youth. A total of 252 high school football players (most from minority and economically disadvantaged backgrounds) took part in the program, which sought to strengthen the academic influence of athletic coaches by providing an academic coach who would assist in creating an environment that would promote positive growth and learning. Results from 2 years of program evaluation showed a marked increase in grade point average (from 2.16 to 2.54, compared to 2.2 for the general school averages) with 98% of the seniors graduating from high school and 83% of that group going on to higher education. While it was concluded that additional data were needed, initial results showed the program to be very effective.

MORAL DEVELOPMENT

For decades, there has been a debate in the literature surrounding the issue of whether or not sport is a domain in which moral character can be developed and fostered. Some have argued that athletics creates a context that requires the use of, and thus promotes the application and enhancement of "virtuous" skills and qualities such as cooperation, courage, fairness, loyalty, teamwork, responsibility, conformity, and acting for the good of others as well as one's self (Kleiber & Roberts 1981; Hodge 1989). In contrast, others have contended that sport is an institution that has overemphasized competition and winning, thus detracting from its ability to build and cultivate moral character (Chandler & Goldberg 1990).

One way in which researchers have attempted to clarify the relationship between sport participation and moral functioning has been to compare the relative moral maturity of athletes with non-athletes. Across several studies, it has been found that non-athletes tend to use significantly higher levels of moral reasoning as assessed by moral dilemmas (both in and outside of sport) than their peers who are involved in sport (Bredemeier & Shields 1986; Shields & Bredemeier 1994; Beller & Stoll 1995). It was suggested that certain demands and structures might influence the impact a specific sport has on moral functioning (e.g., whether or not a sport is contact or non-contact, individual or team, or utilizes closed or open skill sets). Overall, findings like these suggested that sport participation is not an arena conducive to moral development.

With all the factors that have been identified in the research as detracting from moral reasoning and behavior in sport, the belief of sport as a mode of moral functioning has appeared to be supported less and less with time. However, there exists a camp that still remains steadfast in their support for sport as a means of teaching and practicing character. These individuals posit that there are ample opportunities for sport to aid in moral development, and that sport need not be devoid of moral behaviors (Hodge 1989; Chandler & Goldberg 1990). Unfortunately, it has been suggested that the low prevalence of displays of moral actions in sport

today could be attributed to the assumption that participation in sport will automatically build character in its athletes. Another more serious barrier to moral development in sport is that:

> "The prevailing attitude in competitive, organized sport toward morality seems to be one of complacent indifference... acting in a moral sportsmanlike manner seems to be regarded as an expensive luxury when the primary goal is one of winning and beating one's opponent by any means necessary" (Hodge 1989, p. 24).

Therefore, the belief that moral behavior is counterintuitive to the goals of sport must also be addressed.

For sport to become a better provider for moral growth, a perspective shift must occur in which the need for character development is necessary and purposefully fostered (Chandler & Goldberg 1990; Arnold 2001). Parents, coaches, and other authority figures in the athletic environment need to take an active role in providing the opportunities for and actively shaping the moral development of young athletes, as well as modeling these desirable behaviors themselves. In order to aid in character growth most effectively, these influential adults must also examine their own values and motives in sport and daily life to ensure they are in line with the values and models they hope to cultivate in young athletes (Lee 1988).

Chandler and Goldberg (1990) further posit that sport is inherently made of opportunities for character growth as well as character impairment. Thus, it is a matter of significant others influencing the appropriate skills and traits that are available through sport participation (e.g., courage, persistence, and self-control) and de-emphasizing the aspect of too great a focus on winning in sport, that has the potential to conflict with the development of traits such as dignity and integrity.

To assess this opportunity for moral growth through sport, several intervention programs have been run with a variety of populations (Guivernau & Duda 2002). An example of a program aimed at encouraging moral growth through sport was developed by Romance *et al.* (1986). Grade 5 physical education students were divided into an intervention and control group in this field study. All children participated in an 8-week program, playing the same game. However, the intervention group also received specific moral-reasoning strategies that involved discussion of what was moral in different situations. Results revealed that the children in the intervention group demonstrated significantly greater gains in their moral reasoning, both in sport and everyday life, while the control group children did not. These results show that when specifically taught, moral reasoning can be enhanced through physical activity participation.

Gibbons *et al.* (1995) tested a similar moral development program titled Play It Fair. Children in this study (452 children in Grades 4–6) were exposed to various components of the program intended to cultivate moral judgment, reasoning, intention, and pro-social behavior either during physical education, during all academic classes, or not at all. After 7 months of program participation, it was discovered that measures of moral judgment, reasoning, and intention were significantly higher for classrooms who received the intervention than those that did not. With additional support for program effectiveness, individual students who had been exposed to the Play It Fair curriculum scored higher on all four outcome measures than those who did not participate in the program. Again, physical activity was shown as an effective mode for promoting and fostering positive changes in moral development.

Finally, Bredemeier *et al.* (1986) used a summer sport camp as an arena to encourage young athletes' physical performance, sports knowledge, and social skills. One group of campers was exposed to an intervention strategy that emphasized adult modeling reinforcement of moral characteristics and behaviors such as fair play, sharing, and avoidance of aggressive acts. Other campers were encouraged to engage in dialogues with peers to resolve interpersonal disputes as a means of stimulating moral growth. Finally, a third group of campers (control group) did not have instructors who directly emphasized moral issues, but instead were encouraged to obey certain moral standards such as following game rules and safety guidelines. Results from the 6-week intervention demonstrated that there were significant increases in measured moral

understanding and judgments among campers in the two intervention groups, whereas significant changes did not occur in the control group. However, between-group analyses showed that differences in moral growth between the intervention and control groups did not reach significance, which may have been because of the short intervention period. Therefore, it should be recommended that young athletes be continually integrated (not simply trained short term) into an environment that supports morally mature attitudes and actions for complete moral development to occur.

GOAL SETTING

Sport has also been viewed as a viable activity for promoting the use and development of goal setting skills in young athletes. Cultivating this life skill is particularly important in helping individuals identify the successes they achieve, both large and small, so that a positive and realistic view of their competence and overall self can be fostered.

Using sport as an avenue to highlight the potential for and achievement of personal goals is especially practical because "goals in sport are typically tangible, short-term, and easily measured . . . giv[ing] the adolescent a better opportunity to see the value in goal setting and to experience success in setting and achieving goals" (Danish *et al.* 2003, p. 99). Introducing and exercising these same principles in other settings may be less successful because "lifestyle goals" such as those related to school, work, changing maladaptive habits, tend to take more time to achieve. The resulting delay in gratification can lead to loss of interest or confidence in the goal-setting process and frustration on the part of young individuals.

Danish *et al.* have developed a series of programs that use goal setting as a central mode for the development of life skills in young athletes (Danish 1996, 2002; Danish *et al.* 1998). For example, the Sports United to Promote Education and Recreation (SUPER) program was created and aims to deliver the following messages to its young participants:

1 Local student-athletes are available to serve as role models;

2 Development of physical and mental skills are essential for success in sport and in life;

3 Goal setting is key for success in sport and in life;

4 It is possible to overcome obstacles to personal goals; and

5 To be an effective athlete, one must be both healthy and physically fit (Danish 2002).

These themes are addressed in a 25-h, 10-session program that is run similarly to a sport clinic (with a focus on either one or several different sports), with the focus being on learning about and participating in a particular sport or sports and becoming more aware and practicing several life skills (e.g., learning how to learn, communicating with others, managing anger, problem solving, and setting and attaining goals). The SUPER program is primarily run by college (and qualified high school) student-athletes, who serve as effective role models for the young participants and who could arguably develop life skills through their involvement and leadership experiences in the program as well. Since its development, others have successfully implemented the SUPER program and its premises with groups such as young New Zealand Rugby Players (Hodge *et al.* 2000) and youth golfers (S.J. Danish, J. Brunelle, R. Fazio & C. Hogan 2000, unpublished; Danish 2001).

Initial evaluation research on these programs is promising (Brunelle *et al.* 2007), but more research is needed. Studies need to determine if students do increase their knowledge and ability to set goals and whether this knowledge transfers to behavior change in and out of sport.

PERSONAL RESPONSIBILITY

Personal responsibility is considered an important psychosocial skill for youth to develop and the lack of this skill is often seen in underserved youth. For this reason researchers have examined how personal responsibility might be developed through physical activity programs. Based on his work running sports clubs with underserved youth in Chicago, Hellison (1995) has outlined a five-stage model for teaching personal and social responsibility to youth through physical activity. This model contends that youth develop responsibility by moving through five stages:

1 Self-control and respect for others;

2 Effort and participation;

3 Self-direction and goal setting;

4 Caring for others; and

5 Applying these goals outside of the gym.

Practical strategies for implementing this model and helping youth progress through the stages have also been identified.

Evaluation research has been conducted on programs using the personal and social responsibility model. In a recent review of 25 of these studies, Hellison and Walsh (2002) concluded that while none of the studies contained sufficient controls to permit generalizations, evidence provided some support for the utility of teaching responsibility (e.g., respect for the rights of others, effort and teamwork, self-direction and goal setting, and leadership) to these youth through means such as awareness talks, group meetings, and reflection time. It is important to note, however, that these programs were not typical extracurricular sports. Rather, they were specially designed after-school programs for underserved youth that used sport as a setting for social development.

Critical issues and future directions

Need for additional research

If personal development through sport is to advance, more and better research is needed. Research is needed because non-profit and government agencies, who often finance these programs, are calling for greater accountability relative to justifying the spending of program dollars. Saying that sport builds character and keeps kids off the streets may no longer be enough. Agencies are asking for demonstration that such claims are actually happening.

Additional research is also needed to advance theory and practice relative to better identifying and understanding the ways personal development through sport takes place (Fraser-Thomas *et al.* 2005). The bulk of youth sport experiences are supervised by volunteers with little or no training, and when training is provided only short time periods are available. Thus, we need to identify the most effective strategies for promoting youth development through sport and determine how to convey them to volunteers in time efficient, clear, and practical formats.

Both quantitative and qualitative research is needed. Quantitative research is best suited to help determine the scale and scope of personal development through sport issues. For example, knowing the percentage of children who experience specific types of personal gains (e.g., enhanced self-esteem, leadership skills, and work ethic) from the youth sports experience would be very valuable. Additional path analytic research would be extremely valuable in helping tease out important theoretical principles. For example, using this type of research Guest and Sneider (2003) found that the benefits of extracurricular activities differed depending on the social context of the school (high vs. low socio-economic status schools) and concluded that making blanket statements about the benefits of extracurricular sports is too simplistic. Gains will be dependent on the social context and individual difference factors such as a participant's identity.

Longitudinal studies that follow youth across time are also needed, as psychosocial development is a process that unfolds over time. If one really hopes to understand personal development through sport, assessments across time are needed. It is ironic, then, that with the exception of the work of Eccles and her colleagues (e.g., Barber *et al.* 2005), almost all research conducted to date is cross-sectional and provides little information about how one develops personal and social skills in the sport context over time.

More experimental design research is needed, as the bulk of existing studies is correlational in nature and does not allow for the identification of cause and effect relationships. For example, much of the research shows that extracurricular activities, like sports, are associated with developmental gains such as higher levels of initiative, emotional regulation, and attachment to school. Based on this research it is easy to conclude that sport is successful in causing psychologic development in youth. However, the difference might just as likely result from the fact that youth who are drawn to participate in sport are individuals who are more achievement motivated, better regulate their emotions, etc. Thus, findings

might reflect a selection bias more than a program effect.

Experimental or clinical trials type research, such as that conducted by Smith, Smoll and their colleagues (e.g., Smoll *et al.* 1993), allows investigators to show causal links between variables and is essential to advancing knowledge in the area. That is, in these studies, by training one group of coaches and using a matched control with no training and then comparing changes in young athletes' psychologic development across the season, these investigators have shown that coach training was effective in changing coaches' behavior. This behavior change in turn caused changes in athlete psychologic development.

Petitpas *et al.* (2005) have also highlighted the importance of conducting three types of evaluation research on psychologic development through sport. Research on implementation evaluation focuses on examining how programs are implemented. That is, these studies answer the question of whether or not programs are delivered as planned. For example, a national coaching education program was developed for the purpose of training youth coaches how to teach life skills to their players. However, when clinics were observed around the country it was found that many trainers, while experienced and knowledgeable coaches, were not specifically trained in how to deliver the program and failed to deliver it as designed. Because of the failure to implement the program as planned, few conclusions could be drawn about program effectiveness. Focus groups, individual participant interviews, and observational studies might be especially useful implementation research tools.

Outcome evaluation research examines whether program objectives are achieved. For instance, if a program is designed to enhance teamwork and effective group functioning in youth then measures of these key constructs must be used. These assessments might include direct measures of group cohesion or indirect measures thought to be influenced by changes in team cohesion such as fewer observed conflicts in practice.

Finally, process evaluation identifies and examines the specific program features that relate to the personal development outcomes achieved. For instance, if outcome research shows that a program is successful in enhancing moral development and sportsmanship in young athletes, it is important to understand what components of the program are most linked to its success. For example, is it the moral dialogues or discussion a coach has with young athletes in those naturally occurring moral dilemmas that occur in sport that is most critical? Or are other explanations, such as the modeling and social reinforcement of desirable behaviors, or the influence of peers who demonstrate good sportsmanship, that are the most critical aspects of the program.

From a broader youth development perspective, Eccles *et al.* (2003) suggest identity formation, peer group membership, and attachment to caring adults may help explain why youth develop through sport, while Certo *et al.* (2003) emphasize the importance of extracurricular activities creating a sense of belonging for youth. Regardless of the specific mechanism proposed, discovering the process by which personal development takes place in sport and those program aspects and external factors that influence development is essential.

One of the most critical issues for future investigators studying personal development through sport to examine is the transferability of life skills assumption. Most life skill and personal development through sport programs are based on the assumption that those qualities youth develop or enhance through sport carry over and positively influence their actions in other life settings. For example, does what a young person learns about teamwork playing high school basketball transfer to his or her work life in subsequent years? Unfortunately, this assumption is seldom tested.

One of the few studies to test this issue was conducted by Martinek *et al.* (2001). In evaluating an after-school sports club and mentoring program for underserved youth, entitled Project Effort, these investigators used teacher and mentor logs and student exit interviews to determine if participants learned personal and social responsibility and then transferred these skills to academic classroom settings. Results revealed that participants were able to apply the goal of effort to learn what was taught in the sports club to their non-sport classroom settings.

However, the students struggled to transfer goal setting skills learned in the club to the academic realm. These findings are important because they show that certain personal development skills learned in the sport context can be transferred to non-sport settings. However, they also demonstrated that such transfer is not automatic and requires considerable programmatic efforts. Moreover, even with considerable effort to teach for transfer, participants in this program experienced considerable difficulties transferring skills learned through sport to the classroom setting. It is critical that researchers further examine this issue.

Practical implications

While much still needs to be learned about how, when, why, and under what conditions personal development occurs through youth sports participation, the research to date does lead to a number of implications for guiding practice. First, research shows that life skills are taught, not caught through sports participation (Hodge 1988). That is, while some benefits may occur through merely participating in sport (e.g., keep youth off the street during after-school hours when they are most likely to get into trouble), personal development through sport will more systematically and consistently be developed when it is taught through caring and competently trained adults. This concept is best reflected in the moral development and sportspersonship research. In their review of the research, Shields and Bredemier (2001) concluded that merely participating in sports is not associated with enhanced moral development, and, in many instances, has been shown to detract from moral development. However, when moral development is specifically targeted and taught positive changes can occur.

Taken in a broader context, these same sentiments were echoed by Hartmann (2003), who concluded in a case study of Larry Hawkins, a teacher, coach, and youth activist with over 35 years of experience developing youth through sport:

> "While sport can be a powerful force for social intervention, its impacts are not automatically or inevitability positive . . . Thus, sport is better

understood as a tool for social outreach, a hook or instrument whose impact depends upon the ends toward which it is directed, how it is implemented, and the context in which it is deployed." (Hartmann 2003, p. 134).

Thus, sport by itself does not enhance personal development, but rather sport experience—an experience that must be guided by caring and knowledgeable coaches who systematically plan, teach, and facilitate social emotional development.

In terms of strategies for teaching life skills and personal development, the research suggests that these goals are best accomplished by using direct strategies such as coaches contingently reinforcing their players more often or engaging them in moral dialogues. At the same time, a good deal of indirect teaching occurs through modeling and the environment created by the adults involved in these programs. For example, youth sports environments that focus primary attention on sport outcome (social comparison and winning and losing) versus individual improvement result in lower self-esteem, higher levels of stress, and lower levels of intrinsic motivation (Brustad et al. 2001).

As the above suggests, past research also points to the important role adults have in the youth sports process. Their actions have been shown to influence a variety of personal development factors such as motivation, self-esteem, anxiety, and satisfaction. The goals they set, the importance they place on performance, their reinforcement patterns, and their teaching capabilities all influence young athletes' personal development. Moreover, recent youth development research suggests that the nature of mentoring young people is changing. Specifically, Larson (2006) contends that for many years children and adolescents were psychologically viewed as soft clay to be molded by caring adults. They were not viewed as active agents in the developmental process. However, this growth is viewed very differently today. Young people are viewed as being capable and motivated constructive agents of their own development, with adult mentors being more effective when they facilitate and support the young person's own efforts to develop rather than acting in an authoritarian manner. Thus, mentors are not

molding stable clay. In contrast, significant others must support and enable youth to mold themselves by awakening, guiding, and supporting the young individuals' own capabilities for growth. Mentors must help youth activate and sustain their internal motivation, experience ownership in the activities they pursue, and gradually develop self-regulation skills to guide their own development. Agency must also be directed in ways that are constructive and healthy rather than destructive and unhealthy. Coaching educators must consider this shift in orientation as too often coaches take an autocratic, top-down approach to working with young people.

According to Larson (2006), one implication of supporting youth as producers of their own development is what he labels the contractions of helping youth. He contends that it is easier to mold clay than to help the clay mold itself. To effectively mentor youth, adults must find ways to keep ownership for the activity in the hands of the youth, while simultaneously trying to keep the activities and developmental experiences on track. The paradox seems to be finding the right balance of support and challenge. Too much structure and direction from adults can lead to a loss of ownership. However, no challenge and assistance can be equally damaging as young people do not have the self-regulation and problem solving skills needed to move forward towards their goals without any guidance.

Larson (2006) posed a series of day-to-day questions adult mentors must wrestle with in providing the right balance of support and challenge in working with young people. These include: "when to set firm boundaries and when to be flexible?; when to support a child's goals and when to challenge them?; how to grant youth choice and autonomy without putting them at risk?; when to listen and be empathic and when to give one's point of view?; and, when to let youth learn from mistakes?" Sport coaches interested in the personal development of their players must consider these issues.

Petitpas et al. (2005) have also identified a number of implementation concerns that must be considered in guiding practice. Site issues focus on selecting appropriate venues and developing good relationships with program stakeholders. Recruitment and training of individuals who deliver youth development program should also be a carefully involved process. However, in many sport programs, virtually anyone who volunteers is allowed to coach with little or no training taking place. Finally, program providers must monitor the delivery of the program to be sure it is being implemented as planned. Strategies for staff regulation and continuing education are critical.

Finally, Fraser-Thomas *et al.* (2005) emphasize the importance of basing youth sport programs and interventions on the applied research and theory on youth development through sport. Hellison's (2003) responsibility model provides an excellent example in this regard. Fraser-Thomas *et al.* (2005) also propose a more integrated model which considers young individuals' total development, program setting considerations, and development assets.

Conclusions

We began this chapter with de Coubertin's statement that "for each individual, sport is a possible source for inner improvement." Our review of the evidence examining the role sport has in the personal development of young people bears out de Coubertin's belief. Sport can be an effective vehicle for personal and social development. However, the current evidence also reveals that while sport can have positive developmental consequences for youth, it can also have negative outcomes. Key factors that determine whether effects are beneficial or detrimental are program goals and structure, how programs are implemented, the quality and competence of adult leaders, and the context in which the program is deployed. In the end, personal development can occur through the youth sports experience, but is fostered and taught, not caught from mere participation.

References

Arnold, P.J. (2001) Sport, moral development, and the role of the teacher: Implications for research and moral education. *Quest* 53, 135–150.

Barber, B.L., Eccles, J.S. & Stone, M.R. (2001) Whatever happened to the "Jock," the "Brain," and the "Princess?": Young adult pathways linked to adolescent activity involvement and social identity. *Journal of Adolescent Research* 16, 429–455.

Barber, B.L., Stone, M.R., Hunt, J.E. & Eccles, J.S. (2005) Benefits of activity participation: The roles of identity affirmation and peer group norm sharing. In: *Organized Activities as Contexts of Development* (Mahoney, L.L., Larson, R.W. & Eccles, J.S. eds.) Lawrence Erlbaum Associates, Mahwah, NJ: 185–210.

Barnett, N.P., Smoll, F.L. & Smith, R.E. (1992) Effects of enhancing coach–athlete relationships on youth sport attrition. *Sport Psychologist* 6, 111–127.

Beller, J.M. & Stoll, S.K. (1995) Moral reasoning of high school student athletes and general students: An empirical study versus personal testimony. *Pediatric Exercise Science* 7, 352–363.

Bredemeier, B.J. & Shields, D.L. (1986) Moral growth among athletes and non-athletes: A comparative analysis. *Journal of Genetic Psychology* 147, 7–18.

Bredemeier, B.J., Weiss, M.R., Shields, D.L. & Shewchuk, R.M. (1986) Promoting moral growth in a summer sport camp: The implementation of theoretically grounded instructional strategies. *Journal of Moral Education* 15, 212–220.

Brunelle, J., Danish, S.J. & Forneris, T. (2007) The impact of a sports-based life skill program on adolescent prosocial values. *Applied Developmental Science* 11, 43–55.

Brustad, B.J., Babkes, M.L. & Smith, A.L. (2001) Youth in sport: psychological considerations. In: *Handbook of Sport Psychology*, 2nd edn. (Singer, N., Hausenblas, H.A. & Janelle C.M., eds.) John Wiley & Sons, NY: 604–635.

Certo, J.L., Cauley, K.M. & Chafin, C. (2003) Students' perspectives on their high school experience. *Adolescence* 38, 705–724.

Chandler, T.J. & Goldberg, A.D. (1990) Building character through sports: Myth or possibility? *Counseling and Values* 34, 169–176.

Danish, S.J. (1996) Interventions for enhancing adolescents' life skills.

Humanistic Psychologist 24, 365–381.

Danish, S.J. (2001) The First Tee: Teaching youth to succeed in golf and life. In: *Optimizing Performance in Golf* (Thomas, P.R., ed.) Australian Academic Press, Brisbane, Australia: 67–74.

Danish, S.J. (2002) Teaching life skills through sport. In: *Paradoxes of Youth and Sport* (Gatz, M.J., Messner, M.A. & Ball-Rokeach, S.J., eds.) State University of New York Press, Albany, NY: 49–60.

Danish, S., Forneris, T., Hodge, K. & Heke, I. (2004) Enhancing youth development through sport. *World Leisure* 3, 38–49.

Danish, S.J., Meyer, A., Mash, J., *et al.* (1998) *Going for the Goal: Student Activity Book*, 2nd edn. Department of Psychology, Virginia Commonwealth University.

Danish, S.J., Taylor, T.E. & Fazio, R.J. (2003) Enhancing adolescent development through sport and leisure. In: *Blackwell Handbook of Adolescence* (Adams, G.R., ed.) Blackwell Publishing, Malden, MA: 92–108.

Dworkin, J.B., Larson, R. & Hansen, D. (2003) Adolescents' accounts of growth experiences in youth activities. *Journal of Youth and Adolescents* 32, 17–26.

Eccles, J.S. & Barber, B.L. (1999) Student council, volunteering, basketball, or marching band: What kind of extracurricular involvement matters? *Journal of Adolescent Research* **14**, 10–43.

Eccles, J.S., Barber, B.L. & Stone, M. & Hunt, J. (2003) Extracurricular activities and adolescent development. *Journal of Social Issues* **59**, 865–889.

Ewing, M.E., Gano-Overway, L.A., Branta, C.F. & Seefeldt, V.D. (2000) The role of sports in youth development. In: *Paradoxes of Youth and Sport* (Gatz, M.J., Messner, M.A. & Ball-Rokeach, S.J., eds.) State University of New York Press, Albany, NY: 31–47.

Fox, K.R. (2000) Self-esteem, self-perceptions and exercise. *International Journal of Sport Psychology* **31**, 228–240.

Fraser-Thomas, J.L., Cote, J. & Deakin, J. (2005) Youth sport programs: An avenue to foster positive youth development. *Physical Education and Sport Pedagogy* **10**, 19–40.

Gibbons, S.L., Ebbeck, V. & Weiss, M.R. (1995) Fair play for kids: Effects on the moral development of children in physical education. *Research Quarterly for Exercise and Sport* **66**, 247–255.

Gill, D.L. & Perry., J.L. (1979) A case study of leadership in women's intercollegiate softball. *International Review of Sport Sociology* **14**, 83–91.

Gould, D., Collins, K., Lauer, L. & Chung, Y. (2006) Coaching life skills: A working model. *Sport and Exercise Psychology Review* **2**, 10–18.

Gould, D., Collins, K., Lauer, L. & Chung, Y. (2007) Coaching life skills through football: A study of award winning high school coaches. *Journal of Applied Sport Psychology* **19**, 16–37.

Guest, A. & Schneider, B. (2003) Adolescent's extracurricular participation in context: The mediating effects of schools, communities, and identity. *Sociology of Education* **76**, 89–209.

Grusky, O. (1963) The effects of formal structure on managerial recruitment: A study of baseball organization. *Sociometry* **26**, 345–353.

Guivernau, M. & Duda, J.L. (2002) Moral atmosphere and athletic aggressive tendencies in young soccer players. *Journal of Moral Education* **31**, 67–84.

Hansen, D.M., Larson, R.W. & Dworkin, J.B. (2003) What adolescents learn in organized youth activities: A survey of self-reported developmental experiences. *Journal of Research on Adolescence* **13**, 25–55.

Hartmann, D. (2003) Theorizing sport as social intervention: A view from the grassroots. *Quest* **55**, 118–140.

Hellison, D. (1995) *Teaching Responsibility Through Physical Activity*. Human Kinetics, Champaign, IL.

Hellison, D. (2003) *Teaching Responsibility Through Physical Activity*, 2nd edn. Human Kinetics, Champaign, IL.

Hellison, D. & Walsh, D. (2002) Responsibility-based youth programs evaluation: Investigating the investigations. *Quest* **54**, 292–307.

Hodge, K.P. (1988) A conceptual analysis of character development in sport. Dissertation. University of Illinois, Urbana, IL.

Hodge, K.P. (1989) Character building in sport: Fact or fiction? *New Zealand Journal of Sports Medicine* **17**, 23–25.

Hodge, K., Heke, J.I. & McCarroll, N. (2000) The Rugby Advantage Program (RAP). University of Otago, Dunedin, New Zealand.

Holland, A. & Andre, T. (1987) Participation in extracurricular activities in secondary school: What is known, what needs to be known? *Review of Educational Research* **57**, 437–466.

Kleiber, D.A. & Kirshnit, C.E. (1991) Sport involvement and identity formation. In: *Mind–Body Maturity: Psychological Approaches to Sports, Exercise and Fitness* (Diamant, L., ed.) Hemisphere, New York, NY: 193–211.

Kleiber, D.A. & Roberts, G.C. (1981) The effects of sport experience in the development of social character: An exploratory investigation. *Journal of Sport Psychology* **3**, 114–122.

Larson, R. (2000) Toward psychology of positive youth development. *American Psychologist* **55**, 170–183.

Larson, R. (2006) Positive youth development, willful adolescents, and mentoring. *Journal of Community Psychology* **36**, 677–689.

Lee, M. (1988) Values and responsibilities in children's sports. *Physical Education Review* **11**, 19–27.

Loy, J.W. & Sage, J.N. (1970) The effects of formal structure on organizational leadership: An investigation of interscholastic baseball teams. In: *Contemporary Psychology of Sport*, Vol. 3 (Kenyon, G.S. & Grogg, T.M., eds.) Athletic Institute, Chicago, IL: 363–374.

Mahoney, J.L. & Cairns, R.B. (1997) Do extracurricular activities protect against early school dropout? *Developmental Psychology* **33**, 241–253.

Marsh, M.W. (1993) Relations between global and specific domains of self: The importance of individual importance, certainty, and ideals. *Journal of Personality and Social Psychology* **65**, 975–992.

Marsh, M.W. & Kleitman, S. (2003) School athletic participation: Mostly gain with little pain. *Journal of Sport and Exercise Psychology* **25**, 205–228.

Martinek, T., Schilling, T. & Johnson, D. (2001) Transferring personal and social responsibility of underserved youth to the classroom. *Urban Review* **33**, 29–45.

McNeal, R.B. (1995) Extracurricular activities and high school dropouts. *Sociology of Education* **68**, 62–81.

Melnick, M.J. & Loy, J.W. (1996) The effects of formal structure on leadership recruitment: An analysis of team captaincy among New Zealand provincial rugby teams. *International Review of Sociology and Sport* **31**, 91–108.

Mosher, M. & Roberts, D. (1981) The team captain in Canada: Fact or figurehead. *Sports Science Periodical on Research and Technology in Sport* **3**, 1–4.

Patterson, G.D. (1999) Coaching for the development of athlete self-esteem: The relationship between the self-perceptions of junior cricketers and their perceptions of coaching behaviour. *Sociology of Sport Online* **2**.

Petitpas, A.J., Cornelius, A.E., Van Raalte, J.L. & Jones, T. (2005) A framework for planning youth sport programs that foster psychosocial development. *Sport Psychologist* **19**, 63–80.

Petitpas, A.J., Van Raalte, J.L., Cornelius, A.E. & Presbrey, J. (2004) A life skills development program for high school student athletes. *Journal of Primary Prevention* **24**, 325–334.

Romance, T.J., Weiss, M.R. & Bockoven, J. (1986) A program to promote moral development through elementary school physical education. *Journal of Teaching Physical Education* **5**, 126–136.

Shields, D.L.L. & Bredemeier, B.J.L. (1994) *Character Development and Physical Activity*. Human Kinetics, Champaign, IL.

Shields, D.L.L. & Bredemeier, B.J.L. (2001) Moral development and behavior in sport. In: *Handbook of Sport Psychology*, 2nd edn. (Singer, N., Hausenblas, H.A. & Janelle, C.M., eds.) John Wiley & Sons, NY: 585–603.

Smith, R.E., Smoll, F.L. & Barnett, N.P. (1995) Reduction of children's sport performance anxiety through social support and stress-reduction training for coaches. *Journal of Applied Developmental Psychology* **16**, 125–142.

Smith, R.E., Smoll, F.L. & Curtis, B. (1979) Coach effectiveness training: A cognitive–behavioral approach to enhancing relationship skills in youth sport coaches. *Journal of Sport Psychology* **1**, 59–75.

Smoll, F.L., Smith, R.E., Barnett, N.P. & Everett, J.J. (1993) Enhancement of children's self-esteem through social support training for youth sport coaches. *Journal of Applied Psychology* **78**, 602–610.

Snyder, E.E. & Spreitzer, E. (1990) High school athletic participation as related to college attendance among Black, Hispanic, and White males: A research note. *Youth and Society* **21**, 390–398.

Steen, T.A., Kachorek, L.V. & Paterson, C. (2003) Character Strengths among youth. *Journal of Youth and Adolescence* **32**, 5–16.

Terry, J. (2000) Play it again: Notes from the editor. *Community Youth Development (CYD) Journal* **1**, 5.

Tropp, K.J. & Landers, D.M. (1979) Team interaction and the emergence of leadership and interpersonal attraction in field hockey. *Journal of Sport Psychology* **1**, 228–240.

Weinberg, R.S. & Gould, D. (2007) *Foundations of Sport and Exercise Psychology*, 4th edn. Human Kinetics, Champaign, IL.

Whitley, R.L. (1999) Those "dumb jocks" are at it again: A comparison of the educational performances of athletes and non-athletes in North Carolina high school from 1993 through 1996. *High School Journal* **82**, 223–233.

Wright, A. & Côté, J. (2003) A retrospective analysis of leadership development through sport. *Sport Psychologist* **17**, 268–291.

Zimmerman, M.C., Bingenheimer, B. & Nataro, P.C. (2002) Natural mentors and adolescent resiliency: A study of urban youth. *American Journal of Community Psychology* **30**, 221–243.

Chapter 23

Developing Positive Self-Perceptions through Youth Sport Participation

MAUREEN R. WEISS, JENNIFER A. BHALLA, AND MELISSA S. PRICE

Gina and Emily, two 12-year-old girls actively involved in organized youth soccer, show similar performance potential given their years of experience and aptitude for soccer, yet they differ considerably in their attitude and behavior during practices and competitions. Gina exudes a "love of the game," gives all-out effort, and demonstrates relentless persistence, consistent performance, and pride and joy in her accomplishments. By contrast, Emily seems to go through the motions at practice, is prone to giving up on herself when skills and tactics are challenging, does not enjoy but instead shows apathy during play, and performs below her potential during competitions. What might explain why these two girls think, feel, and act in different ways given their similar experiences and skills? One viable reason is differences in their *self-perceptions* or beliefs about their abilities and even in their assessment of personal worth. Self-perceptions of ability are critical to explaining variations in motivation, emotional responses, and actual performance in a specific achievement domain such as sports.

In this chapter we focus on what we know about developing positive self-perceptions in youth sport. Given the critical influence of perceptions of ability on emotional reactions to and motivational consequences of sport participation, understanding how self-perceptions are formed lends itself to strategies for maintaining and enhancing beliefs about physical competence. First, we identify and define self-perceptions such as self-esteem, perceived competence, and self-efficacy. Second, we distinguish among level, accuracy, and sources of perceived competence, and discuss age-related trends in these

constructs. Third, we introduce a conceptual model specifying relationships among self-perceptions and its antecedents (social influence) and consequences (emotional reactions and motivational orientations). This organizing model helps visualize the points of intervention for modifying self-perceptions and desirable developmental outcomes of such change. Fourth, we review relevant literature pertaining to parent, coach, and peer influence on self-perceptions. Fifth, we translate theory and research to provide practical implications for enhancing perceived competence in youth sport settings. Finally, we conclude with several take-home messages about the importance of self-perceptions in contributing to positive psychosocial and behavioral outcomes in sports and physical activities.

Self-perceptions: terminology and definitions

Self-perceptions refer to youths' evaluations or beliefs about themselves in general or their abilities in certain achievement areas (Weiss & Ebbeck 1996; Horn 2004). *Self-esteem* or *self-worth* is an individual's evaluation of his or her worthiness and significance as a person, such as how happy, satisfied, and favorable one is with who they are. Self-esteem is multidimensional, consisting of physical, social, and academic selves, among others. Thus, self-esteem is influenced by individuals' beliefs about their abilities combined with how important it is to be successful in a certain domain. For example, if 15-year-old Sam places high importance on sports success but does not possess a favorable view of his abilities, then self-esteem should be low. However, if ability beliefs are positive then self-esteem should be high (i.e., positive sport ability beliefs plus high importance placed on being successful in sports).

Perceived competence refers to one's beliefs or judgments about abilities in a particular achievement domain (e.g., academics, sports) or subdomain (e.g., math, swimming). Adolescents may view their abilities in sport positively but abilities in social situations negatively, or verbalize confidence in one sport (soccer) while being self-effacing in another sport (swimming). Stronger beliefs about one's competence in sports are related to higher self-esteem, positive affective responses, intrinsic motivation, and continued participation. Because perceived competence is more specific and less stable than global self-evaluations, it is more susceptible to change through intervention; strategies can be recommended for maintaining high or enhancing lower physical competence beliefs. Thus, perceived competence will be the major focus of our chapter given its adaptability to change and strong contribution to thoughts, feelings, and behaviors in sport.

Self-efficacy refers to an individual's belief that he or she can execute a particular behavior to be successful in a situation. For example, 12-year-old Chelsea may understand what is required of her role as point guard in a basketball game but her conviction in being able to carry out this role signifies her self-efficacy. As such, self-efficacy is a form of situation-specific confidence to carry out required behaviors successfully in a given social context. Self-efficacy is the least stable of the self-perceptions discussed, and is predictive of situation-specific behaviors in sport contexts.

Perceived competence: level, accuracy, sources, and age-related trends

Because perceived competence is a powerful predictor of attitudes, emotions, motivation, and participation behavior, it is an important construct highlighted in every theory of motivation (Weiss & Ferrer-Caja 2002). For example, perceived competence is a central determinant of motivational orientations and behavior within competence motivation, self-determination, achievement goal, and

expectancy-value theories, all of which connote practical theories that apply to understanding human behavior in sport and physical activity. In this section, we focus upon developmental trends in level, accuracy, and sources of perceived competence, and their relevance for understanding attitudes and behaviors of youth in sport.

Perceived competence can be assessed in three ways: level, accuracy, and sources of information. *Level* of perceived competence refers to how high or low individuals judge their abilities. For instance, in our opening example Gina is relatively higher and Emily lower in perceived soccer competence. Considerable research has shown a strong linkage between level of perceived physical competence and motivational processes such as intrinsic/extrinsic orientations, effort, persistence, and participation behavior (Weiss *et al.* 1986; Ferrer-Caja & Weiss 2000, 2002; Amorose 2001). Individuals who hold high and favorable perceptions of physical ability enjoy their experiences, and show intensity, sustained effort, and continued involvement in sport and physical activity.

Accuracy of perceived competence refers to whether youth underestimate, accurately estimate, or overestimate their abilities in an achievement domain. This is determined by assessing discrepancy between perceived and actual ability (index of performance or coach rating of skill). A child could be high and accurate in perceived competence, suggesting a close association between favorable self-judgments and objective performance. Conversely, a child could be high and inaccurate by overestimating her actual abilities, or she could be low and inaccurate by underestimating actual ability level. Accuracy of perceived competence is related to achievement cognitions and motivation (Weiss & Horn 1990; Horn & Weiss 1991; Weiss & Amorose 2005). Youth who are high and accurate about their ability use multiple sources of information to determine their ability, and report higher intrinsic motivation, and lower anxiety in sport compared to youth who over- or underestimate physical abilities.

Finally, *sources* of perceived competence align with the question, "How do children and adolescents make judgments about how good they are in a domain?" Sources of information for judging sport competence may include parent feedback, coach evaluation, peer comparison, peer evaluation, performance statistics, skill improvement, ease of learning skills, effort, goal attainment, enjoyment toward learning, and event or game outcome. While all these information sources are available in youth sport environments, children and adolescents may use all or only some of these sources in deriving a sense of how capable they are in sports (Horn 2004).

Research shows age-related differences in level, accuracy, and sources of perceived competence (Horn & Harris 1996; Horn 2004). During early childhood (about 3–6 years), children are very optimistic about their abilities, often much higher than what their actual capabilities suggest. This may be because of their preference for sources such as simple task mastery, parent feedback, and how much effort they exert. In this age range, comparison with peers' abilities for the purpose of calculating their skill is not common; rather, peers are instead used as a source for learning how to do a skill (i.e., observational learning). If they can do a task, their parents tell them they are good, and they try hard, young children will conclude that they are good in sports.

During middle and late childhood (about 7–12 years), characteristics of perceived competence change. Level declines (higher → lower) and accuracy increases (overestimation → accurate estimation of ability) (Horn & Weiss 1991; McKiddie & Maynard 1997). One explanation for these trends is change in the information sources used to determine physical competence. Older children use peer comparison and evaluation, as well as coach feedback and performance outcomes, relatively more than younger children. When youth stack their abilities up to teammates or classmates, turn to credible coaches who directly or indirectly convey information about level of skill, or use performance statistics to judge where they stand relative to others, these sources provide a reality check in terms of where youth stand in athletic competence. Shift in preference from task mastery and parent feedback to peer comparison and coach feedback as sources of competence information helps explain decline in level but increase in accuracy of perceived competence over the childhood years.

Adolescents (ages 13–18 years) also differ in perceived competence level, accuracy, and sources relative to their younger peers (Horn et al. 1993; Horn & Harris 1996; Horn 2004). Level of perceived competence may decline, remain stable, or increase during the adolescent years, while perceptions can now be characterized as accurate because of cognitive and social developmental abilities. Adolescents use self-referenced information (e.g., skill improvement, effort, goal achievement, attraction toward sport) more frequently in comparison with children and also use a wider variety of information sources, including peer comparison and evaluation by adults and peers. An important point is that adolescents develop an internalized set of performance standards that provide a guide for accurately judging how competent they are in a particular domain, whether it is high, medium, or low in level. The variety of information sources that teenagers integrate helps them form an accurate appraisal of high or low abilities in a variety of domains.

Choice of sources of physical competence information may also depend on psychological constructs and not just age. Several studies have shown that use of information sources is related to individuals' psychological characteristics such as level of perceived competence, actual competence, self-esteem, competitive anxiety, perceived control, and achievement goal orientation (Horn & Hasbrook 1987; Williams 1994; Weiss et al. 1997; Weiss & Amorose 2005). For example, youth sport participants who are higher in perceived and actual competence integrate a variety of self- and norm-referenced information sources such as peer comparison, performance improvement, effort, coach feedback, and affect toward learning skills. In addition, Halliburton and Weiss (2002) found that sources of perceived gymnastics competence varied as a function of competitive level and perceived motivational climate. Those at lower levels of competition used effort and enjoyment sources, while those at higher competitive levels relied mostly on spectator feedback, feelings of nervousness prior to performance, and achievement of performance goals. Perceptions of a mastery climate were strongly related to self-referenced sources of competence information (effort/enjoyment, achievement of goals), while higher perceptions of a performance climate were associated with norm-referenced sources (peer evaluation/comparison, competition performance).

In sum, sources of information help explain variations in level and accuracy of perceived competence among youth differing in developmental level (age, level of competition), psychological characteristics (e.g., perceived control), and social environmental influences (e.g., motivational climate). In turn, variations in perceived competence are strongly related to emotional, motivational, and participation outcomes among children and youth in sport. Relationships among sources of perceived competence, self-perceptions of ability, and consequences of self-perceptions are accounted for in almost every theory of motivation applied to youth sport. Situating sources, self-perceptions, and psychosocial and behavioral outcomes within a theoretical framework is useful for highlighting relevant research and recommending practical implications for ensuring positive self-perceptions in youth sport.

A conceptual model for understanding self-perceptions

Harter's (1987, 1999) model of global self-worth provides a practical framework for understanding relationships among self-perceptions and their causes and consequences (Fig. 23.1). The antecedents represent points of intervention for enhancing self-perceptions while the outcomes signify why

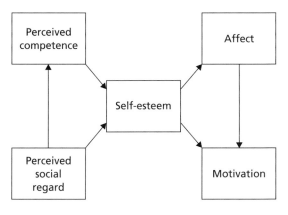

Fig. 23.1 Susan Harter's (1987, 1999) mediational model of global self-worth.

favorable self-perceptions are desirable in valued achievement domains. In addition, the model captures the developmental components of self-perceptions previously described. Harter's model of global self-worth identifies two primary determinants of self-worth—perceptions of competence in domains viewed as important and perceived social regard (reflected appraisals and support) by significant adults and peers—and two correlates or consequences (affect and motivation). In the following paragraphs we elaborate upon key model constructs and research supporting their relationships in sport and physical activity contexts.

In the model, *perceived competence* (domain-specific self-evaluations) represents one determinant of global self-esteem. Children's and adolescents' beliefs about how good they are in sports are directly related to their general self-esteem or how much they like who they are as a person. Harter (1987, 1999) suggests that perceived competence predicts global self-esteem for those achievement domains in which success is deemed important. If being good in sports is important to an individual, then higher perceived physical competence should relate to higher self-esteem while lower competence beliefs will relate to lower self-esteem. Conceptually, if an achievement domain is not important to an individual, their level of perceived competence for that domain (e.g., sports) will not affect their overall feelings of self-worth. Perceived physical competence and importance of being successful in sport (to self, parents, coach, and teammates) were predictive of global self-esteem in youth sport participants (Ebbeck & Stuart 1993, 1996).

Perceived social regard entails reflected appraisals or social support by important adults and peers that influences both perceived competence and general self-esteem (Fig. 23.1). Children and adolescents frequently use feedback by parents and coaches, and peer comparison and evaluation, as sources for judging how athletically skilled they are. If young participants interpret these and other sources of information positively, self-judgments of ability and general self-evaluations are positively affected. *Reflected appraisals* refer to verbal and non-verbal behaviors from significant adults and peers that convey approval or judgment of the child's mastery attempts and performances that, in turn, influence a child's *self-appraisals of ability*. When a coach rolls his eyes following a fielding error, a child is likely to interpret this as disapproval, whereas hand clapping by a parent following the same performance may be viewed as acceptance and encouragement to do better next time. *Social comparison* is the child's attempt to "measure up" or evaluate his or her skills and abilities relative to those of teammates or other peers. Collectively, social influence in the form of feedback and reinforcement by important adults (parents and coaches) and peers (teammates, classmates, close friends) is a powerful determinant of youths' self-perceptions (perceived physical competence and global self-esteem). The research supporting parent, coach, and peer influence on youth self-perceptions is covered extensively in the next section of the chapter.

The outcomes or consequences of self-perceptions are represented in the model by affect and motivation to engage in age-appropriate activities. Affect can include positive (joy, pride, satisfaction, happy, excited) and negative (anxiety, anger, guilt, unhappy) feelings related to participating in sports and physical activities. According to Harter's (1987, 1999) model, higher perceived competence and global self-esteem are associated with greater positive and lower negative affect toward participation. Motivational outcomes include intrinsic and extrinsic reasons for participating in sport as well as behaviors such as continued involvement, intensity of effort, persistence in learning, and performance. Research bolsters the strong relationships among self-perceptions (perceived competence and self-esteem), emotional responses, and motivational orientations and behaviors among youth participating in sport (Weiss *et al.* 1986; Ebbeck & Weiss 1998; Smith 1999).

Finally, the model is consistent with a developmental perspective on self-perceptions. Age differences exist in level and sources of perceived competence, use of adults versus peers to judge competencies and self-worth, and sources of enjoyment in sport and physical activity. Taken together, information on sources and outcomes of self-perceptions within a developmental approach makes this model a practical one from which to recommend age-appropriate strategies to enhance perceived competence and self-esteem. Given the powerful role of significant adults and peers to modify perceptions of competence and self-esteem, we now turn to the empirical research highlighting reflected appraisals (i.e., feedback and reinforcement) and social support (i.e., encouragement, modeling, acceptance) by parents, coaches, teammates, and close friends on youths' perceptions of physical competence and global self-esteem.

Understanding variations in self-perceptions: influence by parents, coaches, and peers

Perceptions of physical competence, global self-worth, enjoyment, and motivation (all components in the conceptual model) are heavily influenced by the beliefs and behaviors of significant adults (parents and coaches) and peers (teammates, close friends). Parent and coach feedback, and comparison to and evaluation by peers, are consistent sources by which youth judge their sport skills. Sources of sport enjoyment consistently point to positive interactions with teammates, acceptance by coaches, and approval by parents (Scanlan & Simons 1992). Predictors of intrinsic motivation and sport commitment include social support, positive feedback, a mastery-oriented climate, and autonomy-supportive style of coaches, parents, and/or peers (Ferrer-Caja & Weiss 2000, 2002; Price & Weiss 2000; Weiss & Weiss 2003, 2006). As such, parents, coaches, and peers reflect *perceived social regard* in the model and a point of intervention to enhance self-perceptions, positive affect, and motivated behavior in youth sport. In the following sections, we review related research on each of these important socializers.

Influence of parents

Parents make a significant impact on children's self-perceptions through the socialization process (for review see Fredricks & Eccles 2004). The socialization process consists of modeling attitudes and behaviors as well as conveying beliefs and expectations about the value of certain domains. Parents' beliefs and behaviors are instrumental in forming and maintaining children's and adolescents' global self-esteem and perceived physical competence. Several studies have demonstrated how parents' beliefs and behaviors operate to influence youths self-perceptions.

Parents affect children's self-perceptions through three main mechanisms of influence:

1 Providing experiences;
2 Interpreting experiences; and
3 Being role models (Fredricks & Eccles 2004).

Parents provide experiences and influence their children's perceived competence by encouraging and supporting skill attempts and performance. As interpreters of experience, parents shape children's perceptions of competence through their beliefs and behaviors regarding their children's ability in sport. Finally, by role modeling sport beliefs and behaviors, parents can help children develop positive perceptions of their competence in sport. These three mechanisms enhance children's self-perceptions when parents remain positive in their beliefs and behaviors regarding their children's involvement in sport. The link between parent beliefs and behaviors and children's self-perceptions can have a lasting effect on children's sport participation. In the following paragraphs, we highlight research that shows how these parental mechanisms of influence relate to youth sport participants' self-perceptions, emotional responses, and motivational outcomes.

As providers of experiences, parents afford children opportunities to participate in sport such as signing them up for sports, transporting to and from practices and competitions, and purchasing necessary equipment and clothing. Providing experiences also includes encouraging and supporting the child's participation, mastery attempts, and performance behaviors. Perceptions of greater parental encouragement and support are associated with youth participants who report more positive self-perceptions and higher enjoyment, intrinsic motivation, and commitment to participate in sport (Brustad 1993, 1996; Leff & Hoyle 1995; Weiss & Hayashi 1995; Green & Chalip 1997; Babkes & Weiss 1999; Weiss & Weiss 2003, 2006; Weiss & Fretwell 2005). By contrast, youth who see their parents as pressuring and controlling report lower

self-perceptions, higher anxiety, and feelings of entrapment in sport (Brustad 1988; Leff & Hoyle 1995; Babkes & Weiss 1999; Weiss & Weiss 2003, 2006; Weiss & Fretwell 2005). It is clear from this research that parents have a huge role in modifying youths' perceptions of sport competence that, in turn, influences enjoyment and motivation to participate.

In their role as interpreters of experience, parents influence children's self-judgments about physical competence as well as their evaluations of performance attempts and outcomes. Parents express beliefs and behaviors about their child's ability and performance, which influences the child's adoption of beliefs and behaviors regarding sport participation. For example, parents' beliefs about their child's ability in sport are strongly related to their children's perceptions of physical competence (Kimiecik et al. 1996; Bois et al. 2002, 2005; Fredricks & Eccles 2002, 2005). Youth who think their parents believe they are good in sports and physical activities and expect they will perform well, report favorable self-judgments of physical competence. Thus, youth may internalize the beliefs their parents hold about their performance potential. Moreover, parents who place importance on being successful in sport are associated with children who report higher athletic competence (Eccles & Harold 1991; Fredricks & Eccles 2002). This parent–child relationship for beliefs about athletic ability is even more important in light of findings that parents' and children's competency beliefs are associated with motivation and participation levels (Dempsey et al. 1993; Babkes & Weiss 1999; Kimiecik et al. 1996; Kimiecik & Horn 1998; Fredricks & Eccles 2005).

Gender of the child may influence how parents convey competency beliefs and behaviors regarding the value of sport participation. A few studies have shown that parents expect lower ability and performance, and value sport less as an achievement domain, for girls than they do for boys (Eccles & Harold 1991; Jacobs & Eccles 1992; Fredricks & Eccles 2002, 2005). Discrepancies in parents' beliefs about competence and importance of sport for daughters and sons are associated with differential encouragement and support by parents (Fredricks & Eccles 2005). If parents think that boys are better in sports and it is more important for them to be successful than girls, they tend to encourage and support boys' interest and involvement in sports to a greater degree. By contrast, other studies indicate no gender differences in parents' competency beliefs and value about sport for their sons and daughters (Kimiecik & Horn 1998; Bois *et al.* 2002). Gender-stereotyped findings imply that parents' differential beliefs and behaviors advantage boys in forming positive self-perceptions and rates of sport participation.

Role modeling is the third parent mechanism for influencing youths' self-perceptions and participation behaviors. By definition, *modeling* refers to changes in attitudes, emotions, and behaviors as a result of observing others; *models* are those individuals whose verbal and non-verbal behaviors serve as cues for observers' subsequent thoughts, feelings, and behaviors (McCullagh & Weiss 2001). Thus, parents as role models may influence their children through behaviors such as participating in sport or physical activity and by demonstrating a positive attitude toward and enjoyment of their activity participation. Parent role modeling has been an important factor related to children's perceptions of physical ability, motivation, and participation behavior (Brustad 1993, 1996; Babkes & Weiss 1999; Bois *et al.* 2005; Weiss & Fretwell 2005). For example, Babkes and Weiss (1999) found that youth soccer players' higher perceived competence, enjoyment, and intrinsic motivation were associated with rating their mothers and fathers as positive exercise role models. However, other research has not shown a link between parent role modeling and children's self-perceptions (Dempsey *et al.* 1993; Kimiecik & Horn 1998). Therefore, all three parent mechanisms—providers of experience, interpreters of experience, and role modeling—should be considered collectively in influencing youths' self-perceptions and participation motivation.

Parents have a crucial role in the lives of children and adolescents (Fredricks & Eccles 2004). Children spend more time with parents at younger ages, thus having more opportunities to be influenced by them. During the childhood years, parents may have the most impact on the development of children's self-perceptions because of their extensive

involvement as providers of experience, interpreters of experience, and as role models. Type of social support changes during the adolescent years but parental influence remains an important contributor to teenagers' self-perceptions, emotional experiences, and motivation (Harter 1999; Weiss & Weiss 2007).

Influence of coaches

Coaches have a central and formative role in youth sport. Not only are coaches important for skill development in young athletes, but they influence how children and adolescents think and feel about their ability to execute skills and strategies during a practice or game. Coaching behaviors are directly linked to the self-perceptions of their athletes and understanding these links will help to foster an environment that enhances self-esteem, perceived competence, and self-efficacy in young athletes.

Smith and Smoll and their colleagues conducted a systematic line of research examining how coaches influence psychosocial development of young athletes (e.g., Smith *et al.* 1979, 1983; Smith & Smoll 1990; Barnett *et al.* 1992; Smoll *et al.* 1993). In one study, Smith *et al.* (1979) found that coaches who were trained to use a positive approach more frequently (i.e., positive reinforcement for desirable behaviors, encouragement and technical instruction following skill errors) had athletes who reported higher perceptions of baseball ability and post-season levels of self-esteem than did athletes who played for untrained coaches. Of particular interest, athletes with lower self-esteem at preseason assessment showed the largest improvement in self-esteem at post-season. These results—that coaches using the positive approach were associated with athletes reporting more favorable self-perceptions—were replicated in several studies (Smith *et al.* 1983; Smith & Smoll 1990; Smoll *et al.* 1993).

Other studies have linked coaching behaviors to perceived competence and self-esteem in youth. Horn (1985) examined how coach feedback and reinforcement influenced the perceived competence of adolescent female softball players. Opposite to results in the Smith and Smoll studies, coaches who provided more frequent positive reinforcement in response to desirable performances were associated with athletes who reported *lower* perceived competence. Moreover, coaches who provided more frequent criticism in response to undesirable performances had athletes who reported *higher* perceived competence. Horn explained these counterintuitive findings relative to the contingency and appropriateness of coaching behaviors.

Contingent reinforcement that is specific to the quality of demonstrated performance conveys precisely to the athlete what was executed correctly and thus contains essential information about the correct technique or strategy. Horn (1985) found that coaches gave positive reinforcement in a general, non-contingent manner (e.g., "way to go," "good"). Athletes receiving more of this type of response may have concluded they were lower in ability, given that the coach was not specific with the praise nor provided technical instruction on how to improve on subsequent attempts. By contrast, criticism that followed unsuccessful performances was constructive by indicating what was incorrect followed by instruction on how to improve (e.g., "Come on Angela, you can kick the ball better than that. Lock your ankle and follow through toward your target"). Thus, athletes receiving more frequent criticism were likely to report higher perceived competence because the coach demonstrated faith in their ability to improve by pairing criticism with corrective instruction. In other words, athletes likely perceived this type of feedback as containing information relevant to improving the next time.

Horn's (1985) interpretation of findings was bolstered by results in a previous study (Horn 1984) in which coaches provided lower ability athletes with more frequent reinforcement and less frequent criticism than higher ability athletes. If lower ability athletes are more prone to receiving non-contingent or inappropriate reinforcement, while higher ability athletes are more frequent recipients of constructive criticism coupled with instruction on how to improve on subsequent efforts, the seemingly counterintuitive findings in Horn (1985) make good sense when combining the results of both studies. Therefore, Horn illustrated that coaches can enhance their athletes' perceptions of competence through the use of feedback and reinforcement that provides appropriate information and is contingent to athletes' skill attempts and performances.

Black and Weiss (1992) extended Horn (1985) by examining the relationship between contingent (specific to performance) coaching behaviors, perceptions of competence, and motivation in 10- to 18-year-old male and female swimmers. Results supported the impact of contingent reinforcement in that athletes who reported their coach as providing more frequent praise and information following desirable performances, and more frequent encouragement plus information following undesirable performances, reported higher levels of perceived competence. Consistent with Horn's (1985) contingency explanation of findings, criticism was negatively related to athletes' perceived competence but only for 15- to 18-year-old swimmers. In other words, when coaches responded with a negative statement, athletes interpreted this response as indicative of lower ability. Similarly, Allen and Howe (1998) found that contingent praise following good performances was associated with higher perceived competence in female adolescent field hockey players. Collectively, these findings support the notion that athletes' perceptions are affected by the *quality* of feedback and reinforcement used by coaches.

Amorose and Weiss (1998) focused on children's perceptions of coaches' evaluative and informational feedback as sources of information about athletic ability. After viewing a performance of hitting a baseball or softball, Amorose and Weiss (1998) asked participants to rate the ability of children who received praise ("great hit"), information ("you kept your eye on the ball"), or a neutral response ("that's right") after successful attempts. Following unsuccessful performance, participants rated the ability of children who received criticism ("that was awful"), information ("you need to keep your eye on the ball"), or a neutral response ("you missed"). Athletes who received praise for success were seen as having higher ability, while those who received information were seen as having lower ability than other groups. For unsuccessful performance, athletes who received criticism were rated as having lower ability, while athletes who received informational feedback were rated as having higher ability than other groups. Findings for positive reinforcement following success and criticism following failure are consistent with previous research. So was the finding for informational feedback following unsuccessful performance, which conveys positive coach expectations to athletes.

The finding that informational feedback following success was associated with *lower* perceived competence was unexpected. Amorose and Weiss (1998) suggested that the *descriptive* nature of feedback following success ("you kept your eye on the ball"), although conveying what was done correctly, may not be viewed as a coach's positive expectancy. By contrast *prescriptive* feedback that followed unsuccessful attempts ("you need to keep your eye on the ball") may be seen as a positive cue of ability in how they can be successful next time. In a follow-up study, Amorose and Smith (2003) divided informational feedback into descriptive and prescriptive. Similar to previous results, athletes who received informational feedback, whether prescriptive or descriptive, following successful performance were rated lower in ability than athletes who received praise or neutral feedback. For unsuccessful attempts, athletes who received descriptive and prescriptive feedback were rated higher in ability than athletes who received criticism or neutral feedback. Collectively, results from these two studies and previous ones highlight that type of feedback coaches provide is important for influencing athletes' perceptions of ability. Contingent praise following success and informational feedback following unsuccessful performance are optimal cues of high ability for young athletes.

Some studies have looked at additional coaching behaviors to feedback and reinforcement in relation to youth athletes' self-perceptions. Price and Weiss (2000) studied how coaches' leadership style, training and instruction, social support, and positive feedback influenced psychological responses of high school soccer players. Coaches who were rated as engaging in more democratic and less autocratic decision making and giving more frequent training and instruction, social support, and positive feedback were associated with athletes who reported higher levels of perceived competence and enjoyment. In other words, athletes felt more proficient

at and liked soccer if their coaches allowed them input on decisions about training sessions, gave them control of their own goals, provided them with frequent skill instruction, showed they cared about athletes as people, and gave praise contingent upon good performances. Similarly, a few studies identified coaching behaviors that relate to athletes' self-efficacy about their sport performances (Gould *et al.* 1989; Weinberg & Jackson 1990; Vargas-Tonsing *et al.* 2004). Coaches and athletes alike felt that coaches who act confidently themselves (i.e., role modeling), encourage their athletes to use positive self-talk, and engage athletes in frequent instruction and hard physical conditioning are effective in contributing to athletes' feelings of self-efficacy.

Consistent with Harter's (1987, 1999) model adopted in this chapter, Amorose (2002, 2003) studied relationships between reflected appraisals of significant others (coaches, parents, teammates) and self-appraisals (perceptions of competence) in middle school through college-age athletes. The key question here is, "Do perceptions of others' ability beliefs about the athlete correspond to the athlete's self-beliefs about sport ability?" Athletes representing several sports rated the extent to which they believed coaches, parents, and teammates thought they were good at their sport as well as how good they thought they were at sports. Results showed that reflected appraisals of coaches were strongly related to athletes' perceptions of competence. Given that coaches make decisions about playing time, provide feedback, and give skill instruction, Amorose stated it is plausible to assume that coaches provide athletes with important information about their abilities. Therefore, the reflected appraisal process between coaches and athletes provides further support for the influence of coaches on athletes' self-perceptions.

Coaching behaviors, such as feedback and reinforcement, social support, and skill instruction, are key ingredients in shaping self-perceptions in youth and adolescent athletes. Given that coaches are a major source of competence information and athletes are constantly interacting with their coaches, it is logical that coaches should be mindful of how to maximize the self-esteem and perceived ability of their athletes. Through quality interactions it is likely that coaches will develop athletes who have positive views of their abilities and themselves.

Influence of peers

Recall that peer comparison and evaluation are important sources of physical competence information for children and especially adolescents. Thus, peer relationships and interactions can have a strong impact on shaping young people's self-evaluations of athletic competence and global self-esteem. We refer to two types of peer relationships—peer group acceptance and close friendship. Peer acceptance entails the degree to which a child is liked or accepted by members of one's peer group, and can range from being rejected (disliked by most peers) to popular (liked by most peers). By contrast, friendship refers to a close, mutual relationship such as a best friend. Hartup (1996) highlights three aspects of friendships that contribute to developmental outcomes:

1 Whether or not one has a close friend (reciprocated affectionate relationship);

2 Who one's friends are (socially adjusted or delinquent); and

3 The quality of one's friendships, such as degree of companionship, esteem, and intimacy support.

Several studies have shown that peer group acceptance and close friendship are important contributors to youth participants' self-perceptions, affective responses, and motivation in sport (Weiss & Stuntz 2004).

Perceptions of greater peer acceptance are associated with favorable perceptions of physical competence (Weiss & Duncan 1992; Smith 1999; Ullrich-French & Smith 2006). Weiss and Duncan (1992) uncovered strong relationships between 8- to 13-year-old participants' perceived and actual sport competence with perceived and actual peer acceptance—those who felt they were good at sports and were athletically skilled felt they were better liked by their peer group and were in fact more popular as rated by their teachers. Smith (1999) found significant relationships between perceptions of peer acceptance and physical self-worth among early adolescents, suggesting that beliefs about fitting in and being liked by one's peers correspond with beliefs about physical competence, fitness, conditioning, and appearance. Ullrich-French and Smith (2006) found that peer acceptance predicted perceived sport competence in 10- to 12-year-old soccer players when father–child relationship quality and friendship quality were high. These findings linking peer acceptance with self-perceptions are especially important in light of our conceptual framework that shows self-perceptions predict emotional and motivational outcomes. In fact, a study by Kunesh et al. (1992) revealed that low ratings of peer acceptance coupled with social exclusion by boys resulted in feelings of anxiety and activity avoidance among 11- to 12-year-old girls. Although self-perceptions were not assessed, it is easy to imagine lowered self-ability beliefs in response to peer rejection leading to negative emotions and unmotivated behavior.

Friendships in sport have also been linked with perceived athletic competence and self-esteem. Duncan (1993) found that greater perceptions of companionship and esteem support from friends in physical education were associated with higher expectancies of success, positive affect, and intrinsic interest to participate in physical activity outside of school. In a series of studies, Weiss et al. showed that self-esteem enhancement and support consistently emerged as a salient dimension of sport friendship quality (Weiss & Smith 1999, 2002; Weiss et al. 1996). Smith (1999) found that having a close friend in sport, in addition to peer acceptance, predicted physical self-worth in adolescent girls and boys. Ullrich-French and Smith (2006) found that higher friendship quality predicted perceived soccer competence when coupled with higher peer acceptance or mother–child relationship quality.

In our organizing model, perceived social regard refers to reflected appraisals of parents, coaches, and peers, which relate to self-appraisals such as perceived competence or self-worth. Harter et al. (1998) found that adolescent girls and boys (14–18 years) displayed "relational self-worth;" that is, reported self-worth varied as a function of the social context (i.e., self-worth around parents, around teachers, and around peers). In turn, social support from parents, teachers, and peers was a better predictor of relational than of global self-worth. The take-home message is that low relational self-worth (e.g., around my teammates) could be addressed by increasing social support from that significant other or by focusing the adolescent's attention on those individuals providing strong validation support (e.g., coach, close friend). Amorose (2002) examined reflected appraisals in sport through the relative influence of mother's, father's, coach's, and teammates' competence beliefs on adolescents' self-appraisals of ability. Reflected appraisals by teammates were most strongly related to athletes' self-appraisals reinforcing the significant role of peer evaluations on adolescents' self-perceptions.

Feeling connected with one's peer group as well as having a close, intimate friend who "is there" in times of need and can boost self-esteem are essential features of well-adjusted children and teenagers. In the sport literature, a great deal of attention has naturally been devoted to the importance of significant adults such as parents and coaches in helping to shape positive experiences for young athletes. We cannot forget, however, that peers are valued equals who youth turn to for a variety of informational and motivational reasons. As such, we must be mindful of peer influence in any intervention for enhancing self-perceptions or for explaining variations in youths' self-evaluations of sport ability.

Enhancing self-perceptions through youth sport experiences

Based on Harter's (1987, 1999) model and the empirical research explaining parent, coach, and peer influence on perceived competence and self-esteem, several practical strategies for enhancing self-perceptions are apparent. Before we translate this knowledge to practical applications for maintaining and enhancing self-perceptions in sport, we first share relevant findings from the few intervention studies that have been conducted to modify domain-specific and general self-evaluations among sport and physical activity participants.

Intervention studies

Field experiments are challenging but necessary to determine if interventions designed to modify self-perceptions are effective. Studies by Smith, Smoll, and colleagues (e.g., Smith *et al.* 1979; Smoll *et al.*

1993) were discussed earlier. In short, training coaches to increase their rate of positive reinforcement following successful attempts and encouragement plus informational feedback following unsuccessful performances, as well as lowering frequency of punitive reinforcement and non-responses following mistakes, resulted in young athletes reporting greater baseball competence and general self-esteem than did control participants (whose coaches did not have the training). These findings were especially effective for athletes who began the season with a low level of self-esteem.

Recently, Coatsworth and Conroy (2006) replicated and extended these studies with young swimmers (7–18 years) over a 7-week intervention. Group differences (trained coaches vs. controls) on self-esteem were assessed at the beginning, middle, and end of the season, and analyses accounted for effects of age, gender, and initial self-esteem. Swimmers 11 years and under who swam for trained coaches reported higher self-esteem over the course of the season in comparison to those who swam for control coaches. In addition, girls with initial low levels of self-esteem who swam for trained coaches reported greater self-esteem over the season than did those who swam for control coaches. It is conceivable that younger swimmers and low self-esteem girls were affected more by coach reinforcement because they look to credible adults such as coaches to glean cues about their abilities. By contrast, older swimmers and those with moderate to high levels of self-esteem use and integrate a broader range of competence information sources.

Marsh and Peart (1988) examined competitive and cooperative climates in promoting physical fitness and perceptions of physical competence and appearance in adolescent girls. The competitive program focused on individualized goals and emphasized performance outcome and favorable comparisons to classmates. The cooperative climate focused upon achieving collective goals and emphasized improvement and mastery of physical fitness and aerobic skills. Both programs resulted in physical fitness gains. However, the cooperative program promoted, and the competitive program hindered, perceptions of physical ability and physical appearance. The program that fostered cooperative learning and goal achievement provided an environment in which adolescent girls thrived in terms of perceived and actual competence, because of shared goals and focus on self-referenced standards of success (i.e., improvement, goal attainment). The competitive program was successful in enhancing physical fitness but ineffective in fostering feelings of improved ability and appearance, attributable to norm-referenced standards imposed for evaluating success (i.e., rankings of classmates, performance outcome).

Ebbeck and Gibbons (1998) also implemented a cooperative-oriented program, focused upon team building through physical challenges, to modify self-perceptions of 10- to 12-year-old physical education students. The intervention lasted 8 months, with one team-building activity conducted twice per month. The challenges were characterized by interdependent goals, mastery of challenges, non-traditional physical activities, and post-activity discussion of their experiences. At the end of 8 months, students in the intervention condition reported higher perceived athletic competence, physical appearance, social acceptance, and global self-worth than did controls. Not only were these differences statistically significant but also the effect sizes were strong, meaning that the intervention effects were meaningful and of practical value.

Collectively, the intervention studies described here occurred within interpersonal contexts that were essential to the success of the interventions (i.e., interactions among coaches/teachers, classmates, and close friends). One might infer that positive changes in self-evaluations were not only because of the skill development focus and physical challenges of the programs, but also because of social interactions and relationships such as interdependent group goals, cooperative rather than competitive activities, coach/instructor and peer support, and coaches'/instructors' evaluative and informational feedback. The findings from these studies, in combination with our conceptual model and previously reported research, shed light on many useful strategies that raise level and accuracy of athletes' perceived competence and self-esteem. Following discussion of general strategies based on our conceptual model and reported research, we provide specific suggestions for parents and coaches.

Provide optimal challenges

An *optimal challenge* is one that matches the difficulty level of skills or activities to the child's capabilities. Thus, children's successful mastery of skills is within reach, but they must exert necessary effort and persistence to attain the goal. We like to think of optimal challenges as "matching the activity to the child, and not the child to the activity." Skills that are too easy in relation to a child's talents are boring and do not allow for realistic goals. Skills that are too difficult invoke anxiety and frustration when persistent efforts are unsuccessful. Because children use mastery of skills, effort expenditure, and self-improvement as salient criteria for determining how physically competent they are, optimal challenges offer children a prime opportunity for developing and demonstrating competence that is at the cutting edge of their capabilities. Teachers, coaches, and parents should ensure developmental progressions in skills and physical activities, collaborate with children in setting realistic goals for physical activity, and modify games or activities to allow for optimal challenges.

Create a mastery motivational climate

Coaches and teachers influence children's beliefs, affective responses, and behaviors by shaping the learning environment or *motivational climate* in which activities take place (Ames 1992). Motivational climate focuses upon how success is defined, how children are evaluated, what is recognized and valued, and how mistakes are viewed. A *mastery* motivational climate is one that promotes learning, effort, and self-improvement, and mistakes are viewed as part of the learning process. Success is self-referenced, and personal improvements are recognized, praised, and emphasized. In contrast, a *performance* climate emphasizes norm-referenced modes of success, and evaluation practices and criteria for recognition that focus upon favorable comparison to peers. The motivational climate that is perceived by participants impacts their perceptions of ability, attraction toward physical activity, and motivation.

The acronym TARGET is used to identify effective strategies for structuring a mastery motivational climate in physical activity contexts (Ames

1992). TARGET stands for dimensions of Task, Authority, Recognition, Grouping, Evaluation, and Time. Task variety and optimal challenges, opportunities for choice and shared decision making, recognition of effort and self-improvement, partner and small-group problem solving tasks, evaluation criteria focused on self-referenced standards, and adequate time for learning and demonstrating skills define the ingredients for maximizing a mastery climate. Rather than focusing on performance outcomes, emphasizing peers' achievements, and recognizing only the most talented youngsters (i.e., a performance climate), significant adults can instead cultivate children's view of sport through rose-colored lenses (i.e., mastery motivational climate). Because a mastery climate emphasizes cooperative learning rather than competition, diverse ability grouping, and recognition based on individual improvement and not peer comparison, this environment is also most conducive for fostering positive peer relationships and enhancing peer acceptance.

Help children help themselves

Mastering skills, achieving personal goals, and progressively improving are salient sources of information children and adolescents use to judge their physical competence. Competence beliefs, in turn, influence levels of self-esteem, enjoyment, motivation, and physical activity levels. Thus, teaching children self-regulated learning strategies such as goal setting and self-monitoring will allow them to adopt self-reliant standards for enhancing their own perceptions of competence (Petlichkoff 2004). Goals that are specific, optimally challenging, and self-referenced will point youth in the right direction for sustaining physical activity motivation. Self-monitoring methods may include the use of goal sheets, logs, or diaries that can be used to compare current to past performance, intensity of effort, and rate of improvement.

Recommendations for parents

ENCOURAGE PARTICIPATION

Parents should continually encourage both boys and girls to participate and achieve in sport because

encouragement enhances children's self-perceptions and motivational processes. Parents should express unbiased beliefs and behaviors toward daughters and sons, because providing more encouragement to boys or girls to participate in sport or a specific sport type may lead to dissimilar self-perceptions, value toward success, and sport participation patterns. Encouragement and support will help children develop and maintain positive self-perceptions in sport, leading to sustained sport participation.

ADOPT HIGH, BUT REALISTIC, EXPECTATIONS

Parents who have high expectations for their children in sport are associated with children who also have high expectations for themselves. Children who believe their parents think they are good develop favorable perceptions of competence and are more likely to remain involved in the sport. However, if parent expectations are unrealistically high, this can lead to undue pressure on the child and negative self-perceptions in sport. Parents who expect realistic outcomes from their children will have children who feel good about themselves and want to remain in sport.

GIVE APPROPRIATE FEEDBACK

Children and teenagers look to parents for feedback and use this information to form judgments about their sport abilities. Parents do not need to praise everything their child does; rather parents need to provide appropriate and contingent feedback to children for performance attempts. This feedback can be in the form of verbal information or encouragement, or through non-verbal behavior (e.g., clapping, smile, thumbs up). By providing feedback that matches the quality of performance (i.e., praise when attempt was successful regardless of outcome, and encouragement when attempt was unsuccessful), parents signify credible sources whereby children can accurately develop perceptions of competence.

BE ACTIVE

Because parents who are active and express joy about their involvement in sport or exercise are associated with children who have higher perceptions of competence and activity levels, parents should express a positive attitude toward physical activity and be physically active themselves. Parents who participate with children (e.g., practicing sports, staying after practice to play) let children know that the activity is important and can influence self-perceptions through their involvement.

Recommendations for coaches

PROVIDE CONTINGENT AND APPROPRIATE FEEDBACK

It is the quality, rather than quantity, of coach feedback that is important for explaining variations in self-perceptions (i.e., contingent and appropriate responses following desirable and undesirable performances). Coaches need to provide feedback that is specific to and directly related to level of performance. Likewise, coaches should avoid providing excessive praise or praise for mediocre performance or simple tasks. Coaches are encouraged to adopt a feedback pattern that focuses on successful performances by "catching kids doing things correctly" and providing praise and specific information as to why performance was desirable. When skill errors occur, coaches should use encouragement and instruction to help athletes know that errors are a part of the learning process and to be successful at future attempts. Feedback and reinforcement should also be based on individualized goals or standards rather than normative standards such as other athletes' performances. Providing athletes with feedback that highlights skill acquisition and improvement allows them to make realistic self-judgments about changes in their level of ability.

MODIFY SPORT SKILLS, GOALS, AND STRATEGIES

Coaches can make modifications to facilities, equipment, and rules to enhance skill development and improvement. For example, using a smaller football will help children be more successful at both passing and catching; such mastery experiences will enhance self-perceptions. Other modifications may include changing the size of the playing area or the rules to allow children to be more successful during early stages of learning. Additionally, the use of skill progressions or "goal ladders" is important for skill development success at each level or "rung" can be seen as short-term goals for children to achieve. For example, a child who moves through a lay-up shooting progression in basketball can see that he or she is able to complete more complex skills moving from shooting a lay-up standing still to shooting a lay-up off the dribble to shooting a lay-up using the non-dominant hand. Achieving each of these short-term goals provides the child with information about ability and can serve as a means to enhance self-perceptions.

CREATE A POSITIVE AND FUN ENVIRONMENT

Coaches can create a positive environment that fosters self-esteem by keeping practices and games fun. Youth find practices fun if they are constantly engaged and active. Optimally challenging activities that are difficult but attainable produce the most fun for learning and improving because such activities are customized to the individual's current skill level. As children make skill gains based on an individualized standard of success, their self-perceptions will increase. Coaches who develop an environment that encourages mastery experiences are also likely to see positive effects in their athletes' self-perceptions. For example, a child learning basic tennis skills and tactics in an environment that focuses on self-improvement rather than teammate comparison will be more likely to learn, improve, and master the sport. When children learn to make evaluations based on their own performance and self-set goals, positive self-perceptions are likely to occur.

Conclusions

The developmental significance of perceived competence and self-esteem means that understanding causes and consequences of self-perceptions is a critical goal for researchers, parents, and practitioners. Theory and research consistently show that youth with higher self-perceptions think, feel, and act in healthier ways compared to youth with lower self-perceptions. Recall our protagonists at the beginning of this chapter—Gina and Emily. Gina, with high perceptions of sport competence, experiences many positive emotions from her soccer involvement, is intrinsically motivated to continue, and exhibits positive performance behaviors such as effort, persistence, and self-regulated strategies. Emily, on the other hand, experiences anxiety and lower motivation because of her lower self-perceptions. How and why do these variations in perceived competence and self-esteem occur? Theory and research also provided insight on antecedents of self-perceptions in the form of reflected appraisals or social support from parents, coaches, and peers. Gina likely experiences approval, support, and high competence beliefs from parents, contingent and appropriate feedback from her coach, and acceptance by teammates and feelings of validation from a close friend. Emily may experience one or more negatives from her significant others. Collectively, the literature provides a wealth of information on how self-judgments are formed, consequences of higher and lower self-perceptions, and effective strategies for modifying perceived competence and self-esteem.

References

Allen, J.B. & Howe, B. (1998) Player ability, coach feedback, and female adolescent athletes' perceived competence and satisfaction. *Journal of Sport & Exercise Psychology* **20**, 280–299.

Ames, C.A. (1992) Achievement goals, motivational climate, and motivational processes. In: *Motivation in Sport and Exercise* (Roberts, G.C., ed.) Human Kinetics, Champaign, IL: 161–176.

Amorose, A.J. (2001) Intraindividual variability of self-evaluations in the physical domain: Prevalence, consequences, and antecedents. *Journal of Sport & Exercise Psychology* **23**, 222–244.

Amorose, A.J. (2002) The influence of reflected appraisals on middle school and high school athletes' self-perceptions of sport competence. *Pediatric Exercise Science* **14**, 377–390.

Amorose, A.J. (2003) Reflected appraisals and perceived importance of significant others' appraisals as predictors of college athletes' self-perceptions of competence. *Research Quarterly for Exercise & Sport* **74**, 60–70.

Amorose, A.J. & Smith, P.J.K. (2003) Feedback as a source of physical competence information: Effects of age, experience and type of feedback. *Journal of Sport & Exercise Psychology* **25**, 341–359.

Amorose, A.J. & Weiss, M.R. (1998) Coaching feedback as a source of information about perceptions of ability: A developmental examination. *Journal of Sport & Exercise Psychology* **20**, 395–420.

Babkes, M.L. & Weiss, M.R. (1999) Parental influence on children's cognitive and affective responses to competitive soccer participation. *Pediatric Exercise Science* **11**, 44–62.

Barnett, N.P., Smoll, F.L. & Smith, R.E. (1992) Effects of enhancing coach-athlete relationships on youth sport attrition. *Sport Psychologist* **6**, 111–127.

Black, S.J. & Weiss, M.R. (1992) The relationship among perceived coaching behaviors, perceptions of ability, and motivation in competitive age-group swimmers. *Journal of Sport & Exercise Psychology* **14**, 309–325.

Bois, J.E., Sarrazin, P.G., Brustad, R.J., Trouilloud, D.O. & Cury, F. (2002) Mothers' expectancies and young adolescents' perceived physical competence: A yearlong study. *Journal of Early Adolescence* **22**, 384–406.

Bois, J.E., Sarrazin, P.G., Brustad, R.J., Trouillard, D.O. & Cury, F. (2005) Elementary schoolchildren's perceived competence and physical activity involvement: The influence of parents' role modeling behaviours and perceptions of their child's competence. *Psychology of Sport and Exercise* **6**, 381–397.

Brustad, R.J. (1988) Affective outcomes in competitive youth sport: The influence of intrapersonal and socialization factors. *Journal of Sport & Exercise Psychology* **10**, 307–321.

Brustad, R.J. (1993) Who will go out and play? Parental and psychological influences on children's attraction to physical activity. *Pediatric Exercise Science* **5**, 210–223.

Brustad, R.J. (1996) Attraction to physical activity in urban schoolchildren: Parental socialization and gender influences. *Research Quarterly for Exercise and Sport* **67**, 316–323.

Coatsworth, J.D. & Conroy, D.E. (2006) Enhancing the self-esteem of youth swimmers through coach training: Gender and age effects. *Psychology of Sport and Exercise* **7**, 173–192.

Dempsey, J.M., Kimiecik, J.C. & Horn, T.S. (1993) Parental influence on children's moderate to vigorous physical activity participation: An expectancy-value approach. *Pediatric Exercise Science* **5**, 151–167.

Duncan, S.C. (1993) The role of cognitive appraisal and friendship provisions in adolescents' affect and motivation toward activity in physical education. *Research Quarterly for Exercise and Sport* **64**, 314–323.

Ebbeck, V. & Gibbons, S.L. (1998) The effect of a team-building program on the self-conceptions of Grade 6 and 7 physical education students. *Journal of Sport & Exercise Psychology* **20**, 300–310.

Ebbeck, V. & Stuart, M.E. (1993) Who determines what's important? Perceptions of competence and importance as predictors of self-esteem in youth football players. *Pediatric Exercise Science* **5**, 253–262.

Ebbeck, V. & Stuart, M.E. (1996) Predictors of self-esteem with youth basketball players. *Pediatric Exercise Science* **8**, 368–378.

Ebbeck, V. & Weiss, M.R. (1998) Determinants of children's self-esteem: An examination of perceived competence and affect in sport. *Pediatric Exercise Science* **10**, 285–298.

Eccles, J.S. & Harold, R.D. (1991) Gender differences in sport involvement: Applying the Eccles' expectancy-value model. *Journal of Applied Sport Psychology* **3**, 7–35.

Ferrer-Caja, E. & Weiss, M.R. (2000) Predictors of intrinsic motivation among adolescent students in physical education. *Research Quarterly for Exercise and Sport* **71**, 267–279.

Ferrer-Caja, E. & Weiss, M.R. (2002) Cross-validation of a model of intrinsic motivation in physical education with students enrolled in elective courses. *Journal of Experimental Education* **71**, 41–65.

Fredricks, J.A. & Eccles, J.S. (2002) Children's competence and value beliefs from childhood through adolescence: Growth trajectories in two male-sex-typed domains. *Developmental Psychology* **38**, 519–533.

Fredricks, J.A. & Eccles, J.S. (2004) Parental influences on youth involvement in sports. In: *Developmental Sport and Exercise Psychology: A Lifespan Perspective* (Weiss, M.R., ed.) Fitness Information Technology, Morgantown, WV: 145–164.

Fredricks, J.A. & Eccles, J.S. (2005) Family socialization, gender, and sport motivation and involvement. *Journal of Sport & Exercise Psychology* **27**, 3–31.

Gould, D., Hodge, K., Peterson, K. & Giannini, J. (1989) An exploratory examination of strategies used by elite coaches to enhance self-efficacy in athletes. *Journal of Sport & Exercise Psychology* **11**, 128–140.

Green, B.C. & Chalip, L. (1997) Enduring involvement in youth soccer: The socialization of parent and child. *Journal of Leisure Research* **29**, 61–77.

Halliburton, A.L. & Weiss, M.R. (2002) Sources of competence information and perceived motivational climate among adolescent female gymnasts varying in skill level. *Journal of Sport & Exercise Psychology* **24**, 396–419.

Harter, S. (1987) The determinants and mediational role of global self-worth in children. In: *Contemporary Topics in Developmental Psychology* (Eisenberg, N., ed.) Wiley, New York: 219–242.

Harter, S. (1999) *The Construction of the Self: A Developmental Perspective*. Guilford, New York.

Harter, S., Waters, P. & Whitesell, N.R. (1998) Relational self-worth: Differences in perceived worth as a person across interpersonal contexts among adolescents. *Child Development* **69**, 756–766.

Hartup, W.W. (1996) The company they keep: Friendships and their developmental significance. *Child Development* **67**, 1–13.

Horn, T.S. (1984) Expectancy effects in the interscholastic athletic setting: Methodological considerations. *Journal of Sport Psychology* **6**, 60–76.

Horn, T.S. (1985) Coaches' feedback and changes in children's perceptions of their physical competence. *Journal of Educational Psychology* **77**, 174–186.

Horn, T.S. (2004) Developmental perspectives on self-perceptions in children and adolescents. In: *Developmental Sport and Exercise Psychology: A Lifespan Perspective* (Weiss, M.R., ed.) Fitness Information Technology, Morgantown, WV: 101–143.

Horn, T.S., Glenn, S.D. & Wentzell, A.B. (1993) Sources of information underlying personal ability judgments in high school athletes. *Pediatric Exercise Science* **5**, 263–274.

Horn, T.S. & Harris, A. (1996) Perceived competence in young athletes: Research findings and recommendations for coaches and parents. In: *Children and Youth in Sport* (Smoll, F.L. & Smith R.E., eds.) Brown & Benchmark, Madison, WI: 309–329.

Horn, T.S. & Hasbrook, C.A. (1987) Psychological characteristics and the criteria children use for self-evaluation. *Journal of Sport Psychology* **9**, 208–221.

Horn, T.S. & Weiss, M.R. (1991) A developmental analysis of children's self-ability judgments. *Pediatric Exercise Science* **3**, 312–328.

Jacobs, J.E. & Eccles, J.S. (1992) The impact of mothers' gender-role stereotypic beliefs on mothers' and childrens' ability perceptions. *Journal of Personality and Social Psychology* **63**, 932–944.

Kimiecik, J.C. & Horn, T.S. (1998) Parental beliefs and children's moderate-to-vigorous physical activity. *Research Quarterly for Exercise and Sport* **69**, 163–175.

Kimiecik, J.C., Horn, T.S. & Shurin, C.S. (1996) Relationships among children's beliefs, perceptions of their parents' beliefs, and their moderate-to-vigorous physical activity. *Research Quarterly for Exercise and Sport* **67**, 324–336.

Kunesh, M.A., Hasbrook, C.A. & Lewthwaite, R. (1992) Physical activity socialization: Peer interactions and affective responses among a sample of sixth grade girls. *Sociology of Sport Journal* **9**, 385–396.

Leff, S.S. & Hoyle, R.H. (1995) Young athletes' perceptions of parental support and pressure. *Journal of Youth and Adolescence* **24**, 187–203.

Marsh, H.W. & Peart, N.D. (1988) Competitive and cooperative physical fitness training programs for girls: Effects on physical fitness and

multidimensional self-concepts. *Journal of Sport & Exercise Psychology* **10**, 390–407.

McCullagh, P. & Weiss, M.R. (2001) Modeling: Considerations for motor skill performance and psychological responses. In: *Handbook of Sport Psychology*, 2nd edn. Singer, R.N., Hausenblas, H.A. & Janelle, C.M., eds.) Wiley, New York: 205–238.

McKiddie, B. & Maynard, I.W. (1997) Perceived competence of schoolchildren in physical education. *Journal of Teaching in Physical Education* **16**, 324–339.

Petlichkoff, L.M. (2004) Self-regulation skills for children and adolescents. In: *Developmental Sport and Exercise Psychology: A Lifespan Perspective* (Weiss, M.R., ed.) Fitness Information Technology, Morgantown, WV: 269–288.

Price, M.S. & Weiss, M.R. (2000) Relationships among coach burnout, coach behaviors, and athletes' psychological responses. *Sport Psychologist* **14**, 391–409.

Scanlan, T.K. & Simons, J.P. (1992) The construct of sport enjoyment. In: *Motivation in Sport and Exercise* (Roberts, G.C., ed.) Human Kinetics, Champaign, IL: 199–215.

Smith, A.L. (1999) Perceptions of peer relationships and physical activity participation in early adolescence. *Journal of Sport & Exercise Psychology* **21**, 329–350.

Smith, R.E. & Smoll, F.L. (1990) Self-esteem and children's reactions to youth sport coaching behaviors: A field study of self-enhancement processes. *Developmental Psychology* **26**, 987–993.

Smith, R.E., Smoll, F.L. & Curtis, B. (1979) Coach effectiveness training: A cognitive–behavioral approach to enhancing relationship skills in youth sport coaches. *Journal of Sport Psychology* **1**, 59–75.

Smith, R., Zane, N., Smoll, F. & Coppel, D. (1983) Behavioral assessment in youth sports: Coaching behaviors and children's attitudes. *Medicine and Sciences in Sports and Exercise* **15**, 208–214.

Smoll, F.L., Smith, R.E., Barnett, N.P. & Everett, J.J. (1993) Enhancement of children's self-esteem through social support training for youth sport coaches. *Journal of Applied Psychology* **78**, 602–610.

Ullrich-French, S. & Smith, A.L. (2006) Perceptions of relationships with parents and peers in youth sport: Independent and combined prediction of motivational outcomes. *Psychology of Sport and Exercise* **7**, 193–214.

Vargas-Tonsing, T.M., Myers, N.D. & Feltz, D.L. (2004) Coaches' and athletes' perceptions of efficacy-enhancing techniques. *Sport Psychologist* **18**, 397–414.

Weinberg, R. & Jackson, A. (1990) Building self-efficacy in tennis players: A coach's perspective. *Journal of Applied Sport Psychology* **2**, 164–174.

Weiss, M.R. & Amorose, A.J. (2005) Children's self-perceptions in the physical domain: Between- and within-age variability in level, accuracy, and sources of perceived competence. *Journal of Sport & Exercise Psychology* **27**, 226–244.

Weiss, M.R., Bredemeier, B.J. & Shewchuk, R.M. (1986) The dynamics of perceived competence, perceived control, and motivational orientation in youth sports. In: *Sport for Children and Youths* (Weiss, M.R. & Gould, D., eds.) Human Kinetics, Champaign, IL: 89–102.

Weiss, M.R. & Duncan, S.C. (1992) The relationship between physical competence and peer acceptance in the context of children's sports participation. *Journal of Sport & Exercise Psychology* **14**, 177–191.

Weiss, M.R. & Ebbeck, V. (1996) Self-esteem and perceptions of competence in youth sport: Theory, research, and enhancement strategies. In: *The Encyclopedia of Sports Medicine: The Child*

and Adolescent Athlete (Bar-Or, O., ed.) Blackwell Science, Oxford, UK: 364–382.

Weiss, M.R., Ebbeck, V. & Horn, T.S. (1997) Children's self-perceptions and sources of competence information: A cluster analysis. *Journal of Sport & Exercise Psychology* **19**, 52–70.

Weiss, M.R. & Ferrer-Caja, E. (2002) Motivational orientations and sport behavior. In: *Advances in Sport Psychology*, 2nd edn. (Horn, T.S., ed.) Human Kinetics, Champaign, IL: 101–183.

Weiss, M.R. & Fretwell, S.D. (2005) The parent-coach/child-athlete relationship in youth sport: Cordial, contentious, or conundrum? *Research Quarterly for Exercise and Sport* **76**, 286–305.

Weiss, M.R. & Hayashi, C.T. (1995) All in the family: Parent–child influences in competitive youth gymnastics. *Pediatric Exercise Science* **7**, 36–48.

Weiss, M.R. & Horn, T.S. (1990) The relationship between children's accuracy estimates of their physical competence and achievement-related behaviors. *Research Quarterly for Exercise and Sport* **61**, 250–258.

Weiss, M.R. & Smith, A.L. (1999) Quality of youth sport friendships: Measurement development and validation. *Journal of Sport & Exercise Psychology* **21**, 145–166.

Weiss, M.R. & Smith, A.L. (2002) Friendship quality in youth sport: Relationship to age, gender, and

motivation variables. *Journal of Sport & Exercise Psychology* **24**, 420–437.

Weiss, M.R., Smith, A.L. & Theeboom, M. (1996) "That's what friends are for": Children's and teenagers' perceptions of peer relationships in the sport domain. *Journal of Sport & Exercise Psychology* **18**, 347–379.

Weiss, M.R. & Stuntz, C.P. (2004) A little friendly competition: Peer relationships and psychosocial development in youth sport and physical activity contexts. In: *Developmental Sport and Exercise Psychology: A Lifespan Perspective* (Weiss, M.R., ed.) Fitness Information Technology, Morgantown, WV: 165–196.

Weiss, W.M. & Weiss, M.R. (2003) Attraction- and entrapment-based commitment among competitive female gymnasts. *Journal of Sport & Exercise Psychology* **25**, 229–247.

Weiss, W.M. & Weiss, M.R. (2006) A longitudinal analysis of commitment among competitive female gymnasts. *Psychology of Sport and Exercise* **7**, 309–323.

Weiss, W.M. & Weiss, M.R. (2007) Sport commitment among competitive female gymnasts; a developmental perspective. *Research Quarterly for Exercise and Sport* **78**, 90–102.

Williams, L. (1994) Goal orientations and athletes' preferences for competence information sources. *Journal of Sport & Exercise Psychology* **16**, 416–430.

Chapter 24

Emotional Stress and Anxiety in the Child and Adolescent Athlete

ROBERT C. EKLUND AND DANIEL GOULD

Participation in highly organized youth sport around the world is extensive—and growing, with tens of millions of children taking part in a wide variety of sports ranging from cricket to rodeo (De Knop *et al.* 1996). The widespread adult support of these endeavors has often been premised on the belief that youth sport participation results in a broad variety of positive outcomes. Clearly, there are potential motoric benefits in learning physical skills and developing performance capacities required by any given youth sport involvement. Positive outcomes are also typically anticipated in the cognitive and affective domains. It is assumed, for example, that young athletes will experience joy and excitement within this setting. Moreover, there is a strong belief that the social interactions inherent in sport will provide opportunities for lessons about competition, important values, and social skills (Estrada *et al.* 1988; Weiss & Smith 2002).

Despite the fact that youth sport has flourished, it does not have a history of being universally embraced as the ideal involvement. Indeed, the rise of highly organized and competitive youth sport structures during the 1920s and 1930s in the USA was greeted with condemnation by US professional physical educators (Wiggins 1996). Competitive stress, in particular, has been a point of central concern throughout the history of youth sport (Berryman 1996) and provocative descriptors such as "psychological trauma" (Smilkstein 1980) and "child abuse" (Tutko & Burns 1979) have been employed to convey concerns on this account.

Although many early beliefs about the effects of competitive sports participation on young athletes were based upon little more than dogma and rhetoric (Wiggins 1996), systematic research efforts have been undertaken in recent decades. Our understanding remains incomplete but these efforts have begun to pay dividends for understanding psychosocial stress and hence have provided information to guide professional practice in the youth sport setting. This review is designed to examine emotional stress and anxiety in the child and adolescent athlete by summarizing this research literature.

For the purposes of this review, participation in competitive sport is defined as athletic involvement where the child attends organized practices in preparation for scheduled competitions under the supervision of an adult leader. Unfortunately, pediatric sport psychology researchers have not characterized young athletes with the same precision as pediatric exercise physiology researchers with regard to the maturational categories such as prepubescent, pubescent, and post-pubescent. Hence, research in this area can only be discussed relative to young athletes' chronologic age.

Competitive stress

One of the major problems confounding common understandings of competitive stress has been the notion that stress is inherently good or bad. Youth sport critics have suggested that stress is always unsatisfactory and potentially harmful to young athletes. On the other hand, advocates have regarded the opportunity to learn how to deal with competitive stress as a developmentally valuable experience for the young athlete. Taken separately, these value-laden perspectives are both inappropriate because stress researchers have shown that stress can have both positive and negative effects (Selye 1974).

Perhaps the most pernicious problem adding confusion to common understandings of competitive stress is that the term itself is informally used in at least two different ways. The first usage invokes stress as a situational demand, something in the environment, which may challenge the response capabilities of an individual (e.g., the stress of a championship game will test Sally's mettle). The second usage invokes the term to reference an affective consequence (e.g., the pressure was intense in the championship game and the stress Fernando was experiencing was evident). The implied meaning of "stress" in each instance is clearly not synonymous—one is an antecedent (or demand) variable while the other is an affective consequence variable (Smith & Smoll 1982). Complicating matters further, there are also a variety of individual differences influencing perceptions of any given stressful demand and the resulting experience of stress. Specifically, not all young athletes perceive championship games as equally stressful (i.e., demanding), and there are substantial differences in the emotional stress experienced as a consequence. Hence, it is important to make a terminologic distinction between potential stressors in the environment and the resultant emotional experience associated with those demands.

Many researchers in this area have adopted a process definition of stress to manage the previously identified problems. In the process conceptualization, "stress" is deemed a cognition or appraisal instead of an environmental demand or an experiential consequence. These appraisals are dynamic assessments of the relative balance (or imbalance)

between environmental demands and personal resources to manage those demands (Lazarus & Folkman 1984). As such, the competitive situation is only stressful (i.e., produces a stress cognitive appraisal) to the extent that the person believes that there is a mismatch between those situational competitive demands and the available personal resources to manage those demands. A particular environment will only provoke a stress-related response (e.g., anxiety) when the individual's cognitive appraisal is that a meaningful imbalance exists between situational demands and available coping resources. Not only does this process conceptualization clarify the causal chain of events between situational demands and the resulting experience, it also helps us to understand that consequences associated with the process may be positive, negative, or neutral.

The stress process

Smith and Smoll (1982) have posited one model of the stress process that has received considerable attention in youth sport literature. As can be observed in Fig. 24.1, the Smith and Smoll (1982) conceptual model is composed of situational, cognitive, physiologic, and coping and task behavior components. Hypothesized relationships between these components are also illustrated. This model illustrates that personality and motivational variables affect and interact with the model components.

SITUATIONAL COMPONENT

In examining stress as a process, neither the particular objective competitive situation that a young athlete encounters (e.g., participating in a championship

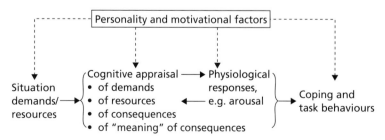

Fig. 24.1 A conceptual model of stress showing hypothesized relationships among situational, cognitive, physiological, and behavioural components. Motivational and personality variables are assumed to affect and interact with each of the components. Redrawn from Smith (1986).

game, playing in front of one's parents) nor the personal or environmental resources available (e.g., the child's sport skill level and social support network) are as important as the interaction between these two sets of factors (Smith & Smoll 1982). Whenever demands are encountered in the competitive environment, resources are mobilized to meet these demands. Stress relates to the relative balance or imbalance between demands and resources. The relative balance between demands and resources determines whether the stress experience is positive, negative, or neutral.

More specifically, stress is unlikely when there is little imbalance between resources and demands (e.g., two evenly matched wrestlers practicing together). If demands slightly exceed resources (e.g., a skilled swimmer facing a slightly better-skilled field of competitors), a young athlete may view a situation as challenging (i.e., a positively valenced stress appraisal associated with effort mobilization). Individuals faced with situations featuring substantial imbalances between demands and coping resources, however, are likely to appraise the situation as stressful. In the case of a substantial imbalance favoring demands (e.g., a backup hockey goal keeper facing league-leading scorers in a championship game), the stress appraisal may be associated with an affective consequence of high levels of nervousness or state anxiety. By contrast, stress also occurs when there is a substantial imbalance favoring resources (e.g., an internationally ranked tennis player confined to local high school competition) and manifested in affective consequences such as boredom.

The balance between situational demands (e.g., opponent, environmental circumstances) and available resources (e.g., personal fitness levels, skill, readiness, availability of suitable equipment) is the central determinant of stress from a process perspective. Nonetheless, Smith and Smoll (1982) emphasize that situational demands can also emanate from within the individual. Personal or motivational factors such as desired goals, performance standards, or even unconscious motives or conflicts contribute to the perception of the competitive situation and influence the salience and interpretation of the array of environmental demands. For

example, perfectionistic young athletes may experience a great deal of stress, without any reference to any particular opponent or competition, purely as a consequence of unrealistic or unobtainable self-expectations. Likewise, memories of past performance, as well as anticipation of future consequences, may interact with the current situation to influence the young athlete's perception of any given setting.

COGNITIVE COMPONENT

The situational component of Smith and Smoll's (1982) model emphasizes that stress is a consequence of an interaction between demands and resources. The second component of this model focuses upon the individual's cognitive appraisal of the situation. The emotional intensity with which individuals respond to situations does not depend upon the actual balance between situational demands and resources, but rather upon what the child believes to be true about the situation. A child's belief, for example, that he or she is outclassed by an opponent is a psychologic reality of much greater importance in the stress process than an objective reality that belies that belief. Clearly, the child's appraisal of demands of the situation and the available resources may or may not be objectively accurate. Personality and motivational factors such as individual differences in self-esteem, confidence, and trait anxiety have an important role in the appraisal process.

Smith and Smoll (1982) have argued that situational appraisals extend beyond the assessment of demands and resources (and their relative balance or imbalance). People also appraise the possible consequences of failure to master the demands and the implications or meaning of such a failure. A situation is more likely to be stressful if a perceived imbalance threatens harm (e.g., injury or embarrassment) or loss of desired goals (e.g., a league championship) than if the outcome is of no consequence (e.g., a loss in practice). There is certainly the possibility of distortion, exaggeration, or underestimation in evaluating the likelihood of potential consequences as well as in the meaning of these consequences. For example, a very skilled young athlete may experience a great deal of self-imposed stress over unfounded concerns about parental rejection over an objectively unlikely potential loss. The objective probability of the particular occurrence or its objective meaning is less important in the stress process than what the individual holds to be true!

As can be seen in Fig. 24.1, the physiologic component of the model is reciprocally related to the cognitive appraisal component of the model. Specifically, it is assumed that cognitive appraisal of threat results in physiologic arousal as a part of the mobilization of resources to deal with situational demands. The resulting physiologic arousal and associated emotion also provides feedback which in turn influences the appraisal of the situation. Hence, there is an ongoing cycle of appraisal and reappraisal influenced by the associated levels of physiologic arousal. For example, a young wrestler's worries about being able to compete with a particular opponent will produce physiologic symptoms of anxiety (e.g., racing heart, increased perspiration). Recognition of and concern about the resulting physiologic symptoms may in turn lead to additional concerns about an inability to perform adequately against the opponent—and so the cycle continues.

BEHAVIORAL COMPONENT

The final component of the Smith and Smoll's (1982) stress process model consists of task-oriented, social, and coping behaviors that occur in response to situational appraisals. The notion is that emitted behaviors are influenced by the individual's stress appraisals of a situation. Performance may suffer or be enhanced and become more pro- or antisocial when individuals experience competitive stress. Athletes will also engage in coping behaviors to manage these appraisals and the associated emotions. The adequacy of these coping behaviors affects the balance between demands and resources as well as the ongoing appraisal process. Successful coping may allow the young athlete to reappraise the balance between situational demands and

available resources more favorably, but coping behaviors are not always effective on this account (Compas 1987). Regardless, the young athlete who perceives his or her responses (sport performance, social and/or coping) as lacking is more likely to experience negative affect. For example, the realization by a young tennis player that his or her passing shots are simply not precise enough to be effective against a particular opponent can have the affective consequence of additional competitive anxiety.

State and trait anxiety

In addition to defining stress itself, state and trait anxiety—terms frequently associated with stress in the scientific literature—must be defined before the stress process and its ramifications can be fully understood. State anxiety is one possible affective byproduct of the stress process and the one with which the negative connotations of stress are most often associated. State anxiety has been defined as "an existing or current emotional state characterized by feelings of apprehension and tension and associated with activation of the organism" (Martens 1977, p. 9). In essence, state anxiety is a negative feeling experienced at a particular moment in time. It is a feeling everyone at some time in their life has noticed, from butterflies experienced a few minutes before an athletic competition to that queasy feeling one might experience in one's stomach before giving a public speech for the first time.

Trait anxiety is defined as "a predisposition to perceive certain environmental stimuli as threatening or non-threatening and to respond to these stimuli with varying levels of state anxiety" (Martens 1977, p. 9). So, trait anxiety is not experienced per se but rather has to do with a dispositional tendency to appraise threat and hence experience (or not) states of anxiety. A young athlete's trait anxiety would be conceptualized within the "personal and motivational factors" component of Smith and Smoll's (1982) process model of stress. As illustrated in Fig. 24.1, individual factors like trait anxiety are hypothesized to influence all four components of the process model. Trait anxiety is important because it has been consistently shown to influence one's level of state anxiety. For example, a high trait anxious child will tend to perceive evaluative environments, such as competition, as very threatening and, as a consequence, experience increases in state anxiety. In contrast, a low trait anxious child placed in the same competitive environment has a lesser tendency to perceive threat and hence is less likely to experience marked increases in state anxiety. Thus, the level of state anxiety a child experiences in evaluative environments is directly related to his or her level of trait anxiety.

Stress research in youth sport

Over the last three decades a number of investigators have examined stress in children's sport and progress has been made toward understanding the stress process as a consequence. Questions of central interest in this research include:

1 Do youth sport participants experience too much stress?
2 What are the consequences of athletic stress?
3 What are the factors related to state anxiety in young athletes?
4 What are the factors related to trait anxiety in young athletes?
5 Do children and adults differ in their perception and responses to stress?

Do youth sport participants experience too much stress?

A fundamental question at issue surrounding youth sport has regarded the desirability of levels of state anxiety experienced by young athletes as a consequence of competitive stress. Critics of youth sport have suggested that competitive stress generates excessive levels of state anxiety that can negatively affect the mental health of the child athlete (Martens 1978). Conversely, youth sport proponents have argued that the very beauty of youth sport is that young athletes do experience stress—but not at excessive levels and in a safe environment that facilitates the development of coping skills to deal with stress successfully. A great deal of energy has been devoted to examining this issue.

Early investigators in the area (Skubic 1955; Hanson 1967; Lowe & McGrath 1971) examined

levels of state anxiety experienced by young athletes using physiologic indices of stress such as heart rate or Galvanic skin response. For example, Skubic (1955), in the earliest study of this issue, assessed physiologic stress in 9- to 15-year-old boys participating in Little League baseball and physical education class softball competitions via Galvanic skin response. Few differences were found between the groups, and it was concluded that the state anxiety experienced during competitive youth baseball was no greater than that experienced in a physical education class competition. In a youth baseball study, Lowe and McGrath (1971) examined respiration rates and heart rate prior to batting under conditions of varying game importance (e.g., based on league standings, won–loss records) and situation criticality (e.g., score, number of outs, position of runners on base). It was found that physiologic state anxiety was positively related to game importance and increased situation criticality. Unfortunately, assessments in non-evaluative circumstances or other forms of competition were not made.

These two example investigations of physiologic indices of state anxiety in youth sport competition illustrate typical findings in the area. These studies suggest that overall either few differences in stress levels exist between youth sport and other competitive environments (e.g., physical education class competitions) or that high, but short-lived, elevations in physiologic stress indices occur during events. Such results must be interpreted with some caution, however, because these sorts of physiologic changes observed may not result from competitive stress appraisals per se, but rather more directly from the physical exertions (cf. Dishman 1989). Notwithstanding this caution, it is important to take note of evidence of a relationship between heightened state anxiety during events and game importance and situation criticality.

Taking a different approach, a number of investigators have asked young athletes (or their parents) to rate the degree of anxiety-related symptoms associated with athletic competition (Skubic 1955; Hale 1961; McPherson et al. 1980; Purdy et al. 1981; Ralio 1982; Gould et al. 1983a; Feltz & Albrecht 1986). In most cases one or two questions on this account were posed as part of a larger youth sport survey project and hence the findings are superficial and somewhat difficult to interpret. However, these results do provide clues about the levels of state anxiety experienced by youth sport participants. Skubic (1955) reported that approximately one-third of the Little League baseball players surveyed reported contest-related sleeping difficulties. Of the youth swimmers surveyed by McPherson *et al.* (1980), 33% of male and 56% of female swimmers reported experiencing some emotional stress. Feltz and Albrect (1986) reported that 41% of their sample of elite young distance runners reported becoming nervous and worried in races (half of these young athletes indicated that this nervousness helped their performance). Interestingly, by contrast, Hale (1961) reported that 97% of the fathers of Little League baseball participants surveyed indicated that their sons were not affected by participation. Despite problems with non-validated instruments and superficiality, these results suggest that some young athletes—but clearly not the majority—engaged in competition experience high levels of competitive state anxiety and associated symptoms.

Finally, a number of investigators have used validated self-report state anxiety instruments to assess levels of state anxiety experienced before, during, and after competitive youth sport events (e.g., Scanlan & Passer 1978, 1979; Simon & Martens 1979; Bump *et al.* unpublished). Simon and Martens (1979) have conducted perhaps the most extensive investigation of state anxiety experienced in competitive and non-competitive sport settings. State anxiety levels of 749 boys (9–14 years) were assessed in practice settings, just prior to required school activities (i.e., classroom tests and physical education class competitions), non-required non-sport competitive activities (i.e., band solos and band group competition), and non-school sports (i.e., baseball, basketball, tackle football, gymnastics, ice hockey, swimming, and wrestling) using the Competitive State Anxiety Inventory for Children (CSAI-C; Martens 1977). Differences between practice and competitive state anxiety levels were examined as well as comparisons between the various competitive activities.

Not surprisingly, precompetitive state anxiety was found to be elevated over practice levels, although the overall change was not excessive. For example, the mean precompetitive state anxiety score for the entire sample was 16.87 (possible scores on the CSAI-C range from 10 to 30). Of particular interest in the Simon and Martens (1979) study was the comparison of state anxiety levels of boys participating in sport to boys participating in other competitive activities not typically the focus of parental concern (i.e., band solos, band group competition). Band solo participation elicited the greatest state anxiety ($M = 21.48$) followed by individual sport participation (M wrestling = 19.52, M gymnastics = 18.52), while physical education competition elicited the lowest levels of anxiety ($M = 14.47$). However, it was noted that substantial individual differences existed. Relatively few of the boys experienced what could be considered extremely high levels of competitive state anxiety (scoring in the upper quartile of possible CSAI-C scores or above 25 out of 30) while the vast majority of boys (82%) scored in the lower half of the scale.

Bump *et al.* (unpublished) also examined state anxiety levels of young athletes by administering the CSAI-C to 112 13- and 14-year-old boys prior to competitive tournament wrestling matches. Similar to the findings of Simon and Martens (1979) for wrestlers, prematch state anxiety levels averaged 18.9 (out of a possible 30). Again, relatively few of the boys reported experiencing extremely high levels of state anxiety with only 9% of the boys scoring in the upper quartile of possible CSAI-C scores (>25). These results are largely consistent with findings from other studies conducted in the area (e.g., Scanlan & Passer 1978, 1979; Hall & Kerr 1997, 1998; Hall *et al.* 1998). Consistently, evidence reveals that the majority of children and adolescents participating in competitive youth sports are not experiencing excessive levels of state anxiety as a result of their competitive experience.

Overall, the results of studies using different approaches to study levels of state anxiety and associated symptoms in young athletes indicate that the vast majority of children involved in competitive sport are not experiencing excessive levels of stress. Critics of organized competitive sport programs for children may be incorrect in their claims about the excessive levels of stress experienced by young athletes. Therefore, concerns about excessive stress should not prevent parents from encouraging their children from becoming involved in sport. Notwithstanding this conclusion, the evidence also shows that a small, but significant, minority of young athletes experience high levels of stress which may be manifested in such symptoms as insomnia and a loss of appetite. If only 5–10% of the youth involved in organized sport—now essentially a worldwide phenomena involving many tens of millions of children and adolescents (De Knop *et al.* 1996)—experience excessive stress, the number of children adversely affected by their involvement is staggering. Efforts need to be made to identify young athletes who are susceptible to heightened state anxiety and the youth sport situations related to heightened anxiety states in young athletes to ensure that the experiences of young athletes are as positive as intended.

What are the consequences of athletic stress on the child?

Excessive competitive stress has been associated with a variety of undesirable outcomes. It has been linked, for example, to sport withdrawal among young athletes (e.g., Gould & Petlichkoff 1988), sport burnout (e.g., Gould *et al.* 1996), performance deterioration (e.g., Scanlan *et al.* 1984; Gould *et al.* 1991), and decreased fun and satisfaction (e.g., Scanlan & Passer 1978, 1979; Scanlan & Lewthwaite 1984). Also identified have been associations with potential health-threatening effects such as a loss of sleep (e.g., Skubic 1955; State of Michigan 1978), loss of appetite (e.g., Skubic 1955), eating disorder risk among adolescent females (e.g., Monsma & Malina 2004), and the incidence or severity of sport injury (e.g., Smith *et al.* 1992; Krasnow *et al.* 1999). Although tentative links have been established in these areas, a great deal of study remains to be carried out before conclusions can be reached with any degree of certainty.

Evidence is accumulating to support the connection between stress and elevations in injury risk—although it would be simplistic to believe that there is a simple deterministic connection (Udry & Andersen 2002). Smith *et al.* (1990), for example, surveyed 451 male and female high school athletes

on 197 life changes (e.g., "getting good grades or progress reports," "pressures or expectations by parents," "getting a driver's license or learner's permit," "parents getting divorced") experienced during the 6 months prior to their high school basketball (boys and girls), wrestling (boys), or gymnastics (girls) season. If an event had been experienced, the athletes indicated whether they perceived it as a positive or negative at the time it occurred. They also classified the event as either a major event with long-term consequences for them, or as a "day-to-day" event that did not. Data were subsequently collected during the season on time lost from their sport due to injury. Smith *et al.* (1990) found no significant relationship between positive or negative life change scores and injury time-loss. When social support and coping variables were considered in conjunction with negative major life changes, however, significant associations were observed. Specifically, high school athletes with low levels of social support and low coping skills who experienced negative stress from major life changes tended to exhibit greater subsequent injury time-loss. Subsequently, Smith *et al.* (1992) found that the relationship between major negative sport-specific life events and ensuing injury time-loss may be most profound for adolescents having a lower dispositional tolerance for arousal (i.e., low sensation seeking athletes).

Evidence is mixed regarding the suggestion that performance deterioration is a consequence of high state anxiety (Scanlan *et al.* 1984; Gould *et al.* 1991). In fact, the assumption that increased state anxiety always negatively influences the performance of the young athlete has received little empirical support. Research with adult athletes (for a review see Gould *et al.* 2002) has shown that increased state anxiety does not always lead to inferior performance but rather can, up to some optimal point anyway, act to enhance performance. This notion is reinforced by findings in youth sport survey literature indicating that substantial percentages of junior elite runners (39%) and wrestlers (50%), ranging in age from 9 to 19 years, identify anxiety and nervousness as facilitating performance (Gould *et al.* 1983a; Feltz & Albrecht 1986).

Critics of youth sport have suggested that an aversion to challenge (i.e., high competitive trait anxiety) may develop among young athletes as a consequence of the experience of excessive levels of stress in youth sport. By contrast, youth sport advocates tend to believe that long-term positive consequences of exposure to competitive stress are more likely than the development of risk aversion. Indeed, Martens (1978) hypothesized that youth sport could act as a sort of "stress vaccination" by stimulating the development of generalizable strategies for coping with stress. Neither of these claims have enjoyed substantive empiricial evaluation and the evidence that does exist on the relationship between participation status and competitive trait anxiety provides no interpretable trends.

Specifically, in various comparisons of competitive trait anxiety, youth sport participants have been found to have:

1 The *same* level as non-participant fourth grade peers (Magill & Ash 1979);

2 *Lower* levels than fifth grade non-participant peers (Magill & Ash 1979); and

3 Slightly *higher* than normative levels for comparable age and gender groups (Feltz & Albrecht 1986). In the only longitudinal study, to our knowledge, reported on this account, Raviv (1981) reported no competitive trait anxiety differences in a 1-year study of 37 matched pairs of Israeli sport club and non-participant children. However, more extensive longitudinal studies controlling for potential moderating variables (e.g., extent of involvement, success level) need to be conducted before definitive conclusions in this area can be reached. Moreover, investigations examining the tenability of Martens' (1978) vaccine stress consequence hypothesis (and related questions such as what might constitute an optimal dosage of stress) remain to be conducted.

Further comprehensive investigation as to the consequences of competitive stress is clearly required. Although appropriate levels of competitive stress are thought to have positive cognitive, affective, and behavioral consequences, there is no clear evidence in this regard. Nonetheless, it can be concluded that excessive competitive stress can have acute negative physical and behavioral consequences on the young athlete. The long-term ramifications of competitive stress are unknown both in terms of the number of children afflicted with negative consequences and

the nature of potential benefits. Lines of systematic research are needed, particularly longitudinal investigations that examine long-term effects of competitive athletic stress on children.

What are the factors related to state and trait anxiety in child and adolescent athletes?

There are a number of reasons why it is imperative that personal and situational factors associated with competitive state and trait anxiety are identified, including:

1 The substantial minority of youth sport participants are at risk of experiencing negative consequences associated with excessive anxiety;

2 Knowledge of such factors provides the basis for intervention efforts; and

3 Identification of such factors helps to ensure that ill-advised efforts do not put additional young participants at risk.

Youth sport researchers have conducted relatively extensive research upon factors related to competitive state and trait anxiety among young athletes (Scanlan & Passer 1978, 1979; Gould *et al.* 1983b, 1991; Passer 1983; Scanlan & Lethwaite 1984; Feltz & Albrecht 1986; Brustad & Weiss 1987; Brustad 1988; Lewthwaite & Scanlan 1989; Hall & Kerr 1997, 1998). Awareness and understanding of these anxiety correlates (Table 24.1) should enable practitioners to better identify children who are susceptible to heightened levels of competitive stress and facilitate effort to ensure that youth sport settings are not excessively stressful.

FACTORS RELATED TO STATE ANXIETY IN CHILD AND ADOLESCENT ATHLETES

The typical approach to identifying factors associated with state anxiety in young athletes has consisted of assessing state anxiety levels immediately prior to and following a competition. Information about various personality factors (e.g., self-esteem), and demographics (e.g., years of experience in sport) collected at a previous non-stressful time (e.g., practice) are used to predict levels of pre- and post-competitive state anxiety. Scanlan (1986) has summarized this research and identified a number

Table 24.1 Anxiety correlates among child and adolescent athletes.

Associated with higher levels of anxiety
Greater tendency to find competition threatening (high competitive trait anxiety)
Higher personal performance expectancies
Greater fear of failure
Perceptions or anticipation of negative social evaluation
Perceptions of high adult expectations and parental pressure
Perfectionism
Ego-oriented achievement goals
Unfavorable game outcome
Perceived game importance
Avoidance behaviors

Associated with lower levels of anxiety
Higher self-esteem
Lower tendency to find competition threatening (low competitive trait anxiety)
Perceptions of personal competence
Perceptions of fun
Perceptions of a socially supportive environment
Satisfaction with participation
Task-oriented achievement goals
Approach behaviors

---

of personal and situational factors associated with competitive state anxiety. These include:

1 Competitive trait anxiety;
2 Self-esteem;
3 Fun;
4 Satisfaction;
5 Personal performance expectancies; and
6 Worries about failure and adult evaluation.

More recent theoretically grounded research has suggested that dispositional tendencies in the way individuals evaluate attainment of achievement goals and their assessments of personal competence must figure prominently in efforts to understand stress appraisals and associated aversive states such as anxiety in youth sport (e.g., Hall & Kerr 1997, 1998; Hall *et al.* 1998; Ntoumanis & Biddle 1998; Williams 1998).

Scanlan (1986) notes that the experience of competitive state anxiety among youth sport participants is reliably predicted by competitive trait anxiety—the young athlete's predisposition to perceive evaluative and competitive environments as

threatening or non-threatening. High trait anxious youth sport participants tend to respond to potentially stressful situations, such as competition, with nervousness or high state anxiety levels. By contrast, low trait anxious participants do not tend to respond to competitive situations with the same levels of state anxiety. Self-esteem also has been reliably associated with state anxiety. Specifically, the lower the young athlete's self-esteem, the higher the state anxiety level experienced in stressful situations.

More recently, evidence on the role of some aspects of dispositional perfectionism in the experience of competitive state anxiety in youth sport has begun to emerge (Gould *et al.* 1996, Hall & Kerr 1997; Hall *et al.* 1998). For example, higher scores on perfectionism relating to concern over mistakes, doubts about one's actions, and personal standards have been reliably related to elevations in state anxiety in high school runners (Hall *et al.* 1998). Similarly, Gould *et al.*'s (1996) study contrasting junior tennis players who burned out (players who lowered or discontinued involvement as result of chronic stress) versus those who did not, found that the perfectionism subscales of parental criticism and expectations, higher need for organization, and greater concern over mistakes differentiated the groups. Thus, dispositional perfectionism has been shown to predict levels of state anxiety experienced in youth sports.

Not surprisingly, youth sport participants perceiving more fun in the game or being more satisfied with their participation tend to experience less state anxiety, even with game outcome controlled for in relationships (Scanlan 1986). State anxiety is also related to the personal and team performance expectancies that young athletes hold. Lower expectancies for team and/or personal performance tend to be associated with a greater experience of state anxiety for the young athlete. Finally, worries about failure, social evaluation, and adult expectations are associated with elevations in state anxiety. For example, in a finding replicated by Gould *et al.* (1991), Scanlan and Lewthwaite (1984) found that increased parental pressure to participate is associated with increased levels of state anxiety among young wrestlers. That is, young wrestlers who believed their participation was important to their parents experienced more state anxiety than athletes who did not perceive parental pressure to participate.

Two readily apparent situational factors have been associated with heightened state anxiety in youth sport participants. The first relates to game outcome (i.e., victory vs. defeat). Young athletes who win games experience less state anxiety than young athletes who lose (Scanlan & Passer 1979). Not surprisingly, young athletes have been consistently found to experience less anxiety in practice settings because the focus is perceived to be less on performance outcomes and more upon learning and mastery (Williams 1998). The second, as Lowe and McGrath's (1971) youth baseball data illustrates, relates to game importance. The greater the importance placed on a particular event, the more stressful the event tends to be perceived by the individual—although there may be some individual differences on this account (Wilson & Raglin 1997). Some young athletes enjoy the "big games" more than those of lesser importance.

Competition is a socially constructed engagement. As such, concerns about how a given performance might be evaluated, in terms of Smith's (1986) stress process model, relate to the individual's appraisal of that socially constructed event. Hence, in this view, it is not the importance of the event (or the presence of social pressure in and of itself) as an objective fact that produces the anxiety experience. Rather, it is the concern that youth may hold about being evaluated negatively that causes anxiety—and events perceived to be more important necessarily involve greater potential for negative evaluation. Those youths having confidence in their ability to "rise to the occasion" are less at-risk, conceptually, of perceiving evaluative threat on those occasions. Nonetheless, evidence does suggest that concerns about negative social evaluation during competition are important contributors to the experience of competitive anxiety (Wilson & Eklund 1998; Prapavessis et al. 2004). Bray et al. (2000), for example, found the state anxiety experienced by young adolescent skiers was significantly associated with their concerns about how others (particularly parents and friends) would evaluate their competitive performance.

A number of stressors for junior elite athletes have been identified. Gould et al. (1983b), for example, examined sources of stress among 400 junior elite wrestlers (13–19 years) at a national tournament. The most frequently experienced stress sources for these junior elite competitors were performing up to their ability, improving on their last performance, participating in championship meets, not performing well, losing, not making weight (probably a sport-specific stressor), and being able to get mentally ready to wrestle. In all these cases, at least 41% of the individuals sampled rated these items as "very important" sources of stress. These findings appear reasonably robust given that other researchers (e.g., Feltz & Albrecht 1986) have found very similar results studying other groups of junior elite sport athletes. Overall, it appears that elite junior competitors (ranging in age from 9 to 19 years) are primarily concerned about fear of failure and performance evaluation issues and related concerns about inabilities to get mentally ready to perform well. Hence, two major stress sources to be recognized when dealing with elite junior level athletes are fear about failure/performance evaluation and feelings of inadequacy.

Some sport scientists (e.g., Hall & Kerr 1997, 1998; Hall et al. 1998; Ntoumanis & Biddle 1998) have employed achievement goal theory to provide an explanatory framework for understanding the stress and state anxiety experienced by young athletes. In achievement goal theory, task-oriented conceptions of success are self-referenced and associated with the belief that hard work and improving and meeting the demands of the task are the primary goals of the activity. Ego-oriented conceptions of success, by contrast, are associated with the belief that superiority over others in the contest (winning) is the primary goal. Hall and Kerr (1997) found that, among young fencers (aged 12.8 ± 1.4 years), ego orientation featured substantial positive relationships with precompetitive cognitive state anxiety among low-perceived ability athletes immediately before performance—and in the 2 days preceding the competition. Some evidence suggests that differential patterns of coping with competitive stress may also be associated with the different motivational orientations (Ntoumanis et al. 1999). For example, emotion-focused strategies such as venting were found to be associated with high ego-orientation athletes (Ntoumanis *et al.* 1999).

In summary, the research on pre- and post-game state anxiety and associated factors has helped to provide a useful profile of personal and situational factors that are associated with heightened state anxiety in organized youth sport settings. Knowledge of these factors can help physicians, parents, and adult leaders identify young athletes who experience high levels of state anxiety in sport and, in turn, take steps toward reducing this stress. Further, such information can be useful in helping to ensure that additional young athletes are not put at risk. For example, perfection is an unattainable performance standard. Competition is bound to be threatening for young athletes who judge their efforts against this standard—or who believe that perfection is the only standard that will satisfy their coaches or parents. Helping these athletes refocus their self-evaluations on personally attainable standards of excellence will help to reduce levels of stress for these athletes. Ensuring that the youth sport social environment emphasizes and reinforces these attainable steps toward personal excellence is also important for creating an optimally "stressful" and enjoyable experience for young athletes.

FACTORS RELATED TO TRAIT ANXIETY IN CHILD AND ADOLESCENT ATHLETES

Several investigators (Passer 1983; Brustad & Weiss 1987; Brustad 1988; Lewthwaite & Scanlan 1989) have examined factors associated with high competitive trait anxiety in young athletes. This is an important area of study because the personality disposition of high competitive trait anxiety has been one of the factors most consistently related to elevated levels of high state anxiety in young athletes. A better understanding of the high trait anxious young athlete and factors related to his or her high trait anxiety should assist youth sport leaders in helping young athletes at-risk to cope with the stress of athletic competition (Gould & Dieffenbach 2003).

Passer (1983) was the first investigator to study the high competitive trait anxious youth sport participant. In particular, he compared 163 high and low competitive trait anxious youth soccer players (10–15 years) on self-esteem, performance expectancies, criticism for failure expectations, perceived competence, and performance- and evaluation-related worries. High trait anxious players reported being worried more frequently about losing, not playing well, and coach, parent, and teammate evaluations than their low anxious peers. It was concluded that high competitive trait anxious young athletes perceived fear of evaluation and failure as major threat sources. Similar findings were reported in investigations extending Passer's work with adolescents participating in baseball (Brustad & Weiss 1987), basketball (Brustad 1988), and wrestling (Lewthwaite & Scanlan 1989). Importantly, Lewthwaite and Scanlan (1989) also observed a behavioral tendency to be associated with trait anxiety in their sample of youth sport wrestlers. Specifically, high trait anxious wrestlers preferred to take a "bye" (an automatic win) against first round opponents to a greater extent than did low trait anxious competitors. Lewthwaite and Scanlan (1989) speculated that this preference might have stemmed from an urge to avoid either the anticipated (and aversive) state anxiety experience or the risk of failure (and the associated potential consequences) perceived by these young athletes.

In a study grounded in achievement goal theory, Voight *et al.* (2000) examined the association between multidimensional trait anxiety and goal orientations in a reasonably large ($n = 176$) sample of adolescent female Mexican-American volleyball players participating in a year-long United States Olympic Committee volleyball training program. Results indicated that being dispositionally ego oriented was substantially associated with higher levels of competitive trait anxiety. Being task oriented, by contrast, was associated with dispositionally lower tendencies to experience these negative aversive states. Importantly, Voight *et al.* (2000) also presented evidence indicating an interaction between ego orientation and self-confidence scores in predicting cognitive aspects of competitive trait anxiety. Hence, young athletes using victory as a primary gauge of personal success in their sporting efforts may be at greater risk of appraising threat in sport competition than those placing a greater priority on improvement and effort—although higher levels of confidence may serve to moderate the risk for the ego-oriented athlete.

Taken together, these results indicate that the emotional aversiveness of competition for some young athletes may be addressed by seeking to reduce evaluation potential, to enhance their low self-esteem, and ensure that they perceive success in their experiences. Further, evidence from recent goal orientation research suggests that efforts to help these young athletes learn to interpret the meaning of success and failure in productive ways may be important. Specifically, high trait anxious young athletes, in particular, need to learn to evaluate their performance from a task orientation (hard work, improving and meeting the demands of the task) while keeping ego-oriented conceptions of success (superiority over others) in perspective.

Do children, adolescents, and adults differ relative to competitive stress in sport?

When we were preparing a chapter for an earlier volume of this *Encyclopaedia, The Child and Adolescent Athlete* (i.e., Gould & Eklund 1996), the editor, Professor Oded Bar-Or queried the extent to which pediatric sport psychologists interested in anxiety and stress had evidence of whether children differ from adolescents and adults in their emotional responses to stressors and, if so, what are the characteristic sport-related responses of the child as compared to the adolescent and/or the adult and, further, are certain stressors unique to children's sports? Despite the importance of these questions, to our knowledge, no investigations have yet been conducted that directly examined whether children, adolescents, and adults differ in their perceptions of and responses to competitive stress in sport. Some investigators (e.g., Scanlan *et al.* 1991; Gould *et al.* 1992) have examined sources of stress in studies of elite (mostly adult) athletic populations and compared their findings with previously discussed studies of stress sources and predictors of state anxiety in young athletes. The conclusions of these comparisons continue to be best summarized by Scanlan *et al.* (1991):

"The results show that elite and youth sport athletes have similar competition-related stressors: namely, worrying about failure, performing poorly, and losing. The extant stress literature's exclusive focus on competition leaves future research to determine whether the elite athlete's stressors outside of competition (e.g., interpersonal conflict, time and financial demands or costs, perfectionism) generalize to youth sport athletes" (Scanlan *et al.* 1991, p. 118).

An area of commonality across child, adolescent, and adult sport participants has been that trait anxiety has consistently been found to be a substantial predictor of state anxiety (Martens *et al.* 1990). That is, high trait anxious athletes, regardless of age, consistently experience higher levels of state anxiety in competition than their low trait anxious counterparts. However, equivocal findings have resulted when levels of trait anxiety have been compared across children and adults in various studies (Martens *et al.* 1990). Specifically, some studies have found younger athletes to exhibit lower trait anxiety than older athletes while other investigations have revealed no such differences. Martens *et al.* (1990) contend that understanding these equivocal findings on the tendency to regard competition as threatening across age groups requires consideration of interrelationship between age and situational factors. For instance, in studies where younger athletes exhibit lower levels of trait anxiety than older athletes, observed differences may result from the fact that younger children have not yet learned to view competition as evaluative threats to their self-esteem. The question remains then, whether age-related trait anxiety differences would exist when the intensity of the competitive situation was controlled.

In summary, the few studies that have been conducted to compare children with adults in their perceptions of and response to anxiety and stress suggest more similarities than differences. Extreme caution must be taken in drawing these conclusions, however, because of the relative paucity of developmentally based studies that simultaneously compare athletes of different development levels and control for potential moderator variables such as the intensity of the competitive situation. This is certainly an area ripe for future research.

Conclusions and recommendations

In this review, the literature on competitive stress accompanying competitive sport participation for the young athlete has been examined. Specifically, we have delineated:

1 The stress process;
2 The levels of state anxiety experienced by young athletes;
3 The consequences of athletic stress;
4 Factors associated with state and trait anxiety; and
5 Comparisons of child and adult perceptions of and responses to anxiety and stress.

Our understanding of the stress process in youth sport is far from complete but, nonetheless, a number of recommendations for guiding practice and future research directions can be forwarded.

Stress, youth sport, and recommendations for practice

The competitive stress experienced by a young athlete results from the complex interplay of situational factors and personal characteristics of that young athlete. Therefore, efforts must be made to consider both types of factors in the youth sport setting rather than simply attributing stress solely to the child or the situation.

Children should not be discouraged from participating in competitive sport because of concerns about competitive stress. The vast majority of youth sport participants do not experience excessive levels of state anxiety nor do they appear to differ from their non-athletic counterparts in trait anxiety.

A significant minority of youth sport participants do suffer from high levels of competitive stress. Efforts must be made to identify and assist these children so that their youth sport involvement is a positive developmental opportunity instead of an onerous aversive struggle. Important clues about how threatening youth sport participants find their involvement can be gleaned from observation of their behaviors before, during, and after practice, and consideration of how they discuss their participation. Do they typically exude interest and enthusiasm about their involvement, or does their participation and verbalization more typically trend more toward aversion, reluctance, and avoidance?

Children with personal characteristics that include high levels of competitive trait anxiety and perfectionism, and/or low self-esteem, are most likely to experience high levels of state anxiety. Also at-risk are children who have low performance expectancies (personal and/or team), experience less fun and satisfaction in the youth sport setting, and worry about failure and adult evaluation. Special attention is warranted with children exhibiting these characteristics (Gould & Dieffenbach 2003) to ensure that the positive possibilities for personal skill development, social interaction, and enjoyment in participation are emphasized and reinforced, rather than winning, social evaluation, and unattainable performance perfection.

Environments laden with social evaluation, where importance is placed upon performance and contest outcome, are most likely to provoke a stress response particularly for young athletes who are uncertain about the expectations of others and his or her ability to perform to those expectations. Efforts to engineer the environment to reduce uncertainty, evaluative components, and importance placed upon contest outcome can help to moderate the situational effects in the stress process.

Although contest outcome is a salient and important aspect of the sport setting, young athletes, particularly high trait anxious young athletes, are likely to benefit by learning to evaluate their performances on the basis of hard work, improvement, and attainment of performance goals, while keeping contest outcome in perspective.

Challenges for future research

Organizational issues producing stress in young athletes need to be examined. Specifically, investigations examining heightened state and trait anxiety in young athletes involved in intensive competition such as league, regional, national, and international championships are needed (Gould et al. 1992). To date, most of the research has not been conducted on young athletes involved in the types of intense training regimens required for competition at these levels.

Developmental investigations of state and trait anxiety, as well as sources of athletic stress, in samples of children, adolescents, and adults are badly needed. In particular, research on the question of whether children differ from adolescents and adults in their emotional responses to stressors is needed (Bar-Or as cited in Gould & Eklund 1996). If so, what are the sport-related typical responses of children versus adolescents versus adult athletes.

Pediatric sport psychology researchers interested in emotional stress may find utility in following the lead of pediatric exercise physiologists in classifying athletes according to developmental or maturational status (i.e., prepubescent, pubescent, and post-pubescent) rather than chronologic age. It has been suggested that children are characterized by separate physical, social-emotional, and intellectual developmental patterns (Martens 1978). Investigations linking anxiety and stress responses to these varying developmental patterns are warranted.

Longitudinal investigations that examine long-term effects of competitive athletic stress on children are warranted.

A need exists to assess potential positive consequences associated with experiencing stress in sport competition. For example, is Martens' (1978) stress vaccine hypothesis tenable? Does youth sport stress exposure prepare or vaccinate a young athlete for handling more severe stress levels later in life? If so, what is the optimal dose of stress needed for such a vaccine effect to occur?

Considerable attention has been paid to identifying sources of stress surrounding athletic competition for children. Elite adult athletes have described non-competitive stressors (e.g., financial costs of participating, time demands) as impacting substantially upon their competitive efforts (Scanlan et al. 1991). A need also exists to evaluate possibilities in this area relative to youth sport athletes.

Qualitative research methods (e.g., in-depth interviews) should be used to examine stress and anxiety responses in young athletes. These methods have potential to be especially useful in examining previously unexplored areas such as the positive consequences of experiencing stress in sport competitions. For example, based on interviews with junior tennis players who burned out, Gould et al. (1997) were able to identify three different, previously identified mechanisms that might lead to stress-induced burnout:

1 A physically driven strain resulting from physical overtraining;
2 A psychologically driven strain resulting from a young athlete having an "at-risk" perfectionist personality predisposing them to burnout; and
3 A psychologic substrain that focused on situational stress, such as coach or parent pressure to participate and perform.

References

Berryman, J.W. (1996) The rise of boys' sports in the United States, 1900 to 1970. In: *Children and Youth in Sport: A Biopsychosocial Perspective* (Smoll, F.L. & Smith, R.E., eds.) Brown & Benchmark, Chicago: 4–14.

Bray, S.R., Martin, K.A. & Widmeyer, W.N. (2000) The relationship between evaluative concerns and sport competition state anxiety among youth skiers. *Journal of Sports Sciences* **18**, 353–361.

Brustad, R.J. (1988) Affective outcomes in competitive youth sport: The influence of intrapersonal and socialization factors. *Journal of Sport & Exercise Psychology* **10**, 307–321.

Brustad, R.J. & Weiss, M.R. (1987) Competence perceptions and sources of worry in high, medium, and low competitive trait-anxious young athletes. *Journal of Sport Psychology* **9**, 97–105.

Compas, B.E. (1987) Coping with stress during childhood and adolescence. *Psychological Bulletin* **101**, 393–403.

De Knop, P., Engstrom, L.M., Skirstad, B. & Weiss, M.R., eds. (1996) *Worldwide Trends in Youth Sport.* Human Kinetics, Champaign, IL.

Dishman, R.K. (1989) Exercise and sport psychology in youth 6 to 18 years of age. In: *Perspectives in Exercise and Sports Medicine. Vol. 2. Youth, Exercise and Sport*

(Gisolfi, C.V. & Lamb, D.R., eds.) Benchmark Press, Indianapolis, IN: 47–97.

Estrada, A.M., Gelfand, D.M. & Hartmann, D.P. (1988) Children's sport and the development of social behaviors. In: *Children in Sport*, 3rd edn. (Smoll, F.L., Magill, R.A. & Ash, M.J., eds.) Human Kinetics, Champaign, IL: 251–262.

Feltz, D.L. & Albrecht, R.R. (1986) Psychological implications of competitive running. In: *Sports for Children and Youth* (Weiss, M.R. & Gould, D., eds.) Human Kinetics, Champaign, IL: 225–230.

Gould, D. & Dieffenbach, K. (2003) Psychological issues in youth sports:

Competitive anxiety, over training and burnout. In: *Youth Sports: Perspectives for a New Century* (Malina, R.M. & Clark, M.A., eds.) Coaches Choice, Monterey, CA: 383–402.

Gould, D. & Eklund, R.C. (1996) Emotional stress and anxiety in the child and adolescent athlete. In: *The Child and Adolescent Athlete* (Bar-Or, O., ed.) Blackwell Science, Oxford, England: 383–398.

Gould, D., Eklund, R.C., Petlichkoff, L., Peterson, K. & Bump, L. (1991) Psychological predictors of state anxiety, and performance in age-group wrestlers. *Pediatric Exercise Science* 3, 198–208.

Gould, D., Greenleaf, C. & Krane, V.I. (2002) Arousal-anxiety and sport behavior. In: *Advances in Sport Psychology*, 2nd edn. (Horn, T., ed.) Human Kinetics, Champaign, IL.

Gould, D., Horn, T. & Spreemann, J. (1983a) Competitive anxiety in junior elite wrestlers. *Journal of Sport Psychology* 5, 58–71.

Gould, D., Horn, T. & Spreemann, J. (1983b) Sources of stress in junior elite wrestlers. *Journal of Sport Psychology* 5, 159–171.

Gould, D., Jackson, S.A. & Finch, L. (1992) Sources of stress experienced by national champion figure skaters. US Olympic Committee Sports Science Grant Final Report.

Gould, D. & Petlichkoff, L. (1988) Participation motivation and attrition in young athletes. In: *Children in Sport*, 3rd edn. (Smoll, F.L., Magill, R.A. & Ash, M.J., eds.) Human Kinetics, Champaign, IL: 161–178.

Gould, D., Udry, E., Tuffey, S. & Loehr, J. (1996) Burnout in competitive junior tennis players. I. A quantitative psychological assessment. *Sport Psychologist* 10, 322–340.

Gould, D., Tuffey, S., Udry, E. & Loehr, J. (1997) Burnout in competitive junior tennis players. III. Individual differences in the burnout experience. *Sport Psychologist* 11, 257–276.

Hale, C.J. (1961) Injuries among 771,810 Little League baseball players. *Journal of Sports Medicine and Physical Fitness* 1, 3–7.

Hall, H.K. & Kerr, A.W. (1997) Motivational antecedents of precompetitive anxiety in youth sport. *Sport Psychologist* 11, 24–42.

Hall, H.K. & Kerr, A.W. (1998) Preddicting achievement anxiety: A social–cognitive perspective. *Journal of Sport & Exercise Psychology* 20, 98–111.

Hall, H.K., Kerr, A.W. & Matthews, J. (1998) Precompetitive anxiety in sport: The contribution of achievement goals and perfectionism. *Journal of Sport & Exercise Psychology* 20, 194–217.

Hanson, D.L. (1967) Cardiac response to participation in Little League baseball competition as determined by telemetry. *Research Quarterly* 38, 384–388.

Krasnow, D., Mainwaring, L. & Kerr, G. (1999) Injury, stress, and perfectionism in young dancers and gymnasts. *Journal of Dance Medicine and Science* 3, 51–58.

Lazarus, R.S. & Folkman, S. (1984) *Stress, Appraisal and Coping*. Springer, New York.

Lewthwaite, R. & Scanlan, T.K. (1989) Predictors of competitive trait anxiety in male youth sport participants. *Medicine and Science in Sports and Exercise* 21, 221–229.

Lowe, R. & McGrath, J.E. (1971) Stress, arousal and performance: Some findings calling for a new theory. Report No. AF1161-67. Air Force Office of Strategic Research, Washington DC.

Magill, R.A. & Ash, M.J. (1979) Academic, psychosocial and motor characteristics of participants and nonparticipants in children's sports. *Research Quarterly* 50, 230–240.

Martens, R. (1977) *Sports Competition Anxiety Test*. Human Kinetics, Champaign, IL.

Martens, R. (1978) *Joy and Sadness in Children's Sports*. Human Kinetics, Champaign, IL.

Martens, R., Vealey, R.S. & Burton, D., eds. (1990) *Competitive Anxiety in Sport*. Human Kinetics, Champaign, IL.

McPherson, B., Martinuk, R., Tihanyi, J. & Clark, W. (1980) The social system of age group swimmers, parents and coaches. *Canadian Journal of Applied Sport Sciences* 4, 142–145.

Monsma, E.V. & Malina, R.M. (2004) Correlates of eating disorders risk among female figure skaters: A profile of adolescent competitors. *Psychology of Sport and Exercise* 5, 447–460.

Ntoumanis, N. & Biddle, S. (1998) The relationship between competitive anxiety, achievement goals, and motivational climates. *Research Quarterly for Exercise and Sport* 69, 176–187.

Ntoumanis, N., Biddle, S. & Haddock, G. (1999) The mediating role of coping strategies on the relationship between achievement motivation and affect in sport. *Anxiety, Stress and Coping* 12, 299–327.

Passer, M.W. (1983) Fear of failure, fear of evaluation, perceived competence and self-esteem in competitive-trait anxious children. *Journal of Sport Psychology* 5, 172–188.

Prapavessis, H., Grove, J.R. & Eklund, R.C. (2004) Self-presentational issues in competition and sport. *Journal of Applied Sport Psychology* 19, 19–40.

Purdy, D.A., Haufler, S.E. & Eitzen, D.S. (1981) Stress among child athletes: Perceptions by parents, coaches and athletes. *Journal of Sport Behavior* 4, 32–44.

Ralio, W.S. (1982) The relationship of sport in childhood and adolescence to mental and social health. *Scandinavian Journal of Sports Medicine Supplement* 29, 135–145.

Raviv, S. (1981) Reactions to frustration, level of anxiety and loss of control of children participating in competitive sports. In: *Children in Sport: Psychosociological Characteristics* (Geron, E., Mashiach, A., Dunkelman, N., Raviv, S., Levin, Z. & Nakash, E., eds.) Wingate Institute, Netanya, Israel: 72–94.

Scanlan, T.K. (1986) Competitive stress in children. In: *Sport for Children and Youth* (Weiss, M.R. & Gould, D., eds.) Human Kinetics, Champaign, IL: 113–118.

Scanlan, T.K. & Lewthwaite, R. (1984) Social psychological aspects of competition for male youth sport participants. I. Predictors of competitive stress. *Journal of Sport Psychology* 6, 208–227.

Scanlan, T.K., Lewthwaite, R. & Jackson, B.L. (1984) Social psychological aspects of competition for male youth sport participants. II. Predictors of performance outcomes. *Journal of Sport Psychology* 6, 422–429.

Scanlan, T.K. & Passer, M. (1978) Factors related to competitive stress among male youth sports participants. *Medicine and Science in Sports* 10, 103–108.

Scanlan, T.K. & Passer, M. (1979) Sources of competitive stress in young female athletes. *Journal of Sport Psychology* 1, 151–159.

Scanlan, T.K., Stein, G.L. & Ravizza, K. (1991) An indepth study of former elite figure skaters. III. Sources of stress. *Journal of Sport & Exercise Psychology* 13, 103–120.

Selye, H. (1974) *Stress Without Distress*. New American Library, New York.

Simon, J. & Martens, R. (1979) Children's anxiety in sport and nonsport evaluative activities. *Journal of Sport Psychology* 1, 160–169.

Skubic, E. (1955) Emotional responses of boys to Little League and Middle League competitive baseball. *Research Quarterly* **26**, 342–352.

Smilkstein, G. (1980) Psychological trauma in children and youth in competitive sport. *Journal of Family Practice* **10**, 737–739.

Smith, R.E. (1986) Toward a cognitive–affective model of athletic burnout. *Journal of Sport Psychology* **8**, 36–50.

Smith, R.E. & Smoll, F.L. (1982) Psychological stress: A conceptual model and some intervention strategies in youth sports. In: *Children in Sport*, 2nd edn. (Magill, R.A., Ash, M.J. & Smoll, F.L., eds.) Human Kinetics, Champaign, IL: 178–195.

Smith, R.E., Ptacek, J.T. & Smoll, F.L. (1992) Sensation seeking, stress, and adolescent injuries: A test of stress-buffering, risk-taking, and coping skills hypotheses. *Journal of Personality and Social Psychology* **62**, 1016–1024.

Smith, R.E., Smoll, F.L. & Ptacek, J.T. (1990) Conjunctive moderator variables in vulnerability and resiliency research: Life stress, social support and coping skills, and adolescent sport injuries. *Journal of Personality and Social Psychology* **58**, 360–370.

State of Michigan (1978) Joint legislative study on youth sports programs: Phase II agency sponsored sports. East Lansing, MI.

Tutko, T. & Burns, W. (1979) The child superstar: A curse or a blessing. *Tennis USA* **March**, 40–48, 56.

Udry, E. & Andersen, M.B. (2002) Athletic injury and sport behavior. In: *Advances in Sport Psychology*, 2nd edn. (Horn, T., ed.) Human Kinetics, Champaign, IL.

Voight, M.R., Callahan, J.L. & Ryska, R.A. (2000) Relationship between goal orientations, self-confidence and multidimensional trait anxiety among Mexican-American femail youth athletes. *Journal of Sport Behavior* **23**, 271–288.

Weiss, M.R. & Smith, A.L. (2002) Friendship quality in youth sport: Relationship to age, gender, and motivation variables. *Journal of Sport & Exercise Psychology* **24**, 420–437.

Wiggins, D.K. (1996) A history of highly competitive sport for American children. In: *Children and Youth in Sport: A Biopsychosocial Perspective* (Smoll, F.L. & Smith, R.E., eds.) Brown & Benchmark, Chicago: 15–30.

Williams, L. (1998) Contextual influences and goal perspectives among female youth sport participants. *Research Quarterly for Exercise and Sport* **69**, 47–57.

Wilson, G.S. & Raglin, J.S. (1997) Optimal and predicted anxiety in 9 to 12 year-old track and field athletes. *Scandinavian Journal of Medicine and Science in Sports* **7**, 253–258.

Wilson, P. & Eklund, R.C. (1998) The relationship between competitive anxiety and self-presentational concerns. *Journal of Sport & Exercise Psychology* **20**, 81–97.

Part 6

Disease and Disability in the Young Athlete

Chapter 25

Exercise Immunology—Basics and Clinical Relevance

BRIAN W. TIMMONS AND HELGE HEBESTREIT

The human immune system is comprised of cellular and soluble factors, which act synergistically to extinguish pathogens, thus contributing to the maintenance of health. Traditional understanding of the immune system separates cellular and soluble factors into specific (i.e., adaptive) and non-specific (i.e., innate) components. Specific immunity, characterized by antigen specificity and "memory", allows the host to mount a stronger and targeted response following repeated exposure to the same antigen, whereas non-specific immunity provides early detection and clearance of pathogens, thus serving as a first-line defense against infection.

Scientific interest in the immunology of exercise was first stimulated by anecdotal evidence from coaches and athletes that intense exercise training resulted in an increased frequency of illness and infection. Consequently, exercise physiologists have been investigating how regular exercise might impact the immune system and its ability to combat infection. In the 1990s, an exponential increase in the number of exercise immunology publications characterized the importance of this area (Nieman & Pedersen 1999), but the number of studies devoted to the pediatric population remains low. Therefore very little is known regarding the interactions of exercise training and immune function in children and adolescents, and advice regarding exercise and infection offered to the young athlete is based on adult data, which may not be accurate or even appropriate. This chapter outlines our current understanding of the impact of acute and chronic exercise on the immune system and the relationship between physical activity (PA) and risk of infection in

children and adolescents. Whenever possible, the findings are discussed in light of child–adult differences and comparisons are made between athletes and non-athletes. Finally, some practical considerations are offered for the young athlete with an infection or recovering from an immune-related disease.

The immune response to acute exercise

An acute bout of exercise transiently affects numerous aspects of the immune system in an intensity- and duration-dependent manner. Furthermore, responses of various immune components to the same exercise stimulus can be quite different. The leukocyte response, for example, shows differential patterns for the various subtypes both in magnitude and direction (Fig. 25.1). Exercise-induced perturbations to cellular and soluble factors are generally short-lived, but when accumulated over time may

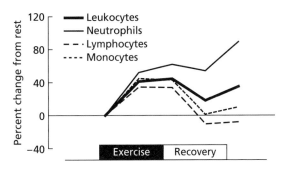

Fig. 25.1 Pattern of leukocyte changes in response to high intensity cycling (70% $\dot{V}O_{2max}$) for 60 min in healthy untrained 12- and 14-year-old boys and girls. Data from Timmons *et al.* (2006b).

337

alter overall immune status. In the following sections, commonly reported aspects of the immune system and their response to acute exercise are discussed.

Salivary immunoglobulin A

Given its anatomic location, salivary immunoglobulin A (sIgA) is an important marker of mucosal immunity and a first-line soluble defense against environmental pathogens. The adult literature is quite consistent in showing depressed sIgA levels following intense exercise (Gleeson 2000). In pediatric studies, however, the picture is less clear. In line with the reports on adult athletes, a number of studies has shown that post-exercise sIgA secretion rate was significantly depressed relative to pre-exercise values in children of both genders (Filaire *et al.* 2004). In the same studies, only young girls (Filaire *et al.* 2004), but not older adolescent girls (Nieman *et al.* 2000; Novas *et al.* 2003) or boys (Nieman *et al.* 2000), experienced significant reductions in sIgA concentration following acute exercise. In contrast, acute bouts of basketball exercise were associated with slight but significant increases in sIgA levels following practice and game situations in pre- and post-pubescent boys (Tharp 1991); however, changes in total salivary protein were not corrected for in this study, nor were secretion rates provided.

It is possible that the above differences in sIgA response to acute exercise between children and adults might be related to the intensity of the exercise. Indeed, exercise intensity is an important determinant of the sIgA response in children in so far as sIgA levels are depressed following high intensity exercise (75% $\dot{V}o_{2max}$), but enhanced following moderate intensity exercise (50% $\dot{V}o_{2max}$) (Dorrington *et al.* 2003), similar to the adult literature. Although no direct comparisons have been made to compare the magnitude of change, there is no strong evidence to suggest that the pattern of sIgA responses to acute exercise in children is any different from that observed in adults. However, repeatedly depressed sIgA levels resulting from regular bouts of acute exercise may have particular relevance for the young athlete's susceptibility to respiratory infections (see below).

Neutrophils

In individuals older than 5 years of age, neutrophils constitute the largest population of the total blood leukocyte pool and during the early stages of inflammation these phagocytes migrate into damaged tissue. Neutrophils can ingest (i.e., phagocytize) microbes and degrade them, thus acting as a first-line cellular defense against infectious agents. During exercise, neutrophils are mobilized into the peripheral circulation, most likely from the bone marrow and other marginated pools (e.g., lungs), resulting in an elevated blood concentration, even when exercise-induced reductions in plasma volume are taken into account. A consistent finding in the adult literature is a sustained neutrophilia for several hours following high intensity exercise (Pedersen & Hoffman-Goetz 2000). While the neutrophil response during exercise is quite comparable in children, adolescents, and adults (Timmons *et al.* 2004a, 2006b), the post-exercise recovery of neutrophil counts is faster in children than in both adolescents (Timmons *et al.* 2006b) and adults (Timmons *et al.* 2004a). Figure 25.2 shows this age effect on recovery

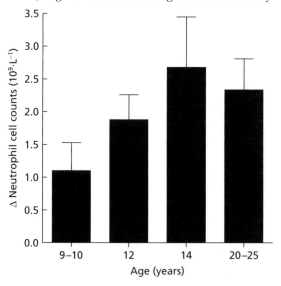

Fig. 25.2 Recovery neutrophilia following 60 min cycling at 70% $\dot{V}o_{2max}$ in children, adolescents, and adults. Data represent the difference (Δ) between recovery and resting neutrophil cell counts. Blood samples were taken before exercise and 60 min into recovery. Data from Timmons *et al.* (2004a, 2006b).

neutrophilia, as the difference between neutrophil counts at rest and counts at recovery. Whether these age differences in the magnitude of the recovery neutrophilia reflect age-related differences in the inflammatory response to muscle damage is unclear. However, these observations do suggest that the inflammatory insult induced by high intensity acute exercise is smaller in young children and are consistent with previous findings that markers of muscle damage during recovery from eccentrically biased exercise are lower in children than in adults (Soares *et al.* 1996; Arnett *et al.* 2000; Marginson *et al.* 2005).

It is also important to note that exercise-induced changes in neutrophil counts do not necessarily reflect simultaneous changes in neutrophil function. Unfortunately, it appears that only one pediatric study has reported the impact of acute exercise on neutrophil function. In this study (Wolach *et al.* 1998a), one aspect of *in vitro* neutrophil function (phorbol myristate acetate [PMA]-induced superoxide anion release), but not other aspects (neutrophil chemotaxis, bactericidal activity, and formylated peptides-induced superoxide anion release) was found to be reduced immediately after a 20-min treadmill run in trained gymnasts and untrained prepubertal girls. In blood samples collected 24-h following the end of the exercise, however, different aspects of neutrophil function (PMA-induced superoxide anion release and neutrophil chemotaxis) were now found to be suppressed relative to pre-exercise values (Wolach *et al.* 1998a). Interestingly, the decline in function in untrained girls was ~64% less than that reported by the same research group for untrained women performing similar exercise (Wolach *et al.* 2000). Thus, there is some evidence that certain aspects of neutrophil function may be better preserved in children than in adults following aerobic-type exercise.

Natural killer cells

Natural killer (NK) cells are a subpopulation of lymphocytes with natural cytotoxicity, which implicates them as key players in antiviral (Biron *et al.* 1999) and anticancer defense mechanisms (Brittenden *et al.* 1996). Similar to adults, NK cells are the most responsive cell type to exercise in most pediatric

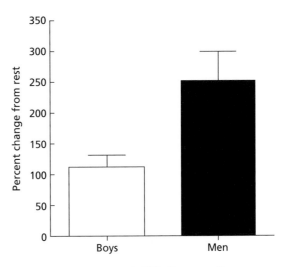

Fig. 25.3 Percent increase in NK cell counts of boys and men in response to 60 min cycling at 70% $\dot{V}o_{2max}$. Data from Timmons *et al.* (2004a).

studies (Boas *et al.* 1996, 2000; Eliakim *et al.* 1997; Shore & Shephard 1998; Wolach *et al.* 1998b; Nieman *et al.* 2000; Perez *et al.* 2001; Nemet *et al.* 2003, 2004; Timmons *et al.* 2004a,b). The magnitude of the NK cell response to endurance exercise, however, is age-dependent, with smaller increases in 9- and 10-year-old boys than in 20- to 25-year-old men (Timmons *et al.* 2004a), as shown in Fig. 25.3. Because NK cells express a high surface density of β-adrenergic receptors, they are particularly susceptible to circulating catecholamines. Therefore, a reasonable explanation for this age difference in NK cell sensitivity, even at the same relative intensity of exercise, is a lower surface density of β-adrenergic receptors on NK cells in children (Reinhardt *et al.* 1984; Galal 1989). Although an older study reported that the epinephrine response to maximal exercise was less in children than in adults, we have not found differences in epinephrine responses to endurance exercise between groups of boys at different stages of puberty, despite differences in their NK cell response to exercise (Timmons *et al.* 2006a). On the one hand, a dampened NK cell response to exercise in children may be beneficial as it might allow the immune system to remain closer to homeostasis in children training and competing on a regular basis. On the other hand, the apparently lower NK cell sensitivity to physiologic stress in children might suggest that any antiviral or anticancer protection offered by exercise is accordingly smaller in youth compared to adults. Given the general belief that the exercise-induced increase in circulating NK cells translates into enhanced immune surveillance, one might consider young children to be less capable of generating an enhanced state of readiness in response to an acute physiologic stressor.

Training status and the immune response to acute exercise

Salivary immunoglobulin A

Whether training status influences sIgA alterations in response to acute exercise in children and adolescents is unknown because direct comparisons between trained and untrained youth are not available.

Neutrophils

Some aspects of post-exercise neutrophil *function* may be better preserved in children than in adults following aerobic-type exercise, at least in the untrained state. This may not hold true, however, in the trained state. The magnitude of reduction in neutrophil chemotaxis reported in young gymnasts, for example, was quite comparable to the reduction observed in trained adults, as reported by the same research group (Wolach *et al.* 2000). There is no strong evidence that the acute effects of exercise on neutrophil counts or function are different in trained and untrained children (Boas *et al.* 1996; Wolach *et al.* 1998a,b). Another approach to determine whether training status impacts the neutrophil response to acute exercise is to measure exercise-induced changes in neutrophils before and after a prescribed exercise program. With this approach, Shore and Shephard (1998) found that 12 weeks of exercise training in healthy children did not influence the acute increase in, or the post-exercise recovery of, neutrophil counts in response to 30 min of cycling. Collectively, the available data do not support the notion that training status modifies the neutrophil response to acute exercise.

Natural killer cells

There is some evidence that training status can modify the responses of NK cell counts and function (i.e., cytotoxicity) to acute exercise. Greater increases in NK cells in response to a 30-s Wingate anaerobic test (WAnT) have been reported for male swimmers vs. non-swimmers (Boas *et al.* 1996). The increase in NK cell cytotoxicity immediately after exercise was also greatest in the male swimmers (Boas *et al.* 1996). At 1 h post-exercise, NK cell cytotoxicity returned to normal levels in the swimmers, but declined below pre-exercise values in the non-swimmers. In contrast, training-related differences in the acute NK cell response to a WAnT between female gymnasts and healthy female controls were not detected (Wolach *et al.* 1998b). Nor did this same research group find differences in NK cell counts between the same groups of subjects in response to a 20-min submaximal treadmill run (Eliakim *et al.* 1997). Consistent with the latter observations, short-term training-induced alterations in the response of NK cell counts to acute exercise were not found (Shore & Shephard 1998). These authors did, however, find that training reduced stimulated NK cell cytotoxicity during recovery from acute exercise (Shore & Shephard 1998), which is contradictory to the findings of Boas *et al.* (1996). Given the mixture of subjects (males vs. females), training history (swimming vs. gymnastics), exercise mode, intensity and duration, and other uncontrolled factors (e.g., diet), it is difficult to draw firm conclusions as to whether training status truly affects the NK cell response to acute exercise in youth. This issue is also clouded in the adult literature by differences among study designs and inconsistent results. Cross-sectional studies comparing trained and untrained adults, for example, have shown that training status does (Kendall *et al.* 1990) and does not (Hong *et al.* 2005) influence the NK cell response to acute exercise. Longitudinal studies (i.e., the same subject tested before and after an exercise training intervention) have reported that responses post-training are larger than the pretraining response to exercise performed at the same relative intensity (Rhind *et al.* 1996).

Training status and immune function at rest

Numerous studies from the adult literature have compared resting immune function in trained and untrained individuals. The general consensus among experts is that the immune system of a trained individual is more similar than dissimilar to that of an untrained individual (Nieman 1996; Shephard 1997; Mackinnon 1999). Although there are few pure pediatric data regarding training and immune function, Table 25.1 provides some comparisons of resting immune status in athletic and non-athletic youth.

Salivary immunoglobulin A

Among young athletes, resting sIgA levels do not seem to be affected by periods of training in young gymnasts (Filaire *et al.* 2004) or tennis players (Novas *et al.* 2003).

Table 25.1 Comparison of immune status in trained and untrained children and adolescents.

Subjects	Sex	Age	Trained vs. untrained comparison	Reference
Neutrophil count				
16 swimmers	M	9.1–17.1	23% lower in swimmers*	Boas *et al.* (1996)
17 non-swimmers	M	9.0–17.0		
7 gymnasts	F	10–12	32% lower in gymnasts	Wolach *et al.* (1998a)
6 controls	F	10–12		
40 swimmers	M/F	12–16	13% lower in swimmers	Santos-Silva *et al.* (2001)
42 controls				
10 healthy children				
Pre-training	M/F	10.3	17% lower following training	Shore & Shephard (1998)
Post-training				
Neutrophil bactericidal activity				
7 gymnasts	F	10–12	32% lower in gymnasts*	Wolach *et al.* (1998a)
6 controls	F	10–12		
Plasma elastase (marker of neutrophil activation)				
40 swimmers	M/F	12–16	63% higher in swimmers*	Santos-Silva *et al.* (2001)
42 controls				
NK cell count				
16 swimmers	M	9.1–17.1	80% lower in swimmers	Boas *et al.* (1996)
17 non-swimmers	M	9.0–17.0		
7 gymnasts	F	10–12	30% higher in gymnasts	Eliakim *et al.* (1997)
6 controls	F	10–12		
11 healthy children				
Pre-training	M/F	10.3	7% lower following training	Shore & Shephard (1998)
Post-training				
NK cell activity				
16 swimmers	M	9.1–17.1	61% lower in swimmers	Boas *et al.* (1996)
17 non-swimmers	M	9.0–17.0		
11 healthy children				
Pre-training	M/F	10.3	43% lower following training	Shore & Shephard (1998)
Post-training				

NK, natural killer.

* Indicates significant difference in trained and untrained comparison, $P < 0.05$.

Neutrophils

One consistent finding among adults seems to be that despite normal neutrophil counts, neutrophil function tends to be lower in athletes than in non-athletes (Nieman 1996; Mackinnon 1999) Smith *et al.* (1990) proposed that this downregulation of neutrophil status may be protective against perpetual chronic inflammation as a result of exercise-induced muscle damage. In children and adolescents, evidence of a training effect on neutrophil function is mixed. While neutrophil cell counts at rest are consistently lower in the trained vs. untrained state (Table 25.1), only one study (Boas *et al.* 1996) found this difference to be statistically significant.

An alternative, indirect approach to the issue of neutrophil status and training status is to identify a statistical correlation between one's resting neutrophil cell count and their maximal aerobic fitness ($\dot{V}O_{2max}$). In this regard, individuals with a higher $\dot{V}O_{2max}$ should also display a lower neutrophil cell count. Based on the data taken from a number of pediatric studies (Shore & Shephard 1998; Boas *et al.* 2000; Nieman *et al.* 2000, 2002; Nemet *et al.* 2003, 2004; Timmons *et al.* 2004a, 2006b), there is little evidence for an association between resting neutrophil cell counts and aerobic fitness in children and adolescents (Fig. 25.4), which is consistent with the conclusion of Nieman *et al.* (2002). Unfortunately, meaningful

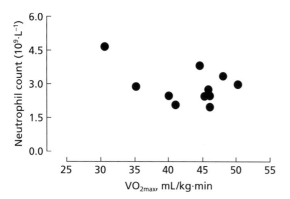

Fig. 25.4 Relationship between resting neutrophil counts and maximal aerobic fitness ($\dot{V}O_{2max}$) in children and adolescents. Each point represents the mean value from one study. Data from Shore & Shephard (1998), Boas *et al.* (2000), Nieman *et al.* (2000), Nieman *et al.* (2002), Nemet *et al.* (2003), Nemet *et al.* (2004), Timmons *et al.* (2004a, 2006b).

insight into whether neutrophil function per se is depressed in the young athlete is lacking because of an insufficient number of studies. Depending on the particular aspect of functional activity assessed, plasma elastase levels can be higher (Santos-Silva *et al.* 2001), bactericidal activity can be lower (Wolach *et al.* 1998a), and chemotaxis (Wolach *et al.* 1998a), along with other markers of cellular activation (Santos-Silva *et al.* 2001), can be similar in the trained vs. untrained state. In light of the antagonism between inflammation and growth (Zoico & Roubenoff 2002), it will be of extreme interest to elucidate further the biologic significance of training-induced alterations in neutrophil status and their potential relationship to exercise-induced muscle damage in the young athlete.

Natural killer cells

Based on the adult literature, NK cell cytotoxicity tends to be higher in athletes compared with non-athletes (Nieman 1996; Mackinnon 1999). Similar training-related differences in NK cell function at rest have not been identified among young swimmers and non-swimmers (Boas *et al.* 1996). Unfortunately, there are no other data to address the issue of chronic exercise training effects on basal NK cell function in children. Short-term (12 weeks) training of healthy but non-athletic children does not significantly influence NK cell counts or cytotoxicity at rest, although post-training cytotoxicity values were non-significantly reduced by 43% compared to pre-training levels (Shore & Shephard 1998). While there is some indirect evidence that resting NK cell counts are positively correlated with $\dot{V}O_{2max}$ when single studies are compiled, other studies have not directly demonstrated such a relationship. Based on the available pediatric data, one must conclude that resting NK cell status of the young athlete is no different from that of their untrained peer.

Relationship between risk of infection and physical activity

The relationship between risk of infection and PA has been of interest for several years. From the adult literature, a J-curve hypothesis of PA and infection risk has been proposed; whereas high intensity, large volume exercise is believed to reduce immune function, and thereby increase the risk of infection, moderate intensities and volumes of activity are believed to enhance immune function, and thereby reduce the risk of infection (Heath *et al.* 1992). Whether a similar relationship exists in children is unclear, as only a few studies have investigated the relationship between risk of infection and PA in youth.

Early studies found that pneumonia at a boy's school occurred most often in athletes (Cowles 1918) and that the risks of enteroviral illness during an outbreak and of the development of aseptic meningitis were greater in members of a high school football team than in the rest of the student population (Baron *et al.* 1982). However, most (Waku *et al.* 1998; Jedrychowski *et al.* 2001; Cieslak *et al.* 2003; Klentrou *et al.* 2003) but not all (Osterback & Qvarnberg 1987) recent studies also find that the incidence of upper respiratory tract infections (URTIs) is inversely associated with PA among children and adolescents. For example, Klentrou *et al.* (2003) found that participation in PA for more than 10 h·week^{-1} vs. less than 10 h·week^{-1} or for more than 3 h/·day^{-1} vs. less than 3 h·day^{-1} (Cieslak *et al.* 2003) was associated with an approximate threefold lower incidence of URTI. In one of these studies (Klentrou *et al.* 2003), the apparent protection of PA against URTI incidence was restricted to male children and was not observed in females.

While these studies are encouraging because they suggest that an active lifestyle protects children from URTIs, they should be interpreted with caution because of the inherent difficulty in accurately measuring PA and because the URTIs were self-reported. To illustrate this conundrum, a J-curve relationship between total daily energy expenditure, assessed by questionnaire, and a URTI symptom index has been reported among young elite female tennis players (Novas *et al.* 2002), suggesting an opposite effect to the findings of Klentrou *et al.* in so far as the most active youngsters experienced the greatest incidence of URTI. In line with this work, a study of over 700 10- to 17-year-old boys and girls (Waku *et al.* 1998) found that the incidence of some symptoms (e.g., sore throat, runny nose, and abdominal pain) were lower in a moderate activity group (3–4 days of sporting activities per week) compared with the control group (no sporting activities). The incidence of

other symptoms (e.g., common cold, cough/sputum, and fever) were higher in the moderate and the highest activity group (>5 days of sporting activities per week), compared with the control group, with no differences for any symptoms between boys and girls. Notwithstanding several studies documenting a protective effect of moderate amounts of PA against the incidence of URTIs, Osterback and Qvarnberg (1987) did not find differences in respiratory infections between children participating in sports and control children over a 12-month period. Given the contrasting findings of the above studies, it is difficult to provide valid interpretation of the results. However, the weight of the evidence would appear to favor a lower risk of URTIs in active children, although the optimal volume and intensity of exercise to achieve this protection is unknown.

Any association between risk of infection and PA might imply a coincident association between immune function and PA. Of the numerous immunologic factors investigated, only sIgA seems to be related to the risk of URTIs in adult athletes (Gleeson 2000). Importantly, a link between depressed sIgA levels and risk of URTI among adult athletes *during* a training season has been demonstrated (Gleeson *et al.* 1999). Among young non-athletic children, resting sIgA levels are not related to PA level (Cieslak *et al.* 2003). In line with these findings, resting sIgA status was not correlated with aerobic fitness (i.e., $\dot{V}o_{2max}$) in a group of untrained children and adolescents (Nieman *et al.* 2002). Repeatedly depressed sIgA levels because of regular bouts of acute exercise may have particular relevance for the young athlete's susceptibility to respiratory infection. This possibility was highlighted when young female tennis players with the greatest exercise-induced reduction in sIgA secretion rate, but not concentration, also had the highest incidence of URTIs (Novas *et al.* 2003). However, this latter study included subjects up to the age of 21 years and therefore cannot be specifically considered to be a pediatric study.

Practical considerations

Team physicians, athletic therapists, and coaches might be called upon to provide advice on whether children and adolescents who are ill should maintain their physical activity routines or what strategies can be implemented to maintain optimal immune health in the face of repeated physiologic stress. Parents of children recovering from a disease (e.g., cancer) may also wonder when is a good time to reintroduce sports participation into their child's life. At present, health care professionals must rely on common sense and some sparse guidelines based solely on the adult literature (Noffsinger 1996) to help navigate through the above issues. Based on our understanding of immune changes in response to exercise performed with and without nutritional supplements, the impact of exercise training on resting immune status, and some historical data, the following sections address some practical considerations for the young athlete.

Nutritional options

In recent years, a large volume of adult research has searched for nutritional strategies to overcome the potentially negative effects of chronic high volume exercise training on immune function and boost resistance to infection (Nieman & Pedersen 2000). Of the many investigated options, few have shown any substantial promise. One of these, vitamin C supplementation, is associated with a lower incidence of URTI during heavy PA in adults (Peters 2000). Among children attending ski schools, vitamin C supplementation (1000 mg·day^{-1}) for 7–9 days was also associated with a reduced incidence of respiratory infections (Bessel-Lorck 1959; Ritzel 1961). This magnitude of vitamin C intake is ~22-fold greater than the current recommended dietary allowance for 9- to 13-year-old children (45 mg·day^{-1}), and is just below the daily tolerable upper intake level (1200 mg) for this same age group (Dietary Reference Intakes 2000). However, given the potential of vitamin C to reduce the incidence of URTI in active children, it would seem prudent to determine whether intakes closer to the recommended dietary allowance would safely reduce the incidence of URTI among young athletes.

Considerable research attention has also focused on carbohydrate (CHO) supplementation, which—when provided in the form of a sports drink during exercise—attenuates the rise in cell number and function and, following exercise, tends to speed the recovery of cells to their pre-exercise concentration

(Nieman 1998). The effects of CHO supplementation, compared with water intake, are generally comparable in children and adolescents to those reported in adults, with some important exceptions (Timmons et al. 2004a). The innate immune system seems to be more sensitive to CHO intake in children than in adults. Attenuation of NK cells was observed following 60 min of exercise in boys, but not in men (Timmons et al. 2004a). In 12-year-old boys (Timmons et al. 2006a) and girls (Timmons et al. 2004b), CHO can blunt the increase in NK cells after 30 min of exercise. Although it has been argued that exercise must be of high intensity (~75–80% $\dot{V}o_{2max}$) and prolonged duration (>2 h) in order to demonstrate an effect of CHO intake (Nieman 2000), this is clearly not the case in children. Likewise, recovery neutrophilia is completely abolished with CHO intake in children compared with adults (Timmons et al. 2004a). In essence, the extra energy provided during exercise minimizes the disruption to immune homeostasis. Unlike vitamin C, however, the acute effects of CHO intake on perturbations to NK cells and other markers of immunity have not yet been linked to a long-term reduction in the incidence of URTI in either children or adults.

Preventing transmissible infections/vaccination

Sports participation—especially with close person–person contact—holds the risk to obtain transmissible infections (Beck 2000). Thus, appropriate medical care must be provided for all athletes with transmissible diseases, including herpes simplex virus, to cure the disease whenever possible. The return-to-sports decision should not only be based on the risk an athlete takes, but must also take into account whether he or she may still be contagious. Furthermore, medical care providers must also check the immunization status of an athlete and—if appropriate—complete missing vaccinations (i.e., against transmissible diseases such as measles, chickenpox, hepatitis B, and against diseases associated with injuries to the skin such as tetanus). A yearly vaccination against influenza has been advocated in athletes by some authors (Beck 2000; Constantini et al. 2001). For athletes traveling to countries with a high prevalence of hepatitis A, a respective immunization may be reasonable.

The young athlete with an infection

Notwithstanding the potential impairment in exercise performance during viral infection (Friman & Ilback 1998), the overall health of the young athlete may be compromised if intense exercise training continues during an infection. From a historical perspective, it was noted that following intense exercise and competitive sport, respiratory infections tended to progress toward pneumonia in boys (Cowles 1918). Moreover, intense PA at the onset of paralytic poliomyelitis in children has been associated with greater severity of disease in a number of studies (Hargreaves 1948; Russell 1949; Horstmann 1950). Acute infectious episodes may also cause increased protein degradation and a temporary negative nitrogen balance (Friman & Ilback 1998). These consequences combined with the energy demands of physical training have obvious implications for growing children. In these cases, children who continue to train during advanced stages of infection may demonstrate a temporary loss of lean muscle tissue. Such scenarios, although unlikely to have long-term detrimental effects, can be easily avoided by complete rest until symptoms resolve. Another example of a potential health implication is if a child exercises and trains with an elevated core body temperature, due to fever. This practice may place added stress on their capacity to thermoregulate efficiently during exercise, particularly in the heat. It is well documented that children are less efficient at thermoregulating under conditions of high heat stress than adults (see Chapter 20). Moreover, for a given level of dehydration, children tend to have a greater rise in core body temperature than adults (Bar-Or et al. 1980). Collectively, these observations suggest that a young athlete who decides to exercise in the heat under febrile conditions could very well increase their risk of heat-related illness.

An athlete's exercise performance is generally reduced during acute illness, and there is some evidence for this in the pediatric age range (Roberts 1985). Whether the impairment in exercise performance is because of true disturbances in energy metabolism and muscle function or because of a reduced psychologic motivation is difficult to ascertain. It would be unethical to experimentally induce illness in the young athlete in order to investigate performance.

However, it might be constructive to determine retrospectively whether decrements in performance can be linked to illness in the young athlete, notwithstanding the methodologic problems with this approach.

Among the general guidelines prepared for adult athletes, most authorities agree upon a "head-and-neck" rule whereby symptoms restricted to above the neck (e.g., common cold, runny nose) should not pose major threats to the individual and that exercise training may continue, albeit at a reduced rate (Roberts 1986; Nieman 1996; Mackinnon 1999). Signs and symptoms of systemic involvement (e.g., fever, body aches) should be taken more seriously, with all PA discontinued. The amount of recovery time necessary before resuming a normal training schedule depends on the severity of the preceding symptoms and any other complications. Unfortunately, recent systematic analyses of responses to exercise after an infection are not available. In the 1960s, Klimt studied the cardiovascular responses to submaximal exercise in previously healthy children recovering from various infectious diseases (summarized in Klimt 1985). He found that exercise responses had normalized after about 4–6 weeks following enteritis, urinary tract infection, and pneumonia, and 8 weeks following URTI. Recovery could require more than 3 months after severe bacterial meningitis. Because of the long periods of immobilization which were part of the medical therapy in those days, the data may not be applicable to young athletes today. For adult athletes, most recommendations regarding return to full training range from 2 weeks (Heath et al. 1992) to 1 month (Roberts 1986). At present, there are no data that would specifically contraindicate the application of these guidelines to the young athlete. If anything, adult guidelines may be over-protective given the overall smaller exercise-induced perturbation to many aspects of the immune system and faster recovery of immune status following exercise in children. However, it is essential that the team physician or family doctor should be consulted and provide consent before the young athlete resumes training and competition.

Children with a disease involving the immune system

Perhaps the most common immune-related disease

among young athletes is bronchial asthma (see Chapter 26). Participation in sport following recovery from other immune-related diseases also deserves some practical considerations. This author has received testimonials that a continued schedule of regular PA during cancer treatment has helped children to beat their disease but empirical evidence for such benefits of exercise is absent. Theoretically, moderate amounts of exercise may help to "boost" the immune system of cancer patients, in particular those with leukemia, and might even improve efficiency of drug–cell interactions, given the cellular mobilization in response to acute exercise. In children with acute lymphoblastic leukemia (ALL), the effects of exercise on the immune system during maintenance chemotherapy (i.e., following induction of remission) have been investigated (Shore & Shephard 1999; Ladha *et al.* 2005). In general, the pattern, magnitude, and direction of exercise-induced leukocytosis are similar between children with ALL and otherwise healthy children. Figure 25.5 depicts acute changes in neutrophil counts in response to 30 min of high intensity cycling in ALL patients and healthy children. To evaluate further the interaction between exercise and the immune system in ALL patients, Shore and Shephard (1999) recruited three patients to exercise train for 12 weeks. Following the training period, many of the measured immune parameters were actually lower than pre-training levels, but none of the differences were statistically significant. One encouraging finding was that NK cell cytotoxicity was nonsignificantly enhanced by ~132%. Although many aspects of this study could have been improved, including the number of subjects, timing of blood sampling relative to administration of chemotherapy, and multiple blood samples to assess "resting" immune function, it is clear that survivors of ALL and cancer in general should be monitored on an individual basis when recommencing regimens of PA.

Challenges for future research

Based on the content of this chapter, the reader should be quite aware that the necessity for studying exercise immunology in active children is immense. Extrapolation of guidelines and principles from the adult literature may not be accurate or even appropriate

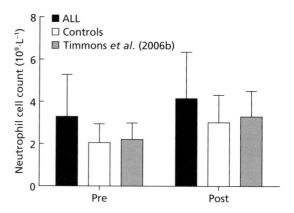

Fig. 25.5 Neutrophil response to 30 min of cycling at 70% $\dot{V}o_{2max}$ in healthy children and children with acute lymphoblastic leukemia (ALL) receiving maintenance chemotherapy. Data are redrawn from Ladha *et al.* (2005) and Timmons *et al.* (2006b).

for the growing athlete. The following list outlines questions for possible areas of future research.

• Are there child–adult differences in the magnitude of exercise-induced changes in salivary immunity, and are these changes predictive of subsequent URTI incidence?

• What impact do puberty and gender have on acute immune changes in response to exercise, and do these factors modify the relationship between risk of infection and PA?

• Does chronic exercise training improve resting immune status in children and adolescents?

• Does exercise training *during* childhood vaccination impact the adequacy and efficiency of the vaccination?

• What nutritional strategies can be offered to the young athlete to maintain immunocompetence during periods of intensive training and competition?

• Compared with adults, are child athletes at greater risk of health complications from training and competing during an infection?

• Can regular exercise be used as a tool to "boost" the immune system of children with cystic fibrosis or those recovering from cancer?

Acknowledgment

B.W. Timmons is supported by a Canadian Institutes of Health Research Industry-partnered (Gatorade Sports Science Institute) Postdoctoral Fellowship.

References

Arnett, M.G., Hyslop, R., Dennehy, C.A. & Schneider, C.M. (2000) Age-related variations of serum CK and CK MB response in females. *Canadian Journal of Applied Physiology* **25**, 419–429.

Bar-Or, O., Dotan, R., Inbar, O., Rotshtein, A. & Zonder, H. (1980) Voluntary hypohydration in 10- to 12-year-old boys. *Journal of Applied Physiology* **48**, 104–108.

Baron, R.C., Hatch, M.H., Kleeman, K. & MacCormack, J.N. (1982) Aseptic meningitis among members of a high school football team: An outbreak associated with echovirus 16 infection. *Journal of the American Medical Association* **248**, 1724–1727.

Beck, C.K. (2000) Infectious diseases in sports. *Medicine and Science in Sports and Exercise* **32** (Supplement), S431–S438.

Bessel-Lorck, C. (1959) Common cold prophylaxis in young people at a ski camp [in German]. *Medizinische* **44**, 2126–2127.

Biron, C.A., Nguyen, K.B., Pien, G.C., Cousens, L.P. & Salazar-Mather, T.P. (1999) Natural killer cells in antiviral defense: Function and regulation by innate cytokines. *Annual Review of Immunology* **17**, 189–220.

Boas, S.R., Danduran, M.J., McColley, S.A., Beaman, K. & O'Gorman, M.R. (2000) Immune modulation following aerobic exercise in children with cystic fibrosis. *International Journal of Sports Medicine* **21**, 294–301.

Boas, S.R., Joswiak, M.L., Nixon, P.A., *et al.* (1996) Effects of anaerobic exercise on the immune system in eight- to seventeen-year-old trained and untrained boys. *Journal of Pediatrics* **129**, 846–855.

Brittenden, J., Heys, S.D., Ross, J. & Eremin, O. (1996) Natural killer cells and cancer. *Cancer* **77**, 1226–1243.

Cieslak, T.J., Frost, G. & Klentrou, P. (2003) Effect of physical activity, body fat and salivary cortisol on mucosal immunity in children. *Journal of Applied Physiology* **95**, 2315–2320.

Constantini, N., Ken-Dror, A., Eliakim, A., *et al.* (2001) Vaccinations in sports and recommendations for immunization against flu, hepatitis A and hepatitis B. *Harefuah* **140**, 1191–1195.

Cowles, W.N. (1918) Fatigue as a contributory cause of pneumonias. *Boston Medical and Surgical Journal* **179**, 555–556.

Dietary Reference Intakes (2000) *Vitamin C, Vitamin E, Selenium, and Carotenoids.*

A Report of the Panel on Dietary Antioxidants and Related Compounds, Subcommittees on Upper Reference Levels of Nutrients and Interpretation and Uses of Dietary Reference Intakes, and the Standing Committee on the Scientific Evaluation of Dietary Reference Intakes, Food and Nutrition Board, Institute of Medicine. National Academy Press, Washington, DC.

Dorrington, M., Gleeson, M. & Callister, R. (2003) Effect of exercise intensity on salivary IgA in children. *Journal of Science and Medicine in Sport* **6**, 46.

Eliakim, A., Wolach, B., Kodesh, E., *et al.* (1997) Cellular and humoral immune response to exercise among gymnasts and untrained girls. *International Journal of Sports Medicine* **18**, 208–212.

Filaire, E., Bonis, J. & Lac, G. (2004) Relationships between physiological and psychological stress and salivary immunoglobulin A among young female gymnasts. *Perceptual and Motor Skills* **99**, 605–617.

Friman, G. & Ilback, N.G. (1998) Acute infection: metabolic responses, effects on performance, interaction with exercise, and myocarditis. *International Journal of Sports Medicine* **19** (Supplement 3), S172–S182.

Galal, O. (1989) [Lymphocytic beta-2-adrenergic receptor density and function in children]. *Monatsschrift fur Kinderheilkunde* **137**, 213–217.

Gleeson, M. (2000) Mucosal immune responses and risk of respiratory illness in elite athletes. *Exercise Immunology Review* **6**, 5–42.

Gleeson, M., McDonald, W.A., Pyne, D.B., *et al.* (1999) Salivary IgA levels and infection risk in elite swimmers. *Medicine and Science in Sports and Exercise* **31**, 67–73.

Hargreaves, E.R. (1948) Poliomyelitis: Effect of exertion during the pre-paralytic stage. *British Medical Journal* **ii**, 1021–1022.

Heath, G.W., Macera, C.A. & Nieman, D.C. (1992) Exercise and upper respiratory tract infections. Is there a relationship? *Sports Medicine* **14**, 353–365.

Hong, S., Johnson, T.A., Farag, N.H., *et al.* (2005) Attenuation of T-lymphocyte demargination and adhesion molecule expression in response to moderate exercise in physically fit individuals. *Journal of Applied Physiology* **98**, 1057–1063.

Horstmann, D.M. (1950) Acute poliomyelitis: Relation of physical activity at the time of onset to the course of the disease. *Journal of the American Medical Association* **142**, 236–241.

Jedrychowski, W., Maugeri, U., Flak, E., Mroz, E. & Bianchi, I. (2001) Cohort study on low physical activity level and recurrent acute respiratory infections in schoolchildren. *Central European Journal of Public Health* **9**, 126–129.

Kendall, A., Hoffman-Goetz, L., Houston, M., MacNeil, B. & Arumugam, Y. (1990) Exercise and blood lymphocyte subset responses: intensity, duration, and subject fitness effects. *Journal of Applied Physiology* **69**, 251–260.

Klentrou, P., Hay, J. & Plyley, M. (2003) Habitual physical activity levels and health outcomes of Ontario youth. *European Journal of Applied Physiology* **89**, 460–465.

Klimt, F. (1985) Infektionserkrankungen. In: *Freistellung vom Sport in Schule und Verein* (Klimt, F., ed.) Thieme Verlag, Stuttgart: 71–85.

Ladha, A.B., Courneya, K.S., Grundy, P., Field, C.J., Robertson, M. & Cuvelier, G.D.E. (2005) Effect of acute exercise on neutrophils in children receiving maintenance treatment for acute lymphblstic leukemia. *Medicine and Science in Sports and Exercise* **37**, S201.

Mackinnon, L.T. (1999) *Advances in Exercise Immunology.* Human Kinetics, Champaign, IL.

Marginson, V., Rowlands, A.V., Gleeson, N.P. & Eston, R.G. (2005) Comparison of the symptoms of exercise-induced muscle damage after an initial and repeated bout of plyometric exercise in men and boys. *Journal of Applied Physiology* **99**, 1174–1181.

Nemet, D., Mills, P.J. & Cooper, D.M. (2004) Effect of intense wrestling exercise on leucocytes and adhesion molecules in adolescent boys. *British Journal of Sports Medicine* **38**, 154–158.

Nemet, D., Rose-Gottron, C.M., Mills, P.J. & Cooper, D.M. (2003) Effect of water polo practice on cytokines, growth mediators, and leukocytes in girls. *Medicine and Science in Sports and Exercise* **35**, 356–363.

Nieman, D.C. (1996) Prolonged aerobic exercise, immune response, and risk of infection. In: *Exercise and Immune Function* (Hoffman-Goetz, L., ed.) CRC Press, Boca Raton, FL: 143–161.

Nieman, D.C. (1998) Influence of carbohydrate on the immune response to intensive, prolonged exercise. *Exercise Immunology Review* **4**, 64–76.

Nieman, D.C. (2000) Carbohydrates and the immune response to prolonged exertion. In: *Nutrition and Exercise Immunology* (Nieman, D.C. & Pedersen, B.K., eds.) CRC Press, Boca Raton, FL: 25–42.

Nieman, D.C., Henson, D.A., Fagoaga, O.R., Nehlsen-Cannarella, S.L., Sonnenfeld, G. & Utter, A.C. (2002) Influence of skinfold sum and peak VO_2 on immune function in children. *International Journal of Obesity and Related Metabolic Disorders* **26**, 822–829.

Nieman, D.C., Kernodle, M.W., Henson, D.A., Sonnenfeld, G. & Morton, D.S. (2000) The acute response of the immune system to tennis drills in adolescent athletes. *Research Quarterly for Exercise and Sport* **71**, 403–408.

Nieman, D.C. & Pedersen, B.K. (1999) Exercise and immune function. Recent developments. *Sports Medicine* **27**, 73–80.

Nieman, D.C. & Pedersen, B.K. (2000) *Nutrition and Exercise Immunology*. CRC Press, Boca Raton, FL.

Noffsinger, J. (1996) Physical activity considerations in children and adolescents with viral infections. *Pediatric Annals* **25**, 585–589.

Novas, A.M.P., Rowbottom, D.G. & Jenkins, D.G. (2002) Total daily energy expenditure and incidence of upper respiratory tract infection symptoms in young females. *International Journal of Sports Medicine* **23**, 465–470.

Novas, A.M.P., Rowbottom, D.G. & Jenkins, D.G. (2003) Tennis, incidence of URTI and salivary IgA. *International Journal of Sports Medicine* **24**, 223–229.

Osterback, L. & Qvarnberg, Y. (1987) A prospective study of respiratory infections in 12-year-old children actively engaged in sports. *Acta Physiologica Scandinavica* **76**, 944–949.

Pedersen, B.K. & Hoffman-Goetz, L. (2000) Exercise and the immune system: regulation, integration, and adaptation. *Physiological Review* **80**, 1055–1081.

Perez, C.J., Nemet, D., Mills, P.J., Scheet, T.P., Ziegler, M.G. & Cooper, D.M. (2001) Effects of laboratory versus field exercise on leukocyte subsets and cell adhesion molecule expression in children. *European Journal of Applied Physiology* **86**, 34–39.

Peters, E.M. (2000) Vitamins, immunity, and infection risk in athletes. In: *Nutrition and Exercise Immunology* (Nieman, D.C. & Pedersen, B.K., eds.) CRC Press, Boca Raton, FL: 109–135.

Reinhardt, D., Zehmisch, T., Becker, B. & Nagel-Hiemke, M. (1984) Age-dependency of alpha- and beta-adrenoceptors on thrombocytes and lymphocytes of asthmatic and nonasthmatic children. *European Journal of Pediatrics* **142**, 111–116.

Rhind, S.G., Shek, P.N., Shinkai, S. & Shephard, R.J. (1996) Effects of moderate endurance exercise and training on *in vitro* lymphocyte proliferation, interleukin-2 (IL-2) production, and IL-2 receptor expression. *European Journal of Applied Physiology and Occupational Physiology* **74**, 348–360.

Ritzel, G. (1961) Critical analysis of the role of vitamin C in the prophylaxis and treatment of the common cold [in German]. *Helvetica Medica Acta* **28**, 63–68.

Roberts, J.A. (1985) Loss of form in young athletes due to viral infection. *British Medical Journal* **290**, 357–358.

Roberts, J.A. (1986) Viral illnesses and sports performance. *Sports Medicine* **3**, 298–303.

Russell, W.R. (1949) Paralytic poliomyelitis: The early symptoms and the effect of physical activity on the course of the disease. *British Medical Journal* **i**, 465–471.

Santos-Silva, A., Rebelo, M.I., Castro, E.M.B., *et al.* (2001) Leukocyte activation, erythrocyte damage, lipid profile and oxidative stress imposed by high competition physical exercise in adolescents. *Clinica Chimica Acta* **306**, 119–126.

Shephard, R.J. (1997) *Physical Activity, Training and the Immune Response*. Cooper, Carmel, IN.

Shore, S. & Shephard, R.J. (1998) Immune responses to exercise and training: A comparison of children and young adults. *Pediatric Exercise Science* **10**, 210–226.

Shore, S. & Shephard, R.J. (1999) Immune responses to exercise in children treated for cancer. *Journal of Sports Medicine and Physical Fitness* **39**, 240–243.

Smith, J.A., Telford, R.D., Mason, I.B. & Weidemann, M.J. (1990) Exercise, training and neutrophil microbicidal activity. *International Journal Sports Medicine* **11**, 179–187.

Soares, J.M., Mota, P., Duarte, J.A. & Appell, H.J. (1996) Children are less susceptible to exercise-induced muscle damage than adults: A preliminary investigation. *Pediatric Exercise Science* **8**, 361–367.

Tharp, G.D. (1991) Basketball exercise and secretory immunoglobulin A. *European Journal of Applied Physiology* **63**, 312–314.

Timmons, B.W., Tarnopolsky, M.A. & Bar-Or, O. (2004a) Immune responses to strenuous exercise and carbohydrate intake in boys and men. *Pediatric Research* **56**, 227–234.

Timmons, B.W., Tarnopolsky, M.A., Snider, D.P. & Bar-Or, O. (2004b) Effects of carbohydrate intake and exercise on circulating natural killer cell phenotypes in 12-yr-old girls. *Canadian Journal of Applied Physiology* **29**, S88.

Timmons, B.W., Tarnopolsky, M.A., Snider, D.P. & Bar-Or, O. (2006a) Puberty effects on NK cell responses to exercise and carbohydrate intake in boys. *Medicine and Science in Sports and Exercise* **38**, 864–874.

Timmons, B.W., Tarnopolsky, M.A., Snider, D.P. & Bar-Or, O. (2006b) Immunological changes in response to exercise: influence of age, puberty, and gender. *Medicine and Science in Sports and Exercise* **38**, 293–304.

Waku, T., Ito, S., Nagatomi, R., Akama, T. & Kono, I. (1998) A prospective study of incidence of infections in 10–12 year old children actively engaged in sports. *Journal of Sports Science* **16**, 525–526.

Wolach, B., Eliakim, A., Gavrieli, R., *et al.* (1998a) Aspects of leukocyte function and the complement system following aerobic exercise in young female gymnasts. *Scandinanvian Journal of Medicine and Science in Sports* **8**, 91–97.

Wolach, B., Falk, B., Gavrieli, R., Kodesh, E. & Eliakim, A. (2000) Neutrophil function response to aerobic and anaerobic exercise in female judoka and untrained subjects. *British Journal of Sports Medicine* **34**, 23–28.

Wolach, B., Falk, B., Kodesh, E., *et al.* (1998b) Cellular immune response to anaerobic exercise among gymnasts and untrained girls. *Pediatric Exercise Science* **10**, 227–235.

Zoico, E. & Roubenoff, R. (2002) The role of cytokines in regulating protein metabolism and muscle function. *Nutrition Reviews* **60**, 39–51.

Chapter 26

Asthma and Sports

DAVID M. ORENSTEIN

Background and historical aspects

Highlights of the historical aspects of asthma are discussed in detail in several sources (McFadden & Ingram 1980; Sakula 1988). Briefly, the relationship between exercise and asthma was recognized at least as far back as the 2nd century AD, when Arateus the Cappadocian observed: "If from gymnastics or other exercise the breathing becomes labored, it is called asthma" (Ghary 1975). In the 17th century, Floyer also recognized exercise-induced asthma (EIA), and differentiated between types of exercise more and less likely to produce it (McFadden & Ingram 1980). The list of activities producing asthma had been modified somewhat by three centuries later (Fitch 1975) but our understanding of the mechanisms underlying EIA had not progressed much and would not do so until the early 1970s, when the role of water and heat loss from the airways began to be elucidated.

Epidemiology

Asthma is the most common chronic illness in childhood, currently affecting 5–15% of children (Gergen et al. 1988). It is increasing in prevalence in American (Akinbami & Schoendorf 2002) and Danish children (Thomsen 2004).

Asthma accounts for some 7.3 million days restricted to bed and 10.1 million days missed from school each year (Taylor & Newacheck 1992). Asthma causes reduced physical activity: 21% of children with asthma were active for less than 30 min·day^{-1}, compared to 9% of their non-asthmatic peers (Lang et al. 2004).

Most experts agree that the incidence of EIA in patients known to have asthma is close to 100%, given the appropriate exercise challenge (McFadden 1987). EIA is not restricted to patients with recognized asthma, as it has also been reported to occur in children with a history of croup (Loughlin & Taussig 1979), allergic rhinitis (Pierson et al. 1972), cystic fibrosis (Silverman et al. 1978), or bronchopulmonary dysplasia (Badger et al. 1987). Perhaps most importantly, EIA has been found to occur in children and adolescents without any other recognized abnormalities, including as many as 9% of high school (Hallstrand et al. 2002) and college athletes (Rice et al. 1985). EIA is especially common in elite cold weather sport competitors, occurring in as many as 50% of the 1998 US Olympic team's cross-country skiers (Wilber et al. 2000). It is also very common among competitive swimmers (Helenius & Haahtela 2000) and other endurance athletes (Helenius et al. 1997). It is considerably more common among these athletes than among their sedentary peers, when other possible contributory factors, such as atopy, are accounted for (Langdeau et al. 2000).

Exercise-induced asthma

Clinical course

EIA presents with cough, wheeze, chest tightness, chest pain, difficulty breathing, or any combination of these symptoms during exercise, or, much more characteristically, shortly following exercise, usually with resolution within 30–90 min. Symptoms may or may not reappear 4–8 h later. The symptoms are

349

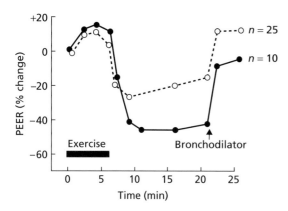

Fig. 26.1 Typical course of exercise-induced asthma in children (open circles) and adults (solid circles), assessed by measurements of peak expiratory flow rate (PEFR). Each point is the mean for the numbers of subjects indicated. Redrawn from Godfrey (1974).

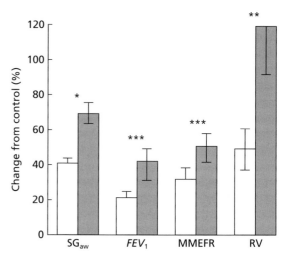

Fig. 26.2 Relative effects of exercise on lung functions while subjects were breathing air at ambient (open bars, $24.5 \pm 1.1°C$) and cold (shaded bars, $-13.5 \pm 2.6°C$) temperatures. The data are expressed as a percentage change from control values. The heights of the bars are mean values, and the vertical lines represent 1 SE of the mean. FEV_1, forced expiratory volume in 1 s; MMEFR, maximal mid-expiratory flow rate; RV, residual volume; SGaw, specific airway conductance. *, $P < 0.001$; **, $P < 0.01$; ***, $P < 0.05$. Redrawn from Strauss et al. (1977).

accompanied by pulmonary function abnormalities consistent with narrowing of intrathoracic airways. Typically, during the exercise session itself, there is little or no difficulty; in fact, expiratory airflows during exercise are actually increased above baseline in most people with asthma (Fig. 26.1) (Jones 1966).

Some authors have used the term exercise-induced bronchospasm (EIB) for this phenomenon. I have employed the term EIA throughout this chapter for two reasons. First, an informal survey of 51 recent articles from the medical literature on the topic revealed 37 that referred to EIA and only 14 that referred to EIB. Second, a more compelling reason is that the term "bronchospasm" may imply that the sole mechanism of airway narrowing is bronchial smooth muscle contraction, while the possible roles of airway inflammation and edema in addition to the smooth muscle contributions are more explicitly included in "asthma."

The exercise most likely to elicit the symptoms of EIA is typically short and intense: bouts 6–10 min long, at an intensity sufficient to raise the subject's heart rate to 80% of its maximum, are the most asthmagenic (Fitch 1975; Godfrey et al. 1975). Shorter sessions are less potent stimuli for EIA (Fitch 1975; Godfrey et al. 1975), and lower intensity exercise will not be as reliable in calling forth the asthmatic response (Fitch 1975, Godfrey et al. 1975). Longer

sessions will not worsen EIA, and may even lessen it—the "run-through" phenomenon (Fitch 1975; Godfrey et al. 1975). Extremely strenuous (supramaximal) brief exercise bouts may provide an even more potent stimulus for the production of EIA (Inbar et al. 1981).

Ambient conditions before, during, and after the exercise session influence the magnitude of the response. It has long been observed that cold air is more asthmagenic than warm air. Haas et al. (1986) cite Salter (1864) as having speculated in 1864 that EIA was caused by "the rapid passage of fresh and cold air over the bronchial mucous membrane." Within the past few decades, experimental evidence has supported the role of cold inspired air as a cause of EIA (Fig. 26.2) (Wells et al. 1960; Strauss et al. 1977; Sakula 1988). It also appears that dry air is more asthmagenic than humidified air (Fig. 26.3) (Bar-Or et al. 1977). Recently, it has been shown that the temperature of the air on the exercising subject's face might be as important as, or even more important

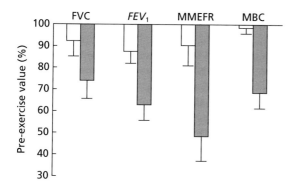

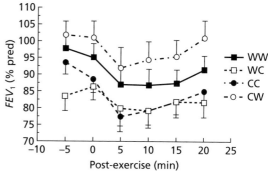

Fig. 26.3 Air humidity and exercise-induced asthma (EIA). Pulmonary functions of 10 6- to 14-year-old girls and boys measured 10 min after each of two treadmill walks. The children were free-breathing in a climatic chamber with air temperature of 25–26°C and humidity 25% ("dry") (open bars) or 90% ("humid") (shaded bars) relative humidity. FEV_1, forced expiratory volume in 1 s; FVC, forced vital capacity; MBC, maximal breathing capacity; MMEFR, maximal mid-expiratory flow rate. Vertical lines denote 1 SE of the mean. Redrawn from Bar-Or (1983). Data originally from Bar-Or *et al.* (1977).

Fig. 26.4 Forced expiratory volume in the 1 s (FEV_1) before and 0, 5, 10, 15, and 20 min after exercise for WW (inhaling warm, exposed to warm air), WC (inhaling warm, exposed to cold air), CC (inhaling cold, exposed to cold air), and CW (inhaling cold, exposed to warm air), as related to the inhaled air temperature and ambient air temperature. Data are presented as mean ± SEM. WC had significantly ($P < 0.001$) lower values than did the other three exposures, and CC was significantly ($P < 0.001$) lower than CW. Redrawn from Zeitoun *et al.* (2004).

than, the temperature of the inspired air (Fig. 26.4) (Zeitoun *et al.* 2004).

Not surprisingly, polluted air also worsens EIA: children who played sports in communities with high ozone levels were much more likely to develop asthma than those who played sports in areas of low ozone (McConnell *et al.* 2002).

The form of exercise seems to influence the amount of airway obstruction that follows it. Several studies in the 1970s suggested that the asthmagenicity of running was greater than cycling, which in turn was greater than arm exercise, and all of these greater than swimming, in inducing an asthmatic response (Fitch 1975). More recent studies indicate that if the volume, temperature, and humidity of the inspired air are held constant among the land-based challenges, the asthmatic response will be equal (Kilham *et al.* 1979). However, several studies have shown that swimming is less asthmagenic than treadmill running, even if minute ventilation and the temperature and humidity of the inspired air are controlled (Inbar *et al.* 1980), indicating that there must be factors other than airway heat and water flux that differentiate swimming from other forms of exercise in regard to initiating EIA (Fig. 26.5).

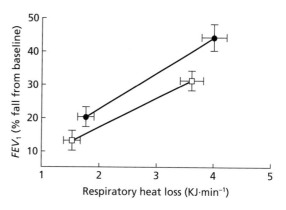

Fig. 26.5 The protective nature of swimming as a function of respiratory heat loss. Thirteen 9- to 17-year-old patients with asthma ran (closed circles) and swam (open squares) while inhaling either dry (8% relative humidity) or humid (98–100% relative humidity) air. Air temperature was 24.5°C and water temperature 31.6°C. Oxygen consumption and minute ventilation were equated in both activities. FEV_1 fall, post-exercise decrease as a percentage of pre-exercise forced expiratory volume in 1 s. Error bars represent SE of the mean. Redrawn from Bar-Or (1983); data from Bar-Yishay *et al.* (1982).

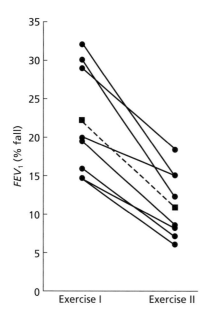

Fig. 26.6 Refractory period in exercise-induced asthma (EIA) showing a smaller decrease in forced expiratory volume in 1 s (FEV_1) after a second exercise challenge performed 60 min after the first challenge. Redrawn from Hamielec *et al.* (1988).

An interesting and important feature of EIA is referred to as the refractory period: a second bout of exercise performed within 1–2 h after the first exercise challenge causes much less airflow obstruction than the initial challenge (Fig. 26.6) (Edmunds *et al.* 1978). This phenomenon will be discussed at greater length in the next section.

Pathophysiology

Centuries after the initial recognition of EIA, there are still many unanswered questions about the pathophysiology of this phenomenon. However, recent work has helped to elucidate underlying mechanisms, and we now understand much more than we did just 20 years ago.

HEAT AND WATER EXCHANGE

It has long been observed that EIA is more likely and more severe in cold air. In the late 1970s and early 1980s, a number of investigators provided experimental evidence to support these observations, and to suggest that airway heat exchange has a central role in the production of EIA, even when the exercise is not in cold environments. Before reviewing these experiments, it is worth considering the mechanisms employed by the airways to condition inspired air (McFadden & Ingram 1979). Air that is cooler than body temperature and less than fully saturated with water vapor is warmed and humidified by transfer of heat and water from the airway mucosa. This heat transfer occurs partly by convection, and once the air is warmed its capacity to hold water increases, allowing for further heat transfer by evaporation from the airway mucosa (McFadden & Ingram 1979). Evaporation occurs even at 37°C, if the inspired air is less than fully saturated with water vapor. This process is usually completed in the upper airway but with large minute ventilation, as is required for vigorous exercise, the heat transfer capacity of the upper airways may be surpassed (particularly if the inspired air is cold and dry), and the heat transfer responsibilities are shared by the intrathoracic airways, perhaps as deep as the tenth generation of airways (McFadden 1987). The corollary of the exchange of heat to the inspired air is the loss of heat from the airways, and the resulting lower than normal temperatures deep within the lung. A temperature probe directly within the anterior segment of the right lower lobe in subjects breathing cold air (–9°C) during exercise has documented temperatures as low as 31°C, compared to 34.6°C at rest (Gilbert *et al.* 1988).

There is considerable evidence that this phenomenon of airway cooling associated with transfer of heat and water to large volumes of inspired air accounts for an important part of EIA. Chen and Horton (1977) showed that asthmatic subjects who exercised breathing warm humidified air had much less EIA than they did when they performed the same exercise breathing dry room air. Deal *et al.* (1979b) duplicated those findings. They then had the patients breathe volumes of cold air, at rest, equal to those they breathed during exercise, and showed a degree of airway obstruction following the hyperpnea equal to that which followed the exercise (Deal *et al.* 1979a). This response was abolished if the inspired air was warmed and

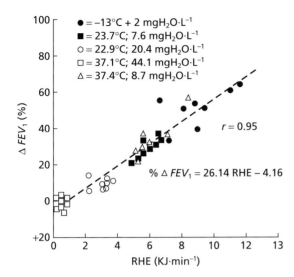

Fig. 26.7 Relationship between respiratory heat exchange (RHE) during exercise and post-exertional percentage change in forced expiratory volume in 1 s (% FEV_1). Redrawn from Deal *et al.* (1979a).

humidified (Deal *et al.* 1979a). These investigators illustrated a close correlation between total respiratory heat exchange and degree of airway obstruction (Fig. 26.7).

Heat exchange within the airways is important in the pathogenesis of EIA, but it is not clear how. In what ways are asthmatic airways different from normal airways in the response to heat flux? Aitken and Morini (1985) reported that both normal and asthmatic subjects experience a fall in airways conductance (which would be expected to cause a fall in expiratory airflow) when their airways extract heat from inspired air, but that the response of the asthmatic subjects 5–10 min afterwards is much greater than that in the normal subject. Furthermore, when heat is added to the airways (via inspiration of large volumes of hot air), the normal subjects increase airway conductance, while the asthmatic subjects show dramatic falls in conductance (Aitken & Morini 1985). As these authors point out, the response in normal airways is consistent with *in vitro* responses of airway smooth muscle strips, which relax (and have diminished constrictor responses to histamine) when warmed (Souhrada & Souhrada 1981). The different response in asthmatic airways is consistent

with McFadden's study that showed post-exercise bronchoconstriction to be related more to the speed and degree of airway rewarming than to the amount of heat loss during exercise (McFadden *et al.* 1986). Lemanske and Henke (1989) speculated that this phenomenon may be an airway analog of the reactive hyperemia seen in skin that is cooled and rapidly rewarmed, "if parallel events occurred in the bronchial vascular bed, engorgement and edema formation in the mucosa and submucosa would result . . . [and] compromise airflow."

It has been suggested that the water content of inspired air is more important than its temperature: "It is the osmotic and not the cooling effects induced by the vaporization of water that is the more important factor determining EIA" (Hahn *et al.* 1984a). The fact that some, but not all, diuretics, when inhaled as an aerosol, block EIA has suggested that electrolyte transport in the airways may somehow be involved in EIA, but the mechanisms are not yet clear (Bianco *et al.* 1988; O'Donnell *et al.* 1992).

MEDIATORS OF INFLAMMATION

One of the explanations for the route by which airway cooling or other exercise-related factors actually cause bronchoconstriction, airway edema, or both, is the elucidation of mediators of inflammation, such as histamine, neutrophil chemotactic factor (NCF—currently labeled interleukin-8, IL-8), and various leukotrienes (Lee *et al.* 1983a, 1984; Manning *et al.* 1990). One of the earliest pieces of evidence that mediators—especially those of mast cell origin—might be important in the pathogenesis of EIA was that sodium cromolyn (a mast cell stabilizer) prevents EIA in a large proportion of asthmatic patients (Godfrey & Konig 1976). Several studies have shown that atopic patients who exercise while they breathe cold dry air experience EIA and have elevated circulating levels of histamine, NCF (IL-8), or both (Anderson *et al.* 1981; Barnes & Brown 1981; Nagakura *et al.* 1983; Lee *et al.* 1984). Of interest, these studies have also shown the absence of these mediators in the circulation following isocapnic hyperventilation, despite equal degrees of airways obstruction (Barnes & Brown 1981; Lee *et al.* 1983a; Nagakura *et al.* 1983). This suggests a possible role for these

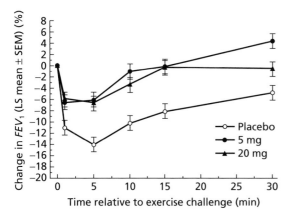

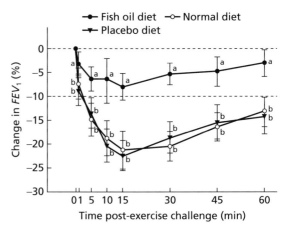

Fig. 26.8 Percent change in FEV_1 (least-squares mean ± SEM) relative to time of exercise challenge immediately before exercise challenge, with pretreatment with placebo or zafirlukast, an antagonist of the receptor for leukotriene D4. Redrawn from Pearlman *et al.* (1999).

Fig. 26.9 The percentage change in FEV_1 from before to after exercise across the three diets (fish oil, normal, placebo). Reductions in $FEV_1 > 10\%$ represent a positive diagnosis of exercise-induced bronchospasm (EIB). Letters a and b refer to comparisons by diet within respective time period. Different letters designate a significant difference ($P < 0.05$). Redrawn from Mickleborough *et al.* (2006).

mediators in EIA, but not in hyperventilation-induced asthma, and also suggests that heat loss alone is not sufficient to release these mediators from mast cells.

Further evidence that mediators of inflammation are important in causing EIA (as opposed to being mere epiphenomena of EIA) comes from studies showing inhibition of EIA by leukotriene antagonists (Fig. 26.8) (Pearlman *et al.* 1999).

Carraro *et al.* (2005) showed exhaled breath condensate to contain significantly higher baseline levels of cysteinyl leukotrienes (CysLT) in asthmatic children with EIA than in asthmatic children without EIA or control subjects. Hallstrand *et al.* (2005) found induced sputum to contain more histamine, tryptase, and CysLT 30 min after EIA than at baseline, and less EIA and reduced histamine and CysLT when patients took the antihistamine and CysLT antagonist, loratadine and montelukast, respectively, prior to exercise.

Fish oil has been shown to decrease the production of proinflammatory leukotrienes and lessen EIA. Mickleborough *et al.* (2006) showed decreased EIA and concentrations of inflammatory mediators (including leukotrienes C_4 and E_4, prostaglandin D_2, interleukin-1β, and tumor necrosis factor-α) in subjects receiving fish oil dietary supplements (Fig. 26.9).

LESSONS FROM THE REFRACTORY PERIOD

Many patients with EIA develop less intense EIA after a second bout of exercise that follows the initial exercise challenge by 2 h or less. It is not yet known why this occurs. The initial challenge need not be severe enough to have caused EIA itself in order to afford protection from the second challenge (Reiff *et al.* 1989; Wilson *et al.* 1990). Furthermore, although either exercise or resting hyperventilation of cool dry air produces a refractory period to a similar challenge (Rosenthal *et al.* 1990), it is not clear that this similarity can be attributed to airway heat loss. Exercise with warm humid air does not cause EIA, but does induce refractoriness to a subsequent exercise challenge (Ben-Dov *et al.* 1982), while resting hyperventilation of warm humid air causes neither asthma nor refractoriness to a subsequent challenge of cold dry air hyperventilation (Bar-Yishay *et al.* 1983). This suggests that something specific about exercise itself is inducing refractoriness.

The possibility that the airway smooth muscle is unable to contract during the refractory period has been disproved, because patients who are refractory to exercise challenge are able to have brisk bronchoconstrictor responses to inhaled histamine (Hahn *et al.* 1984b) or allergen (Weiler-Ravell & Godfrey 1981). It has been suggested that various mediators, including histamine, may help explain the refractory period; with this theory, mediators are released, especially from mast cells, with the initial challenge, and the mediator stores within the mast cells take up to 2 h to be replenished (Edmunds *et al.* 1978).

LATE ASTHMATIC RESPONSE

It has been reported by some investigators that some patients with asthma will suffer not only an immediate but also a late reduction in expiratory airflow, 4–10 h after an exercise challenge, associated with chest tightness, wheezing, or both (Lee *et al.* 1983b). Patients who experience these late responses have been shown to have increased circulating levels of IL-8, while those patients who have only the immediate response have only an initial rise in IL-8.

Other investigators (Boner *et al.* 1992) have been unable to reproduce these results, and point out that a biphasic fall in expiratory flow rates may be characteristic of the diurnal variation seen in some patients, irrespective of prior exercise challenge. These differing findings may possibly be explained by a study in which bronchoscopy and bronchial biopsies were performed 3 h after exercise on 2 separate days (Crimi *et al.* 1992). This study suggested that "exercise may enhance mast cell degranulation and eosinophilic inflammation of the airways, and . . . a delayed bronchoconstriction after exercise is not specific to EIA but is more likely the result of fluctuations in lung function associated with airway inflammation" (Crimi *et al.* 1992).

ENDURANCE TRAINING IN COLD OR CHLORINATED AIR

There is intriguing evidence that exercise training itself—particularly if that training is intense and prolonged, with high minute ventilation, and is carried out in the cold or in indoor swimming pools, with chlorine in the air—might cause changes to the airways, rendering them susceptible to exercise-induced narrowing. Cross-country skiers and competitive swimmers have been found to have evidence of eosinophilic airways inflammation and bronchial hyperresponiveness (Helenius *et al.* 1997). In one study of 162 highly trained athletes and 45 control subjects, the risk of asthma in atopic swimmers was 96 times that of non-atopic non-athletes (Helenius & Haahtela 2000). In another study of 100 high-level athletes in various sports (Langdeau *et al.* 2000), 76% of the swimmers and 52% of the athletes who trained in cold air (cross-country skiers and speed-skaters) had bronchial hyperresponsiveness on methacholine testing, while the other athletes (distance runners and mountain bikers) did not differ from the control subjects in the prevalence of bronchial hyperresponiveness. In a 5-year prospective study of 42 swimmers from the Finnish national team, Helenius *et al.* (2002) showed diminished or even absent airway hyperresponsiveness and asthma, and reduced sputum eosinophilia, in the 26 athletes who stopped their competitive career, while responsiveness, eosinophilia, and symptoms continued in the 16 who continued their competitive careers, suggesting that "athletes' asthma is partly reversible" after the airways are no longer challenged with high volumes of irritants.

Diagnosis

In most cases of children or adolescents with recognized asthma, diagnosing EIA is not challenging: exercise-associated cough, chest pain, or dyspnea can be assumed to be caused by the underlying problem, and to be EIA (Nixon & Orenstein 1988). The most appropriate test in these cases is a therapeutic trial of a regimen designed to block EIA (see below). Only if the symptoms are inordinately severe or worrying to the patient, family, or physician, or if they are not prevented by appropriate treatment, should more testing be carried out. A major exception to this generalization must always be kept in mind; if the sole exercise-related complaint is dyspnea, the culprit may be deconditioning; the young asthmatic patient may be out of breath because of poor conditioning, only indirectly (or not at all) related to his or her asthma. In other cases, even a highly fit child or adolescent might be incorrectly thought to have a problem (commonly EIA) when he or she is noted to be breathing heavily during hard exercise—a response that is completely normal.

Despite the ease of diagnosing EIA in most cases of difficult breathing in children and adolescents with known asthma, there are substantial numbers of youngsters—some with previously diagnosed asthma, and some with no prior respiratory symptoms—who report (or whose parents report) cough, chest pain, difficult breathing, or some combination of these symptoms with exercise, in whom the diagnosis is not as easy. EIA is probably both under- and overdiagnosed in these children. EIA is underdiagnosed because some physicians still insist on wheezing as an absolute diagnostic criterion for asthma, and some driven athletes might hesitate to report problems. It is overdiagnosed because of recent attention to EIA in the lay press, with Olympic champions and other high-profile athletes talking openly about their asthma. The heightened awareness of EIA of course is good, but the degree to which any respiratory symptom (including the normal increase in minute ventilation—heavy breathing—seen with almost any exertion) is labeled as asthma is not as good. EIA is overdiagnosed particularly in athletes; Hallstrand *et al.* (2002) examined 256 high school athletes and found histories suggestive of EIA in 39.5%, but could confirm that diagnosis in only 9.4%. Conversely, a full 45% of the athletes in Hallstrand's sample who had a positive exercise test for EIA had a negative history for asthma, EIA, and allergic rhinitis. Similarly, both Seear *et al.* (2005) and Abu-Hasan *et al.* (2005) found that a high proportion of patients referred to their university specialty practices because of poorly controlled EIA actually had problems other than EIA (Table 26.1).

Of these problems, vocal cord dysfunction (VCD) and deconditioning deserve special mention. I have already discussed deconditioning, and fitness is discussed more fully below. VCD is a condition that consists of paradoxical closing of the vocal cords during inspiration, which causes symptoms of difficulty breathing, air hunger, "choking," throat tightness; there may be wheeze or inspiratory stridor (McFadden & Zawadski 1996; Brugman & Simons 1998). Christopher *et al.* (1983) reported VCD masquerading as asthma more than 20 years ago, but it has only recently been more widely appreciated. Brugman and Simons (1998) have a

Table 26.1 Medical conditions diagnosed in patients with "poorly controlled EIA" in two specialist centers.

	Seear *et al.* (2005) *n* (%)	Abu-Hasan *et al.* (2005) *n* (%)
n	52	142
Confirmed EIA	8 (15.4%)	11 (7.7%)
Unfit (deconditioned)	12 (23.1%)	26 (18.3%)
Vocal cord dysfunction	14 (26.9)	13 (9.2%)
Habit cough	7 (13.5%)	–
"Restrictive abnormality"		15 (10.6%)
Normal	11 (21.1%)	74 (52.1%)

EIA, exercise-induced asthma.

helpful table distinguishing VCD from EIA (Table 26.2). Complicating the diagnosis of VCD as the principal cause of a patient's difficult breathing is the fact that as many as 50% of athletes with VCD also have EIA (Rundell & Spiering 2003).

Part of the problem in diagnosing EIA based on history is that children's and parents' perception of the children's exercise-related symptoms are surprisingly poor and have either minimal or no correlation with objectively measured airway obstruction (Panditi & Silverman 2003). Even in elite Olympic-caliber athletes (age 22 ± 4.4 years), self-reported symptoms of EIA were of no use in distinguishing those with demonstrable fall in pulmonary function (PFT) after exercise from those with no PFT change (Rundell *et al.* 2001). The authors of this study concluded: "The use of self-reported symptoms for EIA diagnosis in

Table 26.2 Features of vocal cord dysfunction (VCD) and exercise-induced asthma (EIA) compared. From Brugman & Simons (1998).

Feature	VCD	EIA
Female preponderance	+	–
Chest tightness	+/–	+
Throat tightness	+	–
Stridor	+	–
Usual onset of symptoms after beginning exercise (min)	<5*	>5–10
Recovery period (min)	5–10	15–60
Refractory period	–	+
Late-phase response	–	+
Response to β-agonist	–	+

* Onset can be variable.

this population will likely yield high frequencies of both false positive and false negative results."

In evaluating the otherwise healthy youngster with atypical presentation of asthma, such as exercise-associated chest pain (Wiens *et al.* 1992), exercise-related symptoms not responsive to appropriate EIA preventive treatment (see below), cough or dyspnea in the absence of other evidence of asthma, an exercise challenge test may be helpful.

Exercise test

Challenge tests for diagnosing EIA should take into account some important features of its pathophysiology and clinical course. EIA is most likely following 6–10 min of exercise intense enough to raise the heart rate to 80% of its maximum (about 170 beats·min^{-1} for most pediatric tests) (Godfrey *et al.* 1975). Cold dry air heightens and warm humid air diminishes EIA (Deal *et al.* 1979b), therefore testing should be carried out in a setting with relatively stable ambient conditions, ideally with dry air (most hospital and clinical settings ordinarily have dry air). The mode of exercise should also be considered. Given the appropriate intensity, the form of dry-land exercise (cycle ergometer, treadmill, "free-range" running) probably does not matter, but swimming is not an appropriate challenge (except in the very special case of a youngster with symptoms that are difficult to understand during or after swimming), because it seems to be less asthmagenic

than other forms of exercise (Inbar *et al.* 1980; Bar-Yishay *et al.* 1982; Bar-Or & Inbar 1992).

EIA responses peak 3–20 min after exercise (Cropp 1975). Therefore, it makes sense to measure pulmonary function before the exercise challenge for a baseline value, and again at roughly 3-min intervals, beginning immediately afterwards, until about 20 min after exercise. Different investigators have used different pulmonary function parameters as their preferred measurement and different degrees of change in those parameters for diagnosing EIA. Table 26.3 shows Cropp's criteria for diagnosing mild, moderate, and severe EIA, based on values expressed as a percentage of pre-exercise values (Cropp 1979). In our laboratory, we prefer to see forced vital capacity (FVC) relatively unchanged after exercise, because that reassures us that a decreased forced expiratory flow (FEF) of 25–75% of vital capacity, for example, is not simply a reflection of fatigue, or a poorer effort after a tiring session on the exercise cycle or treadmill. Some investigators suggest comparing the lowest post-exercise pulmonary function values with the best values—either during exercise (Silverman & Anderson 1972) or after bronchodilator inhalation (Jones 1966)—rather than just with the pre-exercise baseline. We routinely administer bronchodilator (salbutamol, by metered-dose inhaler) after the 20-min post-exercise pulmonary function measurement, and compare the lowest post-exercise value with the highest value, which is usually the immediate post-bronchodilator value.

Table 26.3 Criteria for the diagnosis of mild, moderate and severe exercise-induced asthma (EIA). Adapted from Cropp (1979).

PFT parameter	Post-exercise measurement		
	Mild EIA (% predicted)	Moderate EIA (% predicted)	Severe EIA (% predicted)
SGaw	51–70	30–50	<30
PEFR	61–75	40–60	<40
FEF$_{25-75}$	61–75	40–60	<40
FEV$_1$	66–80	50–65	<50
FVC	81–90	70–80	<70

FEF$_{25-75}$, forced expiratory flow between 25 and 75% of vital capacity, also referred to as maximal mid-expiratory flow rate; *FEV*$_1$, forced expiratory volume in 1 s; FVC, forced vital capacity; PEFR, peak expiratory flow rate; PFT, pulmonary function; SGaw, specific airway conductance. FEF$_{25-75}$ is thought to reflect the status of the small bronchi, while the other measurements are more related to the large airways.

Whatever test is chosen and whatever parameters are used, false negative tests are common (Nixon & Orenstein 1988), and some investigators suggest repeat testing within a week (Godfrey 1974) if the first test is negative. Even on repeat testing the tests are not as sensitive as some of the literature would suggest, and false negative tests, or tests with smaller decrements in expiratory flow rates than in Table 26.3, even in children with known EIA, are reasonably common (Orenstein 1993). One cannot interpret these tests in a clinical vacuum; rather, the whole history and, in many cases, the patient's response to a trial of pre-exercise β_2-agonist, cromolyn or nedocromil (see under Prevention below) help confirm the diagnosis.

COLD AIR CHALLENGE

Some laboratories substitute a cold air challenge for the more traditional exercise challenge in their attempts to diagnose EIA (Zach *et al.* 1984). In these tests, patients at rest breathe cold (typically <3°C) dry air for 3–7 min at a minute ventilation comparable to that which they would have used during exercise —approximately 20 times the forced expiratory volume in 1 s (FEV_1) (Strauss *et al.* 1977), or two-thirds of the predicted maximum voluntary ventilation (Deal *et al.* 1980). Pulmonary function measurements are made before and at 3-min intervals after the challenge, just as with the standard EIA tests (McLaughlin & Dozor 1983). During these tests, end-tidal carbon dioxide tensions must be monitored, and carbon dioxide occasionally added to the inspired air, in order to prevent the bronchoconstriction caused by hypocapnia (McFadden *et al.* 1977). Another approach sometimes employed is to have the patient breathe cold dry air during an exercise challenge (Orenstein 1993).

DIAGNOSING VOCAL CORD DYSFUNCTION

Diagnosing VCD can be difficult. In some competitive athletes with this problem, symptoms have been reproducible only in the competitive setting (McFadden & Zawadski 1996). When VCD is in the differential diagnosis, the exercise test should probably include measurement of flow–volume loops

during the exercise test. The telltale finding is felt by some to be flattening of the inspiratory limb of the flow–volume loop (Fig. 26.10), while others

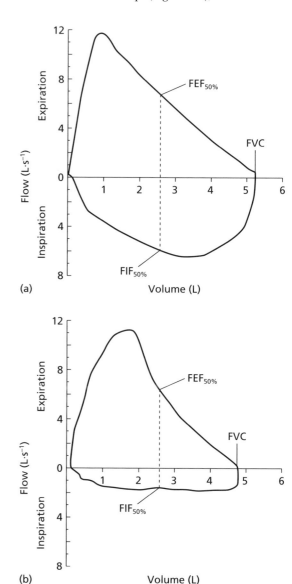

Fig. 26.10 (a) A normal flow–volume loop. (b) Extrathoracic airflow obstruction with truncation of the inspiratory loop. This is consistent with symptomatic vocal cord dysfunction (VCD) but may be seen in other laryngeal diseases. FEF_{50}, forced expiratory flow at 50% forced vital capacity; FIF_{50}, forced inspiratory flow at 50% forced vital capacity; FVC, forced vital capacity. Redrawn from Perkner *et al.* (1998).

(Rundell & Spiering 2003) have pointed out that this is not always seen, and point instead to different findings on pulmonary function testing (Heimdal *et al.* 2006). The gold standard is likely direct visualization of the vocal cords by fiberoptic laryngoscopy during exercise (Heimdal *et al.* 2006), a procedure that is not readily carried out in most clinical exercise laboratories.

Fitness

FITNESS LEVELS

Most (Cropp & Tanakawa 1977; Clark & Cochrane 1988; Strunk *et al.* 1988; Garfinkel *et al.* 1992), but not all (Ingemann-Hansen *et al.* 1980; Fink *et al.* 1993; Thio *et al.* 1996), studies have shown that patients with asthma have lower aerobic fitness than their non-asthmatic peers. This is not surprising, because exercise can induce an asthma attack, and because airway obstruction would be expected to limit exercise tolerance. However, the fascinating and important fact emerging from recent studies is that the limited fitness in patients with asthma seems not to be related very closely to their degree of airway obstruction (Strunk *et al.* 1988; Garfinkel *et al.* 1992; Fink *et al.* 1993), but to be much more closely related to their levels of habitual activity (Fig. 26.11) (Garfinkel *et al.* 1992; Fink *et al.* 1993) or their perceptions of competence in physical activity (Pianosi & Davis 2004). Nevertheless, between half and two-thirds of the patients in one study reported that they did not exercise more because they "get short of breath/wheeze" when they exercise, a finding not corroborated by objective testing in the laboratory after the inhalation of a single dose of a β-agonist (Garfinkel *et al.* 1992; Schwartzenstein 1992).

Exercise conditioning

The beneficial effects of exercise conditioning programs in young patients with asthma have been noted for some time (Petersen & McElhenney 1965; Bar-Or 1985; Nickerson *et al.* 1983; Orenstein *et al.* 1985; Varray *et al.* 1991; Bar-Or & Inbar 1992; Matsumoto *et al.* 1999). These benefits have ranged from the very subjective:

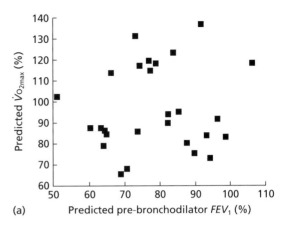

(a)

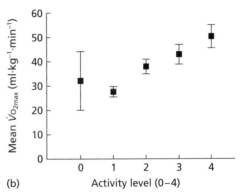

(b)

Fig. 26.11 Relationships between fitness and resting pulmonary function (a) and habitual activity level (b) in a group of patients with asthma. There is no relationship between fitness (expressed as percent predicted maximum oxygen consumption $\dot{V}_{O_{2max}}$) and degree of pulmonary dysfunction, whereas there is a relationship between fitness and habitual activity. Redrawn from Garfinkel *et al.* (1992).

1 Improved ability to participate in activities, including school and church programs and sports;
2 Acceptance by peers;
3 Decrease in emotional upset, and recognition that sickness need not be a way of life (Bar-Or 1983); and
4 Decrease in the intensity of wheezing attacks (Varray *et al.* 1991);
to the objective:
1 Increased running performance (Nickerson *et al.* 1983); and
2 Increased peak oxygen consumption (Orenstein *et al.* 1985; Varray *et al.* 1991),

indicating increased aerobic fitness, and increased oxygen pulse (Orenstein *et al.* 1985), suggesting increased cardiac stroke volume which is also consistent with improved aerobic fitness, and increased ventilatory threshold (the point at which minute ventilation abruptly increases out of proportion to changes in oxygen consumption) (Varray *et al.* 1991; Matsumoto *et al.* 1999) (see Chapter 32). The types of training have varied, and have included swimming (Varray *et al.* 1991; Matsumoto *et al.* 1999) and jogging (Nickerson *et al.* 1983; Orenstein *et al.* 1985). Not all studies have included the use of inhalers (see Prevention, below) prior to conditioning sessions, but some have (Orenstein *et al.* 1985), and it seems prudent to do so (Schwartzstein 1992). The now well-known successes of asthmatic athletes in the past several Olympiads highlights the potential for patients with asthma to respond to exercise conditioning programs, and the possibility of engaging in an active lifestyle, including competitive sports: 117 (16.7%) of the 699 athletes who competed for the USA in the 1996 Olympics had asthma (Weiler *et al.* 1998). Some 45% of the cyclists and mountain bikers, 26% of the swimmers, but none of the divers and weight lifters had active asthma. The athletes with asthma won medals in about the same proportions as those without asthma.

Effect of conditioning

Although early reports suggested that exercise programs diminish airway obstruction in the patient in response to exercise (Oseid & Haaland 1978), these early reports failed to control for changes in minute ventilation. That is, patients were challenged with a workload after their conditioning programme equal to the preconditioning challenge, and most often were found to have a smaller EIA response.

However, if the patients became more aerobically fit, it is expected that their ventilatory threshold would have increased, and therefore a vigorous work rate which might have been above the ventilatory threshold prior to conditioning might well be below the ventilatory threshold after conditioning. By definition of the ventilatory threshold, this means that the patient would have a lower minute ventilation at this same work rate after having become more fit with the conditioning program. Breathing a smaller volume of air puts less stress on the air conditioning capacity of the airways, and thus provides a smaller stimulus for EIA (see above) (Carroll & Sly 1999). Most studies that have taken this principle into consideration (Nickerson *et al.* 1983; Fitch *et al.* 1986) have concluded that exercise conditioning does not diminish EIA. There is one very carefully performed study (Haas *et al.* 1986) that does suggest that the EIA response may be smaller after training. No studies suggest worsened EIA after conditioning, and it seems unlikely that improved aerobic fitness would worsen EIA, yet there is now reason to be concerned about repetitive training in cold air or poorly ventilated natatoriums (see Endurance training in cold or chlorinated air). No doubt there is something of a dose relationship when considering training intensity. In the Matsumoto study (1999), children swam for 15 min, rested for 10 min, then swam for 15 min more, covering a total of something under 900 m·day^{-1}, for 6 weeks. This compares with something like 5486–7315 m·day^{-1} (6000–8000 yards·day^{-1}) for most of the calendar year for swimmers competing at an elite level (Trappe *et al.* 2001). For the sedentary child, the Matsumoto training schedule is adequate for improving aerobic fitness, and probably not intense enough to bring about the changes described for elite swimmers.

Prevention

Pharmacotherapy

Pharmacotherapy for EIA has been reviewed (Hansen-Flaschen & Schotland 1998; Milgrom & Taussig 1999). The main classes of drugs that may have some use in preventing EIA are β-adrenergic agonists, cromolyn sodium (and its analogs), corticosteroids, and leukotriene antagonists.

β-ADRENERGIC AGONISTS

Among cell membrane receptors, the β-adrenergic receptors are important in the control of intestinal motility, the rate and intensity of cardiac contractions, relaxation or contraction of bronchial smooth muscle and arterial smooth muscle. Stimulation of the β_1-receptors increases cardiac rate and contractility and influences intestinal motility, while stimulation of β_2-receptors dilates bronchial smooth muscle. Recent years have seen the development of relatively selective β_2-agonists, which have potent bronchial smooth muscle relaxant effect, with little cardiac stimulation. These agents, including albuterol (USA) or salbutamol (rest of the world), metaproterenol, terbutaline, bitolterol, formoterol, and salmeterol, are the mainstay in the treatment of the bronchospastic component of asthma, be it chronic or acute, including EIA. These were the first-line drugs for both prevention and treatment of asthma until recently, when the primary role of airways inflammation in the pathogenesis of asthma became appreciated, and when concern has been raised about the possible dangers of these agents when used as maintenance therapy for chronic asthma (Sears *et al.* 1990; Spitzer *et al.* 1992). The β_2-agonists are still accepted as very safe and effective for symptomatic relief of asthma and prevention of EIA. When inhaled 10–20 min prior to exercise, these agents block EIA in virtually all subjects. Their protective effect ranges between 1 h (metaproterenol), 2 h (terbutaline), and 4 h (salbutamol) (Lemanske & Henke 1989). The combination of cromolyn and terbutaline increases the length of time of protection from EIA from 2 h for each agent alone to 4 h (Woolley *et al.* 1990). Most of these drugs are available in oral or inhaled form (metered-dose inhaler or nebulizer solution), the inhaled route being preferable because of speed and potency of action and lack of side effects. Currently, a β_2-agonist delivered by metered-dose inhaler 15 min prior to exercise is probably the most potent and reliable means of preventing EIA in the largest number of subjects (Morton & Fitch 1992).

Tolerance to long-term use of β_2-agonists

Unfortunately, regular use of β_2-agonists blunts their effectiveness in preventing EIA. Hancox *et al.* (2002) had subjects take salbutamol or placebo inhalations q.i.d. for 1 week, and then cross over to the other preparation, and found worse EIA after 1 week of regular salbutamol. The salbutamol continued to provide bronchodilator effect when it was given after the exercise challenge, but after a week of salbutamol, the FEV_1 never returned to the values seen after a week of placebo (Fig. 26.12). Inman and O'Byrne (1996) had demonstrated a lower resting FEV_1 and a similar blunting of the protective effect of pre-exercise salbutamol after 8 days of salbutamol q.i.d. compared with placebo, but pointed out that the pre-exercise salbutamol still did provide protection against EIA (albeit less than it did when the subjects had not been taking it on a regular basis).

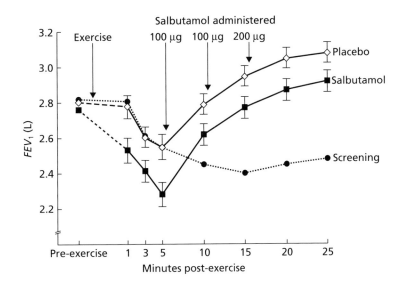

Fig. 26.12 FEV_1 changes before and after exercise and during the dose–response to salbutamol in patients after 1 week of salbutamol q.i.d. or placebo. Error bars represent 95% confidence intervals. For comparison the FEV_1 changes from the prerandomization screening challenge are shown to illustrate the spontaneous changes in FEV_1 following exercise. Redrawn from Hancox *et al.* (2002).

The protection against EIA with pre-exercise salbutamol is often less than 2.5 h (Anderson *et al.* 1991), hardly adequate for a child who might be active periodically through the day or an athlete with heats and finals spread over a several hour period.

Long-acting β₂-agonists

Formoterol is a long-acting β_2-agonist that affords protection against EIA as long as 8 h (and perhaps as long as 12 h) after a single inhalation (Pearlman *et al.* 2006). It has been very helpful for those with EIA. Its onset of action is as rapid as that of the short-acting β_2-agonists, but its duration of protection is much longer. Formoterol has faster onset of action than salmeterol (another long-acting β_2-agonist) and—unlike salmeterol and the short-acting β_2-agonists—does not seem to show diminishing effects after subjects have been taking it on a regular basis (Nelson *et al.* 1998).

CROMOLYN SODIUM

Cromolyn is a disodium salt, developed in the 1960s. It is useful in chronic asthma, particularly in those patients with an allergic component to their asthma. In the chronic asthmatic, cromolyn may take weeks before its effects are seen. Therefore it is perhaps surprising that it is also very effective acutely in blocking EIA, if administered 15–20 min prior to exercise. It may block EIA completely in 40% of subjects, and partly in more than 70% of subjects (Godfrey & Konig 1976). Its effects are dose related (Morton *et al.* 1992a). Cromolyn is unique, or nearly so, among therapeutic agents, for its lack of side effects. Its mode of action is not completely clear, but most clinicians credit its effect to its apparent ability to stabilize mast cell membranes (Morton *et al.* 1992), and thus inhibit the release of chemical mediators (Cox & Altounyan 1970). It may also act by inhibiting phosphodiesterase activity, inhibiting reflex mechanisms or modifying calcium flux across cell membranes (Lemanske & Henke 1989). The protective effect of cromolyn lasts about 2 h, but in combination with terbutaline, protection lasts twice as long (Woolley *et al.* 1990). Cromolyn sodium is available in three forms: a powder contained within a capsule (20 mg per capsule), inhaled via a Spinhaler,

a metered-dose inhaler (1 mg per puff) and a nebulizer solution (20 mg per ampulla). Nedocromil sodium is a compound related to cromolyn sodium, with comparable potency and efficacy, and comparable freedom from toxicity (Morton *et al.* 1992).

CORTICOSTEROIDS

Corticosteroids are extremely effective in preventing and treating airways inflammation and edema in chronic asthma. Inhaled steroids, with very little systemic absorption, have become the first-line maintenance drug in adults and children with asthma (Expert Panel 2002). Inhaled steroids may have some ability to block EIA in children who have been taking the medication for 1–3 weeks (Fig. 26.13) (Henriksen & Dahl 1983; Lemanske & Henke 1989), probably by attenuating bronchial reactivity.

However, their importance lies more in their role in controlling baseline airway inflammation. When these agents are taken regularly, they can help maintain optimal airway patency, thereby reducing the effect of any subsequent narrowing following exercise (or allergen challenge), and can also increase the effectiveness of a low dose pre-exercise β_2-agonist aerosol in preventing EIA in children (Henriksen & Dahl 1983).

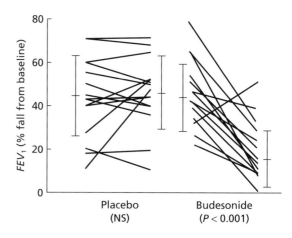

Fig. 26.13 Individual percentage falls in forced expiratory volume in 1 s (FEV_1) induced by exercise before and after 3 weeks of treatment with budesonide aerosol and placebo. Means and SD are shown. Redrawn from Henriksen and Dahl (1983).

LEUKOTRIENE RECEPTOR ANTAGONISTS

These are the newest drugs in the fight against EIA, and show great promise. Pearlman *et al.* (1999) showed substantial protection against EIA 4 h after a single oral dose of zafirlukast, compared with placebo (Fig. 26.8). Unlike the β_2-agonists, leukotriene antagonists do not seem to bring about tolerance to their protective effects; montelukast gave as good protection against EIA after 4, 8, or 12 weeks of a once-daily oral dose (about 47% inhibition). The only bad news here is that, while 23% of the patients had complete protection from EIA (less than 10% decline in FEV_1 after exercise), another 25% had little or no protection (less than 30% decline in FEV_1) (Leff *et al.* 1998).

One possible way around these limitations is to combine a leukotriene antagonist and a long-acting β_2-agonist, as Coreno *et al.* (2005) did in a cold/dry air challenge, and found considerable additive effect of the two agents in preventing airway narrowing in response to the exercise substitute (Fig. 26.14).

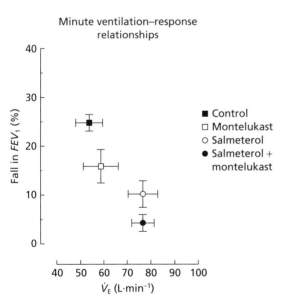

Minute ventilation–response relationships

■ Control
□ Montelukast
○ Salmeterol
● Salmeterol + montelukast

Fig. 26.14 The effect of treatment with a combination of a long-acting β_2-agonist and a leukotriene antagonist on the relationship between (minute ventilation $\dot{V}_E$) and the degree of airway obstruction. The ordinate is the drop in FEV_1 and the abscissa, the $\dot{V}_E$ in L·min^{-1}. The symbols represent mean values, and the brackets represent 1 SEM. Redrawn from Coreno *et al.* (2005).

ANTICHOLINERGIC AGENTS

Because vagal input increases resting bronchomotor tone, anticholinergic agents such as atropine may cause bronchodilatation in some people. Ipratropium bromide (Atrovent) is a quarternary ammonium derivative of atropine, and when taken by metered-dose inhaler, is absorbed only poorly, thus reducing atropine-like side effects (e.g., dry mouth, visual problems). Ipratropium bromide has become a useful agent for some patients, but has only moderate effectiveness in preventing EIA (Lemanske & Henke 1989).

METHYL XANTHINES

Theophylline was for many years the preferred drug for treatment of chronic asthma in the USA. More recently, the availability of agents with better anti-inflammatory action (corticosteroids, leukotriene antagonists, cromolyn) and better bronchodilator effect (β_2-agonists) has relegated theophylline to the third or fourth tier in the classification of helpful drugs for asthma. Theophylline is effective in preventing EIA in about 80% of subjects (Ellis 1984), but its rather narrow therapeutic window, considerable toxicity, and slow onset of action have made it a poor choice for young athletes with EIA (Lemanske & Henke 1989).

CALCIUM-CHANNEL BLOCKERS

These agents are finding use in many different medical settings. As Lemanske and Henke (1989) and Middleton (1984) point out, the pathologic processes in the airways of patients with asthma are calcium-dependent: "excitation–contraction coupling in smooth muscle, stimulus–secretion coupling in mast cells and mucous glands . . . and the movement and activation of inflammatory cells." The calcium-channel blockers nifedipine and verapamil have been shown to be effective in blocking EIA, while diltiazem has not (Lemanske & Henke 1989).

Legal and banned asthma drugs in competitive sport

The list of allowed and disallowed medications is different for each school, and therefore I will not attempt to categorize these drugs for young athletes. For competition under the aegis of the International Olympic Committee, the World Anti-Doping Agency (http://www.wada-ama.org/en/index.ch2) establishes and maintains the policies and lists legal and banned drugs. Table 26.4 lists most of the drugs relevant to asthma, and is adapted and updated from Morton *et al.* (1992b).

SPECIFIED SUBSTANCES

" 'Specified substances' are those with general availability in medicinal products . . . [and] less likely to be successfully abused as doping agents . . . A doping violation . . . *may* result in a reduced sanction provided that the Athlete can establish that use . . . was not intended to enhance sport performance."

These "specified substances" include all inhaled β_2-agonists except clenbuterol, and all glucocorticoids. Additionally, certain medications used for allergic conditions, such as antihistamines, ephedrine, pseudoephedrine, phenylephrine, and phenylpropanolamine are no longer prohibited.

ERGOGENIC PROPERTIES OF ANTI-ASTHMA DRUGS

Some of the agents used in treating and preventing asthma have properties that might theoretically give a boost to muscular performance: aminophylline has been shown to increase the contractility of the diaphragm (Aubier *et al.* 1981) and of cardiac muscle (Matthay & Mahler 1986), while certain selective β-agonists have been associated with increases in

Table 26.4 Drugs commonly used for exercise-induced asthma (EIA), their route of administration, effectiveness, whether they are legal or banned for intercollegiate and international competition, and whether they are used prophylactically, for treatment, or both.

Medication	Route of administration	Effectiveness in EIA	Legal, prohibited, or TUE*	Prophylaxis (P); therapeutic (T)
Cromolyn	Aerosol	Good	Legal	P
Nedocromil	Aerosol	Good	Legal	P
β_2-Agonists				
Salbutamol	Aerosol	Excellent	TUE*	P,T
	Oral	Fair	Prohibited	P,T
Terbutaline	Aerosol	Excellent	TUE*	P,T
	Oral	Fair	Prohibited	P,T
Formoterol	Aerosol	Excellent	TUE*	P,T
Salmeterol	Aerosol	Very good	TUE*	P,T
Clenbuterol	Aerosol	Excellent	Prohibited	P,T
Ipratropium	Aerosol	Fair	Legal	T
Theophylline	Oral	Good	Legal	P,T
Corticoids				
Budesonide	Aerosol	Good	TUE*	P
Prednisone	Oral	?	TUE*	T
Prednisolone	Oral	?	TUE*	T
Leukotriene antagonists				
Montelukast	Oral	Good	Legal	P
Safirlukast	Oral	Good	Legal	P

* All β_2-agonists are prohibited, except inhaled formoterol, salbutamol, salmeterol, and terbutaline, which can be legal with a therapeutic use exemption (TUE).
All glucocorticoids are prohibited, but can be allowed with a TUE. The criteria for a TUE are:
• The athlete would experience significant health problems without taking the prohibited substance or method;
• The therapeutic use of the substance would not produce significant enhancement of performance; and
• There is no reasonable therapeutic alternative to the use of the otherwise prohibited substance or method (http://www.wada-ama.org/en/exemptions.ch2).

muscle mass in farm animals (Baker *et al.* 1984). Yet, the preponderance of evidence seems to indicate that neither theophylline (Morton *et al.* 1989), salbutamol (Meeuwisse *et al.* 1992; Morton *et al.* 1992; Signorile *et al.* 1992), salmeterol (Sue-Chu *et al.* 1999), nor monteleukast (Rundell *et al.* 2004) influences power output or athletic performance in non-asthmatic athletes or non-athletes. It seems that the main effect of these drugs is to relieve the abnormal narrowing of the asthmatic athlete's bronchi, thus allowing him or her to compete on an equal footing (equal breathing) with the athlete not burdened with an abnormal bronchial tree. Other β-agonists, including clenbuterol, may indeed have ergogenic properties, and are appropriately banned.

Non-pharmacologic means

It is possible to take advantage of our understanding of the pathophysiology of EIA to employ non-pharmacologic means that can be successful in preventing or attenuating EIA.

WARM INSPIRED AIR

As simple a procedure as wrapping a scarf around the face, or using a simple mask over the nose and mouth, can increase the temperature and humidity of the inspired air by mixing inspired air with exhaled air. This reduces the stimulus to EIA and the likelihood of an attack (Fig. 26.15) (Brenner *et al.* 1980; Schachter *et al.* 1981).

WARM-UP EXERCISE

It is possible to take advantage of the refractory period by exercising in the 30–90 min prior to competition. The first (warm-up) session need not be vigorous enough to induce EIA itself in order to block EIA (Reiff *et al.* 1989). It is not clear whether short sprints or longer, less intense, warm-ups are better. The best warm-up for preventing EIA and not interfering with performance is best determined by the individual based on experience, and will likely vary from athlete to athlete, and perhaps from sport to sport.

SELECT THE APPROPRIATE SPORT

Because the stimulus that is most likely to cause EIA is non-swimming exercise vigorous enough to raise the heart rate to 170 beats·min^{-1} or so for 6–10 min, especially in cold air, this knowledge can in some cases help to direct the aspiring asthmatic athlete towards a sport or event of relatively low asthmagenicity, such as swimming, or events that are shorter or longer in duration, such as sprints or distance running or cycling. (Directing the aspiring athlete to a competitive career in swimming is no longer as clearly beneficial in terms of least likelihood of asthma as it once was.) Stop-and-go sports may also be included and be of low asthmagenicity. Lifting, throwing, or jumping events are not likely to provoke much difficulty. Of course, the physician, coach, or parent does not always have the luxury of

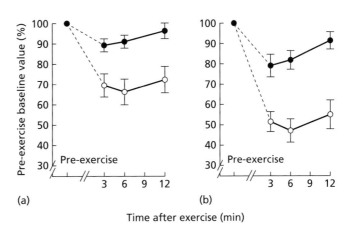

Fig. 26.15 Average pulmonary function indices, (a) FEV_1 and (b) maximal mid-expiratory flow rate, while breathing room air (open circles) and with mask (filled circles) at 3, 6, and 12 min after exercise, expressed as percent of baseline value (mean ± SE for 10 subjects). Redrawn from Brenner *et al.* (1980).

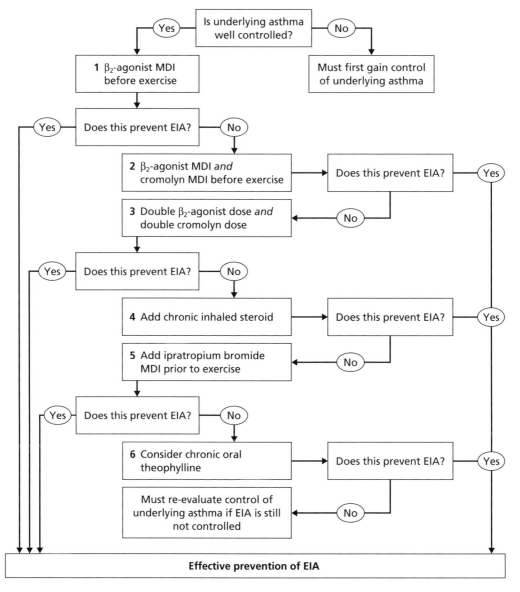

Fig. 26.16 Flow chart for selecting drugs to prevent exercise-induced asthma (EIA). MDI, metered dose inhaler. Adapted from Morton *et al.* (1992).

being able to steer the young athlete towards an "appropriate" sport; instead the young runner may have trouble during her or his event, and wants help with that event. The cross-country skiier will not appreciate being advised to take up the shot put.

MISCELLANEOUS

Hypnosis has been shown to help block EIA in some subjects (Ben-Zvi *et al.* 1982), perhaps through influencing resting bronchomotor tone via vagal routes, or perhaps by altering ventilation. Acupuncture has been shown in one study (Fung *et al.* 1986) to be more helpful than sham acupuncture in attenuating EIA, while another study could not confirm any benefit for laser acupuncture (Gruber *et al.* 2002).

Practical approach to the young athlete with asthma

In most cases, diagnosing a youngster with EIA will be straightforward. If a child or adolescent already carries the diagnosis of asthma, then exercise-related symptoms of chest pain, shortness of breath, cough, or wheeze can generally be assumed to be related to the underlying reactive airways, and as part of the evaluation can be treated as such. Lack of a quick response to appropriate EIA prevention should prompt further investigation. Exercise testing to determine the youngster's level of fitness should be carried out, as many people with asthma will have restricted their own activity, or had it restricted by physicians, parents, teachers, or coaches, to the point of substantial deconditioning. The poorly fit individual might well suffer shortness of breath with an aerobic or anaerobic challenge beyond his or her capabilities. In these cases, more exercise, in a rational conditioning program is indicated. It is important that asthmatic athletes have excellent care for and control of their asthma, with special attention being paid to the underlying airways inflammation. Only when the asthma, and the airway inflammation, is well-controlled will the exercise-related component be readily prevented. Then, non-pharmacologic approaches, such as wearing a face mask or scarf while exercising in cold weather, may help. If this proves ineffective, pretreatment with a β_2-agonist inhaler should be tried. If inadequate, the dose can be doubled. The next step should be the addition of inhaled cromolyn sodium. If these are not completely successful, the cromolyn dose can be doubled. A final pharmacologic addition can be ipratropium bromide. Finally, if these are all unsuccessful, it is important to review again the state of control of the underlying airways inflammation, and perhaps to conduct exercise tests in the laboratory setting with the various medications. Figure 26.16 gives a schematic approach to the child athlete with asthma.

It is fortunate that the vast majority of youngsters with asthma are able to engage in a normal active life, including competitive athletics. Caring for these young athletes is truly one of the most satisfying activities a physician can engage in.

Challenges for future research

Much has been learned about asthma and sports over the past several hundred years, especially the past two decades. Yet there are still some unknown areas, particularly concerning pathogenesis. What precisely is the role of water and heat loss in causing EIA? What is it about exercise itself beyond the respiratory heat exchange that leads the susceptible airway to become narrower? Where do the various mediators of inflammation fit in? How can the fact that swimming is less asthmagenic than other forms of exercise be explained: is it body position, water immersion, or another as yet undefined factor? Finally, what of treatment? Do the β_2-agonists have ergogenic properties, or are there important differences among them that would make one member of the class "fair" and another unfair?

References

Abu-Hasan, M., Tannous, B. & Weinberger, M. (2005) Exercise-induced dyspnea in children and adolescents: if not asthma then what? *Annals of Allergy, Asthma & Immunology* **94**, 366–371.

Aitken, M. & Morini, J. (1985) Effect of heat delivery and extraction on airway conductance in normal and in asthmatic subjects. *American Review of Respiratory Disease* **131**, 357–361.

Akinbami, L.J. & Schoendorf, K.C. (2002) Trends in childhood asthma: prevalence, health care utilization, and mortality. *Pediatrics* **110**, 315–322.

Anderson, S. (1983) Current concepts of exercise induced asthma. *Allergy* **38**, 289–302.

Anderson, S., Bye, P., Schoeffel, R., Seale, J., Taylor, K. & Ferris, L. (1981) Arterial plasma histamine levels at rest and during and after exercise in patients with asthma: effects of terbutaline aerosol. *Thorax* **36**, 259–267.

Anderson, S., Rodwell, L., DuToit, J. & Young, I. (1991) Duration of protection by inhaled salmeterol in exercise-induced asthma. *Chest* **100**, 1254–1260.

Aubier, M., Troyer, A., Sampson, M., Macklem, P. & Roussos, C. (1981) Aminophylline improves diaphragmatic contractility. *New England Journal of Medicine* **305**, 249–252.

Badger, D., Ramos, A., Lew, C., Platzker, A., Stabile, M. & Keens, T. (1987) Childhood sequelae of infant lung disease: exercise and pulmonary function abnormalities after bronchopulmonary dysplasia. *Journal of Pediatrics* **110**, 693–699.

Baker, P., Dalrymple, R., Ingle, D. & Ricks, C. (1984) Use of an adrenergic agent to alter muscle and fat deposition in lambs. *Journal of Animal Science* **59**, 1256–1261.

Barnes, P.J. & Brown, M.J. (1981) Venous plasma histamine in exercise- and hyperventilation-induced asthma in man. *Clinical Science* **61**, 159–162.

Bar-Or, O. (1983) Pediatric Sports Medicine for the Practitioner. In: *Physiologic Principles to Clinical Applications*. Springer-Verlag, New York: 88–109.

Bar-Or, O. (1985) Physical conditioning in children with cardiorespiratory disease. *Exercise and Sport Sciences Reviews* **13**, 305–334.

Bar-Or, O. & Inbar, O. (1992) Swimming and asthma. Benefits and deleterious effects. *Sports Medicine* **14**, 397–405.

Bar-Or, O., Neuman, I. & Dotan, R. (1977) Effects of dry and humid climates on exercise-induced asthma in children and preadolescents. *Journal of Allergy and Clinical Immunology* **60**, 163–168.

Bar-Yishay, E., Ben-Dov, I. & Godfrey, S. (1983) Refractory period after hyperventilation-induced asthma. *American Review of Respiratory Disease* **127**, 572–574.

Bar-Yishay, E., Gur, I., Inbar, O., *et al.* (1982) Differences between swimming and running as stimuli for exercise-induced asthma. *European Journal of Applied Physiology* **48**, 387–397.

Ben-Dov, I., Bar-Yishay, E. & Godfrey, S. (1982) Refractory period after exercise-induced asthma unexplained by respiratory heat loss. *American Review of Respiratory Disease* **125**, 530–534.

Ben-Zvi, Z., Spohn, W.A., Young, S.H. & Kattan, M. (1982) Hypnosis for exercise-induced asthma. *American Review of Respiratory Disease* **125**, 392–395.

Bernard, A., Carbonnelle, S., Michel, O., *et al.* (2003) Lung hyperpermeability and asthma prevalence in schoolchildren: unexpected associations with the attendance at indoor chlorinated swimming pools. *Occupational and Environmental Medicine* **60**, 385–394.

Bianco, S., Vaghi, A., Robuschi, M. & Pasargiklian, M. (1988) Prevention of exercise-induced bronchoconstriction by inhaled frusemide. *Lancet* **2**(8605), 252–255.

Boner, A., Vallone, G., Chiesa, M., Spezia, E., Fambri, L. & Sette, L. (1992)

Reproducibility of late phase pulmonary responses to exercise and its relationship to bronchial hyperreactivity in children with chronic asthma. *Pediatric Pulmonology* **14**, 156–159.

Brenner, A.M., Weiser, P.C., Krogh, L.A. & Loren, M.L. (1980) Effectiveness of a portable face mask in attenuating exercise-induced asthma. *Journal of the American Medical Association* **244**, 2196–2198.

Brugman, S. & Simons, S. (1998) Vocal cord dysfunction: don't mistake it for asthma. *Physician and Sportsmedicine* **26**, 63–85.

Carraro, S., Corradi, M., Zanconato, S., *et al.* (2005) Exhaled breath condensate cysteinyl leukotrienes are increased in children with exercise-induced bronchoconstriction. *Journal of Allergy and Clinical Immunology* **115**, 764–770.

Carroll, N. & Sly, P. (1999) Exercise training as an adjunct to asthma management? *Thorax* **54**, 190–191.

Chen, W.Y. & Horton, D.J. (1977) Heat and water loss from the airways and exercise-induced asthma. *Respiration* **34**, 305–313.

Christopher, K., Wood, R., Eckert, R., Blager, F., Raney, R. & Souhrada, J. (1983) Vocal-cord dysfunction presenting as asthma. *New England Journal of Medicine* **308**, 1566–1570.

Clark, C.J. & Cochrane, L.M. (1988) Assessment of work performance in asthma for determination of cardiorespiratory fitness and training capacity. *Thorax* **43**, 745–749.

Coreno, A., Skowronski, M., West, E., El-Ekiaby, A. & McFadden, E. Jr. (2005) Bronchoprotective effects of single doses of salmeterol combined with montelukast in thermally induced bronchospasm. *Chest* **127**, 1572–1578.

Cox, J.S. & Altounyan, R.E. (1970) Nature and modes of action of disodium cromoglycate (Lomudal). *Respiration* **27** (Suppl), 292–309.

Crimi, E., Balbo, A., Milanese, M. *et al.* (1992) Airway inflammation and occurrence of delayed bronchoconstriction in exercise-induced asthma. *American Review of Respiratory Disease* **146**, 507–512.

Cropp, G.J. (1975) Grading, time course, and incidence of exercise-induced airway obstruction and hyperinflation in asthmatic children. *Pediatrics* **56**(Suppl), 868–879.

Cropp, G.J. (1979) The exercise bronchoprovocation test:

standardization of procedures and evaluation of response. *Journal of Allergy and Clinical Immunology* **64**, 627–633.

Cropp, G. & Tanakawa, N. (1977) Cardiorespiratory adaptations of normal and asthmatic children to exercise. In: *Muscular Exercise and the Lung* (Dempsey, J. & Reed, C., eds.) University of Wisconsin Press, Madison, WI: 265–278.

Deal, E. Jr., McFadden, E. Jr. & Ingram, R. Jr. (1979a) Hyperpnea and heat flux: initial reaction sequence in exercise-induced asthma. *Journal of Applied Physiology: Respiratory, Environmental and Exercise Physiology* **46**, 476–483.

Deal, E. Jr., McFadden, E. Jr., Ingram, R. Jr., Breslin, F. & Jaeger, J. (1980) Airway responsiveness to cold air and hyperpnea in normal subjects and in those with hay fever and asthma. *American Review of Respiratory Disease* **121**, 621–628.

Deal, E., Mcfadden, E., Ingram, R. Jr., Strauss, R. & Jaeger, J. (1979b) Role of respiratory heat exchange in production of exercise-induced asthma. *Journal of Applied Physiology* **46**, 467–475.

Edmunds, A., Tooley, M. & Godfrey, S. (1978) The refractory period after exercise-induced asthma: its duration and relation to the severity of exercise. *American Review of Respiratory Disease* **117**, 247–254.

Ellis, E. (1984) Inhibition of exercise-induced asthma by theophylline. *Journal of Allergy and Clinical Immunology* **73**, 690–692.

Expert Panel of the National Heart, Lung and Blood Institute (2002) National Asthma Program. Guidelines for the diagnosis and management of asthma. Update of Selected Topics 2002 Available at: http://www.nhlbi.nih. gov/guidelines/asthma/ asthmafullrpt.pdf

Fink, G., Kaye, C., Blau, H. & Spitzer, S. (1993) Assessment of exercise capacity in asthmatic children with various degrees of activity. *Pediatric Pulmonology* **15**, 41–43.

Finnerty, J., Wood-Baker, R., Thomson, H. & Holgate, S. (1992) Role of leukotrienes in exercise-induced asthma. Inhibitory effect of ICI 204219, a potent leukotriene D4 receptor antagonist. *American Review of Respiratory Disease* **145**, 746–749.

Fitch, K. (1975) Comparative aspects of available exercise systems. *Pediatrics* **56** (Supplement), 904–907.

Fitch, K.D., Blitvich, J.D. & Morton, A.R. (1986) The effect of running training on exercise-induced asthma. *Annals of Allergy* **57**, 90–94.

Fung, K.P., Chow, O.K. & So, S.Y. (1986) Attenuation of exercise-induced asthma by acupuncture. *Lancet* **2**, 1419–1422.

Garfinkel, S., Kesten, S., Chapman, K. & Rebuck, A. (1992) Physiologic and nonphysiologic determinants of aerobic fitness in mild to moderate asthma. *American Review of Respiratory Disease* **145**, 741–745.

Gergen, P., Mullaly, D. & Evans, R. (1988) National survey of prevalence of asthma among children in the United States, 1977–80. *Pediatrics* **81**, 1–7.

Geubelle, F., Ernould, C. & Jovanovich, M. (1971) Working capacity and physical training in asthmatic children, at 1800 m altitude. *Acta Paediatrica Scandinavica Supplement* **217**, 93–98.

Ghary, J. (1975) Exercise and asthma: overview and clinical impact. *Pediatrics* **56** (Supplement), 844–846.

Gilbert, I., Fouke, J. & McFadden, E. Jr. (1988) Intra airway thermodynamics during exercise and hyperventilation in asthmatics. *Journal of Applied Physiology* **64**, 2167–2174.

Godfrey, S. (1974) *Exercise Testing in Children*. W.B. Saunders, Philadelphia.

Godfrey, S. & Konig, P. (1976) Inhibition of exercise induced asthma by different pharmacological pathways. *Thorax* **31**, 137–143.

Godfrey, S., Silverman, M. & Anderson, S. (1975) The use of the treadmill for assessing exercise-induced asthma and the effect of varying the severity and duration of exercise. *Pediatrics* **56** (Supplement), 893–898.

Gruber, W., Eber, E., Malle-Scheid, D., *et al.* (2002) Laser acupuncture in children and adolescents with exercise induced asthma. *Thorax* **57**, 222–225.

Haas, F., Levin, N., Pasierski, S., Bishop, M. & Axen, K. (1986) Reduced hyperpnea-induced bronchospasm following repeated cold air challenge. *Journal of Applied Physiology* **61**, 210–214.

Hahn, A., Anderson, S., Morton, A., Black, J. & Fitch, K. (1984a) A reinterpretation of the effect of temperature and water content of the inspired air in exercise-induced asthma. *American Review of Respiratory Disease* **130**, 575–579.

Hahn, A., Nogrady, S., Tumilty, D., Lawrence, S. & Morton, A. (1984b) Histamine reactivity during the refractory period after exercise-induced asthma. *Thorax* **39**, 919–923.

Hallstrand, T., Curtis, J., Koepsell, T., *et al.* (2002) Effectiveness of screening examinations to detect unrecognized exercise-induced bronchoconstriction. *Journal of Pediatrics* **141**, 343–349.

Hallstrand, T.S., Moody, M.W., Aitken, M.L. & Henderson, W.R. Jr. (2005) Airway immunopathology of asthma with exercise-induced bronchononstriction. *Journal of Allergy and Clinical Immunology* **116**, 586–593.

Hamielec, C.M., Manning, P.J. & O'Byrne, P.M. (1988) Exercise refractoriness after histamine inhalation in asthmatic subjects. *American Review of Respiratory Disease* **138**, 794–798.

Hancox, R., Subbarao, P., Kamada, D., Watson, R., Hargreave, F. & Inman, M. (2002) β₂-Agonist tolerance and exercise-induced bronchospasm. *American Journal of Respiratory Critical Care Medicine* **165**, 1068–1070.

Hansen-Flaschen, J. & Schotland, H. (1998) New treatments for exercise-induced asthma (Editorial). *New England Journal of Medicine* **339**, 192–193.

Heimdal, J.-H., Roksund, O., Halvorsen, T., Skadberg, B. & Olofsson, J. (2006) Continuous laryngoscopy exercise test: a method for visualizing laryngeal dysfunction during exercise. *Laryngoscope* **116**, 52–57.

Helenius, I.J., Tikkanen, H.O. & Haahtela, T. (1997) Association between type of training and risk of asthma in elite athletes. *Thorax* **52**, 157–160.

Helenius, I., Rytilä, P., Metso, T., Haahtela, T., Venge, P. & Tikkanen, H. (1998) Respiratory symptoms, bronchial responsiveness and cellular characteristics of induced sputum in elite swimmers. *Allergy* **53**, 346–352.

Helenius, I. & Haahtela, T. (2000) Allergy and asthma in elite summer sport athletes. *Journal of Allergy and Clinical Immunology* **106**, 444–452.

Helenius, I., Rytila, P., Sarna, S., *et al.* (2002) Effect of continuing or finishing high-level sports on airway inflammation, bronchial hyperresponsiveness, and asthma: a 5-year prospective follow-up study of 42 highly trained swimmers. *Journal of Allergy and Clinical Immunology* **109**, 962–968.

Henriksen, J. & Dahl, R. (1983) Effects of inhaled budesonide alone and in combination with lowdose terbutaline in children with exercise-induced asthma. *American Review of Respiratory Disease* **128**, 993–997.

Inbar, O., Alvarez, D. & Lyons, H. (1981) Exerciseinduced asthma: a comparison between two modes of exercise stress. *European Journal of Respiratory Disease* **62**, 160–167.

Inbar, O., Dotan, R., Dlin, R., Neuman, I. & Bar-Or, O. (1980) Breathing dry or humid air and exercise induced asthma during swimming. *European Journal of Applied Physiology and Occupational Physiology* **44**, 43–50.

Ingemann-Hansen, T., Bundgaard, A., HalkjaerKristensen, J., Siggaard-Andersen, J. & Weeke, B. (1980) Maximal oxygen consumption rate in patients with bronchial asthma: the effect of i32-adrenoreceptor stimulation. *Scandinavian Journal of Clinical and Laboratory Investigation* **40**, 99–104.

Inman, M.D. & O'Byrne, P.M. (1996) The effect of regular inhaled albuterol on exercise-induced bronchoconstriction. *American Journal of Respiratory and Critical Care Medicine* **153**, 65–69.

Israel, E., Dermarkarian, R., Rosenberg, M., *et al.* (1990) The effects of a 5-lipoxygenas, inhibitor on asthma induced by cold, dry air. *New England Journal of Medicine* **323**, 1740–1744.

Jones, R. (1966) Assessment of respiratory function in the asthmatic child. *British Medical Journal* **2**, 297–295.

Kilham, H., Tooley, M. & Silverman, M. (1979) Running, walking, and hyperventilation causing asthma in children. *Thorax* **34**, 582–586.

Lang, D., Butz, A., Duggan, A. & Serwint, J. (2004) Physical activity in urban school-aged children with asthma. *Pediatrics* **113**, e341–e346.

Langdeau, J.-B., Turcotte, H., Bowie, D., Jobin, J., Desgagné, P. & Boulet, L.-P. (2000) Airway hyperresponsiveness in elite athletes. *American Journal of Respiratory Critical Care Medicine* **161**, 1479–1484.

Lee, T., Assoufi, B. & Kay, A. (1983a) The link between exercise, respiratory heat exchange, and the mast cell in bronchial asthma. *Lancet* **i**, 520–522.

Lee, T., Nagakura, T., Papageorgiou, N., Cromwell, O., Iikura, Y. & Kay, A. (1984) Mediators in exercise-induced asthma. *Journal of Allergy and Clinical Immunology* **73**, 634–639.

Lee, T., Nagakura, T., Papageorgiou, N., Ikura, Y. & Kay, A. (1983b) Exercise-induced late asthmatic reactions with neutrophil chemotactic activity. *New England Journal of Medicine* **308**, 1502–1505.

Lee, T., Hoover, R., Williams, J., *et al.* (1985) Effect of dietary enrichment with eicosapentaenoic and docosahexaenoic acids on *in vitro* neutrophil and monocyte leukotriene generation and neutrophil function. *New England Journal of Medicine* **312**, 1217–1224.

Leff, J., Busse, W., Pearlman, D., *et al.* (1998) Montelukast, a leukotriene-receptor antagonist, for the treatment of mild asthma and exercise-induced bronchoconstriction. *New England Journal of Medicine* **339**, 147–152.

Lemanske, R. Jr. & Henke, K. (1989) Exercise-induced asthma. In: (Gisolfi, C. & Lamb, D., eds.) *Youth, Exercise, and Sport. Perspectives in Exercise Science and Sports Medicine.* Benchmark Press, Indianapolis, IN: 465–511.

Loughlin, G. & Taussig, L. (1979) Pulmonary function in children with a history of laryngotracheobronchitis. *Journal of Pediatrics* **94**, 365–369.

McConnell, R., Berhane, K., Gilliland, F., *et al.* (2002) Asthma in exercising children exposed to ozone: a cohort study. *Lancet* **359**, 386–391.

McFadden, E. (1987) Exercise-induced asthma. Assessment of current etiologic concepts. *Chest* **91**, 151S–157S.

McFadden, E. & Ingram, R. Jr. (1979) Exercise-induced asthma. Observations on the initiating stimulus. *New England Journal of Medicine* **301**, 763–769.

McFadden, E. & Ingram, R.J. (1980) Asthma: perspectives, definition, and classification. In: *Pulmonary Diseases and Disorders*, 1st edn. (Fishman, A., ed.) McGraw-Hill, New York: 562–566.

McFadden, E.J., Lenner, A. & Strohl, K. (1986) Postexertional airway rewarming and thermally induced asthma. New insights into pathophysiology and possible pathogenesis. *Journal of Clinical Investigation* **78**, 18–25.

McFadden, E. Jr., Stearns, D., Ingram, R. Jr. & Leith, D. (1977) Relative contributions of hypocarbia and hyperpnea as mechanisms in post-exercise asthma. *Journal of Applied Physiology* **42**, 22–27.

McFadden, E. Jr. & Zawadski, D. (1996) Vocal cord dysfunction masquerading as exercise-induced asthma: a physiologic cause for "choking" during athletic activities. *American Journal of Respiratory Critical Care Medicine* **153**, 942–947.

McLaughlin, F. & Dozor, A. (1983) Cold air inhalation challenge in the diagnosis of asthma in children. *Pediatrics* **72**, 503–509.

Manning, P., Watson, R., Margolskee, D., Williams, V., Schwartz, J. & O'Byrne, P. (1990) Inhibition of exercise-induced bronchoconstriction by MK-571, a potent leukotriene D4-receptor antagonist. *New England Journal of Medicine* **323**, 1736–1739.

Matsumoto, I., Araki, H., Tsuda, K., *et al.* (1999) Effects of swimming training on aerobic capacity and exercise induced bronchoconstriction in children with bronchial asthma. *Thorax* **54**, 196–201.

Matthay, R. & Mahler, D. (1986) Theophylline improves global cardiac function and reduces dyspnea in chronic obstructive lung disease. *Journal of Allergy and Clinical Immunology* **78**, 793–799.

McConnell, R., Berhane, K., Gilliland, F., *et al.* (2002) Asthma in exercising children exposed to ozone: a cohort study. *Lancet* **359**, 386–391.

Meeuwisse, W., McKenzie, D., Hopkins, S. & Road, J. (1992) The effect of salbutamol on performance in elite nonasthmatic athletes. *Medicine & Science in Sports & Exercise* **24**, 1161–1166.

Mickleborough, T., Lindley, M., Ionescu, A. & Fly, A. (2006) Protective effect of fish oil supplementation on exercise-induced bronchoconstriction in asthma. *Chest* **129**, 39–49.

Middleton, E. Jr. (1984) Airway smooth muscle, asthma, and calcium ions. *Journal of Allergy and Clinical Immunology* **73**, 643–650.

Milgrom, H. & Taussig, L. (1999) Keeping children with exercise-induced asthma active. *Pediatrics* **104**, e38.

Morton, A.R., Ogle, S.L. & Fitch, K.D. (1992a) Effects of nedocromil sodium, cromolyn sodium, and a placebo in exercise-induced asthma. *Annals of Allergy* **68**, 143–148.

Morton, A., Papalia, S. & Fitch, K. (1992b) Is salbutamol ergogenic? The effects of salbutamol on physical performance in high-performance nonasthmatic athletes. *Clinical Journal of Sports Medicine* **2**, 93–97.

Morton, A., Scott, C. & Fitch, K. (1989) The effects of theophylline on the physical performance and work capacity of well-trained athletes. *Journal of Allergy and Clinical Immunology* **83**, 55–60.

Nagakura, T., Lee, T., Assoufi, B., Newman-Taylor, A., Denison, D. & Kay, A. (1983) Neutrophil chemotactic factor in exercise- and hyperventilationinduced asthma. *American Review of Respiratory Disease* **128**, 294–296.

Nelson, J., Strauss, L., Skowronski, M., Ciufo, R., Novak, R. & McFadden, E. (1998) Effect of long-term salmeterol treatment on exercise-induced asthma.

New England Journal of Medicine **339**, 141–146.

Nickerson, B., Bautista, D., Namey, M., Richard, W. & Keens, T. (1983) Distance running improves fitness in asthmatic children without pulmonary complications or changes in exercise-induced bronchospasm. *Pediatrics* **71**, 147–152.

Nixon, P. & Orenstein, D. (1988) Exercise testing in children. *Pediatric Pulmonology* **5**, 107–122.

O'Donnell, W., Rosenberg, M., Niven, R., Drazen, J. & Israel, E. (1992) Acetazolamide and furosemide attenuate asthma induced by hyperventilation of cold, dry air. *American Review of Respiratory Disease* **146**, 1518–1523.

Orenstein, D. (1993) Assessment of exercise pulmonary function. In: *Pediatric Laboratory Exercise Testing: Clinical Guidelines* (Rowland, T., ed.) Human Kinetics, Champaign, IL: 141–163.

Orenstein, D., Reed, M., Grogan, F. & Crawford, L. (1985) Exercise conditioning in children with asthma. *Journal of Pediatrics* **106**, 556–560.

Oseid, S. & Haaland, K. (1978) Exercise studies on asthmatic children before and after regular physical training. In: *Swimming Medicine*, Vol. IV (Eriksson, B. & Furberg, B., eds.) University Park Press, Baltimore: 32–41.

Panditi, S. & Silverman, M. (2003) Perception of exercise induced asthma by children and their parents. *Archives of Diseases in Childhood* **88**, 807–811.

Pearlman, D., Milgrom, H., Till, D. & Ziehmer, B. (2006) Effect of formoterol fumarate treatment on exercise-induced bronchoconstriction in children. *Annals of Allergy, Asthma and Immunology* **97**, 382–388.

Pearlman, D., Ostrom, N., Bronsky, E., Bonuccelli, C. & Hanby, L. (1999) The leukotriene D4-receptor antagonist zafirlukast attenuates exercise-induced bronchoconstriction in children. *Journal of Pediatrics* **134**, 273–279.

Perkner, J., Fennelly, K., Balkissoon, R., *et al.* (1998) Irritant-associated vocal cord dysfunction. *Journal of Occupational & Environmental Medicine* **40**, 136–143.

Petersen, K. & McElhenney, T. (1965) Effects of a physical fitness program upon asthmatic boys. *Pediatrics* **35**, 295–299.

Pianosi, P. & Davis, H. (2004) Determinants of physical fitness in children with asthma. *Pediatrics* **113**, e225–e229.

Pierson, W., Bierman, W., Kawabori, L. & Van Arsdel, P. (1972) The incidence of exercise-induced bronchospams in 'normal' and 'atopic' children. *Journal of Allergy and Clinical Immunology* **49**, 129A–130A.

Reiff, D., Choudry, N., Pride, N. & Ind, P. (1989) The effect of prolonged submaximal warm-up exercise on exercise-induced asthma. *American Review of Respiratory Disease* **139**, 479–484.

Rice, S., Bierman, C., Shapiro, G., Furukawa, C. & Pierson, W. (1985) Identification of exercise-induced asthma among intercollegiate athletes. *Annals of Allergy* **55**, 790–793.

Rosenthal, R., Laube, B., Hood, D. & Norman, P. (1990) Analysis of refractory period after exercise and eucapnic voluntary hyperventilation challenge. *American Review of Respiratory Disease* **141**, 368–372.

Rundell, K., Im, J., Mayers, L., Wilber, R., Szmedra, L. & Schmitz, H. (2001) Self-reported symptoms and exercise-induced asthma in the elite athlete. *Medicine & Science in Sports & Exercise* **33**, 208–213.

Rundell, K. & Spiering, B. (2003) Inspiratory stridor in elite athletes. *Chest* **123**, 468–474.

Rundell, K., Spiering, B., Baumann, J. & Evans, T. (2004) Montelukast has no ergogenic effect on cycle ergometry in cold temperature. *Medicine & Science in Sports & Exercise* **36**, 1847–1851.

Rupp, N., Guill, M. & Brudno, D. (1992) Unrecognized exercise-induced bronchospam in adolescent athletes. *American Journal of Diseases of Children* **146**, 941–944.

Sakula, A. (1988) A history of asthma. The FitzPatrick Lecture 1987. *Journal of the Royal College of Physicians of London* **22**, 36–43.

Salter, H. (1864) *On Asthma: Its Pathology and Treatment*. Blanchard & Lea, Philadelphia.

Schachter, E., Lach, E. & Lee, M. (1981) The protective effect of a cold weather mask on exercise-induced asthma. *Annals of Allergy* **46**, 12–16.

Schwartzstein, R.M. (1992) Asthma: to run or not to run? *American Review of Respiratory Disease* **145**, 739–740.

Sears, M., Taylor, D., Print, C., *et al.* (1990) Regular inhaled beta-agonist treatment in bronchial asthma. *Lancet* **336**, 1391–1396.

Seear, M., Wensley, D. & West, N. (2005) How accurate is the diagnosis of exercise induced asthma among Vancouver school children? *Archives of Diseases in Childhood* **90**, 898–902.

Sheppard, D., Saisho, A., Nadel, J. & Boushey, H. (1981) Exercise increases sulfur dioxide-induced bronchoconstriction in asthmatic subjects. *American Review of Respiratory Disease* **123**, 486–591.

Signorile, J., Kaplan, T., Applegate, B. & Perry, A. (1992) Effects of acute inhalation of the bronchodilator, albuterol, on power output. *Medicine & Science in Sports & Exercise* **24**, 638–642.

Silverman, M. & Anderson, S. (1972) Standardization of exercise tests in asthmatic children. *Archives of Diseases in Childhood* **47**, 882–889.

Silverman, M., Hobbs, F., Gordon, I. & Carswell, F. (1978) Cystic fibrosis, atopy and airways lability. *Archives of Diseases in Childhood* **53**, 873–877.

Souhrada, M. & Souhrada, J. (1981) The direct effect of temperature on airway smooth muscle. *Respiration Physiology* **44**, 311–323.

Spitzer, W., Saissa, S., Ernst, P., *et al.* (1992) The use of j3-agonists and the risk of death and near death from asthma. *New England Journal of Medicine* **326**, 501–506.

Strauss, R., McFadden, E., Ingram, R. Jr. & Jaeger, J. (1977) Enhancement of exercise-induced asthma by cold air. *New England Journal of Medicine* **297**, 743–747.

Strunk, R., Rubin, D., Kelly, L. & Sherman, B. (1988) Determination of fitness in children with asthma. *American Journal of Diseases of Children* **142**, 940–944.

Sue-Chu, M., Sandsun, M., Helgerud, J., Reinertsen, R. & Bjermer, L. (1999) Salmeterol does not affect physical performance in highly-trained nonasthmatic cross country skiers. *Scandinavian Journal of Medicine & Science in Sports* **9**, 48–52.

Taylor, W. & Newacheck, P. (1992) Impact of childhood asthma on health. *Pediatrics* **90**, 657–662.

Thio, B., Nagelkerke, A., Ketel, A., van Keeken, B. & Dankert-Roelse, J.E. (1996) Exercise-induced asthma and cardiovascular fitness in asthmatic children. *Thorax* **51**, 207–209.

Thomsen, S.F., Ulrik, C.S., Larsen, K. & Backer, V. (2004) Change in prevalence of asthma in Danish children and adolescents. *Annals of Allergy, Asthma & Immunology* **92**, 506–511.

Trappe, S., Costill, D. & Thomas, R. (2001) Effect of swim taper on whole muscle and single muscle fiber contractile properties. *Medicine & Science in Sports & Exercise* **33**, 48–56.

Varray, A., Mercier, J., Terral, C. & Prefaut, C. (1991) Individualized aerobic and high intensity training for asthmatic children in an exercise readaptation program. Is training always helpful for better adaptation to exercise? *Chest* **99**, 579–586.

Weiler, J., Layton, T. & Hunt, M. (1998) Asthma in United States Olympic athletes who participated in the 1996 Summer Games. *Journal of Allergy and Clinical Immunology* **102**, 722–726.

Weiler-Ravell, D. & Godfrey, S. (1981) Do exercise and antigen-induced asthma utilize the same pathways? *Journal of Allergy and Clinical Immunology* **67**, 391–397.

Wells, R.J., Walker, J. & Hiclder, R. (1960) Effects of cold air on respiratory airflow resistance in patients with respiratory-tract disease. *New England Journal of Medicine* **263**, 268–273.

Wiens, L., Sabath, R., Ewing, L., Gowdamarajan, R., Portnoy, J. & Scagliotti, D. (1992) Chest pain in otherwise healthy children and adolescents is frequently caused by exercise-induced asthma. *Pediatrics* **90**, 350–353.

Wilber, R., Rundell, K.L., Szmedra, L., Jenkinson, D., Im, J. & Drake, S. (2000) Incidence of exercise-induced bronchospasm in Olympic winter sport athletes. *Medicine & Science in Sports & Exercise* **32**, 732–737.

Wilson, B., Bar-Or, O. & Seed, L. (1990) Effects of humid air breathing during arm or treadmill exercise on exercise-induced bronchoconstriction and refractoriness. *American Review of Respiratory Disease* **142**, 349–352.

Woolley, M., Anderson, S. & Quigley, B. (1990) Duration of protective effect of terbutaline sulfate and cromolyn sodium alone and in combination on exercise-induced asthma. *Chest* **97**, 39–45.

Zach, M., Polgar, G., Kump, H. & Kroisel, P. (1984) Cold air challenge of airway hyper-reactivity in children: practical application and theoretical aspects. *Pediatric Research* **18**, 469–478.

Zeitoun, M., Wilk, B., Matsuzaka, A., Knöpfli, B., Wilson, B. & Bar-Or, O. (2004) Facial cooling enhances exercise-induced bronchoconstriction in asthmatic children. *Medicine & Science in Sports & Exercise* **36**, 767–771.

Chapter 27

Type 1 Diabetes Mellitus and Sport

KATHERINE E. ISCOE AND MICHAEL C. RIDDELL

Treatment for the child with type 1 diabetes mellitus (DM), formally insulin-dependent or juvenile diabetes, has improved dramatically since the discovery of insulin in 1921, in both biologic and technological terms. Nevertheless, a number of important clinical management issues are needed for the active child with diabetes to ensure proper health and prevention of long-term complications from the disease. Some evidence suggests that optimal metabolic control maximizes physical performance in youth with diabetes, although more studies are needed to confirm this suggestion. With the increasing prevalence of childhood obesity, the importance of physical activity to help prevent type 2 diabetes in youth is of more recent consideration. For all children and adolescents, regular exercise can increase insulin sensitivity, decrease fat mass, increase lean mass, improve blood lipid profile, and lower arterial blood pressure. Importantly, large-scale epidemiologic studies suggest that modest amounts of regular exercise (i.e., 30 min·day^{-1} walking) reduce the risk of developing type 2 diabetes from a state of impaired glucose tolerance, at least in adulthood, by approximately 60% (Knowler *et al.* 2002).

For youth with diabetes who are engaged in sport, control must go beyond the typical regimen of diet and insulin treatment to obtain optimal performance and prevent metabolic complications that can occur both during and after exercise. Adolescence presents additional concerns for these patients, as hormonal changes during growth and maturation create a temporary state of insulin resistance. In addition, many adolescents maintain some

endogenous insulin secretion just after diagnosis, which can make metabolic control particularly challenging. Other behavioral issues may make for a difficult task of educating and counseling them on their disease. This chapter focuses on both the physiologic and clinical aspects of diabetes management in the adolescent athlete and highlights the beneficial effects of regular exercise for the child with diabetes mellitus.

Classification, diagnosis, and management

Definition

Diabetes mellitus is a group of five disorders that express either absolute or relative insulin deficiency. Clinical manifestations typically include hyperglycemia (fasting glucose levels >7.1 mmol·L^{-1} and/or post-load glucose >11.1 mmol·L^{-1}) and glycosuria. The most common of these disorders are type 1 and type 2 DM. A wide (over 400-fold) variation exists in worldwide incidence rates of type 1 diabetes in youth, with the highest occurring in Finland (over 45 per 100,000 under the age of 15 years) and the lowest in parts of China (Silink 2002). The incidence of type 2 DM is increasing more rapidly than type 1 DM and type 2 DM is occurring at younger ages, including adolescence and childhood. In the USA, approximately one-third of the newly diagnosed cases of type 2 DM are in the adolescent age group (Alberti *et al.* 2004). Among Japanese school children, type 2 DM is seven times more common than type 1 DM (Rosenbloom *et al.* 1999). The prevalence of type 2 DM is increasing largely because of the detrimental effects of obesity caused by a positive energy balance (Botero & Wolfsdorf 2005), with type 2 DM rates in children and adolescents rising from 2–4% of all individuals with DM to a staggering 8–45% in various geographical regions (Rosenbloom *et al.* 1999). Treatment of type 2 DM may or may not include insulin therapy and usually includes regular exercise and weight loss.

Education and management

Effective glucose management in the active child can occur only through proper education; the formal component may take as little as a few days or weeks but should be ongoing to maintain optimal health. Unfortunately, the impact of physical activity on blood glucose management is often misunderstood and sometimes not emphasized in the educational experience. Allowing the child more interaction with his or her treatment team results in superior self-management, a factor of increasing importance as the child develops and spends more time away from his or her parents (Pyorala 2004). Thankfully, children and adolescents with type 1 diabetes appear to spend more time in sporting activity than their healthy siblings, especially in spare time (Raile *et al.* 1999).

Treatment should reflect the age and maturity of the child. Often, the parent will take over the child's daily regimen, rendering the child somewhat dependent. Diabetic camps that include physical activity are an effective means to provide education and allow the child to interact and bond with other children with diabetes.

The Diabetes Control and Complications Trial (DCCT) shows that intensive blood glucose management helps to prevent long-term complications from the disease both in adults (DCCT Research Group 1993) and in children with diabetes (DCCT Research Group 1994). During adolescence blood glucose control may be "relaxed" as the risk of hypoglycemia increases threefold with intensive insulin therapy (DCCT Research Group 1994), and is even more prevalent in very active children (see below). Reasonable glycemic goals for diabetes management, based on recommendations by the US Department of Health and Human Services, National Institutes of Health and the Centers for Disease Control and Prevention (National Diabetes Education Program 2006) are shown in Table 27.1.

Insulin therapy

Insulin is a key regulatory hormone for fuel metabolism during rest and exercise. In persons without diabetes insulin levels increase following a meal to allow for substrate storage. During a fasted state and during endurance exercise, insulin secretion is lowered to help mobilize fuel and maintain euglycemia (i.e., blood glucose of 4–7 $mmol \cdot L^{-1}$) in the face of increased glucose disposal. The child with type 1 DM relies solely on exogenous insulin for the regulation of fuel metabolism. Because of the imperfections associated with determining precise

Table 27.1 Plasma blood glucose and HbA1C goals for type 1 diabetes mellitus by age group which also apply to young athletes.

Values by age	Plasma blood glucose goal range ($mmol \cdot L^{-1}$)		
	Before meals	Bedtime/overnight	HbA1C
Toddlers and preschoolers (<6 years)	5.6–10	6.1–12.2	<8.5% (but >7.5%)
School age (6–12 years)	5–10	5.6–10	<8%
Adolescents and young adults (13–19 years)	5–130	5–8.3	<7.5%*

Goals should be individualized and lower blood glucose levels may be reasonably based on a risk–benefit assessment. Blood glucose goals should be higher than those listed above in children with frequent hypoglycemia or hypoglycemia unawareness.
* A lower goal (<7.0%) is reasonable if it can be achieved without excessive hypoglycemia.

insulin needs, which may change from minute to minute, the child is often exercising in either an over- or underinsulinized state, resulting in hypo- and hyperglycemia, respectively. Various types of insulin may be administered by syringe, pen, or pump, each having different pharmacologic profiles (Perkins & Riddell 2006). Weight gain has typically been associated with intensive insulin therapy that includes multiple daily injections or continuous insulin infusion systems (DCCT Research Group 1988). Regular physical activity allows for a lowering in daily insulin needs (see below for recommendations) and a reduction in fat mass gains.

Exercise benefits and guidelines

Research has improved our understanding of the various biochemical and metabolic aspects of diabetic pathology and the impact of exercise on diabetes control. Through such research, specific prescriptions of physical activity can be made to optimize health and fitness benefits. Although somewhat dependent on intensity and duration, advantages include a decline in resting heart rate and blood pressure, an improved lean muscle mass to fat ratio and weight control. Additional benefits specific to diabetes include improved insulin sensitivity, a reduction in daily insulin needs, and a diminished glycemic response to a meal.

Most children with diabetes attain the recommended daily activity levels and individuals in certain age groups even exceed the levels of activity of their non-diabetic counterparts, possibly because of intensive health care education (Raile *et al*. 1999). Unfortunately, the endorsement of exercise may be difficult in teenagers because hormonal changes during puberty may complicate glucose management increasing susceptibility to hypoglycemia (Raile *et al*. 1999).

A positive association between glycemic control and $\dot{V}O_{2max}$ (Ludvigsson 1980; Huttunen *et al*. 1984, 1989; Poortmans *et al*. 1986) or between glycemic control and reported physical activity (Sackey & Jefferson 1996; Horgan 2005) in youth with type 1 DM has been observed. This suggests that either increased aerobic capacity improves glycemic control or that proper metabolic control maximizes aerobic capacity. In support of the former notion,

when subjects are stratified according to their level of participation, metabolic control is significantly better in those who exercise frequently, regardless of the type of activity (Huttunen *et a*l. 1989). Despite the positive associations between $\dot{V}O_{2max}$ and glycemic control in the above cross-sectional studies, the influence of exercise training on glycemic control, based on longitudinal studies, is unclear. Indeed, the influence of regular exercise on improving blood glucose control in children and adolescents with type 1 DM is equivocal; some studies show an improvement in blood glucose control (Dahl-Jorgensen *et al*. 1980; Campaigne *et al*. 1984; Stratton *et al*. 1987) but others show no effect (Larsson *et al*. 1962, 1964; Landt *et al*. 1985; Rowland *et al*. 1985). Based on these studies, training may decrease HbA1c levels and fasting glycemia in some adolescents, particularly if they are in poor glycemic control initially (i.e., HbA1c >10%). It is likely that carbohydrate ingestion to prevent or treat hypoglycemia may counter the beneficial effects of exercise on glycemic control in some individuals. Clearly, the goal of regular exercise should be to increase insulin sensitivity and to improve the overall cardiovascular and psychologic profile of the child with type 1 DM, regardless of any putative benefits to blood glucose management.

Adolescents with type 1 DM who undergo aerobic training appear to improve cardiorespiratory endurance and muscle strength at least as much as their non-diabetic peers (Larsson *et al*. 1964; Huttunen *et al*. 1989; Mosher *et al*. 1998). In addition, youth who attend camps that feature increased regular physical activities, along with education about how to modify dietary intake or daily insulin dosage to prevent hypoglycemia, show improved metabolic control and fitness (Akerblom *et al*. 1980; Braatvedt *et al*. 1997).

Impact of diabetes on fitness and performance

Children and adolescents with type 1 DM may have some impaired fitness-related components and alterations in their cardiorespiratory responses to exercise. Most studies indicate that maximal aerobic power ($\dot{V}O_{2max}$) (Larsson *et al*. 1962, 1964; Persson & Thoren 1980; Baran & Dorchy 1982; Poortmans *et al.* 1986; Baraldi *et al.* 1992; Niranjan *et al.* 1997; Komatsu *et al.* 2005) and physical work capacity (Sterky 1963; Huttunen *et al.* 1984; Baraldi *et al.* 1992; Austin *et al.* 1993; Barkai *et al.* 1996) are impaired in young people with type 1 DM, especially if they are in fair to poor metabolic control. Inactivity may contribute to decreased performance in some children with diabetes because, when matched for age, body size, and habitual activity, adolescents with type 1 DM have cardiac function and $\dot{V}o_{2max}$ levels similar to those in healthy adolescents (Rutenfranz *et al.* 1968; Hagan *et al.* 1979; Dahl-Jorgensen *et al.* 1980; Rowland & Cunningham 1992).

Children with type 1 DM have higher systolic blood pressure (Persson & Thoren 1980; Nordgren *et al.* 1994), lower O_2 pulse ($\dot{V}o_2$/heart rate) (Baraldi *et al.* 1992), a thickening of capillary basal membrane in skeletal muscle (Raskin *et al.* 1983; Sosenko *et al.* 1984), and impairments in the regulation of skeletal muscle blood flow (Ewald *et al.* 1981; Ewald & Tuvemo 1985; Kobbah *et al.* 1985). In addition, adolescent boys with type 1 DM, who exercise at a relative intensity similar to that of controls, have elevated ratings of perceived exertion (Riddell *et al.* 2000a) and an impaired rate of carbohydrate utilization (Riddell *et al.* 2000b). In young adults, skeletal muscle strength appears normal but nerve conduction speed and endurance capacity may be diminished (Almeida *et al.* 2005). Thus, cardiorespiratory, metabolic, neuromuscular, and perceptual effort may be altered in individuals with diabetes if they are poorly controlled and these factors may impair their exercise performance. Nonetheless, well-motivated youth with diabetes, who are in good metabolic control, may be able to compete equally with their peers. In point of fact, individuals with type 1 DM can achieve world-class excellence in sports and an international organization pays tribute to these remarkable individuals (www. diabetes-exercise.org/).

Sports selection

Recommended sporting activities have traditionally been those with stable energy expenditures that are spread out over long periods (Dorchy 1989; Hough 1994) and these may be relevant for those attempt-

ing to determine caloric expenditures and carbohydrate and insulin adjustments for exercise. Most sports, however, have unpredictable energy demands, such as those with short but intense periods of exertion and children's activities that are often spontaneous and of an unpredictable duration. As such, metabolic control may be more challenging for the active child, yet still should be an attainable goal. It is particularly important that coaches, teachers, supervisors, and parents be made aware of the child's condition and are knowledgeable about how to treat hypoglycemia (see below).

With adequate education and insulin therapy, the child with diabetes should be encouraged to participate in any sport they wish. Using self-blood glucose monitoring (SBGM) prior to, during, and after the activity, he or she should feel confident and understand how to control glucose fluctuations by changing insulin and carbohydrate intake to prevent acute complications (see below for recommendations). Newly developed continuous blood glucose monitoring devises allow minute-by-minute measures of glucose concentrations and an enhancement in glycemic control in youth (Chase *et al.* 2001). As an advantage, some of these devises provide patients with "real time" directional changes in blood glucose, which tend to be sudden during vigorous exercise (Iscoe *et al.* 2006).

Fuel metabolism and mechanisms of glucose regulation during exercise

To understand the possible metabolic responses to exercise in children with diabetes, it is useful to first briefly describe the mechanisms of glucose regulation in non-diabetic youth.

Non-diabetic children and adolescents

At rest, the body uses primarily free fatty acids (FFA) delivered from adipose tissue. During the transition to exercise, muscles draw upon a complex mixture of circulating FFA, muscle triglycerides, muscle glycogen, and blood glucose derived from liver glycogen. Fuel metabolism during exercise is under complex neuroendocrine control and includes the hormones insulin, glucagon, catecholamines, growth hormone, and cortisol (Camacho *et al.* 2005). The proportions of the substrates listed above depend on the intensity and duration of the activity. At low to moderate intensities, plasma-derived FFA predominate, while both plasma glucose and muscle glycogen make up the majority of fuel as the exercise intensifies. During heavy exercise, total glucose utilization may be as much as 1.0–1.5 g·kg body mass^{-1}·h^{-1} in healthy adolescents and in adolescents with diabetes (Riddell *et al.* 2000b). As the exercise duration increases, there is a greater reliance on fuels from outside of the muscle, including plasma FFA and blood glucose. This greater dependence on fuels from outside the muscle can have dramatic effects on blood glucose levels, particularly for the child with type 1 DM. Compared with adults, children and adolescents oxidize more fat and less carbohydrates during exercise performed at the same relative intensity (Martinez & Haymes 1992; Mahon *et al.* 1997), possibly because they have lower muscle glycogen stores. In support of a reduced glycogen availability, children utilize more exogenous carbohydrate (i.e., ingested sports beverage) during exercise than adults (Timmons *et al.* 2003). Hypo- and hyperglycemia are rare in exercising healthy children who do not have diabetes because insulin secretion is lowered with increasing muscle glucose uptake and counterregulatory hormones are elevated which cause glucose production to match glucose disposal.

Children and adolescents with type 1 diabetes

The mix of fuel utilization during exercise in youth with type 1 DM appears to be similar to those without diabetes, except that the former may rely slightly more on fat and less on carbohydrates even if well insulinized (Raguso *et al.* 1995; Riddell *et al.* 2000b). In individuals with type 1 DM, the pancreas does not regulate insulin levels in response to exercise, making blood glucose regulation nearly impossible. Moreover, there may be deficiencies in the release of the counterregulatory hormones epinephrine and glucagon which would normally help facilitate glucose production and release by the liver (Camacho *et al.* 2005; Tansey *et al.* 2006). As patients soon discover, they may have either

increases or decreases in blood glucose levels during exercise. The following sections outline the typical problems of over- and underinsulinization during exercise that can contribute to the development of acute metabolic complications.

Intensive insulin therapy, overinsulinization, and hypoglycemia

Many find that intensive insulin therapy helps with glucose management during exercise, because it allows for frequent changes in insulin dosages, particularly if they use an insulin pump. However, the move toward more aggressive insulin therapy increases the risk of exercise-associated hypoglycemia for some active people with diabetes, especially young patients (DCCT Research Group 1994). Indeed, hypoglycemia is the most severe acute complication of intensive insulin treatment, with exercise being a frequent cause (Wasserman *et al.* 2002). Nonetheless, such aggressive insulin therapy should be considered for active youth because it helps to prevent long-term complications from the disease and because physical performance and aerobic capacity are related to the degree of metabolic control (see above).

Most children and adolescents with type 1 DM who exercise for prolonged periods (i.e., >30 min) experience a significant drop in blood glucose levels (Persson & Thoren 1980; Sills & Cerny 1983; Schiffrin & Parikh 1985; McNiven-Temple *et al.* 1995; Riddell *et al.* 1999; Tansey *et al.* 2006). Hypoglycemia is not restricted to those individuals who begin exercise with lower glycemic levels as there appears to be a strong positive correlation between the drop in glycemia and the pre-exercise value (Riddell *et al.* 1999). Severe post-exercise late-onset hypoglycemia (up to 36 h after exercise) is particularly common in active children with type 1 DM (MacDonald 1987; Aman *et al.* 1989; Bell & Cutter 1994; Shehadeh *et al.* 1998; Tupola *et al.* 1998), possibly because proper strategies are not adopted to replace muscle and liver glycogen stores. The maximal risk of post-exercise hypoglycemia appears to be 6–10 h after the cessation of exercise. A recent multicentre trial of children with type 1 DM found that 75 min of late afternoon intermittent exercise causes more frequent episodes of nighttime hypoglycemia (26% of the time) than a night where no exercise was performed (6% of the time) (Tsalikian *et al.* 2005). Those who exercised regularly or participated in sports typically had more episodes of nocturnal hypoglycemia. Therefore, patients and parents should be particularly cautious if exercise is performed in the late afternoon or early evening. Strategies to limit the possibility of hypoglycemia caused by exercise are provided under Practical considerations below.

In addition to intensive insulin therapy, there are other factors that contribute to overinsulinization and hypoglycemia during exercise:

1 The absorption of injected insulin increases with exercise. The increase in subcutaneous tissue and skeletal muscle blood flow is associated with a concurrent increase in insulin absorption and accelerated hypoglycemia (Zinman *et al.* 1977). In addition, the rise in body temperature and the massage-like effect of exercise increases insulin absorption rate (Koivisto *et al.* 1981).

2 Plasma insulin levels do not decrease, and may even increase (see above), during exercise. A failure in the ability to lower insulin levels during exercise, as would normally occur in an individual without diabetes, causes a relative hyperinsulinemia that impairs hepatic glucose production and, as a result, glucose levels drop (Schiffrin & Parikh 1985; Riddell *et al.* 1999; Tansey *et al.* 2006).

3 Exercise causes enhanced glucose disposal via increased activation of contraction-mediated glucose transporters. The dramatic increase in non-insulin mediated glucose disposal considerably reduces the need for circulating insulin (Dorchy *et al.* 1976). Because the increase in insulin sensitivity persists after the end of exercise in children (Dorchy *et al.* 1976), likely to help replenish muscle and liver glycogen stores, patients are at increased risk of hypoglycemia after the completion of exercise.

Counterregulatory failure

Hypoglycemia during exercise has recently been reported to result from impaired release of glucose-counterregulatory hormones caused by previous exposure to either exercise or hypoglycemia (Wasserman *et al.* 2002). The mechanisms for impaired

counterregulation are unclear but repeated episodes of either hypoglycemia or exercise appears to degrade the body's ability to mount a counterregulatory response to either stressor (Sandoval *et al.* 2004; Camacho *et al.* 2005). The main impairment is a blunted catecholamine response to exercise, which occurs even in intensively treated patients with no clinical evidence of diabetic autonomic neuropathy (Schneider *et al.* 1991). This finding of a blunted counterregulatory response to exercise is similar to the scenario that occurs in intensively treated patients with diabetes who develop defects in counterregulatory responses to hypoglycemia (Dagogo-Jack *et al.* 1993). During intermittent exercise, children with type 1 DM have insufficient increases in glucose counterregulatory hormones to prevent exercise-associated hypoglycemia (Tansey *et al.* 2006).

Underinsulinization and hyperglycemia

Not all forms of exercise are associated with hypoglycemia and some patients frequently report hyperglycemia just after heavy exercise, likely because of an inability to secrete insulin to compensate for elevations in catecholamine levels (Purdon *et al.* 1993). Indeed, intermittent high-intensity exercise, which reflects field and team sports, does not appear to increase the risk of immediate post-exercise hypoglycemia in patients with type 1 DM, likely because of increases in catecholamine levels (Guelfi *et al.* 2005).

In individuals with poor metabolic control, exercise can cause an additional increase in blood glucose and ketoacidosis (Berger *et al.* 1977). The rise in blood glucose is caused by exaggerated hepatic glucose production and impairment in exercise-induced glucose utilization. Increased ketone body production results from elevated FFA release from adipocytes and possibly from an increase in intra-hepatic ketogenic efficiency (Wahren *et al.* 1984). Hyperglycemia and ketosis during exercise is particularly undesirable because it causes dehydration and may decrease blood pH, both of which impair exercise performance. Heavy exercise (i.e., >60–70% $\dot{V}_{O_{2max}}$ or >75–85% of maximal heart rate) may particularly aggravate this condition, because increases in catecholamines and glucocorticoids will further exaggerate the elevations in glucose concentrations and ketone production (Marliss & Vranic 2002).

High intensity exercise and hyperglycemia

High intensity exercise may be defined as activities above the "lactate threshold", which is approximately 60–70% $\dot{V}_{O_{2max}}$ or 85–90% maximal heart rate. This threshold coincides with dramatic elevation in catecholamines which increase hepatic glucose release, FFA, and ketone levels, and impairs glucose utilization by skeletal muscle. Even those individuals treated with intensive insulin therapy may have increases in blood glucose levels during and after high intensity exercise (Mitchell *et al.* 1988; Purdon *et al.* 1993; Bussau *et al.* 2006). The rise in glucose concentration is usually transient and tends to last only as long as there are elevations in counterregulatory hormones (i.e., 30–60 min). Although some individuals can easily correct the elevations in stress hormones with an insulin bolus, particularly if they take rapid acting insulin analogs, others may be reluctant to take additional insulin after exercise because there will be greater risk of late-onset post-exercise hypoglycemia.

Competition stress, heat stress, and hyperglycemia

The psychologic stress of competition is frequently associated with increases in blood glucose levels even though the pre-exercise glucose concentrations may be normal. Those pursuing vigorous aerobic exercise may find that on regular training or practice days they become hypoglycemic but on the day of competition they develop hyperglycemia. Although empirical data do not exist for patients with type 1 DM, excessive increases in glucose counterregulatory hormones likely occur just before exercise when anticipatory stress is high. It is also probable that the stress during competition can further increase blood glucose levels. Individuals may find that training or competing in warm and humid environments also elevates blood glucose levels, likely because of excessive increases in circulating plasma catecholamines, glucagon, cortisol, and growth hormone (Hargreaves *et al.* 1996).

Practical considerations for the clinical management of type 1 diabetes mellitus in athletic youth

The major challenge for active youth with type 1 DM is to balance food, insulin, and exercise in order to limit blood glucose excursions. Some of the factors affecting blood glucose levels during exercise are baseline blood glucose levels; circulating plasma insulin levels; the timing, composition and quantity of food ingested; the intensity and duration of the exercise; the type of sport performed; and the prevailing concentrations of the glucose counterregulatory hormones. To a lesser extent, other variables also influence the metabolic responses to exercise: age, gender, level of metabolic control, and the level of aerobic fitness. Even if a number of these variables are taken into consideration, the glycemic response appears to vary greatly between individuals (McNiven-Temple *et al.* 1995; Riddell *et al.* 1999). Fortunately, blood glucose changes during exercise have some degree of reproducibility within an individual, as long as the exercise conditions and pre-exercise insulin and diet are consistent (McNiven-Temple *et al.* 1995). Because of the variability between individuals, no precise guidelines are available to prevent fluctuations in glucose levels during exercise, although some general strategies do exist. A well-organized plan should be developed and conveyed to the child's coaches, teachers, friends, guardians, and siblings. Children and adolescents should delay participation in physical activity if blood glucose levels are below 3.5 mmol·L^{-1} or above 15.0 mmol·L^{-1} with detectable urine ketones. Practical recommendations to help prevent hypo- and hyperglycemia are provided below and are summarized in Table 27.2.

Blood glucose monitoring

Regular blood glucose monitoring, coupled with activity and nutritional logs, is essential for developing insulin strategies to prevent hypo- and hyperglycemia. Prior to and during activity, measurements should be taken every 30 min to map glucose trends, as a single assessment will not determine the direction of change. Post-exercise monitoring can be less frequent (every 2 h) but is imperative

Table 27.2 Practical guidelines to limit glucose excursions before, during and after exercise.

Before exercise
1 Determine the timing, mode, duration, and intensity of exercise
2 Eat a carbohydrate rich meal 2–3 h prior to exercise (i.e., 55–65% of calories from carbohydrate) with either usual insulin dosage or a 50% reduction in insulin. Note: reducing the amount of insulin may place the child at risk of pre-exercise hyperglycemia
3 Assess metabolic control:
(a) If blood glucose is <5.0 mmol·L^{-1} and levels are decreasing, extra calories may be needed
(b) If blood glucose is 5–14 mmol·L^{-1}, extra calories may not be needed, depending on the duration of exercise and the individual responses to exercise
(c) If blood glucose is >14 mmol·L^{-1} and urine or blood ketones are present, delay exercise until levels are normalized with insulin administration
4 If the activity is aerobic, estimate the energy expenditure and determine if insulin or additional carbohydrate will be needed based on the peak insulin activity
(a) If insulin dose is to be changed for long duration—moderate to high intensity activities—try a 50% pre-meal reduction 1 h prior to exercise. Dosages can be altered on subsequent exercise days, based on the measured individual responses. Insulin should always be injected into a site away from the exercising muscles and into subcutaneous tissue
(b) If carbohydrate intake is to be increased, try 1.0 g·kg body mass^{-1}·h^{-1} of moderate to high intensity exercise performed during peak insulin activity and less carbohydrate as the duration because insulin injection increases. Refer to tables of exercise exchanges for sport-specific recommendations and children weighing 20–60 kg (Riddell & Iscoe 2006). The amount of carbohydrate can be altered on subsequent exercise days, based on the measured individual responses. The total dose of carbohydrate should be divided equally and consumed at 20-min intervals
5 If the exercise is anaerobic or during heat or competition stress, than an increase in insulin may be needed
6 Consider fluid intake to maintain hydration (~250 mL 20 min prior to exercise) and every 20 min during exercise lasting longer than 30 min

to avoid late-onset hypoglycemia. As nocturnal hypoglycemia is common in children and frequently asymptomatic, we recommend that blood glucose concentrations be monitored once during the night if there is a major change in exercise, insulin, or carbohydrate intake. The lowest glucose level is usually between midnight and 3 AM (Tsalikian *et al.* 2005), typically because of the timing of peak insulin activity and the low levels of circulating counter-regulatory hormones. An alarm may be useful for waking the child for occasional glucose monitoring during the night to determine if he or she is being exposed to asymptomatic hypoglycemia. Automated alarm systems are useful in detecting dysglycemia, particularly during sleep, in continuous glucose monitoring systems (see below).

Patients and parents should be told that "body awareness" and symptoms of hypo- or hyper-glycemia (Table 27.3) do not translate into quantitative estimation of a child's blood glucose levels. Indeed, a poor correlation exists between estimated and measured blood glucose in exercising youth with diabetes (Riddell & Bar-Or 2002). Because

frequent monitoring may be impractical in some sports, the convenience of continuous glucose monitoring devices (e.g., Continuous Glucose Monitoring Systems, Medtronic) coupled with insulin pump therapy can be ideal for youth (Chase *et al.* 2001).

Insulin modification

Because exercise is one of the most common causes of hypoglycemia, children may be prevented from participating in physical activities out of fear and lack of knowledge by caregivers. Such a preventable situation is frustrating for the child and is not helpful in addressing the growing problem of obesity in the adolescent population.

Before any adjustments can be made to an insulin regimen, a history of proper self-monitoring and a log of blood glucose measurements should be present. Specific modifications to insulin management depend on a combination of factors, including the type, duration, and intensity of exercise, as well as the child's nutrient intake and fitness. Because it is impossible to predict the exact insulin reduction

Hypoglycemia	Hyperglycemia
Shakiness	Excessive thirst
Dizziness	Fatigue, weakness
Sweating	Frequent urination
Hunger	Blurred vision
Headache	Shortness of breath
Pale skin color	Breath that smells fruity
Sudden moodiness or behavior changes,	Nausea and vomiting
(i.e. crying for no apparent reason)	Dry mouth
Clumsy or jerky movements	
Seizure	
Difficulty paying attention, or confusion	
Tingling sensations around the mouth	

Table 27.3 Typical symptoms of hypo- and hyperglycemia.

Many of the symptoms of hypo- and hyperglycemia are masked by exercise. Exercise may lower blood glucose levels in the child who is hyperglycemia prior to exercise. However, if blood glucose is above ~14 mmol·L^{-1} with urine ketones, patients should *not* exercise.

needed, individuals should use records of previous experiences as a guideline and always have additional carbohydrates available. Reductions in insulin dose can be as low as 10% for light activities (e.g., brisk walking) and as high as 90% for prolonged vigorous activities (e.g., marathon). Indeed, several elite athletes with diabetes will remove their insulin pump altogether for sport and competition to dramatically reduce circulating insulin levels (Perkins & Riddell 2006).

Based on limited published studies with children, patients often become hypoglycemic within 45 min of starting strenuous exercise when the activity is performed 2 h after a typical meal and their usual insulin (Schiffrin & Parikh 1985; Riddell et al. 1999; Tansey et al. 2006). Exercise performed just after a meal may cause a greater risk of hypoglycemia because plasma insulin levels are elevated two- to threefold (Riddell et al. 1999). The route of insulin delivery (pump vs. multiple daily injections) does not appear to influence the frequency of hypoglycemia in children and the complete removal of an insulin pump does prevent exercise-associated hypoglycemia or late-onset hypoglycemia (Admon et al. 2005). In those on multiple daily insulin injections, the reduction in blood glucose during exercise can be attenuated by a 30–50% reduction in premeal bolus insulin (Schiffrin & Parikh 1985). For more prolonged activities, a greater reduction in insulin is

warranted (Rabasa-Lhoret et al. 2001). As an example, cross-country skiers with type 1 DM were able to exercise for several hours without becoming hypoglycemic if the insulin dose was reduced by 80% (Sane et al. 1988). If the insulin dose is reduced by only 50%, these same athletes could exercise for only 90 min. In general, higher aerobic exercise intensities that are prolonged elicit a greater drop in blood glucose and a greater need for reduced insulin dosage. In contrast, exercise performed in the fasted or post-absorptive state (i.e., >3 h after insulin analog administration and meal) may be performed with no reduction in bolus insulin (Schiffrin et al. 1984; Nathan et al. 1985). Insulin adjustments based on semi-quantitative estimates of energy expenditures during various sports and an individual's insulin to carbohydrate ratios are provided by Perkins and Riddell (2006).

Because muscular contractions accelerate insulin absorption, the site of injection should be away from working muscles (i.e., abdomen) to minimize risk of hypoglycemia (Koivisto & Felig 1978) and fast-acting carbohydrates should be made available to treat hypoglycemia. For example, a runner should not inject into the leg, particularly because the amount of subcutaneous fat may be small in this area. Patients should be advised and instructed as to how to inject their reduced insulin dose into subcutaneous fat and not to inadvertently inject directly into skeletal muscle, because insulin absorption rates may be dramatically increased in the latter location.

General nutrition

The general nutrition of pediatric athletes with type 1 DM is not different from those of other athletes. Adolescents who are endurance athletes require 37–41 kcal·kg^{-1}·day^{-1} for moderate intensity training, while strength training requires 34–50 kcal·kg^{-1}·day^{-1} to help support muscle growth (Petrie *et al.* 2004). It is generally recommended that carbohydrate (CHO) should be 60% of the total daily caloric intake, with the majority in the complex form (e.g., whole grains, beans). These low glycemic foods limit post-meal hyperglycemia and elevated needs for insulin. Although recommendations are not readily available for active children with diabetes, endurance athletes should ingest ~8–10 g CHO·kg body weight^{-1}·day^{-1} (Franz 2002; Petrie *et al.* 2004). Sport beverages containing simple carbohydrates in a 6% solution may be useful in providing extra energy and fluid availability during exercise. The amount of carbohydrate supplement will vary according to body size and the intensity of the activity (Riddell & Iscoe 2006). Protein requirements (12–15% of total daily calories) can easily be met by a normal diet, preferably from lean meats and vegetable sources rather than those high in saturated fats. Protein intake ranges for young athletes are recommended to be 1.2–1.4 g·kg^{-1} for general endurance sports to 1.6–1.7 g·kg body weight^{-1} for strength training (Petrie *et al.* 2004). Approximately 20–25% of daily caloric intake should be derived from fat, with no more than 10% obtained from saturated sources (e.g., animal fat).

FLUID

Hydration levels will substantially affect performance in the child athlete and as little as a 1% reduction in body weight from dehydration will increase fatigue (Petrie *et al.* 2004). Fluid loss in children and adolescents is exacerbated by increased sweating rates in hot or humid environments (Hernandez *et al.* 2000). Those with diabetes may be at particular risk because a prior bout of hyperglycemia reduces hydration levels. Fluid requirements have been extrapolated from adult needs (Leiper *et al.* 1996) and are estimated to be ~1.6 L·day^{-1} for basic requirements and an additional 0.5–1.0 L·day^{-1} during physical activity (Petrie *et al.* 2004). On average, fluid intake should be approximately 250 mL for every 20 min of moderate to heavy intensity exercise and the first drink should precede exercise by 20 min (Riddell & Bar-Or 2002).

Competition strategies

Frequent glucose monitoring and proper insulin and nutritional strategies are essential to ensure optimal performance and the prevention of glucose excursions. Although refinements in carbohydrate and insulin can be made just prior to exercise, nutritional adjustments well before, during, and after competition are essential for long-term success.

PRE-COMPETITION

A meal containing carbohydrates, fats, and protein should be consumed roughly 3–4 h prior to competition to allow for digestion and a maximizing of endogenous energy stores. Glycogen stores can be enhanced with a carbohydrate beverage (1–2 g CHO·kg^{-1}) approximately 1 h prior; this also helps to supplement energy stores and provide adequate fluids for hydration. A beverage containing 6% simple sugar (i.e., sucrose, fructose, glucose) provides optimal absorption compared to other more concentrated beverages such as juice or carbonated drinks which delay gastric absorption and cause stomach upset. Nutritionally complete fluids that contain fat and protein may be effective in preventing late-onset post-exercise hypoglycemia if they are consumed immediately after the activity (Hernandez *et al.* 2000).

DURING COMPETITION

Carbohydrate ingestion rate during exercise depends upon the intensity and duration of the activity, as well as the age and gender of the individual, and the timing of the last insulin injection.

In general, approximately 1.0–1.5 g CHO·kg body weight^{-1}·h^{-1} should be consumed during exercise performed during peak insulin action in young adults with diabetes (Wasserman *et al.* 2002). Tables of exercise exchanges that estimate carbohydrate utilization may be helpful in determining the carbohydrate intake regimen for younger individuals (Riddell & Iscoe 2006). To treat hypoglycemia, 15 g fast-acting carbohydrate (e.g., 3 glucose tablets, 1/2 cup of fruit juice, or 5–6 pieces of hard candy) is recommended and a retest of blood glucose level is needed about 15 min after the carbohydrate intake and prior to resuming exercise. Because symptoms of hypo- or hyperglycemia (Table 27.3) may be masked by exercise, frequent monitoring is necessary and patients should be advised to err on the side of treating hypoglycemia if in doubt about his or her symptoms and if blood glucose monitoring is unavailable.

POST-COMPETITION

Carbohydrates are not only required for energy during activity, but also to replace the energy derived from liver and muscle glycogen stores. Because insulin sensitivity remains elevated for up to 24–36 h post-exercise, carbohydrate stores must be replenished quickly to lower the risk of hypoglycemia during the first few hours post-activity. For patients who tend to experience post-exercise late-onset hypoglycemia during the night, a complex carbohydrate (e.g., uncooked corn starch), or a mixed snack containing fat and protein may be particularly beneficial at bedtime (Kalergis *et al.* 2003). Alternatively, nutritionally complete fluids that contain fat and protein may be effective in preventing late-onset post-exercise hypoglycemia if they are consumed during and immediately after the activity (Hernandez *et al.* 2000).

Conclusions and future research directions

Regular physical activity should be considered an important component in the clinical management of youth with diabetes. Research has provided some understanding of the physiologic responses to exercise in the child with diabetes and, as a result, there are some general guidelines for the modification of insulin and diet to limit excursions in blood glucose levels. The goal for all children with diabetes should be to learn their individual glycemic responses to exercise and sport and to control glucose fluctuations by modifying insulin dosage and diet appropriately. Few limitations should be placed on active youth with diabetes so that they may compete on equal ground with their peers so that they can derive the social, psychologic, and physiologic benefits of a physically active lifestyle.

Future investigations should determine:
1 If the drop in blood glucose associated with exercise is more dramatic in children than in adults because of the apparent immature glycogenolytic system.
2 If carbohydrate intake matched with total carbohydrate utilization prevents post-exercise late-onset hypoglycemia.
3 The appropriate adjustments in basal insulin dosage to limit nocturnal hypoglycemia associated with exercise.
4 The effects of intermittent high intensity sport on blood glucose levels in youth.
5 If the effects of regular exercise help to limit long-term complications from DM.

References

Admon, G., Weinstein, Y., Falk, B., *et al.* (2005) Exercise with and without an insulin pump among children and adolescents with type 1 diabetes mellitus. *Pediatrics* **116**, e348–e355.

Akerblom, H.K., Koivukangas, T. & Ilkka, J. (1980) Experiences from a winter camp for teenage diabetics. *Acta Paediatrica Scandinavica Supplement* **283**, 50–52.

Alberti, G., Zimmet, P., Shaw, J., Bloomgarden, Z., Kaufman, F. & Silink, M. (2004) Type 2 diabetes in the young: the evolving epidemic: the international diabetes federation consensus workshop. *Diabetes Care* **27**, 1798–1811.

Almeida, S., Riddell, M.C. & Cafarelli, E. (2005) Motor unit firing rate and nerve conduction velocity in type 1 diabetes in response to a fatigue protocol. *Medicine and Science in Sports and Exercise* **37**, S108–S109.

Aman, J., Karlsson, I. & Wranne, L. (1989) Symptomatic hypoglycaemia in childhood diabetes: a population-based questionnaire study. *Diabetic Medicine* **6**, 257–261.

Austin, A., Warty, V., Janosky, J. & Arslanian, S. (1993) The relationship of physical fitness to lipid and lipoprotein(a) levels in adolescents with IDDM [see comments]. *Diabetes Care* **16**, 421–425.

Baraldi, E., Monciotti, C., Filippone, M., *et al.* (1992) Gas exchange during exercise in diabetic children. *Pediatric Pulmonology* **13**, 155–160.

Baran, D. & Dorchy, H. (1982) Physical fitness in diabetic adolescents. *Bulletin Europeen de Physiopathologie Respiratoire* **18**, 51–58.

Barkai, L., Peja, M. & Vamosi, I. (1996) Physical work capacity in diabetic children and adolescents with and without cardiovascular autonomic dysfunction. *Diabetic Medicine* **13**, 254–258.

Bell, D.S. & Cutter, G. (1994) Characteristics of severe hypoglycemia in the patient with insulin-dependent diabetes. *Southern Medical Journal* **87**, 616–620.

Berger, M., Berchtold, P., Cuppers, H.J., *et al.* (1977) Metabolic and hormonal effects of muscular exercise in juvenile type diabetics. *Diabetologia* **13**, 355–365.

Botero, D. & Wolfsdorf, J.I. (2005) Diabetes mellitus in children and adolescents. *Archives of Medical Research* **36**, 281–290.

Braatvedt, G.D., Mildenhall, L., Patten, C. & Harris, G. (1997) Insulin requirements and metabolic control in children with diabetes mellitus attending a summer camp. *Diabetic Medicine* **14**, 258–261.

Bussau, V.A., Ferreira, L.D., Jones, T.W. & Fournier, P.A. (2006) The 10-s maximal sprint: a novel approach to counter an exercise-mediated fall in glycemia in individuals with type 1 diabetes. *Diabetes Care* **29**, 601–606.

Camacho, R.C., Galassetti, P., Davis, S.N. & Wasserman, D.H. (2005) Glucoregulation during and after exercise in health and insulin-dependent diabetes. *Exercise and Sport Sciences Reviews* **33**, 17–23.

Campaigne, B.N., Gilliam, T.B., Spencer, M.L., Lampman, R.M. & Schork, M.A. (1984) Effects of a physical activity program on metabolic control and cardiovascular fitness in children with insulin-dependent diabetes mellitus. *Diabetes Care* **7**, 57–62.

Chase, H.P., Kim, L.M., Owen, S.L., *et al.* (2001) Continuous subcutaneous glucose monitoring in children with type 1 diabetes. *Pediatrics* **107**, 222–226.

Dagogo-Jack, S.E., Craft, S. & Cryer, P.E. (1993) Hypoglycemia-associated autonomic failure in insulin-dependent diabetes mellitus. Recent antecedent hypoglycemia reduces autonomic responses to, symptoms of, and defense against subsequent hypoglycemia. *Journal of Clinical Investigation* **91**, 819–828.

Dahl-Jorgensen, K., Meen, H.D., Hanssen, K.F. & Aagenaes, O. (1980) The effect of exercise on diabetic control and hemoglobin A1 (HbA1) in children. *Acta Paediatrica Scandinavica Supplement* **283**, 53–56.

DCCT Research Group (1988) Weight gain associated with intensive therapy in the diabetes control and complications trial. *Diabetes Care* **11**, 567–573.

DCCT Research Group (1993) The effect of intensive treatment of diabetes on the development and progression of long-term complications in insulin-dependent diabetes mellitus. The Diabetes Control and Complications Trial Research Group. *New England Journal of Medicine* **329**, 977–986.

DCCT Research Group (1994) Effect of intensive diabetes treatment on the development and progression of long-term complications in adolescents with insulin-dependent diabetes mellitus: Diabetes Control and Complications Trial. *Journal of Pediatrics* **125**, 177–188.

Dorchy, H. & Poortmans, J. (1989) Sport and the diabetic child. *Sports Medicine* **7**, 248–262.

Dorchy, H., Ego, F., Baran, D. & Loeb, H. (1976) Effect of exercise on glucose uptake in diabetic adolescents. *Acta Paediatrica Belgica* **29**, 83–85.

Ewald, U. & Tuvemo, T. (1985) Reduced vascular reactivity in diabetic children and its relation to diabetic control. *Acta Paediatrica Scandinavica* **74**, 77–84.

Ewald, U., Tuvemo, T. & Rooth, G. (1981) Early reduction of vascular reactivity in diabetic children detected by transcutaneous oxygen electrode. *Lancet* **1**, 1287–1288.

Franz, M.J. (2002) Nutrition, physical activity, and diabetes. In: *Handbook of Exercise in Diabetes* (Ruderman, N., Devlin, J.T., Schneider, S.H. & Kriska, A., eds.) American Diabetes Association, Alexandria, VA: 321–338.

Guelfi, K.J., Jones, T.W. & Fournier, P.A. (2005) Intermittent high-intensity exercise does not increase the risk of early postexercise hypoglycemia in individuals with type 1 diabetes. *Diabetes Care* **28**, 416–418.

Hagan, R.D., Marks, J.F. & Warren, P.A. (1979) Physiologic responses of juvenile-onset diabetic boys to muscular work. *Diabetes* **28**, 355–365.

Hargreaves, M., Angus, D., Howlett, K., Conus, N.M. & Febbraio, M. (1996) Effect of heat stress on glucose kinetics during exercise. *Journal of Applied Physiology* **81**, 1594–1597.

Hernandez, J.M., Moccia, T., Fluckey, J.D., Ulbrecht, J.S. & Farrell, P.A. (2000) Fluid snacks to help persons with type 1 diabetes avoid late onset postexercise hypoglycemia. *Medicine and Science in Sports and Exercise* **32**, 904–910.

Horgan, G. (2005) Healthier lifestyles series: 1. Exercise for children. *Journal of Family Health Care* **15**, 15–17.

Hough, D.O. (1994) Diabetes mellitus in sports. [Review]. *Medical Clinics of North America* **78**, 423–437.

Huttunen, N.P., Kaar, M.L., Knip, M., Mustonen, A., Puukka, R. & Akerblom, H.K. (1984) Physical fitness of children and adolescents with insulin-dependent diabetes mellitus. *Annals of Clinical Research* **16**, 1–5.

Huttunen, N.P., Lankela, S.L., Knip, M., *et al.* (1989) Effect of once-a-week training program on physical fitness and metabolic control in children with IDDM. *Diabetes Care* **12**, 737–740.

Iscoe, K.A., Campbell, J., Jamnik, V., Perkins, B.A. & Riddell, M.C. (2006) Efficacy of continuous real time blood glucose monitoring during and after prolonged high intensity cycling exercise in Type 1 diabetes: spinning with CGMS. *Diabetes Technologies and Therapeutics* **8**, 627–635.

Kalergis, M., Schiffrin, A., Gougeon, R., Jones, P.J. & Yale, J.F. (2003) Impact of bedtime snack composition on prevention of nocturnal hypoglycemia in adults with type 1 diabetes undergoing intensive insulin management using lispro insulin before meals: a randomized, placebo-controlled, crossover trial. *Diabetes Care* **26**, 9–15.

Knowler, W.C., Barrett-Connor, E., Fowler, S.E., *et al.* (2002) Reduction in the incidence of type 2 diabetes with lifestyle intervention or metformin. *New England Journal of Medicine* **346**, 393–403.

Kobbah, M., Ewald, U. & Tuvemo, T. (1985) Vascular reactivity during the first year of diabetes in children. *Acta Paediatrica Scandinavica Supplement* **320**, 56–63.

Koivisto, V.A. & Felig, P. (1978) Effects of leg exercise on insulin absorption in diabetic patients. *New England Journal of Medicine* **298**, 79–83.

Koivisto, V.A., Fortney, S., Hendler, R. & Felig, P. (1981) A rise in ambient temperature augments insulin absorption in diabetic patients. *Metabolism* **30**, 402–405.

Komatsu, W.R., Gabbay, M.A., Castro, M.L., *et al.* (2005) Aerobic exercise capacity in normal adolescents and those with type 1 diabetes mellitus. *Pediatric Diabetes* **6**, 145–149.

Landt, K.W., Campaigne, B.N., James, F.W. & Sperling, M.A. (1985) Effects of exercise training on insulin sensitivity in adolescents with type I diabetes. *Diabetes Care* **8**, 461–465.

Larsson, Y., Persson, B., Sterky, G. & Thoren, C. (1964) Functional adaptation to vigorous training and exercise in diabetic and nondiabetic adolescents. *Journal of Applied Physiology* **19**, 629–635.

Larsson, Y.A.A., Sterky, G.C.G., Ekengren, K.E.K. & Möller, T.G.H.O. (1962) Physical fitness and the influence of training in diabetic adolescent girls. *Diabetes* **11**, 109–117.

Leiper, J.B., Carnie, A. & Maughan, R.J. (1996) Water turnover rates in sedentary and exercising middle aged men. *British Journal of Sports Medicine* **30**, 24–26.

Ludvigsson, J. (1980) Physical exercise in relation to degree of metabolic control in juvenile diabetics. *Acta Paediatrica Scandinavica Supplement* **283**, 45–49.

MacDonald, M.J. (1987) Postexercise late-onset hypoglycemia in insulin-dependent diabetic patients. *Diabetes Care* **10**, 584–588.

Mahon, A.D., Duncan, G.E., Howe, C.A. & Del, C.P. (1997) Blood lactate and perceived exertion relative to ventilatory threshold: boys versus men. *Medicine and Science in Sports and Exercise* **29**, 1332–1337.

Marliss, E.B. & Vranic, M. (2002) Intense exercise has unique effects on both insulin release and its roles in glucoregulation: implications for diabetes. *Diabetes* **51** (Supplement 1), S271–S283.

Martinez, L.R. & Haymes, E.M. (1992) Substrate utilization during treadmill running in prepubertal girls and women. *Medicine and Science in Sports and Exercise* **24**, 975–983.

McNiven-Temple, M.Y., Bar-Or, O. & Riddell, M.C. (1995) The reliability and repeatability of the blood glucose response to prolonged exercise in adolescent boys with IDDM. *Diabetes Care* **18**, 326–332.

Mitchell, T.H., Abraham, G., Schiffrin, A., Leiter, L.A. & Marliss, E.B. (1988) Hyperglycemia after intense exercise in IDDM subjects during continuous subcutaneous insulin infusion. *Diabetes Care* **11**, 311–317.

Mosher, P.E., Nash, M.S., Perry, A.C., LaPerriere, A.R. & Goldberg, R.B. (1998) Aerobic circuit exercise training: effect on adolescents with well-controlled insulin-dependent diabetes mellitus. *Archives of Physical Medicine and Rehabilitation* **79**, 652–657.

Nathan, D.M., Madnek, S.F. & Delahanty, L. (1985) Programming pre-exercise snacks to prevent post-exercise hypoglycemia in intensively treated insulin-dependent diabetics. *Annals of Internal Medicine* **102**, 483–486.

National Diabetes Education Program (2006) National Diabetes Education Program: Blood glucose goals. www.ndep.nih.gov/diabetes/youth/youth_FS.htm#Goals.

Niranjan, V., McBrayer, D.G., Ramirez, L.C., Raskin, P. & Hsia, C.C. (1997) Glycemic control and cardiopulmonary function in patients with insulin-dependent diabetes mellitus. *American Journal of Medicine* **103**, 504–513.

Nordgren, H., Freyschuss, U. & Persson, B. (1994) Blood pressure response to physical exercise in healthy adolescents and adolescents with insulin-dependent diabetes mellitus. *Clinical Science* **86**, 425–432.

Perkins, B.A. & Riddell, M.C. (2006) Type 1 Diabetes and Exercise. Part 2: Using the Insulin Pump to Maximum Advantage. *Canadian Journal of Diabetes* **30**, 72–80.

Persson, B. & Thoren, C. (1980) Prolonged exercise in adolescent boys with juvenile diabetes mellitus. Circulatory and metabolic responses in relation to perceived exertion. *Acta Paediatrica Scandinavica Supplement* **283**, 62–69.

Petrie, H.J., Stover, E.A. & Horswill, C.A. (2004) Nutritional concerns for the child and adolescent competitor. *Nutrition* **20**, 620–631.

Poortmans, J.R., Saerens, P., Edelman, R., Vertongen, F. & Dorchy, H. (1986) Influence of the degree of metabolic control on physical fitness in type I diabetic adolescents. *International Journal of Sports Medicine* **7**, 232–235.

Purdon, C., Brousson, M., Nyveen, S.L., *et al.* (1993) The roles of insulin and catecholamines in the glucoregulatory response during intense exercise and early recovery in insulin-dependent diabetic and control subjects. *Journal of*

Clinical Endocrinology and Metabolism **76**, 566–573.

Pyorala, E. (2004) The participation roles of children and adolescents in the dietary counseling of diabetics. *Patient Education and Counseling* **55**, 385–395.

Rabasa-Lhoret, R., Bourque, J., Ducros, F. & Chiasson, J.L. (2001) Guidelines for premeal insulin dose reduction for postprandial exercise of different intensities and durations in type 1 diabetic subjects treated intensively with a basal-bolus insulin regimen (ultralente-lispro). *Diabetes Care* **24**, 625–630.

Raguso, C.A., Coggan, A.R., Gastaldelli, A., Sidossis, L.S., Bastyr, E.J. & Wolfe, R.R. (1995) Lipid and carbohydrate metabolism in IDDM during moderate and intense exercise. *Diabetes* **44**, 1066–1074.

Raile, K., Kapellen, T., Schweiger, A., *et al.* (1999) Physical activity and competitive sports in children and adolescents with type 1 diabetes [Letter]. *Diabetes Care* **22**, 1904–1905.

Raskin, P., Pietri, A.O., Unger, R. & Shannon, W.A.J. (1983) The effect of diabetic control on the width of skeletal-muscle capillary basement membrane in patients with Type I diabetes mellitus. *New England Journal of Medicine* **309**, 1546–1550.

Riddell, M.C. & Bar-Or, O. (2002) Children and adolescents. In: *Handbook of Exercise in Diabetes* (Ruderman, N., Devlin, J.T. & Schneider, S.H., eds.) American Diabetes Association, Alexandria, VA: 547–566.

Riddell, M.C., Bar-Or, O., Ayub, B.V., Calvert, R.E. & Heigenhauser, G.J.F. (1999) Glucose ingestion matched with total carbohydrate utilization attenuates hypoglycemia during exercise in adolescents with IDDM. *International Journal of Sport Nutrition* **9**, 24–34.

Riddell, M.C., Bar-Or, O., Gerstein, H.C. & Heigenhauser, G.J. (2000a) Perceived exertion with glucose ingestion in adolescent males with IDDM. *Medicine and Science in Sports and Exercise* **32**, 167–173.

Riddell, M.C., Bar-Or, O., Hollidge-Horvat, M., Schwarcz, H.P. & Heigenhauser, G.J. (2000b) Glucose ingestion and substrate utilization during exercise in boys with IDDM. *Journal of Applied Physiology* **88**, 1239–1246.

Riddell, M.C. & Iscoe, K.E. (2006) Physical activity, sport, and pediatric diabetes. *Pediatric Diabetes* **7**, 60–70.

Rosenbloom, A.L., Joe, J.R., Young, R.S. & Winter, W.E. (1999) Emerging epidemic of type 2 diabetes in youth. *Diabetes Care* **22**, 345–354.

Rowland, T.W. & Cunningham, L.N. (1992) Oxygen uptake plateau during maximal treadmill exercise in children [see comments]. *Chest* **101**, 485–489.

Rowland, T.W., Swadba, L.A., Biggs, D.E., Burke, E.J. & Reiter, E.O. (1985) Glycemic control with physical training in insulin-dependent diabetes mellitus. *American Journal of Diseases of Children* **139**, 307–310.

Rutenfranz, J., Mocellin, R., Bauer, J. & Herzig, W. (1968) [Studies on the physical working capacity of healthy and sick adolescents. II. The physical working capacity of children and adolescents with diabetes mellitus]. *Zeitschrift fur Kinderheilkunde* **103**, 133–156.

Sackey, A.H. & Jefferson, I.G. (1996) Physical activity and glycaemic control in children with diabetes mellitus. *Diabetic Medicine* **13**, 789–793.

Sandoval, D.A., Guy, D.L., Richardson, M.A., Ertl, A.C. & Davis, S.N. (2004) Effects of low and moderate antecedent exercise on counterregulatory responses to subsequent hypoglycemia in type 1 diabetes. *Diabetes* **53**, 1798–1806.

Sane, T., Helve, E., Pelkonen, R. & Koivisto, V.A. (1988) The adjustment of diet and insulin dose during long-term endurance exercise in type I (insulin-dependent) diabetic men. *Diabetologia* **31**, 35–40.

Schiffrin, A. & Parikh, S. (1985) Accommodating planned exercise in type I diabetic patients on intensive treatment. *Diabetes Care* **8**, 337–342.

Schiffrin, A., Parikh, S., Marliss, E. & Desrosiers, M.M. (1984) Metabolic response to fasting exercise in adolescent insulin-dependent diabetic subjects treated with continuous subcutaneous insulin infusion and intensive conventional therapy. *Diabetes Care* **7**, 255–260.

Schneider, S.H., Vitug, A., Ananthakrishnan, R. & Khachadurian, A.K. (1991) Impaired adrenergic response to prolonged exercise in type I diabetes. *Metabolism* **40**, 1219–1225.

Shehadeh, N., Kassem, J., Tchaban, I., *et al.* (1998) High incidence of hypoglycemic episodes with neurologic manifestations in children with insulin dependent diabetes mellitus. *Journal of Pediatric Endocrinology and Metabolism* **11** (Supplement 1), 183–187.

Silink, M. (2002) Childhood diabetes: a global perspective. *Hormone Research* **57** (Supplement 1), 1–5.

Sills, I.N. & Cerny, F.J. (1983) Responses to continuous and intermittent exercise in healthy and insulin-dependent diabetic children. *Medicine and Science in Sports and Exercise* **15**, 450–454.

Sosenko, J.M., Miettinen, O.S., Williamson, J.R. & Gabbay, K.H. (1984) Muscle capillary basement-membrane thickness and long-term glycemia in type I diabetes mellitus. *New England Journal of Medicine* **311**, 694–698.

Sterky, G. (1963) Physical work capacity in diabetic schoolchildren. *Acta Paediatrica Scandinavica* **52**, 1–10.

Stratton, R., Wilson, D.P., Endres, R.K. & Goldstein, D.E. (1987) Improved glycemic control after supervised 8-week exercise program in insulin-dependent diabetic adolescents. *Diabetes Care* **10**, 589–593.

Tansey, M.J., Tsalikian, E., Beck, R.W., *et al.* (2006) The effects of aerobic exercise on glucose and counterregulatory hormone concentrations in children with type 1 diabetes. *Diabetes Care* **29**, 20–25.

Timmons, B.W., Bar-Or, O. & Riddell, M.C. (2003) Oxidation rate of exogenous carbohydrate during exercise is higher in boys than in men. *Journal of Applied Physiology* **94**, 278–284.

Tsalikian, E., Mauras, N., Beck, R.W., *et al.* (2005) Impact of exercise on overnight glycemic control in children with type 1 diabetes mellitus. *Journal of Pediatrics* **147**, 528–534.

Tupola, S., Rajantie, J. & Maenpaa, J. (1998) Severe hypoglycaemia in children and adolescents during multiple-dose insulin therapy. *Diabetic Medicine* **15**, 695–699.

Wahren, J., Sato, Y., Ostman, J., Hagenfeldt, L. & Felig, P. (1984) Turnover and splanchnic metabolism of free fatty acids and ketones in insulin-dependent diabetics at rest and in response to exercise. *Journal of Clinical Investigation* **73**, 1367–1376.

Wasserman, D.H., Davis, S.N. & Zinman, B. (2002) Fuel metabolism during exercise in health and diabetes. In: *Handbook of Exercise in Diabetes* (Ruderman, N., Devlin, J.T., Schneider, S.H. & Kriska, A., eds.) American Diabetes Association, Alexandria, VA: 63–100.

Zinman, B., Murray, F.T., Vranic, M., *et al.* (1977) Glucoregulation during moderate exercise in insulin treated diabetics. *Journal of Clinical Endocrinology and Metabolism* **45**, 641–652.

Chapter 28

The Young Athlete with a Motor Disability

PATRICIA E. LONGMUIR

The 21st century offers almost limitless possibilities to young athletes with motor disabilities. From "A" (e.g., aerobics) to "Z" (e.g., Zen yoga), the array of sport opportunities and the number of young athletes with motor disabilities has never been greater (Patel & Greydanus 2002). This tremendous growth in sport opportunities and participation is cause for celebration, given the strong connection between sports participation, self-concept, motor development, childhood growth and development, and physical and psychologic health (Thoren 1978; Lai *et al*. 2000; Ayyangar 2002; Wind *et al*. 2004).

Historically, the term "athlete with a motor disability" was viewed as a contradiction, because athletic success is predicated on optimal motor performance. However, the athletic prowess of young and adult athletes with motor disabilities is now showcased through elite international competitions, such as the Paralympic Games and headline grabbing feats of physical performance (Fig. 28.1). Through these events, young athletes with motor disabilities can connect with high performance role models, such as Chantal Petitclerc, Canada (track), Ragnhild Myklebust, Norway (cross-country skiing), or Mayumi Narita, Japan (swimming), all of whom won five or more gold medals at the most recent Paralympic Games. These outstanding individuals demonstrate that "athlete" and "motor disability" truly belong in the same phrase.

The most significant influence on the sport participation of children with motor disabilities is the manner in which the title of this chapter is interpreted by the adults involved in providing the sport opportunity (i.e., parents, coaches, teachers,

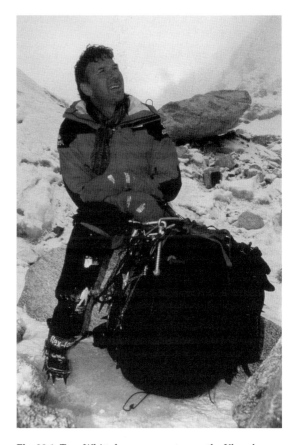

Fig. 28.1 Tom Whittaker, an amputee, on the Khumbu glacier shortly after his successful bid to reach Mount Everest's 29,035 foot summit, May 27, 1998. Photo © Howard Kelley. Citation: Howard Kelly/Tom Whittaker Collection.

managers). For most adults, the chapter title would be read as "The Young Athlete *with a Motor Disability*", with a very strong and prominent emphasis on the presence of a disability. In contrast, optimal athletic success requires that the chapter title be read as "*The Young Athlete* with a Motor Disability." Keeping the focus squarely on "the young athlete" is essential to successful participation because the differences associated with an athlete with a disability are few relative to the common ground that all child athletes share.

A concept of disability for the 21st century

The International Classification of Functioning, Disability and Health (ICF; World Health Organization 2002) clearly describes the concept of disability in the 21st century. It includes three categories: body structure and function; activity and participation; and environment and context (Fig. 28.2). Individuals are considered to have a disability if their ability to perform activities, either alone or with others, is limited either by a difference in body

structure (an impairment) or societal restrictions (a handicap). The key lessons to be learned from the ICF in terms of young athletes with motor disabilities are twofold:

1 The same system of analyzing or classifying motor function applies to all individuals, with and without disabilities;

2 A disability occurs as often from societal factors (e.g., environmental constraints, societal expectations) as it does through changes to the structure or function of the body.

Abilities-based approach

The abilities-based approach enables a coach to optimize the sport participation of each athlete, with or without a disability, by analyzing both the demands of the activity and the abilities of the athlete. It has the individual as the central focus, is critically influenced by the attitude of the coach or physical activity professional, and can be used for all types of sports and with athletes of all ages and abilities (Emes *et al.* 2002). Based on the concept of task analysis, the abilities-based approach (Longmuir

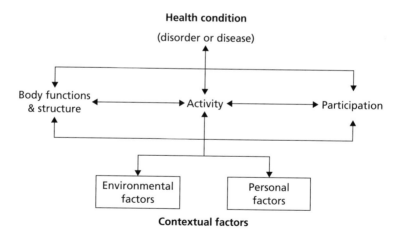

Fig. 28.2 World Health Organization International Classification of Functioning, Disability and Health. Body functions are physiologic functions of body systems (including psychologic functions). Body structures are anatomic parts of the body such as organs, limbs, and their components. Impairments are problems in body function or structure such as a significant deviation or loss. Activity is the execution of a task or action by an individual. Participation is involvement in a life situation. Activity limitations are difficulties an individual may have in executing activities. Participation restrictions are problems an individual may experience in life situations. Environmental factors make up the physical, social, and attitudinal environment in which people live and conduct their lives. Reprinted with permission of the World Health Organization (WHO), and all rights are reserved by the Organization.

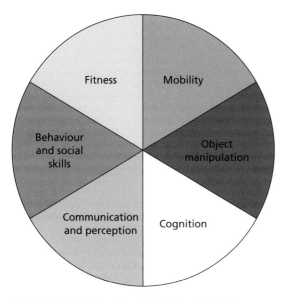

Fig. 28.3 Abilities-based model for physical activity participation. From Steadward *et al.* (2003).

2003) defines physical activity participation in terms of six categories: mobility; object manipulation; behavior and social skills; communication and perception; cognition; and fitness (Fig. 28.3). Optimal participation occurs when there is maximum overlap between the activity demands and the participant's abilities. Coaches can look at changing the demands of the

activity to enhance participation as well as the more traditional approach of modifying the athlete's abilities. For athletes with motor disabilities, "mobility", "object manipulation," and "fitness" categories will be the most relevant, although a motor disability may influence any or all aspects of the abilities-based approach.

Consider the athletic interests and abilities of a 13-year-old female named Nathalie (Table 28.1). Nathalie is keenly interested in basketball, which requires substantial mobility, object manipulation, and cognitive skills. However, a fused knee makes it difficult for Nathalie to run. If the sport club in her area offered only "standing" basketball, Nathalie would have a significant disability (i.e., limited ability to participate). Nathalie could have the object manipulation, cognitive, communication and perception, fitness, and behavior and social skills needed for participation in basketball but her mobility skills would limit her success. Using the abilities-based approach, enhancing Nathalie's participation could be achieved in two ways. The first approach, which is also most typical, would be to work with Nathalie to enhance her mobility skills. The second approach, which is often overlooked, would be to modify the demands of the activity so they more closely match Nathalie's abilities. For example, requiring players to be stationary when they are in possession of the ball (a drill often used to develop passing skills) or

Table 28.1 Case study: Nathalie plays basketball.

Abilities-based approach	Nathalie's abilities	Basketball demands
Mobility	Difficulty running and jumping Straight leg limits crouching, propulsion and impact abatement	Sprinting and quick turns Jumping
Object manipulation	Unaffected	Catching and throwing Dribbling
Cognition	Unaffected	Strategy of team Comprehension of rules
Communication and perception	Unaffected	Communication with team Perception of team's and opponents' movements Tracking of ball position
Behavior and social skills	Unaffected	Team cooperation Behavior according to rules
Fitness	Unaffected	Repeat sprinting during game Maintenance of arm strength for throwing and catching

offering a wheelchair basketball program would allow Nathalie to compete on an equal basis even if she is unable to change her mobility skills.

Understanding childhood motor disabilities and sport

The motor disabilities that most commonly occur during childhood can be summarized within the following categories.

• *Altered coordination.* Changes in coordination, balance, and agility most commonly occur because of cerebral palsy or traumatic brain injury. In both cases, the motor control center of the brain is damaged, making the control and coordination of muscular movements difficult. Coordination difficulties can also occur in children with disabilities even in the absence of a coordination-related diagnosis.

• *Loss of strength, movement, and/or sensation.* Various forms of muscular dystrophy or muscular atrophy are the primary causes of decreased muscle strength in children. Because, in children, most of these conditions are progressive, the loss of strength and movement will increase with age. In older youth it is common for the loss of strength to prevent voluntary movement (i.e., the muscles can no longer move the weight of the limb). Spina bifida and traumatic spinal cord injuries are the most common reasons for a total loss of movement or sensation in

children. Polio remains a common cause of loss of movement in some regions of the world. The extent of the paralysis is dependent on the area of damage to the spinal cord.

• *Bone loss and/or changes.* Bone loss in children can occur because of a traumatic amputation or because of altered prenatal bone growth. Changes to bone structure in children most commonly result from juvenile arthritis or scoliosis. Osteogenesis imperfecta is a relatively rare congenital condition that results in decreased bone strength and a greatly increased risk of fracture.

Table 28.2 provides examples of literature reviews on sport and exercise for children with different types of motor disability. The sport implications of each type of disability are highly variable, making it virtually impossible to define the implications based only on the medical diagnosis. For example, a child "with cerebral palsy" may have only a slight limp that is barely detectable or almost no control of voluntary movement. Coaches should strive to obtain specific information about each athlete's abilities from the athlete, his or her parents, and the family physician. For example, less than half of child amputees experience phantom limb pain, and for those who do, exercise is a common trigger (Wilkins *et al.* 1998). The coach should consider medical information in light of their own knowledge of physiology and anatomy to determine the specific

Table 28.2 Literature reviews of sport and children with motor disabilities.

Commonalities for sport among children with different disabilities	Dec *et al.* 2000; Patel & Greydanus 2002; Geist *et al.* 2003; Wind *et al.* 2004
Disabilities that alter coordination	
Cerebral palsy	Bar-Or 1996; Rimmer 2001; Wind *et al.* 2004
Brain injury	Sullivan *et al.* 1990 (adults); Cronin 2001
Disabilities that result in a loss of movement, strength or sensation	
Muscular dystrophy	Bar-Or 1996; Kilmer 2002; McDonald 2002
Spinal cord injury	Slater & Meade 2004 (adults)
Spina bifida	Wind *et al.* 2004
Disabilities that result in bone loss or change	
Amputation	Webster *et al.* 2001; Wind *et al.* 2004
Juvenile arthritis	Klepper 2003; LeBovidge *et al.* 2003; Wind *et al.* 2004
Scoliosis	Hawes 2003
Osteogenesis imperfecta	Engelbert *et al.* 1998

Table 28.3 Overview of physical activity research with children with motor disabilities. *Continued on facing page.*

Disabilities that alter coordination

Aerobic capacity	↓ Peer	Rimmer 2001; Sullivan *et al.* 1990
	↑ Train	Sullivan *et al.* 1990; Bar-Or 1996; Hutzler *et al.* 1998; van den Berg-Emons *et al.* 1998
Mechanical efficiency	↓ Peer	Rose *et al.* 1993; Duffy *et al.* 1996; Bowen *et al.* 1999; Suzuki *et al.* 2001; Detrembleur *et al.* 2003; Littlewood *et al.* 2004
	↑ Train	Bar-Or 1996; Mossberg *et al.* 2002
Muscular endurance	↓ Peer	Bar-Or 1996; Rossi & Sullivan 1996; Unnithan *et al.* 1998
Muscular strength	↓ Peer	Bar-Or 1996; Rossi & Sullivan 1996; Wiley & Damiano 1998; Rimmer 2001; Buckon *et al.* 2002
	No	Buckon *et al.* 2002
	↑ Train	Bar-Or 1996; Damiano & Abel 1998; Rimmer 2001; Blundell *et al.* 2003; Dodd *et al.* 2003
Flexibility	↓ Peer	Rossi & Sullivan 1996; Cronin 2001
Agility and balance	↓ Peer	Kuhtz-Buschbeck *et al.* 2003; Gagnon *et al.* 2004
	↑ Train	Kozhevnikova 2005
Body composition	↓ Peer	Berg 1970; Thommessen *et al.* 1991; Dahl & Gebremed-hin 1993; Cronk & Stallings 1997
	No	Bar-Or *et al.* 1976
	↑ Train	van den Berg-Emons *et al.* 1998
Bone density	↓ Peer	Apkon 2002; Henderson *et al.* 2002
	↑ Train	Chad *et al.* 1999; Apkon 2002
Motor skill, memory and control	↓ Peer	Rossi & Sullivan 1996; Cronin 2001; Kuhtz-Buschbeck *et al.* 2003; Tilton 2003
	↑ Train	Bloswick *et al.* 1996; Dursun *et al.* 2004

Disabilities that result in a loss of movement, strength, or sensation

Aerobic capacity	↓ Peer	Bar-Or 1986; Kilmer 2002; McDonald 2002; Slater & Meade 2004
	↑ Train	Andrade *et al.* 1991; Bar-Or 1996; Kilmer 2002; Slater & Meade 2004
Mechanical efficiency	↓ Peer	Bar-Or *et al.* 1976; Williams *et al.* 1983; Luna-Reyes *et al.* 1988; Duffy *et al.* 1996
	No	Bowen *et al.* 1999
	↑ Train	Bar-Or 1996
Muscular endurance	↓ Peer	Bar-Or 1996; Matecki *et al.* 2001; McDonald 2002
	No	Sharma *et al.* 1995
	↑ Train	Mccool & Tzelepis 1995; Topin *et al.* 2002
Muscular strength	↓ Peer	Brussock *et al.* 1992; Araujo *et al.* 1995; McDonald *et al.* 1995; Bar-Or 1996; McDonald 2002
	No	Russman *et al.* 1992
	↑ Train	Andrade *et al.* 1991; Bar-Or 1996; Gozal & Thiriet 1999

↑ Peer, improved relative to healthy peers; ↓ Peer, decreased relative to healthy peers; No, not affected; ↑ Train, improved with training.

physical activity implications of the disability and any particular issues of concern.

The previous physical activity experience of the child also has a strong influence on the observed motor skills and fitness. Table 28.3 provides an overview of research into the physical activity capabilities of children with motor disabilities. It is important to keep in mind that these studies are based on assessments of performance, not physical capacity. Even where research has established a correlation between decreased performance and type of disability, coaches must remember that a correlation does not necessarily imply causation. The

decreased performance observed may or may not result from the physical limitations imposed by the motor disability. It must also be recognized that there is very little research on which to base sport training recommendations for many childhood motor disabilities.

Type of physical activity setting

Childhood sport opportunities occur in a wide variety of settings, such as school physical education, community recreation programs, or competitive venues, which can influence the participation of

Table 28.3 *(cont'd)*

Flexibility	↓ Peer	McDonald *et al.* 1995; McDonald 2002; Wind *et al.* 2004
Body composition	↑ Peer	Dahl & Gebre-Medhin 1993; Leroy-Willig *et al.* 1997; McDonald 2002
	↓ Peer	McDonald *et al.* 1995
	No	Bar-Or *et al.* 1976
Bone density	↓ Peer	Apkon 2002; McDonald 2002; Wind *et al.* 2004
Motor skill, memory and control	↓ Peer	Tilton 2003

Disabilities that result in bone loss or change

Aerobic capacity	↓ Peer	Kearon *et al.* 1993; Upadhyay *et al.* 1993; Ferrari *et al.* 1997; Klepper 2003; Takken *et al.* 2004; Wind *et al.* 2004
	No	Hebestreit *et al.* 1998
	↑ Train	Binder *et al.* 1993; Athanasopoulos *et al.* 1999; Klepper 2003; Wind *et al.* 2004
Mechanical efficiency	↓ Peer	Bar-Or 1986; Herbert *et al.* 1994
	No	Durmala *et al.* 2002; Klepper 2003
Muscular endurance	No	Klepper 2003
	↑ Train	Klepper 2003
Muscular strength	↓ Peer	Engelbert *et al.* 1998; Mooney *et al.* 2000; Klepper 2003; Takken *et al.* 2004
	No	Burd *et al.* 2002
	↑ Train	Binder *et al.* 1993; Engelbert *et al.* 1998; Mooney *et al.* 2000; Klepper 2003; Wind *et al.* 2004
Flexibility	↑ Peer	Binder *et al.* 1984; Engelbert *et al.* 1998
	↓ Peer	Binder *et al.* 1993; Engelbert *et al.* 1998
	No	Burd *et al.* 2002
	↑ Train	Binder *et al.* 1984; Engelbert *et al.* 1998; Klepper 2003; Wind *et al.* 2004
Agility and balance	↑ Train	Wind *et al.* 2004
Bone density	↓ Peer	Binder *et al.* 1984; Engelbert *et al.* 1998
	↑ Train	Binder *et al.* 1984; Wind *et al.* 2004
Motor skill, memory and control	↓ Peer	Engelbert *et al.* 1998
	No	Burd *et al.* 2002
	↑ Train	Gerber *et al.* 1990; Wind *et al.* 2004

↑ Peer, improved relative to healthy peers; ↓ Peer, decreased relative to healthy peers; No, not affected; ↑ Train, improved with training.

children with motor disabilities. For example, children who have undergone spinal surgery for scoliosis are typically allowed to resume physical education and recreational activities, but many are prohibited from competitive sports involving body contact (Rubery & Bradford 2002). Regardless of setting, the impact of a lack of opportunity can never be underestimated. A lack of accessible facilities, restrictions on program participation or a dearth of coaches who are willing to work with athletes with disabilities are just a few of the many factors that make the availability (or lack thereof) of physical activity and sport opportunities a very critical factor influencing the sport participation of children with motor disabilities.

It is often assumed that children with disabilities participate equally in school physical activity opportunities because they are now educated primarily within the regular school setting. However, research indicates that this assumption is often incorrect (Simeonsson *et al.* 2001), particularly for students with motor disabilities. Classroom teachers, who often feel ill-prepared to teach physical education to students without disabilities, can be overwhelmed by the prospect of including students with motor disabilities into the class (Steadward & Wheeler 1996). Children with motor disabilities also frequently report that they are allowed to "opt out" of physical education in exchange for remedial learning activities or physical therapy.

Approaches to provide recreational sport opportunities have varied widely over time and from one country to another. In North America, the development of the International and North American Federations for Adapted Physical Activity, and in particular the adapted physical activity certification offered in the USA, have placed a strong focus on the need for specialized training and leadership. Fortunately, the segregated programs of the past are gradually being replaced by more inclusive settings through the resources and training opportunities provided by programs such as Moving to Inclusion (Active Living Alliance for Canadians with a Disability 1994). In contrast to North America, countries in Scandinavia and Australia (http://www.ausport.gov.au/dsu/index.asp) have been particularly progressive in adopting a "sport for all" (http://www.olympic.org/uk/organisation/commissions/sportforall/index_uk.asp) approach to physical activity for all children, including those with motor disabilities. It must also be recognized that in many developing countries, participation in physical activity is of relatively low importance for families struggling to ensure that their children have food, shelter, and a basic education (United Nations 2005).

Competitive sport opportunities for children with motor disabilities have expanded tremendously in recent years (Patel & Greydanus 2002). For example, an Internet search for "junior paralympians" identifies over 6500 websites with information about a wide range of sports. Although most coaches of children's sports recognize the need to include children with disabilities, a large percentage still express concern about their lack of training related to athletes with disabilities (Kozub & Porretta 1998). The increased opportunities now available reflect our increased understanding of the importance of childhood physical activity, the athletic potential of children with motor disabilities, and the need for athletes to be highly trained in order to achieve international success.

Depending on the level of competition (local, national, international) and the country in which the athlete lives, competitive sport opportunities may be offered within the sport system serving all amateur athletes or through a segregated system specific to disability sport. For example, Canadian wheelchair basketball teams can use players with and without disabilities at the local, regional, and national level, whereas international competitions require all players to have a disability. At the regional level, allowing athletes with and without disabilities to compete together is an effective way of increasing sport opportunities for athletes with disabilities in rural areas where getting enough children with disabilities together to form a team may be difficult.

At the elite level, the Paralympic Games offer international "Olympic level" competition to athletes who meet the disability classification criteria. The Paralympic Games (International Paralympic Committee 2005) have grown from a sport festival for 400 athletes from 23 countries competing in eight different sports (Rome, 1960) to a showcase of athletic talent for over 3800 athletes from 136 countries who compete in 19 different sports (Athens, 2004). Traditionally, Paralympic competitors are drawn from six groups of athletes: amputee, cerebral palsy, visual impairment, spinal cord injury, intellectual disability, and a group that includes all those that do not fit into the aforementioned groups (les autres). Classification systems, analogous to the weight classifications used in boxing or weightlifting, are used to ensure that athletes competing against one another have similar abilities. Each of the 21 summer and 4 winter Paralympic sports has its own classification system based on the sport-specific skills required. For example, archery has three classes: ARST (archery standing); ARW1 (wheelchair with arm and leg disabilities); and ARW2 (wheelchair with leg disabilities). Regardless of the cause of the disability, all athletes with disabilities who do archery from a standing position would compete in the ARST class. More detailed information about the Paralympic sport classification system is available on the website of the International Paralympic Committee (www.paralympic.org/release/Main_Sections_Menu/Classification).

Hypoactivity

For all children with motor disabilities, there is an increased risk of a sedentary lifestyle (Longmuir & Bar-Or 2000). For some children, decreased capacity for physical activity results from the disability

(Bar-Or 1986), such as the paralysis resulting from muscular dystrophy or an increased oxygen cost of movement (Maltais *et al.* 2005). Research also suggests that decreased physical activity is more common among children with more severe disabilities (Johnson *et al.* 2004). However, in many cases, the hypoactivity observed among children with motor disabilities does not result from the disability but from decreased opportunities for participation (Johnson *et al.* 2004) that lead to decreased fitness and motor skill. The desire to avoid embarrassment with one's peer group and the increased energy demands of participation from someone who is less skilled or less fit leads to a self-perpetuating downward spiral of decreased motivation for and participation in physical activity. It is critically important that coaches be able to clearly distinguish the actual limits imposed by the disability from the impacts of a sedentary lifestyle or the lack of opportunities for the development of motor skills and physical fitness. Except for the small percentage of children with progressive motor disabilities (e.g., Duchenne muscular dystrophy), the impact of the disability for the majority of children will have clearly defined limits and will remain stable over time. Access to quality coaching and sport opportunities can be used to overcome all of the limitations on physical activity participation except those that result specifically from the disability.

Training principles

The training principles for athletes with motor disabilities are the same as those used for children without disabilities (Steadward & Wheeler 1996). Frequency, intensity, and duration of training sessions should follow age-appropriate guidelines. Overload, progression, and periodization of the training program should be based on competitive opportunities and the athlete's skills and abilities. Historically, many children with motor disabilities were discouraged from exercise and athletic training because of concerns that the impact of the disability would be increased (Wind *et al.* 2004). However, Vignos and Watkins (1966) stated that regular training was appropriate for children with muscular dystrophy and others (Richter *et al.* 1996;

Klepper 2003) have subsequently shown that there is no negative impact from strenuous physical training for children with other motor disabilities.

Coaches also need to understand the influence of assistive devices used by the athlete (e.g., prostheses, braces, wheelchair). The specific impact of each device will vary, depending on the make and model of device used, the athlete's experience and expertise in device use, and the athlete's abilities without the device. For example, the type of prosthesis or orthotic can have a significant impact on the energy cost of physical activity (Katz *et al.* 1997; Hafner *et al.* 2002). Coaches should work closely with the athlete and device providers to ensure that the assistive device chosen will allow the athlete optimal performance.

As with all athletes, those with disabilities should be educated on the health and ethical issues related to performance enhancement. Coaches should be vigilant in looking for signs of inappropriate training methods, such as the use of performance-enhancing substances. Coaches of athletes with cervical or high thoracic spinal cord injury should also be aware of autonomic dysreflexia (Long *et al.* 1997). Autonomic dysreflexia is a very risky and potentially fatal enhancement of the body's response to exercise, particularly a dramatic increase in blood pressure, which results from an exaggerated nervous system response to noxious stimuli (e.g., pain, over-extended bladder). The lack of sensation resulting from the spinal cord injury means that the athletes do not feel any of the pain or negative effects that would normally force the person to remove the noxious stimuli. Research indicates that virtually all (>90%) athletes with high level spinal cord injuries have experimented with using autonomic dysreflexia to boost their performance. Autonomic dysreflexia poses a particular problem for sport officials because it effectively increases performance without the use of any "foreign" or introduced substance that could be detected through athlete drug testing.

Athlete assessment

Assessment procedures for athletes with motor disabilities should generally parallel those used for child athletes without disabilities, although the specific mode of exercise may be different. Preparticipation medical screening should be provided to all athletes, including those with a disability. There are no "special" preparticipation guidelines necessary for child athletes with motor disabilities (Patel & Greydanus 2002). The Sports-Medical Assessment Protocol (SMAP; Jacob & Hutzler 1998) is an in-depth preparticipation assessment designed for athletes with disabilities, but research is needed to determine whether the additional resources required to conduct the SMAP provide significant additional benefits (Lai et al. 2000). The preparticipation examination should include a detailed medical history as well as consideration of the impact of any prosthetics, orthotics, or other assistive devices that the child may use. It is important that the medical screening be carried out by physicians who are familiar with the child's disability so that they will be knowledgeable about any potential risks or special considerations (Patel & Greydanus 2002). For example, contact sports are usually contraindicated for athletes with internal shunts or metal rods. It is equally important that the physician ensures that common medical issues are not overlooked because of a focus on the disability and its implications.

A wide variety of fitness and performance assessment protocols have been developed for athletes with motor disabilities. These include protocols for the assessment of aerobic capacity and power, anaerobic threshold or power, muscular strength, balance, flexibility, and body composition (Bar-Or 1993; Campbell 1996; Steadward & Wheeler 1996; van den Berg-Emons et al. 1996, 1998; Van Mil et al. 1996). It is important that the assessment procedures selected are well suited to the physical size, mental capacity, and emotional maturity of the child and relevant to the child's athletic performance (Bar-Or 1993, 1996). Athletes should be thoroughly familiar with the activities to be performed and the familiarization period may need to be more extensive for athletes with more severe disabilities. In general, direct measures of exercise capacity are preferred to estimations of performance from indirect measures (e.g., heart rate prediction of $\dot{V}_{O_{2max}}$) because many types of disability influence the exercise response (Keefer et al. 2004) and prediction equations have seldom been validated for athletes

with disabilities. It is also important to keep in mind the specificity of training, the impact of the disability, and the athlete's method of ambulation when choosing the type of assessment equipment. For example, athletes who use a wheelchair for ambulation obtain higher measures of aerobic capacity using a wheelchair ergometer. Bicycle ergometry may be a more effective mode of assessment for those who walk for ambulation (Bhambhani et al. 1992). Similarly, athletes with cerebral palsy have lower levels of energy consumption when exercising with the least-affected limbs (Piskorz & Klimek-Piskorz 1998).

The type of assistive device used by the athlete can also have a significant influence on test results. For example, if an athlete changes from a static to a flexible pylon or ankle in a prosthetic leg there may be significant changes to the physiology or biomechanics of exercise (Colborne et al. 1992; Coleman et al. 2001). It is also important to consider the speed of movement required by the assessment protocol for athletes with disabilities that affect motor coordination. For example, testing at 30 rev·min^{-1} on an arm crank ergometer may be more efficient for athletes with cerebral palsy than lower or higher pedaling speeds (Maltais et al. 2000).

As for any child athlete, the need for assessment should be considered in light of why the tests are being carried out, how valuable the results will be, whether repeat assessments will be possible, and whether the athlete will be safe throughout the test procedure (Steadward & Wheeler 1996). Of particular importance to the assessment of a child athlete with a motor disability is the question of repeat assessments. Because the presence of a motor disability almost always precludes the use of standardized normative data or prediction equations, the ability to repeat the assessment procedures is critical in order to understand the impact of training on performance. For the same reason, it is seldom possible to predict athletic success or athlete suitability for a particular sport based on single-session assessments. However, repeat assessments at appropriate intervals can provide valuable information that will enable the coach to more effectively monitor the impact of the training program in light of the athlete's disability.

Athletic injury

The injury patterns, prevalence of sports-related pain, and need for sports medicine treatment are similar for athletes with and without motor disabilities (Wilson & Washington 1993; Dec *et al.* 2000; Ferrara & Peterson 2000; Patel & Greydanus 2002; Bernardi *et al.* 2003). However, there also may be specific training implications associated with the disability. For example, athletes with paralysis must be vigilant for bladder problems or pressure sores and soft tissue injuries (Peck & McKeag 1994) which may go undetected because of the lack of sensation. Similarly, a spinal cord injury, spina bifida, or cerebral palsy can affect thermoregulation making these athletes more susceptible to both hyper- and hypo-thermia (Wilson & Washington 1993; Lai *et al.* 2000; Patel & Greydanus 2002; Maltais *et al.* 2004).

Athletes with motor disabilities often have an increased risk for overuse injuries (Dyson-Hudson & Kirschblum 2004). As a result of the disability, most athletes tend to rely heavily on the least-affected limbs for day-to-day and physical activities (Engsberg *et al.* 1993; Steadward & Wheeler 1996; Nolan *et al.* 2003). For example, a child whose legs are paralyzed will rely on his or her arms for mobility. Similarly, a child with a prosthetic arm will rely primarily on the unaffected arm for most tasks. These already high levels of daily use put the least-affected limbs at a much higher risk for overuse injury when the demands of a sport-training regime are superimposed. Coaches, trainers, and athletes must always be alert to the heightened risk for overuse injuries and the associated loss of independence for essential daily functions. Because the disability already imposes some degree of limitation, the impact of an overuse injury may be more significant than for athletes without a disability. For example, the impact of "tennis elbow" or shoulder injuries will be much greater for the athlete whose legs are paralyzed because it will not only affect sport training but also any type of independent mobility. Needless to say, it is critically important that athletes with motor disabilities have access to sports medicine personnel who have experience and expertise in relation to the child's disability. Too often, the child athlete with a motor disability is referred to a rehabilitation or disability specialist (e.g., physiatrist), who has no knowledge or experience in sports medicine, for the treatment of a sport-related injury. In contrast, child athletes without disabilities are routinely referred to sports medicine personnel for the care and therapeutic treatment of sport-related injuries. It is not appropriate for the care of athletic injuries for athletes with motor disabilities to be the responsibility of rehabilitation or disability specialists, unless that specialist also has training in sports medicine or athletic training. The use of injury assessment tools suitable for athletes with motor disabilities is also important (Jacob & Hutzler 1998).

Coaches and athletes should also keep up-to-date on innovations in assistive technology (e.g., wheelchairs, braces, prosthetic limbs) to ensure that the technologies that provide optimal performance with minimal additional load are used whenever possible. For example, the type of prosthetic foot used by an amputee athlete can significantly affect the energy cost of physical activity (Schneider *et al.* 1993). The training regime itself may also influence the athlete's risk for injury. For example, the increased stress of running rather than walking can magnify the negative effects of altered gait patterns. Research indicates that volume of training is positively related to sports-related pain for athletes with disabilities (Bernardi *et al.* 2003). Exercise training equipment that is not suitable for ensuring an optimal training regime can also be a cause of injury. For example, athletes with a below knee amputation often have difficulty strengthening the hamstring and quadricep muscles of the affected leg because the absence of the lower leg limits their use of strengthening machines designed for that purpose. Research into the prevalence of upper limb nerve entrapments (i.e., carpal tunnel syndrome) among elite wheelchair racers indicates that these athletes are not automatically more susceptible, and indeed may be less susceptible to overuse injuries when an appropriate training program is followed (Boninger *et al.* 1996).

MIXING SPORT WITH MEDICINE AND THERAPY

The sport participation of children with motor

disabilities is often influenced by a variety of medical factors. For example, the additional time required to complete medical or self-care and therapy requirements may significantly reduce the leisure time available for physical activity (Ayyangar 2002). Similarly, the time required for medical appointments and the perceived need to split time equally between all siblings can limit parental availability to support the recreational activities of the child with a disability (Field & Oates 2001; Taanila *et al.* 2002). Historically, it has also been common for sport programs for children with disabilities to be segregated and taught by a medical or therapy professional using institutional facilities (Bernard *et al.* 1981; Reid 2003) or for sports, such as horseback riding, to be offered as a form of therapy (Haskin *et al.* 1974). As the inclusion of children with disabilities in community-based sport opportunities increases, the frequency of medically based programs is decreasing but remains a significant source of physical activity opportunities for up to 25% of children with motor disabilities (Field & Oates 2001).

Therapists often define their interventions in terms of the exercises performed (e.g., strength or flexibility activities) (Siegel 1978; Weiss & Weiss 2002), which may lead parents and teachers to equate the therapy session with physical education or sport participation. Parents are often unaware of the sport opportunities available to their child and most feel that available opportunities are inadequate or that there are significant barriers to their child's participation (Field & Oates 2001). Meaningful participation in physical education is also often seen as impossible for the child with a motor disability (Bernard *et al.* 1981). As a result, teachers and parents often agree to have a child with a motor disability attend a physical therapy session in lieu of physical education. It is essential that the adults who can influence the participation of a child with a motor disability be educated on the need for physically active play and physical education as separate and distinct from medical or therapeutic treatments. Sport and physical activity offer many benefits, such as teamwork, socialization, fitness, and the development of lifelong skill and activity interests, that are not provided through physical therapy.

Nutrition

Nutrition is a key component of athletic performance, and no less so for athletes with motor disabilities. In general, dietary requirements are similar to child athletes without disabilities. For athletes with disabilities that result in an increased energy cost for activities, additional attention should be paid to the maintenance of appropriate body composition. For example, children with moderate to severe cerebral palsy have an increased risk of feeding problems which result in a higher risk of poor nutritional status (Fung *et al.* 2002). Surprisingly, despite reporting problems such as constipation or vomiting, over 60% of children with cerebral palsy have never had a nutritional assessment (Sullivan *et al.* 2000). Coaches should consult with the child athlete and family to determine whether additional nutritional considerations or referral to a dietitian are necessary to ensure sufficient energy for the demands of sport participation (Steadward & Wheeler 1996). Unfortunately, the availability of dietitian's experienced in managing child athletes with disabilities is often limited (Hartley & Thomas 2003). Coaches of athletes with motor disabilities should also be vigilant for eating disorders or the use of ergogenic aids (Patel & Greydanus 2002), just as they would for all of their athletes.

Psychologic factors

Most children with motor disabilities are the same as child athletes without disabilities in terms of their psychosocial adjustment and response to sport psychology techniques (Tyc 1992; Edwards Beckett 1995). However, factors such as societal attitudes towards disability and limited previous life experiences mean that psychosocial sequelae may be more commonly observed among children with motor disabilities (Lavigne & Faier-Routman 1992; Varni & Setoguchi 1992; McDermott *et al.* 1996; Zurmohle *et al.* 1998; LeBovidge *et al.* 2003; Witt *et al.* 2003). The risk of psychosocial problems is higher for children who have disabilities affecting the brain (Geist *et al.* 2003), that result from traumatic injuries (e.g., motor vehicle accidents) that may result in undiagnosed closed head injuries (Povolny & Kaplan 1993), that change over time (e.g., remitting-relenting conditions; Patterson & Blum 1996), or those that do not have strong social support from parents and peers (Wallander & Varni 1989; Antle 2004).

Children who have recently acquired a disability or are living with a degenerative condition may face additional psychologic obstacles. Typically, there is an adjustment period when a disability is acquired during which the child may be very hesitant to become involved in physical activity because of his or her uncertainties about their new life and abilities. For a child with a degenerative condition, these periods of adjustment to new levels of decreased function may occur almost continuously, depending on the speed of deterioration. Coaches working with athletes in these situations should be particularly sensitive to the child's psychologic needs and highly supportive of their physical activity participation. It is important that the coaches are realistic in their praise, but they must also educate themselves, the child, and others (e.g., parents, teammates) about the positive benefits of seemingly small to non-existent changes in performance. For example, the maintenance of muscular strength at previous levels may actually represent a tremendous fitness gain for a child with a degenerative disability (e.g., Duchenne muscular dystrophy).

Research indicates that perceived physical competence is strongly associated with perceived social competence among children with disabilities, and that peers have a strong influence on these beliefs (Armstrong et al. 1992). Therefore it is not surprising that children with motor disabilities who participate in high level sport have a decreased risk for psychologic sequelae (Sherrill et al. 1990) and that involvement in physical activity and sport can improve the self-concept of children with motor disabilities (Andrade et al. 1991).

FEAR AND OVERPROTECTION

"Ethically and morally, the child with a disability should not be denied access to any programs" (Steadward & Wheeler 1996). However, in reality, fear and overprotection are just two of the many barriers to physical activity that children with disabilities must overcome. For children, the concept of overprotection is most often associated with parental overprotection. Therapists have identified family factors (e.g., support to child, expectations) as one of four factors influencing the acquisition of motor skills for children with cerebral palsy (Bartlett & Palisano 2002). Research also suggests that overprotection may be more common among parents who regularly provide physical therapy treatments to a child with a disability (Sarimski & Hoffmann 1993). This raises the question of whether overprotection is a significant factor for most athletes with disabilities, or only a subset of athletes who receive ongoing therapy services (who presumably have more severe disabilities). The influence of overprotection from other sources, such as medical personnel, teachers, or the children themselves, must also be considered (Steadward & Wheeler 1996).

Societal attitudes towards people with disabilities, and expectations for their participation in sport, continue to be a very significant barrier (Lindström 1992). For many adults, the concept of being responsible for a child with a disability is enough to discourage them from volunteering to coach or organize a physical activity opportunity (Steadward & Wheeler 1996). Our relative lack of knowledge and experience in identifying what constitutes "reasonable practice" related to the sport participation of children with disabilities also results in a perception that the liability and possibility of litigation could be substantially increased for organizations and individuals offering such programs. Therefore it is not surprising that the majority of child athletes with disabilities report that their coach is a family member, therapist, or another athlete (Wilson & Washington 1993). The very high level of sport performance achieved by some athletes with disabilities suggests that psychosocial factors, such as the influence of fear and overprotection, may be very significant influences on the decreased sport performance observed among many children with motor disabilities.

Challenges for future research

The importance of physical activity to childhood

development and lifelong health makes it critical that sport opportunities be available to children with motor disabilities. Future research efforts should be encouraged across the full spectrum of sport and physical activity realms, including efforts to address the following issues.

• *Full inclusion.* Research is needed to identify interventions that will effectively influence society's attitudes and expectations so that the full participation of children with motor disabilities is expected and supported. Full inclusion can only occur when all sport opportunities are designed to welcome children of all abilities, whether or not any children with disabilities actually participate.

• *Physical activity and child development.* Research is needed to establish clearly the benefits of sport participation for childhood development and lifelong health. In addition, the applicability and relevance of these benefits to children with motor disabilities must be clearly established.

• *Optimal training.* More detailed information on the optimal training principles for children with different types of disability is required. Increased knowledge of optimal training levels and activity intensities will help to address issues of liability, fear, and overprotection.

• *Injury prevention and treatment.* Given the increased impact of overuse injuries, research into effective injury prevention and treatment strategies is very important for children with motor disabilities. Efforts to educate medical personnel in providing appropriate support for sport and physical activity participation by child athletes with motor disabilities are also required.

• *Ethical concerns.* Historically, the importance of ethical issues has been underestimated in disability sport. The tendency to "marvel" at the abilities of athletes with motor disabilities has often overshadowed the need to be vigilant to issues such as performance enhancement. Greater research is required to clarify the use of performance-enhancing substances and techniques as well as the implications of elite sport training for children with a motor disability. The development and implementation of an appropriate code of ethics, as previously suggested by Rutenfranz (1985), that includes the participation of child athletes with motor disabilities should be considered (Steadward & Wheeler 1996).

References

Active Living Alliance for Canadians with a Disability (1994) *Moving to Inclusion. Active Living Through Physical Education: Maximizing Opportunities for Students with a Disability.* Ottawa.

Andrade, C.K., Kramer, J., Garber, M. & Longmuir, P. (1991) Changes in self-concept, cardiovascular endurance and muscular strength of children with spina bifida aged 8 to 13 years in response to a 10-week physical-activity programme: a pilot study. *Child: Care, Health and Development* **17**, 183–196.

Antle, B.J. (2004) Factors associated with self-worth in young people with physical disabilities. *Health & Social Work* **29**, 167–175.

Apkon, S.D. (2002) Osteoporosis in children who have disabilities. *Physical Medicine and Rehabilitation Clinics of North America* **13**, 839–855.

Araujo, A.P.Q.C., Duro, L.A., Araujo, A.Q.C. & Penque, G.M.C.A. (1995) Myometry assessment in patients with Duchenne muscular-dystrophy. *Arquivos de Neuro-Psiquiatria* **53**, 233–237.

Armstrong, R.W., Rosenbaum, P.L. & King, S. (1992) Self-perceived social function among disabled-children in regular classrooms. *Journal of Developmental and Behavioral Pediatrics* **13**, 11–16.

Athanasopoulos, S., Paxinos, T., Tsafantakis, E., Zachariou, K. & Chatziconstantinou, S. (1999) The effect of aerobic training in girls with idiopathic scoliosis. *Scandinavian Journal of Medicine and Science in Sports* **9**, 36–40.

Ayyangar, R. (2002) Health maintenance and management in childhood disability. *Physical Medicine and Rehabilitation Clinics of North America* **13**, 793–821.

Bar-Or, O. (1986) Pathophysiological factors which limit the exercise capacity of the sick child. *Medicine and Science in Sports and Exercise* **18**, 276–282.

Bar-Or, O. (1993) Noncardiopulmonary pediatric exercise tests. In: *Pediatric Laboratory Exercise Testing* (Rowland, T.W., ed.) Human Kinetics, Springfield, IL: 165–185.

Bar-Or, O. (1996) Role of exercise in the assessment and management of neuromuscular disease in children. *Medicine and Science in Sports and Exercise* **28**, 421–427.

Bar-Or, O., Inbar, O. & Spira, R. (1976) Physiological effects of a sports rehabilitation program on cerebral palsied and post-poliomyelitic adolescents. *Medicine and Science in Sports and Exercise* **8**, 157–161.

Bartlett, D.J. & Palisano, R.J. (2002) Physical therapists' perceptions of factors influencing the acquisition of motor abilities of children with cerebral palsy: implications for clinical reasoning. *Physical Therapy* **82**, 237–248.

Berg, K. (1970) Body composition and nutrition of school children with cerebral palsy. *Acta Paediatrica Scandinavica* **204** (Supplement), 41–52.

Bernard, B., Creswell, J., Erickson, V., Ivey, J., Johnston, B. & Alexander, L.S. (1981) Exercise for children with physical disabilities. *Issues in Comprehensive Pediatric Nursing* **5**, 99–107.

Bernardi, M., Castellano, V., Ferrara, M.S., Sbriccoli, P., Sera, F. & Marchetti, M. (2003) Muscle pain in athletes with locomotor disability. *Medicine and Science in Sports and Exercise* **35**, 199–206.

Bhambhani, Y.N., Holland, L.J. & Steadward, R.D. (1992) Maximal aerobic power in cerebral-palsied wheelchair athletes: validity and reliability. *Archives of Physical Medicine and Rehabilitation* **73**, 246–252.

Binder, H., Conway, A., Hason, S., *et al.* (1993) Comprehensive rehabilitation of the child with osteogenesis imperfecta. *American Journal of Medical Genetics* **45**, 265–269.

Binder, H., Hawks, L., Graybill, G., Gerber, N.L. & Weintrob, J.C. (1984) Osteogenesis imperfecta: rehabilitation approach with infants and young children. *Archives of Physical Medicine and Rehabilitation* **65**, 537–541.

Bloswick, D.S., Brown, D., King, E.M., Howell, G. & Gooch, J.R. (1996) Testing and evaluation of a hip extensor tricycle for children with cerebral palsy. *Disability and Rehabilitation* **18**, 130–136.

Blundell, S.W., Shepherd, R.B., Dean, C.M., Adams, R.D. & Cahill, B.M. (2003) Functional strength training in cerebral palsy: a pilot study of a group circuit training class for children aged 4–8 years. *Clinical Rehabilitation* **17**, 48–57.

Boninger, M.L., Robertson, R.N., Wolff, M. & Cooper, R.A. (1996) Upper limb nerve entrapments in elite wheelchair racers. *American Journal of Physical Medicine & Rehabilitation* **75**, 170–176.

Bowen, T.R., Miller, F. & Mackenzie, W. (1999) Comparison of oxygen consumption measurements in children with cerebral palsy to children with muscular dystrophy. *Journal of Pediatric Orthopaedics* **19**, 133–136.

Brussock, C.M., Haley, S.M., Munsat, T.L. & Bernhardt, D.B. (1992) Measurement of isometric force in children with and without Duchenne's muscular dystrophy. *Physical Therapy* **72**, 105–114.

Buckon, C.E., Thomas, S.S., Harris, G.E., Piatt, J.H., Aiona, M.D. & Sussman, M.D. (2002) Objective measurement of muscle strength in children with spastic diplegia after selective dorsal rhizotomy. *Archives of Physical Medicine and Rehabilitation* **83**, 454–460.

Burd, T.A., Pawelek, L. & Lenke, L.G. (2002) Upper extremity functional assessment after anterior spinal fusion via thoracotomy for adolescent idiopathic scoliosis: Prospective study of twenty-five patients. *Spine* **27**, 65–71.

Campbell, S.K. (1996) Quantifying the effects of interventions for movement disorders resulting from cerebral palsy. *Journal of Child Neurology* **11** (Supplement 1), S61–S70.

Chad, K.E., Bailey, D.A., McKay, H.A., Zello, G.A. & Snyder, R.E. (1999) The effect of a weight-bearing physical activity program on bone mineral content and estimated volumetric density in children with spastic cerebral palsy. *Journal of Pediatrics* **135**, 115–117.

Colborne, R.G., Naumann, S., Longmuir, P.E. & Berbrayer, D. (1992) Analysis of mechanical and metabolic factors in the gait of congenital below knee amputees: a comparison of the SACH and Seattle feet. *American Journal of Physical Medicine & Rehabilitation* **71**, 272–278.

Coleman, K.L., Boone, D.A., Smith, D.G. & Czerniecki, J.M. (2001) Effect of trans-tibial prosthesis pylon flexibility on ground reaction forces during gait. *Prosthetics and Orthotics International* **25**, 195–201.

Cronin, A.F. (2001) Traumatic brain injury in children: issues in community function. *American Journal of Occupational Therapy* **55**, 377–384.

Cronk, C.E. & Stallings, V.A. (1997) Growth in children with cerebral palsy. *Mental Retardation and Developmental Disabilities Research Reviews* **3**, 129–137.

Dahl, M. & Gebre-Medhin, M. (1993) Feeding and nutritional problems in children with cerebral palsy and myelomeningocele. *Acta Paediatrica* **82**, 816–820.

Damiano, D.L. & Abel, M.F. (1998) Functional outcomes of strength training in spastic cerebral palsy. *Archives of Physical Medicine and Rehabilitation* **79**, 119–125.

Dec, K.L., Sparrow, K.J. & McKeag, D.B. (2000) The physically-challenged athlete: medical issues and assessment. *Sports Medicine* **29**, 245–258.

Detrembleur, C., Dierick, F., Stoquart, G., Chantraine, F. & Lejeune, T. (2003) Energy cost, mechanical work, and efficiency of hemiparetic walking. *Gait & Posture* **18**, 47–55.

Dodd, K.J., Taylor, N.F. & Graham, H.K. (2003) A randomized clinical trial of strength training in young people with cerebral palsy. *Developmental Medicine and Child Neurology* **45**, 652–657.

Duffy, C.M., Hill, A.E., Cosgrove, A.P., Corry, I.S. & Graham, H.K. (1996) Energy consumption in children with spina bifida and cerebral palsy: a comparative study. *Developmental Medicine and Child Neurology* **38**, 238–243.

Durmala, J., Dobosiewicz, K., Jendrzejek, H. & Pius, W. (2002) Exercise efficiency of girls with idiopathic scoliosis based on the ventilatory anaerobic threshold. *Studies in Health Technology and Informatics* **91**, 357–360.

Dursun, E., Dursun, N. & Alican, D. (2004) Effects of biofeedback treatment on gait in children with cerebral palsy. *Disability and Rehabilitation* **26**, 116–120.

Dyson-Hudson, T.A. & Kirshblum, S.C. (2004) Shoulder pain in chronic spinal cord injury. Part I: Epidemiology, etiology, and pathomechanics. *Journal of Spinal Cord Medicine* **27**, 4–17.

Edwards Beckett, J. (1995) Parental expectations and child's self-concept in spina-bifida. *Childrens Health Care* **24**, 257–267.

Emes, C., Longmuir, P. & Downs, P. (2002) An abilities-based approach to service delivery and professional preparation in adapted physical activity. *Adapted Physical Activity Quarterly* **19**, 403–419.

Engelbert, R.H.H., Pruijs, H.E.H., Beemer, F.A. & Helders, P.J.M. (1998) Osteogenesis imperfecta in childhood: treatment strategies. *Archives of Physical Medicine and Rehabilitation* **79**, 1590–1594.

Engsberg, J.R., Lee, A.G., Tedford, K.G. & Harder, J.A. (1993) Normative ground reaction force data for able-bodied and trans-tibial amputee children during running. *Prosthetics and Orthotics International* **17**, 83–89.

Ferrara, M.S. & Peterson, C.L. (2000) injuries to athletes with disabilities: identifying injury patterns. *Sports Medicine* **30**, 137–143.

Ferrari, K., Goti, P., Sanna, A., *et al.* (1997) Short-term effects of bracing on exercise performance in mild idiopathic thoracic scoliosis. *Lung* **175**, 299–310.

Field, S.J. & Oates, R.K. (2001) Sport and recreation opportunities for children with spina bifida and cystic fibrosis. *Journal of Science and Medicine in Sport* **4**, 71–76.

Fung, E.B., Samson-Fang, L., Stallings, V.A., *et al.* (2002) Feeding dysfunction is associated with poor growth and health status in children with cerebral palsy. *Journal of the American Dietetic Association* **102**, 361–373.

Gagnon, I., Swaine, B., Friedman, D. & Forget, R. (2004) Children show decreased dynamic balance after mild traumatic brain injury. *Archives of Physical Medicine and Rehabilitation* **85**, 444–452.

Geist, R., Grdisa, V. & Otley, A. (2003) Psychosocial issues in the child with chronic conditions. *Best Practice and Research in Clinical Gastroenterology* **17**, 141–152.

Gerber, L.H., Binder, H., Weintrob, J., *et al.* (1990) Rehabilitation of children and infants with osteogenesis imperfecta. A program for ambulation. *Clinical Orthopaedics and Related Research* **251**, 254–262.

Gozal, D. & Thiriet, P. (1999) Respiratory muscle training in neuromuscular disease: long-term effects on strength and load perception. *Medicine and Science in Sports and Exercise* **31**, 1522–1527.

Hafner, B.J., Sanders, J.E., Czerniecki, J.M. & Fergason, J. (2002) Transtibial energy-storage-and-return prosthetic devices: a review of energy concepts and a proposed nomenclature. *Journal of Rehabilitation Research and Development* **39**, 1–11.

Hartley, H. & Thomas, J.E. (2003) Current practice in the management of children with cerebral palsy: a national survey of paediatric dietitians. *Journal of Human Nutrition and Dietetics* **16**, 219–224.

Haskin, M.R., Erdman, W.J., Bream, J. & Mac Avoy, C.G. (1974) Therapeutic horseback riding for the handicapped. *Archives of Physical Medicine and Rehabilitation* **55**, 473–474.

Hawes, M.C. (2003) The use of exercises in the treatment of scoliosis: an evidence-based critical review of the literature. *Pediatric Rehabilitation* **6**, 171–182.

Hebestreit, H., Müller-Scholden, J. & Huppertz, H.I. (1998) Aerobic fitness and physical activity in patients with HLA-B27 positive juvenile spondyloarthropathy that is inactive or in remission. *Journal of Rheumatology* **25**, 1626–1633.

Henderson, R.C., Lark, R.K., Gurka, M.J., *et al.* (2002) Bone density and metabolism in children and adolescents with moderate to severe cerebral palsy. *Pediatrics* **110**, e5.

Herbert, L.M., Engsberg, J.R., Tedford, K.G. & Grimston, S.K. (1994) A comparison of oxygen-consumption during walking between children with and without below-knee amputations. *Physical Therapy* **74**, 943–950.

Hutzler, Y., Chacham, A., Bergman, U. & Szeinberg, A. (1998) Effects of a movement and swimming program on vital capacity and water orientation skills of children with cerebral palsy. *Developmental Medicine and Child Neurology* **40**, 176–181.

International Paralympic Committee (2005) Paralympic Games. [On-line] Available at: http://www.paralympic. org/release/Main_Sections_Menu/ Paralympic_Games.

Jacob, T. & Hutzler, Y. (1998) Sports-medical assessment for athletes with a disability. *Disability and Rehabilitation* **20**, 116–119.

Johnson, K.A., Klaas, S.J., Vogel, L.C. & McDonald, C. (2004) Leisure characteristics of the pediatric spinal cord injury population. *Journal of Spinal Cord Medicine* **27** (Supplement 1), S107–S109.

Katz, D.E., Haideri, N., Song, K. & Wyrick, P. (1997) Comparative study of conventional hip-knee-ankle-foot orthoses versus reciprocating-gait orthoses for children with high-level paraparesis. *Journal of Pediatric Orthopedics* **17**, 377–386.

Kearon, C., Viviani, G.R. & Killian, K.J. (1993) Factors influencing work capacity in adolescent idiopathic thoracic scoliosis. *American Review of Respiratory Disease* **148**, 295–303.

Keefer, D.J., Tseh, W., Caputo, J.L., Apperson, K., McGreal, S. & Morgan, D.W. (2004) Comparison of direct and indirect measures of walking energy expenditure in children with hemiplegic cerebral palsy. *Developmental Medicine and Child Neurology* **46**, 320–324.

Kilmer, D.D. (2002) Response to aerobic exercise training in humans with neuromuscular disease. *American Journal of Physical Medicine and Rehabilitation* **81**, S148–S150.

Klepper, S.E. (2003) Exercise and fitness in children with arthritis: evidence of benefits for exercise and physical activity. *Arthritis and Rheumatism: Arthritis Care and Research* **49**, 435–443.

Kozhevnikova, V.T. (2005) Vertical stability of schoolchildren with spastic diplegia before and after complex physical rehabilitation. *Meditsinskaia Tekhnika* **2**, 42–45.

Kozub, F.M. & Porretta, D.L. (1998) Interscholastic coaches' attitudes toward integration of adolescents with disabilities. *Adapted Physical Activity Quarterly* **15**, 328–344.

Kuhtz-Buschbeck, J.P., Hoppe, B., Golge, M., Dreesmann, M., Damm-Stunitz, U. & Ritz, A. (2003) Sensorimotor recovery in children after traumatic brain injury: analyses of gait, gross motor, and fine motor skills. *Development Medicine and Child Neurology* **45**, 821–828.

Lai, A.M., Stanish, W.D. & Stanish, H.I. (2000) The young athlete with physical challenges. *Clinics in Sports Medicine* **19**, 793–819.

Lavigne, J.V. & Faier-Routman, J. (1992) Psychological adjustment to pediatric physical disorders: a meta-analytic review. *Journal of Pediatric Psychology* **17**, 133–157.

LeBovidge, J.S., Lavigne, J.V., Donenberg, G.R. & Miller, M.L. (2003) Psychological adjustment of children and adolescents with chronic arthritis: A meta-analytic review. *Journal of Pediatric Psychology* **28**, 29–39.

Leroy-Willig, A., Willig, T.N., Henry-Feugeas, M.C., *et al.* (1997) Body composition determined with MR in patients with Duchenne muscular dystrophy, spinal muscular atrophy, and normal subjects. *Magnetic Resonance Imaging* **15**, 737–744.

Lindström, H. (1992) Integration of sport for athletes with disabilities into sport programming for able-bodied athletes. *Palaestra* **4**, 19–23.

Littlewood, R.A., Davies, P.S., Cleghorn, G.J. & Grote, R.H. (2004) Physical activity cost in children following an acquired brain injury: a comparative study. *Clinical Nutrition* **23**, 99–104.

Long, K., Meredith, S. & Bell, G.W. (1997) Autonomic dysreflexia and boosting in wheelchair athletes. *Adapted Physical Activity Quarterly* **14**, 203–209.

Longmuir, P.E. (2003) Creating inclusive physical activity opportunities: an abilities-based approach. In: *Adapted Physical Activity* (Steadward, R.D., Watkinson, E.J. & Wheeler, G.D., eds.) University of Alberta Press, Edmonton: 363–382.

Longmuir, P.E. & Bar-Or, O. (2000) Factors affecting the physical activity levels of youths with physical and sensory disabilities. *Adapted Physical Activity Quarterly* **17**, 40–53.

Luna-Reyes, O.B., Reyes, T.M., So, F.Y., Matti, B.M.S. & Lardizabal, A.A. (1988) Energy cost of ambulation in healthy and disabled Filipino children. *Archives of Physical Medicine and Rehabilitation* **69**, 946–949.

Maltais, D., Kondo, I. & Bar-Or, O. (2000) Arm cranking economy in spastic cerebral palsy: effects of different speed and force combinations yielding the same mechanical power. *Pediatric Exercise Science* **12**, 258–269.

Maltais, D., Wilk, B., Unnithan, V. & Bar-Or, O. (2004) Responses of children with cerebral palsy to treadmill walking exercise in the heat. *Medicine and Science in Sports and Exercise* **36**, 1674–1681.

Maltais, D.B., Pierrynowski, M.R., Galea, V.A., Matsuzaka, A. & Bar-Or, O. (2005) Habitual physical activity levels are associated with biomechanical walking economy in children with cerebral palsy. *American Journal of Physical Medicine and Rehabilitation* **84**, 36–45.

Matecki, S., Topin, N., Hayot, M., *et al.* (2001) A standardized method for the evaluation of respiratory muscle endurance in patients with Duchenne muscular dystrophy. *Neuromuscular Disorders* **11**, 171–177.

Mccool, F.D. & Tzelepis, G.E. (1995) Inspiratory muscle training in the patient with neuromuscular disease. *Physical Therapy* **75**, 1006–1014.

McDermott, S., Coker, A.L., Mani, S., *et al.* (1996) A population-based analysis of behavior problems in children with cerebral palsy. *Journal of Pediatric Psychology* **21**, 447–463.

McDonald, C.M. (2002) Physical activity, health impairments, and disability in neuromuscular disease. *American Journal of Physical Medicine and Rehabilitation* **81**, S108–S120.

McDonald, C.M., Abresch, R.T., Carter, G.T., *et al.* (1995) Profiles of neuromuscular diseases. *American Journal of Physical Medicine and Rehabilitation* **74**, S70–S92.

Mooney, V., Gulick, J. & Pozos, R. (2000) A preliminary report on the effect of measured strength training in adolescent idiopathic scoliosis. *Journal of Spinal Disorders* **13**, 102–107.

Mossberg, K.A., Kuna, S. & Masel, B. (2002) Ambulatory efficiency in persons with acquired brain injury after a rehabilitation intervention. *Brain Injury* **16**, 789–797.

Nolan, L., Wit, A., Dudzinski, K., Lees, A., Lake, M. & Wychowanski, M. (2003) Adjustments in gait symmetry with walking speed in trans-femoral and trans-tibial amputees. *Gait & Posture* **17**, 142–151.

Patel, D.R. & Greydanus, D.E. (2002) The pediatric athlete with disabilities. *Pediatric Clinics of North America* **49**, 803–827.

Patterson, J. & Blum, R.W. (1996) Risk and resilience among children and youth with disabilities. *Archives of Pediatrics and Adolescent Medicine* **150**, 692–698.

Peck, D.M. & McKeag, D.B. (1994) Athletes with disabilities: removing medical barriers. *Physician and Sportsmedicine* **22**, 59–62.

Piskorz, C. & Klimek-Piskorz, E. (1998) Cardiorespiratory responses to graded upper or lower limb exercise applied to boys with diparetic cerebral palsy. *Biology of Sport* **15**, 113–118.

Povolny, M.A. & Kaplan, S.P. (1993) Traumatic brain injury occurring with spinal cord injury: significance for rehabilitation. *Journal of Rehabilitation* **59**, 23–37.

Reid, G. (2003) Defining adapted physical activity. In: *Adapted Physical Activity* (Steadward, R.D., Watkinson, E.J. & Wheeler, G.D., eds.) University of Alberta Press, Edmonton: 11–25.

Richter, K.J., GaeblerSpira, D. & Mushett, C.A. (1996) Sport and the person with spasticity of cerebral origin. *Developmental Medicine and Child Neurology* **38**, 867–870.

Rimmer, J.H. (2001) Physical fitness levels of persons with cerebral palsy. *Developmental Medicine and Child Neurology* **43**, 208–212.

Rose, J., Haskell, W.L. & Gamble, J.G. (1993) A comparison of oxygen pulse and respiratory exchange ratio in cerebral palsied and nondisabled children. *Archives of Physical Medicine and Rehabilitation* **74**, 702–705.

Rossi, C. & Sullivan, S.J. (1996) Motor fitness in children and adolescents with traumatic brain injury. *Archives of Physical Medicine and Rehabilitation* **77**, 1062–1065.

Rubery, P.T. & Bradford, D.S. (2002) Athletic activity after spine surgery in children and adolescents: results of a survey. *Spine* **27**, 423–427.

Rutenfranz, J. (1985) Long-term effects of excessive training procedures on young athletes. In: *Children and Exercise: International Series on Sports Sciences* (Binkhorst, R.A., Kemper, C.G. & Saris, W.H.M., eds.) Human Kinetics, Champaign, IL: 354–357.

Russman, B.S., Iannacone, S.T., Buncher, C.R., *et al.* (1992) Spinal muscular atrophy: new thoughts on the pathogenesis and classification schema. *Journal of Child Neurology* **7**, 347–353.

Sarimski, K. & Hoffmann, I.W. (1993) Compensatory processes in parental coping with physical therapy. *Zeitschrift fur Kinder-und Jugendpsychiatrie und Psychotherapie* **21**, 109–114.

Schneider, K., Hart, T., Zernicke, R.F., Setoguchi, Y. & Oppenheim, W. (1993) Dynamics of below-knee child amputee gait: SACH foot versus Flex foot. *Journal of Biomechanics* **26**, 1191–1204.

Sharma, K.R., Mynhier, M.A. & Miller, R.G. (1995) Muscular fatigue in Duchenne muscular dystrophy. *Neurology* **45**, 306–310.

Sherrill, C., Hinson, M., Gench, B., Kennedy, S.O. & Low, L. (1990) Self-concepts of disabled youth athletes. *Perceptual and Motor Skills* **70**, 1093–1098.

Siegel, I.M. (1978) The management of muscular dystrophy: a clinical review. *Muscle and Nerve* **1**, 453–460.

Simeonsson, R.J., Carlson, D., Huntington, G.S., McMillen, J.S. & Lytle Brent, J. (2001) Students with disabilities: a national survey of participation in school activities. *Disability and Rehabilitation* **23**, 49–63.

Slater, D. & Meade, M.A. (2004) Participation in recreation and sports for persons with spinal cord injury: review and recommendations. *Neurorehabilitation* **19**, 121–129.

Steadward, R.D. & Wheeler, G.D. (1996) In: *The Child and Adolescent Athlete* (Bar-Or, O., ed.) Blackwell Science, Oxford: 493–520.

Steadward, R.D., Wheeler, G.D. & Watkinson, E.J. (2003) *Adapted Physical Activity*. University of Alberta Press, Edmonton.

Sullivan, P.B., Lambert, B., Rose, M., Ford-Adams, M., Johnson, A. & Griffiths, P. (2000) Prevalence and severity of feeding and nutritional problems in children with neurological impairment: Oxford Feeding Study. *Developmental Medicine and Child Neurology* **42**, 674–680.

Sullivan, S.J., Richer, E. & Laurent, F. (1990) The role of and possibilities for physical conditioning programmes in the rehabilitation of traumatically brain-injured persons. *Brain Injury* **4**, 407–414.

Suzuki, N., Oshimi, Y., Shinohara, T., Kawasumi, M. & Mita, K. (2001) Exercise intensity based on heart rate while walking in spastic cerebral palsy. *Bulletin of the Hospital for Joint Diseases* **60**, 18–22.

Taanila, A., Syrjala, L., Kokkonen, J. & Jarvelin, M.R. (2002) Coping of parents with physically and/or intellectually disabled children. *Child Care, Health and Development* **28**, 73–86.

Takken, T., Terlingen, H.C., Helders, P.J., Pruijs, H., Van der Ent, C.K. & Engelbert, R.H. (2004) Cardiopulmonary fitness and muscle strength in patients with osteogenesis imperfecta type I. *Journal of Pediatrics* **145**, 813–818.

Thommessen, M., Heiberg, A., Kase, B.F., Larsen, S. & Riis, G. (1991) Feeding problems, height and weight in different groups of disabled children. *Acta Paediatrica Scandinavica* **80**, 527–533.

Thoren, C. (1978) Exercise testing in children. *Paediatrician* **7**, 100–115.

Tilton, A.H. (2003) Approach to the rehabilitation of spasticity and neuromuscular disorders in children. *Neurologic Clinics* **21**, 853–881.

Topin, N., Matecki, S., Le, Bris, S., *et al.* (2002) Dose-dependent effect of individualized respiratory muscle training in children with Duchenne muscular dystrophy. *Neuromuscular Disorders* **12**, 576–583.

Tyc, V.L. (1992) Psychosocial adaptation of children and adolescents with limb deficiencies: a review. *Clinical Psychology Review* **12**, 275–291.

United Nations (2005) Sport for Development and Peace Working Group. [On-line] Available at: http://www.un.org/sport2005/newsroom/international_working_group.html.

Unnithan, V.B., Clifford, C. & Bar-Or, O. (1998) Evaluation by exercise testing of the child with cerebral palsy. *Sports Medicine* **26**, 239–251.

Upadhyay, S.S., Ho, E.K.W., Gunawardene, W.M.S., Leong, J.C.Y. & Hsu, L.C.S. (1993) Changes in residual volume relative to vital capacity and total lung capacity after arthrodesis of the spine in patients who have adolescent idiopathic scoliosis. *Journal of Bone and Joint Surgery (American)* **75A**, 46–52.

van den Berg-Emons R.J., van Baak, M.A., de Barbanson, D.C., Speth, L. & Saris, W.H. (1996) Reliability of tests to determine peak aerobic power, anaerobic power and isokinetic muscle strength in children with spastic cerebral palsy. *Developmental Medicine and Child Neurology* **38**, 1117–1125.

van den Berg-Emons R.J., van Baak, M.A. & Westerterp, K.R. (1998) Are skinfold measurements suitable to compare body fat between children with spastic cerebral palsy and healthy controls? *Developmental Medicine and Child Neurology* **40**, 335–339.

Van Mil, E., Schoeber, N., Calvert, R.E. & Bar-Or, O. (1996) Optimization of force in the Wingate Test for children with a neuromuscular disease. *Medicine and Science in Sports and Exercise* **28**, 1087–1092.

Varni, J.W. & Setoguchi, Y. (1992) Screening for behavioral and emotional problems in children and adolescents with congenital or acquired limb deficiencies. *American Journal of Diseases of Children* **146**, 103–107.

Vignos, P.J. Jr. & Watkins, M.P. (1966) The effect of exercise in muscular dystrophy. *Journal of the American Medical Association* **197**, 843–848.

Wallander, J.L. & Varni, J.W. (1989) Social support and adjustment in chronically ill and handicapped children. *American Journal of Community Psychology* **17**, 185–201.

Webster, J.B., Levy, C.E., Bryant, P.R. & Prusakowski, P.E. (2001) Sports and recreation for persons with limb deficiency. *Archives of Physical Medicine and Rehabilitation* **82**, S38–S44.

Weiss, H.R. & Weiss, G. (2002) Curvature progression in patients treated with scoliosis in-patient rehabilitation:

a sex and age matched controlled study. *Studies in Health Technology and Informatics* **91**, 352–356.

Wiley, M.E. & Damiano, D.L. (1998) Lower extremity strength profiles in spastic cerebral palsy. *Developmental Medicine and Child Neurology* **40**, 100–107.

Wilkins, K.L., McGrath, P.J., Finley, G.A. & Katz, J. (1998) Phantom limb sensations and phantom limb pain in child and adolescent amputees. *Pain* **78**, 7–12.

Williams, L.O., Anderson, A.D., Campbell, J., Thomas, L., Feiwell, E. & Walker, J.M. (1983) Energy cost of walking and of wheelchair propulsion by children with myelodysplasia: comparison to normal children. *Developmental Medicine and Child Neurology* **25**, 617–624.

Wilson, P.E. & Washington, R.L. (1993) Pediatric wheelchair athletics: sports injuries and prevention. *Paraplegia* **31**, 330–337.

Wind, W.M., Schwend, R.M. & Larson, J. (2004) Sports for the physically challenged child. *Journal of the American Academy of Orthopaedic Surgeons* **12**, 126–137.

Witt, W.P., Riley, A.W. & Coiro, M.J. (2003) Childhood functional status, family stressors, and psychosocial adjustment among school-aged children with disabilities in the United States. *Archives of Pediatrics and Adolescent Medicine* **157**, 687–695.

World Health Organization (2002) *Towards a Common Language for Functioning, Disability and Health ICF.* WHO, Geneva.

Zurmohle, U.M., Homann, T., Schroeter, C., Rothgerber, H., Hommel, G. & Ermert, J.A. (1998) Psychosocial adjustment of children with spina bifida. *Journal of Child Neurology* **13**, 64–70.

Chapter 29

The Young Athlete with a Mental Disability

BO FERNHALL

Mental retardation (MR) is the most common developmental disorder in industrialized societies with an estimated prevalence of 3% of the total population (Fernhall 1997). In order to fulfill the criteria, MR must be evident before age 18 years. Traditionally, MR was defined solely by IQ scores and individuals were classified into four categories: mild, moderate, severe, and profound (Rimmer 1994). However, today individuals are classified into two categories (mild and severe/profound) based on significant subaverage intelligence (2 standard deviations below the mean or an IQ <70 for mild MR, <35 for severe/ profound MR) plus related limitations in two or more adaptive skills areas such as communication, self-care, home living, social skills, community use, self-direction, health and safety, functional academics, leisure and work, and the level of care the individual requires (American Association on Mental Retardation 2002; Fernhall 1997). It is estimated that over 90% of all persons with MR would be classified with mild MR (Fernhall 1997; Auxter et al. 2001). Although MR is developmental in nature, it is not a static, non-changeable condition. Instead, MR is a fluid condition, and with early intervention some individuals may progress to the point where they would no longer be classified as having MR (Auxter et al. 2001).

There are many potential causes of mental retardation, but frequently there is no specifically known cause. Some of the identified contributing factors to MR include genetic and maternal disorders, birth trauma, and infectious diseases. It is also believed that behavioral or societal factors such as poverty, malnutrition, maternal drug and alcohol use, as well as severe stimulus deprivation can contribute

to MR (Fernhall 1997; Auxter et al. 2001). The most common cause of MR in industrialized nations is fetal alcohol syndrome with an incidence rate of 1 in 100 births. The second leading known cause of MR is Down syndrome, or trisomy 21, with an incidence rate of 1 in 800–1000 births (Krebs 1990; Auxter et al. 2001). Most children with MR live at home and attend either special schools for children with developmental disabilities, or regular schools in a special education or main streamed environment. Consequently, many children with MR participate in various school and after-school activities, including competitive sports.

Tests of aerobic fitness in children with mental retardation

The gold standard for a measurement of aerobic fitness is maximal oxygen uptake ($\dot{V}o_{2max}$), typically measured in a laboratory setting. However, in populations with MR, the validity of maximal testing has been questioned (Seidl et al. 1987; Pitetti et al. 1993) because of limitations such as task understanding, motivation, and poor physical function in many children with MR. In an early study, Bar-Or et al. (1971) showed that 15% of the children with MR tested were unable to complete a maximal treadmill protocol satisfactorily. Also, in adult women with MR, Seidl et al. (1987) were forced to alter a standard step protocol in order to collect acceptable data. However, neither study utilized familiarization protocols typically used in more recent studies (Fernhall & Tymeson 1987; Pitetti et al. 1993). With the development of proper familiarization protocols which typically include several familiarization sessions, treadmill testing has been shown to be both valid and reliable in children with MR (Fernhall et al. 1996a,b, 1998; Pitetti et al. 2000). In fact, in one study most children were able to produce a plateau in $\dot{V}O_2$, considered the best indicator of "true" $\dot{V}O_{2max}$ (Teo-Koh & McCubbin 1999), and other studies have shown that the children were able to obtain very high respiratory quotients, above 1.1 (Fernhall et al. 2000; Pitetti et al. 2000), also considered an objective marker of maximal effort. The reliability of maximal effort tests is also high in children with MR, usually with a reliability coefficient above 0.9 (Fernhall et al. 1990, 1996a,b; Pitetti et al. 2000). Thus, following established protocols, maximal exercise testing is both valid and reliable in children with MR. However, it is important to note that only treadmill testing has been shown to be both valid and reliable in children with MR, and cycle ergometry is not an accepted mode for measurement of aerobic fitness in this population (Fernhall & Pitetti 2001), as it is not reliable and no data exist to show whether true maximal efforts can be reached (McCubbin et al. 1997; Fernhall & Pitetti 2001).

The most common form of exercise testing to evaluate aerobic fitness in persons with MR is various types of field tests. Field tests are attractive because they provide information on work capacity and $\dot{V}O_{2max}$ without the need for expensive laboratory based testing, and many field tests tend to be submaximal in nature. The most commonly used field test in children with MR is the 300-yard run/walk, but this test has never been validated for use in children with MR nor is it used in non-disabled children, thus making comparisons difficult. Recently, the 600-yard run, 1-mile Rockport Walking Fitness

Test (RPWFT), and 20-m shuttle run have been assessed for their applicability in children and adolescents with MR (Fernhall et al. 1998, 2000; Teo-Koh & McCubbin 1999). These tests have been found to be both valid and reliable for use with this population. Formulae are available for these tests to predict $\dot{V}O_{2max}$ from the field test performance. These formulae for children and adolescents with MR differ from the prediction formulae for their non-disabled peers; thus, it is important that these population specific formulae are used (Table 29.1). Furthermore, the individual variability of the estimated $\dot{V}O_{2max}$ is much greater in children and adolescents with MR than in non-disabled populations, suggesting that although predicting the $\dot{V}O_{2max}$ of groups of children with MR may be reasonably accurate, individual predictions are less accurate and may not be useful (Fernhall et al. 1996b, 2000).

Another interesting aspect of using run/walk tests in children with MR is that leg strength also contributes to endurance run performance in this population (Fernhall et al. 2000). This is very different from findings in non-disabled children. In the study by Fernhall et al. (2000), the relationship between leg strength and run performance was similar to that of $\dot{V}O_{2max}$ and run performance, suggesting that leg strength and $\dot{V}O_{2peak}$ were equal contributors. Both leg strength and $\dot{V}O_{2max}$ were included as significant predictors of run performance, explaining approximately 65% of the variance. However, the beta weights indicated that the relative contribution of leg strength was greater than that of $\dot{V}O_{2max}$. The partial correlation between leg strength and run performance was still significant (r = −0.62) even after controlling for $\dot{V}O_{2max}$, body mass index (BMI), and gender, clearly suggesting an

---

Table 29.1 Formulae for predicting $\dot{V}O_{2max}$ from field test performance in children with mental retardation.

20-m shuttle run (Fernhall et al. 1998)
$\dot{V}O_{2max}$ (mL·kg^{-1}·min^{-1}) = 0.35 (number of 20-m laps) − 0.59 (BMI) − 4.5 (gender: 1 boy, 2 girls) + 50.8

600-yard run/walk (Fernhall et al. 1998)
$\dot{V}O_{2max}$ (mL·kg^{-1}·min^{-1}) = −5.24 (600-yard run time in min) − 0.37 (BMI) − 4.61 (gender: 1 boy, 2 girls) + 73.64

1-mile Rockport Walk Fitness Test (Teo-Koh & McCubbin 1999)
$\dot{V}O_{2max}$ (mL·min^{-1}) = −0.18 (walk time in min) + 0.03 (body weight in kg) + 2.90

independent contribution of leg strength to field test performance in children with MR. This may have important implications for the design of endurance training programs in this population.

Aerobic capacity of children with mental retardation

Data on aerobic capacity of children and adolescents with MR show considerable variation. Early data on boys and girls 6–16 years of age (Bar-Or *et al.* 1971) showed $\dot{V}O_{2max}$ varied from 43 to 47 mL·kg^{-1}·min^{-1} for girls and from 48 to 52 mL·kg^{-1}·min^{-1} for boys. This is well within normal limits and very similar to the reported mean for a similar aged sample of children and adolescents without MR (Cureton *et al.* 1995). However, this study (Bar-Or *et al.* 1971) included subjects with an IQ of 90 or below, thus many of their subjects would not be classified with MR based on current standards. Maksud and Hamilton (1974) reported much lower $\dot{V}O_{2max}$ values (39 mL·kg^{-1}·min^{-1}) in 62 boys with MR. However, they used cycle ergometry which is not a valid mode testing in this population and also yields lower $\dot{V}O_{2max}$ values than treadmill testing in general. Even so, in support of these findings, Yoshizawa *et al.* (1975) reported $\dot{V}O_{2peak}$ values for boys and girls 12–16 years of age, of 42 and 33 mL·kg^{-1}·min^{-1}, respectively, using cycle ergometry. Because these subjects were not particularly physically active, these $\dot{V}O_{2max}$ values would still be considered within normal limits.

Some recent studies on aerobic capacity in children with MR have shown very low $\dot{V}O_{2max}$ values. Fernhall *et al.* (1996b) reported aerobic capacities of 32 and 26 mL·kg^{-1}·min^{-1} for boys and girls with MR, respectively, and similar values have been reported in other studies (mean for boys and girls of 35 and 36 mL·kg^{-1}·min^{-1}) by the same group of researchers (Pitetti & Fernhall 1997; Fernhall *et al.* 1998). However, other studies have found higher $\dot{V}O_{2max}$ values. Mean $\dot{V}O_{2max}$ was 39.4 mL·kg^{-1}·min^{-1} in 17 children with MR (nine boys and eight girls) in a recent study (Fernhall *et al.* 2000) and four of the boys exhibited $\dot{V}O_{2peak}$ values above 50 mL·kg^{-1}·min^{-1}. Teo-Koh and McCubbin (1999) reported similar values (41 mL·kg^{-1}·min^{-1}). A comparison of children

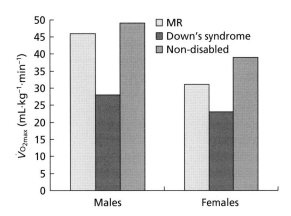

Fig. 29.1 $\dot{V}O_{2max}$ of individuals with and without mental retardation (MR). There is little difference between boys with MR and non-disabled boys, but boys with Down syndrome exhibit very low levels of $\dot{V}O_{2max}$. Girls with MR have lower levels of $\dot{V}O_{2max}$ compared to girls without disabilities, and girls with Down syndrome have the lowest levels of $\dot{V}O_{2max}$. Based on data from Fernhall *et al.* (1998); Fernhall & Pitetti (2001); Pitetti & Fernhall (2000).

with MR and an age-matched control group reported normal values in boys with MR (46 mL·kg^{-1}·min^{-1}) but girls with MR exhibited lower levels of $\dot{V}O_{2max}$ (31 mL·kg^{-1}·min^{-1}) than their peers without MR (Pitetti *et al.* 2000). A comparison of $\dot{V}O_{2max}$ values between boys and girls with and without MR is shown in Fig. 29.1. The much lower $\dot{V}O_{2max}$ in girls with MR is probably explained by higher levels of obesity. The girls with MR had a BMI of 23.4 kg·m^2 compared to a BMI of 19.9 kg·m^2 for the girls without disabilities, whereas the boys with MR exhibited slightly lower BMI than their peers without disabilities (18.1 vs. 19.5 kg·m^2, respectively).

Based on the available laboratory data on $\dot{V}O_{2max}$ in individual children and adolescents with MR, these children have either lower than expected or close to expected levels of $\dot{V}O_{2max}$. In most instances, the differences between children with MR and their peers without MR are more exaggerated in girls than in boys. However, there are several individual case reports of high $\dot{V}O_{2max}$ values in this population, suggesting that under the right circumstances high $\dot{V}O_{2max}$ values can be attained by children and adolescents with MR.

Performance on aerobic field tests by children with MR is unexpectedly poor, more so than would be predicted from their $\dot{V}O_{2max}$ values. For instance, the expected performance on a 20-m shuttle run for a non-disabled child is over 41 laps (Cureton 1994), whereas the mean performance of a group of adolescents of similar age with MR was 15.5 laps (Fernhall *et al.* 1998). Also, adolescents with MR exhibited a mean run time for a 0.5-mile run of just over 7 min (Fernhall *et al.* 1996b), which is the expected run time for a 1-mile run in a non-disabled adolescent of the same age (Cureton *et al.* 1995). Thus, run performance in children and adolescents with MR is about 50% or less of that of their non-disabled peers, but their $\dot{V}O_{2max}$ measured in the laboratory was only about 25% lower than that of their non-disabled peers (Fernhall *et al.* 1996b, 1998; Fernhall & Unnithan 2002). Consequently, the relationship between $\dot{V}O_{2max}$ and run time is altered in children with MR, and the amount of work they perform for a given level of $\dot{V}O_{2max}$ is lower than in non-disabled children. It is not known if this is a physiologic or a behavioral phenomenon.

Another interesting phenomenon in children with MR is that run performance does not change with maturation along the same path as in their non-disabled peers (Fig. 29.2) (Pitetti *et al.* 2001). Both boys and girls with MR change run performance very little between ages of 8 and 18 years, whereas there are considerable changes in non-disabled children. Although the adolescents with MR had

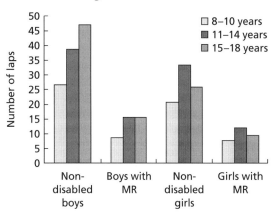

Fig. 29.2 Performance on the 20-m shuttle run of three different age groups of boys and girls with and without MR. Boys and girls with MR do not exhibit the same developmental trajectory as boys and girls without MR. Based on data from Pitetti *et al.* (2001).

slightly higher BMI compared to their non-disabled peers, BMI did no explain the difference in run performance (Pitetti *et al.* 2001). Thus, in boys and girls with MR, run performance is very low from childhood through adulthood. The current data also suggest that run performance starts to decline in early adolescence. The reason for the different developmental path in performance of children with MR compared to their peers without MR is not known at this time.

Muscle strength in children with mental retardation

Muscle strength of individuals with MR has consistently been shown to be very low, using a variety of different measurement tools such as exercise machines, hand grip dynamometry, hand held dynamometry, leg and back dynamometry, and isokinetic dynamometry (Pitetti *et al.* 1992b; Pitetti & Boneh 1995; Croce *et al.* 1996; Horvat *et al.* 1997, 1999; Pitetti & Fernhall 1997; Suomi 1998; Fernhall & Pitetti 2000; Guerra *et al.* 2000). Reported strength levels of individuals with MR are typically 50–70% of those reported for their non-disabled peers (Pitetti *et al.* 1992b; Pitetti & Boneh 1995; Horvat *et al.* 1997, 1999). These differences in muscle strength between individuals with MR and their non-disabled peers are present in childhood (Pitetti & Fernhall 1997; Horvat *et al.* 1999; Fernhall & Pitetti 2000) and persist into adulthood (Pitetti *et al.* 1992b; Croce *et al.* 1996; Horvat *et al.* 1997; Suomi 1998). Even individuals with MR who were aerobically fit ($\dot{V}O_{2max}$ >50 mL·kg^{-1}·min^{-1}) and who were very active, exhibited low levels of muscle strength (about 25% lower) compared with age and activity matched subjects without MR (Frey *et al.* 1999).

Pitetti and Yarmer (2002) recently evaluated the developmental trajectory of muscle strength in a large sample of children and adolescents with ($n = 269$) and without ($n = 449$) MR. They showed that for each age group, leg and back strength was lower in children and adolescents with MR compared to their non-disabled peers. This difference could not be explained by body size. However, the developmental trajectory of muscle strength was similar between boys and girls with and without MR (Fig. 29.3).

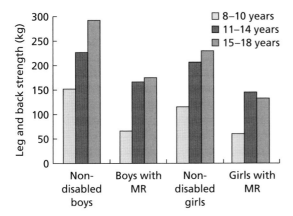

Fig. 29.3 Leg and back muscle strength of three different age groups of boys and girls with and without MR. Boys and girls with MR exhibit lower levels of muscle strength but a similar developmental trajectory compared to their peers without MR. Based on data from Pitetti & Yarmer (2002).

The only exception was the group of adolescent girls with MR, who exhibited an unexpected decline in muscle strength during late compared to early adolescence. These data show most children with MR increase muscle strength in an expected manner from childhood through late adolescence; however, the absolute level of muscle strength was still approximately 30–50% below the muscle strength of their non-disabled peers.

The low level of muscle strength in children with MR is of considerable concern. Muscle strength may be an important prerequisite for adequate performance and participation in recreational activities (Horvat & Croce 1995) and for vocational activities later in life (Horvat & Croce 1995; Fernhall 2004). Also, because muscle strength is a significant contributor to both aerobic capacity and run performance in children with MR (Pitetti & Fernhall 1997; Fernhall & Pitetti 2000), these low levels of muscle strength may present a significant impediment to high level athletic performance in children and adolescents with MR.

Physical activity levels in children with MR

The data on physical activity levels in children with MR are very limited. Data exist using direct observation, physical activity recall interviews, heart rate monitoring, activity monitoring, and doubly labeled water (Sharav & Bowman 1992; Luke *et al.* 1994; Lorenzi *et al.* 2000; Horvat & Franklin 2001). It has been suggested that children with MR participate less in active play and as a result they are less physically active than children without disabilities (Fernhall & Pitetti 2001). Consequently, the perception that children with MR are more sedentary than their peers without MR is well accepted (Fernhall 1993; Fernhall & Pitetti 2001). However, direct observation studies of physical activity during school recess periods do not support this notion. During school recess periods, children with MR have been shown to exhibit similar play behavior to children without MR (Lorenzi *et al.* 2000; Horvat & Franklin 2001). Furthermore, Horvat and Franklin (2001) recently showed that heart rates and activity counts during the recess periods were high enough to classify the activity as moderate to vigorous physical activity.

Physical activity recall questionnaires have been used to compare physical activity between children with Down syndrome (DS) and their siblings without disabilities (Sharav & Bowman 1992). Because of the limitations in cognitive abilities and communication skills, parents were asked to rate their children's physical activity and no information was obtained directly from the subjects studied. Children with DS were perceived as being less physically active than their siblings, and the mean number of hours spent playing outdoors was also reported to be lower in children with DS.

Data on energy expenditure in children with DS, measured through doubly labeled water, do not support the parental perceptions reported above (Luke *et al.* 1994). The energy expenditure resulting from physical activity and the thermic effect of food was almost identical in children with DS and their non-disabled peers (Luke *et al.* 1994), at 751 vs. 733 kcal·day^{-1}, respectively. However, children with DS had lower resting metabolic rates compared to their non-disabled peers. Thus, unless the energy cost of movement or the thermic effect of food was significantly greater in children with DS, this group of children exhibited similar levels of physical activity as their peers without disabilities.

Objective data on physical activity patterns in children with MR show they are no less active than their non-disabled peers. However, all the investigations to date have limited sample sizes and there are also a limited number of studies.

Effect of exercise training on children with MR

There are many reports of the impact of various exercise training programs on children with MR, but most have not employed appropriate methodologies (Fernhall 1993; Pitetti *et al*. 1993). The major weaknesses were usually failure to use validated tests or lack of control groups, and very few have used a randomized controlled design. Nevertheless, the data are remarkably consistent, showing improvements in field test performance and submaximal exercise performance (Kasch & Zasueta 1971; Beasley 1982; Bundschuh & Cureton 1982; Fernhall *et al*. 1988; Millar *et al*. 1993).

Kasch and Zasueta (1971) were able to show substantial improvements in $\dot{V}O_{2max}$ in children with MR, but they only tested $\dot{V}O_{2max}$ in 6 of their 41 children with MR and did not include a control group. Similar findings have also been shown in adults with MR (Pitetti & Tan 1991). The best designed study was conducted by Millar *et al*. (1993). This was a randomized controlled trial, but the number of subjects was small. They showed that a 10-week endurance training program following standard exercise prescription guidelines did not change $\dot{V}O_{2max}$ in adolescents with DS, although treadmill performance significantly increased. However, because this study included only adolescents with DS, it is difficult to generalize the findings to the overall population of children and adolescents with MR, because individuals with DS constitute a very unique population that is physiologically different from their peers with MR but without DS (Fernhall & Pitetti 2001).

It is clear that exercise training data are lacking for children with MR. The currently available data suggest that appropriately designed exercise training programs will increase muscle endurance, possible increase run performance, and may improve $\dot{V}O_{2max}$. However, because the research design was not optimal in most of the studies to date, concrete conclusions are not possible at this time.

Individuals with Down syndrome— a special case

Individuals with DS exhibit several physical and physiologic characteristics that could impact the exercise response. Characteristics such as small stature, short limbs and digits, digital malformations (especially common are malformations of the feet and toes), small mouth and nasal cavities with a large protruding tongue can create problems with exercise performance because of gait and breathing abnormalities (Fernhall 1997). Persons with DS also typically present with joint laxity, which is especially important because of the common occurrence of atlanto-axial instability (Fernhall 1997; Fernhall & Pitetti 2001). It has also been reported that young children with DS exhibit skeletal muscle hypotonia and it is possible that some individuals may exhibit pulmonary hypoplasia (Roizen & Patterson 2003). Up to 40% of individuals born with DS have congenital heart disease, most of which is now surgically corrected early in life. Most individuals with DS exhibit reduced immune function, and are at higher than normal risk of developing leukemia (Krebs 1990; Fernhall 1997; Roizen & Patterson 2003).

Both children and adults with DS have very low $\dot{V}O_{2max}$ values. Findings on individuals with DS are also much more uniform than in persons with MR but without DS and the variation in $\dot{V}O_{2max}$ is remarkably small. Children, adolescents, and young adults with DS show $\dot{V}O_{2peak}$ values of 18–25 mL·kg^{-1}·min^{-1}, with little influence of age (Fernhall *et al*. 1996a, 1989; Pitetti *et al*. 1992a; Millar *et al*. 1993). Recent data on trained young adults with DS showed they exhibited higher aerobic capacity than their untrained counterparts, but their $\dot{V}O_{2peak}$ values were still below 40 mL·kg^{-1}·min^{-1}, even though many trained as much as 10 h·week^{-1} (Guerra *et al*. 2000). These data are consistent with training studies, showing that individuals with DS do not improve as much as expected with exercise training (Millar *et al*. 1993; Varela *et al*. 2001). Thus, DS appears to negatively affect aerobic capacity. The low levels of $\dot{V}O_{2peak}$ reported cannot be explained by the high incidence of congenital heart disease in this population as none of the studies to date have included persons with congenital heart disease. Consequently, the real work capacity in the population (with DS) as a whole including individuals with congenital heart disease is expected to be even lower (Fernhall 1997).

There is also a disconnect between field test run performance and $\dot{V}o_{2max}$ in children with DS. Contrary the findings in children with MR but without DS, $\dot{V}o_{2max}$ is not related to run performance in children with DS (Fernhall *et al*. 2002).

A major contributor to the low work capacity of individuals with DS is a much lower than expected maximal heart rate. In a large multicenter study, Fernhall *et al*. (1998) showed that individuals with DS exhibited maximal heart rates that were 30 beats·min^{-1} lower than those of the non-disabled control group. Consistent with this notion, most studies on children with DS show that maximal heart rates rarely exceed 180 beats·min^{-1} in any individual during treadmill testing, and maximal heart rate typically averages 168–175 beats·min^{-1} in children and adolescents with DS regardless of age (Fernhall & Pitetti 2001). Guerra *et al*. (2003) recently showed that the heart rate response to exercise of individuals with DS can be classified as true chronotropic incompetence, based on both the maximal heart rate response and the chronotropic response index. Furthermore, it has been shown that the low maximal heart rate accounts for the difference in $\dot{V}o_{2max}$ between individuals with MR with and without DS (Fernhall *et al*. 1996a). The low maximal heart rate in this population shows a consistent decrease with age at a similar rate to non-disabled controls (Fernhall *et al*. 1998) and does not change with exercise training (Millar *et al*. 1993). A recent study also showed that obesity did not impact maximal heart rate in children with DS, in contrast to children with MR without DS (Fernhall 2003).

Furthermore, Fernhall and Otterstetter (2003) showed that subjects with DS exhibited reduced heart rate and blood pressure responses to isometric handgrip exercise and cold pressor testing. The reduced responses are at least partially brought about by reduced vagal withdrawal during the

perturbation (Figueroa *et al*. 2005) but reduced sympathetic stimulation cannot be ruled out. Other recent data also show reduced heart rate responses to upright tilt in persons with DS (Fernhall *et al*. 2005) and this is probably caused by alterations in baroreceptor function (Iellamo *et al*. 2005). Alterations in baroreceptor function during hand grip exercise has also been shown in this population (Heffernan *et al*. 2005). Thus, it is likely that autonomic dysfunction contributes to the altered heart rate response to exercise and the low $\dot{V}o_{2max}$ values found in children with DS (Fernhall & Otterstetter 2003; Fernhall *et al*. 2005; Figueroa *et al*. 2005).

Potential for high level athletic performance in children with MR

Although it is clear that the average child with MR has normal to low levels of physical fitness, it is not unusual for children and adolescents with MR to compete in youth sport programs and school sport programs with their non-disabled peers. Several subjects included in the author's studies have competed at a high level in high school varsity sports within the particular state high school system. Thus, reasonably high level performance can be expected of some children and adolescents with MR provided they have the right opportunities and the right setting.

There are no data available on elite performance in children and adolescents with MR. However, adults with MR participated in the Paralympics in Sydney, Australia and some insight regarding the potential for elite performance may be gleaned from those performances. For example, the winning time in the 100 m sprint (males) was 10.85 s, and the winning time in the 1500 m was under 4 min. These times would certainly suggest that some individuals with MR can produce outstanding athletic performances. However, the winning toss in the shot-put was only 13.1 m, a relatively poorer performance compared with the running events. This would support the research data, showing that muscle strength is decreased even in well-trained individuals with MR (Frey *et al*. 1999).

The available information certainly suggests that some individuals with MR can produce very high level sports performance. It is likely that if this population was provided with more opportunities to train and compete, in conjunction with excellent coaching, more high level performances would occur. The exception might be individuals with DS. None of the high level performances to date have been produced by a person with DS, and the research data suggest that this population has a physiologic disadvantage for high level performances. However, little is known regarding physical potential of this population and future research may show different results. It is certainly clear that more opportunities for training, competing, and being physically active are needed for all children and adolescents with MR.

Potential risks of sport participation in children with MR

For most children with MR without DS, there are few physical risks for sports participation. However, because individuals with MR sometimes have poor gross motor function and coordination, careful instruction and coaching are needed to ensure these children avoid injuries associated with sport participation. Also, some children with MR may be taking medications that can affect heart rate and blood pressure. which need to be considered when designing training programs. Because many children with MR will have short attention spans and may exhibit behavioral problems, these psychologic and behaviorial aspects probably present the greatest challenge. This requires careful planning to avoid potential hazardous situations caused by the child athlete not paying attention or not following instructions.

Considering that almost half of the children with DS will also have congenital heart disease, it is important to conduct a careful history and evaluation of all children with DS. If the child has a history of congenital heart disease, it is imperative that a physician evaluation be conducted before participation, and physician clearance for participation should always be obtained. In addition, because there is a high incidence of atlanto-axial instability, all children with DS need to be screened before participation in "high-risk" sports (Pizzutillo &

Herman 2005). In general, contact sports are deemed inappropriate for children with this condition, which also include sports that are not traditionally thought of as contact sports, such as the high jump. Children with DS may also be on medication, and the concerns regarding psychologic or behavioral issues apply to this population as well. For all children with MR, including those with DS, it is essential that the child has an opportunity to become familiarized with the tasks, ensure they understand the tasks, and provide an opportunity for the child to learn the skills and the sport at their own pace.

Challenges for future research

Although it is well established that aerobic capacity is lower than expected in children with MR, the contributors to these lower levels are not well understood. Chronotropic incompetence clearly contributes in children with DS but it does not explain all the variance. Chronotropic incompetence is an inconsistent finding in children with MR without DS, and does not contribute a great deal to the lower aerobic capacity in children without DS. Virtually nothing is known regarding the contribution of peripheral compared to cardiac or autonomic control factors to the lower aerobic capacity. We also do not know why girls with MR have lower aerobic capacity than boys with MR, compared to their non-disabled peers.

The importance of muscle strength has received some attention, but it is not understood why children with MR exhibit poor muscle strength. It is not known if improving muscle strength will improve both run performance and $\dot{V}o_{2max}$. Furthermore, the reason for the altered relationship between run performance and $\dot{V}o_{2max}$ is unknown, and the potential influence of muscle strength needs to be investigated. Finally, the incongruence between developmental aspects of muscle strength, $\dot{V}o_{2max}$ and run performance needs to be investigated.

Recent investigations have provided a great deal of information regarding the normal and expected response to endurance training in non-disabled children. However, we know very little about the response to training in children with MR, and nor do we know which factors may contribute to improvements. This may be especially important in children with DS, because it appears that $\dot{V}o_{2max}$ is not improved with exercise training in this group of children with MR.

Only a few studies have investigated physical activity patterns in children with MR. Little is known what factors might contribute to physical activity in this population, and we do not know whether and how physical activity is related to physical fitness and obesity in children with MR. There are also no data on physical activity based interventions, nor do we know anything about the potential health effects of such interventions in children with MR.

References

American Association on Mental Retardation (2002) Classification in Mental Retardation. Washington, DC.

Auxter, D., Pfyfer, J. & Huettig, C. (2001) *Principles and Methods of Adapted Physical Education and Recreation.* McGraw-Hill, New York, NY: 428–460.

Bar-Or, O., Skinner, J., Bergsteinova, V., *et al.* (1971) Maximal aerobic capacity of 6–15 year old girls and boys with subnormal intelligence quotients. *Acta Paediatrica Scandinavica Supplement* **217**, 108–113.

Beasley, C.R. (1982) Effects of a jogging program on cardiovascular fitness and work performances of mentally retarded persons. *American Journal on Mental Deficiency* **86**, 609–613.

Bundschuh, E. & Cureton, K. (1982) Effect of bicycle ergometer conditioning on the physcial work capacity of mentally retarded adolescents. *American Corrective Therapy Journal* **36**, 159–163.

Croce, R.V., Pitetti, K.H., Horvat, M., *et al.* (1996) Peak torque, average power, and hamstring/quadriceps ratios in non-disabled adults and adults with mental retardation. *Archives of Physical Medicine and Rehabilitation* **77**, 369–372.

Cureton, J.K., Sloniger, M.A., O'Bannon, J.P., *et al.* (1995) A generalized equation for prediction of $\dot{V}o_2$ peak from 1-mile run/walk performance. *Medicine and Science in Sports and Exercise* **27**, 445–451.

Cureton, K. (1994) Aerobic capacity. In: Fitnesgram Technical Reference Manual (Morrow, J.R., Falls, H., Kohl, H., eds.) Cooper Institute of Aerobics, Dallas: 33–56.

Fernhall, B. (1993) Physical fitness and exercise training of individuals with mental retardation. *Medicine and Science in Sports and Exercise* **25**, 442–450.

Fernhall, B. (1997) Mental retardation. *ACSM's Exercise Management for Persons with Chronic Disease and Disability.* Human Kinetics, Champaign, IL: 221–226.

Fernhall, B. (2003) Mental retardation. In: *ACSM's Exercise Management for Persons with Chronic Diseases and Disabilities,* 2nd edn. (Durstine, J. & Moore, G., eds.) Human Kinetics, Champaign, IL: 304–310.

Fernhall, B. (2004) Mental retardation. In: *Clinical Exercise Physiology: Application and Physiological Principles* (LeMura, L. & von Duvillard, S., eds.) Lippincott Williams & Williams, Philadelphia, PA: 617–627.

Fernhall, B., Figueroa, A., Collier, S. *et al.* (2005) Blunted heart rate response to upright tilt in individuals with Down syndrome. *Archives of Physical Medicine and Rehabilitation* **86**, 813–818.

Fernhall, B., Figueroa, A., Giannopoulou, I., *et al.* (2002) Chronotropic incompetence and autonomic dysfunction in individuals with Down syndrome. *Medicine and Science in Sports and Exercise* **S47**.

Fernhall, B., Millar, A.L., Tymeson, G., *et al.* (1990) Maximal exercise testing of mentally retarded adolescents and adults: Reliability study. *Archives of Physical Medicine and Rehabilitation* **71**, 1065–1068.

Fernhall, B. & Otterstetter, M. (2003) Attenuated responses to sympathoexcitation in individuals with Down syndrome. *Journal of Applied Physiology* **94**, 2158–2165.

Fernhall, B. & Pitetti, K. (2000) Leg strength is related to endurance run performance in children and adolescents with mental retardation. *Pediatric Exercise Science* **12**, 324–333.

Fernhall, B. & Pitetti, K. (2001) Limitations to work capacity in individuals with intellectual disabilities. *Clinical Exercise Physiology* **3**, 176–185.

Fernhall, B., Pitetti, K., Millar, A.L., *et al.* (2000) Cross validation of the 20 m shuttle run in children with mental retardation. *Adapted Physical Activity Quarterly* **17**, 402–412.

Fernhall, B., Pitetti, K., Rimmer, J.H., *et al.* (1996a) Cardiorespiratory capacity of individuals with mental retardation including Down syndrome. *Medicine and Science in Sports and Exercise* **28**, 366–371.

Fernhall, B., Pitetti, K., Stubbs, N., *et al.* (1996b) Validity and reliability of the 1/2 mile run-walk as an indicator of aerobic fitness in children with mental retardation. *Pediatric Exercise Science* **8**, 130–142.

Fernhall, B., Pitetti, K.H., Vukovich, M.D., *et al.* (1998) Validation of cardiovascular fitness field tests in children with mental retardation. *American Journal of Mental Retardation* **102**, 602–612.

Fernhall, B. & Tymeson, G. (1987) Graded exercise testing of metally retarded adults: a study of feasibility. *Archives of Physical Medicine and Rehabilitation* **63**, 363–365.

Fernhall, B., Tymeson, G., Millar, A.L., *et al.* (1989) Cardiovascular fitness testing and fitness levels of adolescents and adults with mental retardation including Down syndrome. *Education and Training in Mental Retardation* **68**, 363–365.

Fernhall, B., Tymeson, G. & Webster, G. (1988) Cardiovascular fitness of mentally retarded adults. *Adapted Physical Activity Quarterly* **5**, 12–28.

Fernhall, B. & Unnithan, V. (2002) Physical activity, metabolic issues, and assessment. *Physical Medicine and Rehabilitation Clinics of North America* **13**, 925–947.

Figueroa, A., Collier, S., Baynard, T., *et al.* (2005) Impaired vagal modulation of heart rate in individuals with Down syndrome. *Clinical Autonomic Research* **15**, 45–50.

Frey, G., McCubbin, J.A., Hannigan-Downs, S., *et al.* (1999) Physical fitness of trained runners with and without mild mental retardation. *Adapted Physical Activity Quarterly* **16**, 126–137.

Guerra, M., Llorens, N. & Fernhall, B. (2003) Chronotropic incompetence in persons with Down syndrome. *Archives of Physical Medicine and Rehabilitation* **84**, 1604–1608.

Guerra, M., Roman, B., Geronimo, C., *et al.* (2000) Physical fitness levels of sedentary and active individuals with Down syndrome. *Adapted Physical Activity Quarterly* **17**, 310–321.

Heffernan, K., Baynard, T., Goulopoulou, S., *et al.* (2005) Baroreflex sensitivity during static exercise in individuals with Down syndrome. *Medicine and Science in Sports and Exercise* **12**, 2025–2031.

Horvat, M. & Croce, R. (1995) Physical rehabilitation of individuals with mental retardation: physical fitness and information processing. *Critical Critical Reviews in Physical Rehabilitation Medicine* **7**, 233–252.

Horvat, M., Croce, R., Pitetti, K.H., *et al.* (1999) Comparison of isokinetic peak force and work parameters in youth with and without mental retardation. *Medicine and Science in Sports and Exercise* **31**, 1190–1195.

Horvat, M. & Franklin, C. (2001) The effect of the environment on physical activity patterns of children with mental retardation. *Research Quarterly for Exercise and Sport* **72**, 189–195.

Horvat, M., Pitetti, K.H. & Corce, R. (1997) Isokinetic torque, average power, and flexion/extension ratios in nondisabled adults and adults with mental retardation. *Journal of Orthopaedic and Sports Physical Therapy* **6**, 395–399.

Iellamo, F., Galante, A., Legremante, J.M., *et al.* (2005) Altered autonomic cardiac regulation in individuals with Down syndrome. *American Journal of Physiology. Heart and Circulatory Physiology* **289**, H2387–H2391.

Kasch, F. & Zasueta, S. (1971) Physical capacities of mentally retarded children. *Acta Paediatrica Scandinavica* **217**, 217–218.

Krebs, P. (1990) Mental retardation. In: *Adapted Physical Education and Sport* (Winnick, J., ed.) Human Kinetics, Champaign, IL: 153–176.

Lorenzi, D., Horvat, M. & Pellegrini, A. (2000) Physical activity of children with

and without mental retardation in inclusive recess settings. *Education and Training in Mental Retardation/ Developmental Disability* **35**, 160–167.

Luke, A., Rozien, N.J., Sutton, M., *et al.* (1994) Energy expenditure in children with Down syndrome: Correcting metabolic rate for movement. *Journal of Pediatrics* **125**, 829–838.

Maksud, M. & Hamilton, L. (1974) Physiological responses of EMR children to strenuous exercise. *American Journal of Mental Deficiency* **79**, 32–38.

McCubbin, J., Rintala, P. & Frey, G. (1997) Correlational study of three cardiorespiratory fitness tests for men with mental retardation. *Adapted Physical Activity Quarterly* **14**, 43–50.

Millar, A.L., Fernhall, B., Burkett, L.N. *et al.* (1993) Effect of aerobic training in adolescents with Down syndrome. *Medicine and Science in Sports and Exercise* **25**, 260–264.

Pitetti, K. & Fernhall, B. (1997) Aerobic capacity as related to leg strength in youths with mental retardation. *Pediatric Exercise Science* **9**, 223–236.

Pitetti, K. & Yarmer, D. (2002) Lower body strength of children and adlescents with and without mild mentl retardation: a comparison. *Adapted Physical Activity Quarterly* **19**, 68–81.

Pitetti, K.H. & Boneh, S. (1995) Cardiovascular fitness as related to leg strength in adults with mental retardation. *Medicine and Science in Sports and Exercise* **27**, 423–428.

Pitetti, K.H., Climstein, M., Campbell, K.D., *et al.* (1992a) The cardiovascular capacities of adults with Down syndrome: A comparative study. *Medicine and Science in Sports and Exercise* **24**, 13–19.

Pitetti, K.H., Climstein, M., Mays, M.J., *et al.* (1992b) Isokinetic arm and leg strength of adults with Down syndrome: A comparative study. *Archives of Physical Medicine and Rehabilitation* **73**, 847–850.

Pitetti, K.H., Millar, A.L. & Fernhall, B. (2000) Reliability of peak performance treadmill test for children and adolescents with and without mental retardation. *Adapted Physical Activity Quarterly* **17**, 322–332.

Pitetti, K.H., Rimmer, J.H. & Fernhall, B. (1993) Physical fitness and adults with mental retardation: An overview of current research and future directions. *Sports Medicine* **16**, 23–56.

Pitetti, K.H. & Tan, D.M. (1991) Effects of a minimally supervised exercise program for mentally retarded adults. *Medicine and Science in Sports and Exercise* **23**, 594–601.

Pitetti, K.H., Yarmer, D.A. & Fernhall, B. (2001) Cardiovascular fitness and body composition of youth with and without mental retardation. *Adapted Physical Activity Quarterly* **18**, 127–141.

Pizzutillo, P. & Herman, M. (2005) Cervical spine issues in Down syndrome. *Journal of Pediatric Orthopedics* **25**, 253–259.

Rimmer, J. (1994) *Fitness and Rehabilitation Programs for Special Populations.* Brown and Benchmark, Dubuque, IA: 247–294.

Roizen, N.J. & Patterson, D. (2003) Down's syndrome. *Lancet* **361**, 1281–1289.

Seidl, L., Reid, G. & Montgomery, D.L. (1987) A critique of cardiovascular fitness testing with mentally retarded persons. *Adapted Physical Activity Quarterly* **4**, 106–116.

Sharav, T. & Bowman, T. (1992) Dietary practices, physical activity, and body mass index in a selected population of Down syndrome children and their siblings. *Clinical Pediatrics* **June**, 341–344.

Suomi, R. (1998) Self directed strength training: Its effect on leg strength in men with mental retardation. *Archives of Physical Medicine and Rehabilitation* **79**, 323–328.

Teo-Koh, S.M. & McCubbin, J.A. (1999) Relationship between peak $\dot{V}o_2$ and 1-mile walk test performance of adolescents with mental retardation. *Pediatric Exercise Science* **11**, 144–157.

Varela, A.M., Sardinha, L. & Pitetti, K.H. (2001) Effects of aerobic rowing training in adults with Down syndrome. *American Journal of Mental Retardation* **106**, 135–144.

Yoshizawa, S., Tadatoshi, T. & Honda, H. (1975) Aerobic work capacity of mentally retarded boys and girls in junior high school. *Journal of Human Ergology* **4**, 15–26.

Part 7

Methodology

Chapter 30

Body Composition Assessment in the Young Athlete

TIMOTHY G. LOHMAN, SCOTT B. GOING, AND BRADLEY R. HERRIN

Regular assessment of body composition is a vital aspect of monitoring the health and physical development of child and adolescent athletes. While physical activity is undoubtedly critical for optimal growth, the demands of training for competition are not without some risks. In developing girls, for example, the risks of the female athlete "triad" on bone and possibly muscle development are well documented (Eliakim & Beyth 2003). The health and growth consequences of "weight cycling" in adolescent wrestlers has also received considerable attention (Tipton & Oppliger 1984) and recommendations for weight loss based on percent body fat have been developed (Medicine 1997).

Regular body composition assessments are critical to detecting potentially harmful changes in body weight and composition as a result of inappropriate nutritional practices, excessive training, or illness, and to relate body composition status to performance. Body mass and body composition are surely factors in competitive success. However, the multitude of factors involved make it difficult to give precise recommendations, although descriptive studies provide ranges for various components that are associated with success in different sports (Going & Mullins 2000).

Body composition is also clearly associated with disease risks. There have been numerous reports of an association between excess fat and elevated risk factors for cardiovascular disease and type 2 diabetes in children and adolescents. Given that body fatness tends to track into adulthood (Srinivasan et al. 1996; Gordon-Larsen et al. 2004), adolescents with excess body fat are at increased risk for adult obesity and its attendant comorbidities. While active children are likely protected, and presumably few would be overweight or obese, there are some sports where higher mass is an advantage, and it is important to monitor body fat to be sure children and adolescents stay within a healthy range.

Methods are available to assess body composition on atomic, chemical, cellular, and tissue and/or system levels of analysis (Wang et al. 1992). While only indirect, non-destructive methods are suitable for application in children and adolescents, many options exist. By necessity, indirect methods are based on models reflecting expected relationships between various body compartments, and are only as accurate as the underlying assumptions. Field methods are typically validated against indirect laboratory methods and thus are doubly indirect, susceptible to errors in both the field and criterion method. It is essential that methods be applied that were validated against an appropriate method and, ideally, cross-validated in additional studies. In this chapter we review the most feasible and accurate methods and methods with historical significance, beginning with the models that underlie them.

Two component and multicomponent models

Historically, the most often used methods (e.g., densitometry and hydrometry) have been ones based on a two-component (2C) model that defines the body as composed of fat (FM) and fat-free masses (FFM). In this approach it is only necessary to estimate one compartment accurately and the other is found by difference. Thus, the measurement burden is fairly low, the instrumentation is affordable, and the methods are feasible in many situations. The equations that are used to estimate FM and FFM are derived from assumed relationships between the components comprising these compartments and thus their accuracy is limited by the validity of the underlying assumptions. The inherent inaccuracies of using 2C methods in developing children and adolescents, especially when based on equations derived from adult data, have been widely noted (Lohman 1989, 1992). With the application of age- and maturation-specific models, the errors are substantially reduced, although not eliminated because they do not account for the interindividual variation found at any age. Fortunately, significant work has been carried out in recent years to improve child and adolescent models (Lohman 1986), although athlete-specific equations are rare (Stout *et al.* 1995; Modlesky *et al.* 1996; Prior *et al.* 2001; Heyward & Wagner 2004).

The errors inherent in the 2C approach model can be avoided by using multicomponent models (Going 2005). Although more complex models have been described, three- and four-component (3C and 4C) models are adequate (Table 30.1). Application of these models requires a combination of measurements (e.g., body density and body water or mineral).

By measuring more components, fewer assumptions are required and hence validity is improved. However, measurement burden and cost are increased, there is the potential for greater technical error, and the assessment is typically not feasible outside the laboratory. Multicomponent approaches are particularly useful as criterion methods in validation and cross-validation studies to avoid propagation of errors from the criterion method to the method being developed. When choosing a method or equation, it is important, if possible, to select one that was validated against a multicomponent model.

The advantages of 3C and 4C models are illustrated in Table 30.2. In this example, the 2C equation based on an adult data set significantly overestimates fatness in children. Application of an equation based on a 3C model combining body density and body water dramatically improves the accuracy of estimating percent fat, and with the addition of body mineral, a small additional improvement is evident. In this example, the major improvement is brought about by accounting for body water, as it typically is a larger source of variation in adolescents then bone mineral. However, ultimately, the best model depends on which component is expected to vary most in the population of interest. When estimation of body fatness cannot be based on a 3C or 4C model, a 2C model with adjustments for age- and

Table 30.1 Equations for estimating % fat based on 2-, 3-, and 4-comparment models of body composition (based on data collected in adults)

Model	Equation	Reference
2C	$\% \text{ Fat} = (\frac{4.95}{D_b} - 4.50)\,100$	Siri (1956)
	$\% \text{ Fat} = (\frac{4.570}{D_b} - 4.142)\,100$	Brožek *et al.* (1963)
3C	$\% \text{ Fat} = (\frac{2.118}{D_b} - 40.78W - 1.354)\,100$	Siri (1961)
	$\% \text{ Fat} = (\frac{6.386}{D_b} - 3.96M - 6.090)\,100$	Lohman (1986)
4C	$\% \text{ Fat} = (\frac{2.747}{D_b} - 0.714W + 1.146B - 2.0503)\,100$	Selinger (1977)

B, osseous mineral as a fraction of body weight, D_b, body density; M, mineral (osseous + non-osseous) as a fraction of body weight; W, total body water as a fraction of body weight.

Table 30.2 Application of a three-component (3C) and 4C system to body fat estimates in a hypothetical child at three levels of chemical maturation.

	Water (%)	Bone mineral (%)	Body density (g·mL^{-1})	Fat* (%)	Fat[†] (%)	Fat[‡] (%)
Reference child						
10 years of age	64.9	4.5	1.0513	15.1	15.4	20.8
Advanced	64.0	5.0	1.0553	15.1	15.4	19.1
Delayed	66.0	4.0	1.0450	15.1	15.8	23.7
Reference adult	62.4	5.9	1.064	15.3	15.0	15.3

B, osseous mineral as a fraction of body weight; D_b, body density; W, total body water as a fraction of body weight.

* Percent fat = $(2.747/D_b - 0.714W + 1.146B - 2.0503)\,100$ (Selinger 1977).

[†] Percent fat = $(2.118/D_b - 0.78W - 1.354)\,100$ (Siri 1961).

[‡] Percent fat = $(4.95/D_b - 4.50)\,100$ (Siri 1956).

Table 30.3 Age- and sex-specific constants for body density, water, and potassium which allow improved predictions of percent fat in children and adolescents compared with equations based only on adult data (see also Fig. 30.1). From Lohman (1986).

	Fat-free body mass (FFM) composition*							
	Density (% FFM)		Water (% FFM)		Potassium (% FFM)		Mineral (% FFM)	
Age (years)	Male	Female	Male	Female	Male	Female	Male	Female
7–9	1.081	1.079	76.8	77.6	2.40	2.32	5.1	4.9
9–11	1.084	1.082	76.2	77.0	2.45	2.34	5.4	5.2
11–13	1.087	1.086	75.4	76.6	2.53	2.36	5.7	5.5
13–15	1.084	1.092	74.7	75.5	2.56	2.38	6.2	5.9
15–17	1.096	1.094	74.2	75.0	2.61	2.40	6.5	6.1
17–20	1.0985	1.095	74.0	74.8	2.63	2.41	6.6	6.0
20–25	1.100	1.096	73.8	74.5	2.66	2.42	6.8	6.2

gender-related variation in the density of FFM may be used (Tables 30.3 and 30.4).

The impact of physical activity on the chemical maturation of children and adolescents, and on estimates of body composition through effects on body mineral, hydration, and muscularity, remains uncertain. Thus, the constants given in Table 30.3 may not be as applicable to the athletic population. Indeed, there is mounting evidence that high resistance (e.g., weightlifting) and impact (e.g., gymnastics, jumping) activities increase bone mass, but few studies have derived independent estimates of FFM to assess the effect of activity on the mineral fraction of FFM or the ratios among other FFM constituents. While it seems likely that the effect of physical activity on FFM constituents would be greater in post-pubescent than prepubescent athletes, there are opposing points of view and data supporting both opinions. The effects of activity on FFM density are complicated by potential increases in muscle mass which may accompany increases in mineral. Muscle mass, having a density lower than FFM density, would decrease FFM density, countering the effect of increased mineral, which has a density higher than FFM density.

These competing influences of water and bone density variation in FFM have been quantified in the college-age wrestling population. Stout *et al.* (1995) showed for this population that equations developed in the non-athlete population may not provide accurate estimates of body fat. Systematic investigations of the effects of different training programs on FFM composition and density as a function of age, gender, and maturation have yet to be undertaken;

Table 30.4 Equations for estimating percent fat from body density based on age and gender. (Reprinted from Lohman, T.G. (1989) Assessment of body composition in children. *Pediatric Exercise Science* 1, 19–30. Copyright 1989 by Human Kinetics, Champaign, IL, with permission.)

Age (years)	Males		Females	
	C_1	C_2	C_1	C_2
1	5.72	5.36	5.69	5.33
1–2	5.64	5.26	5.65	5.26
3–4	5.53	5.14	5.58	5.20
5–6	5.43	5.03	5.53	5.14
7–8	5.38	4.97	5.43	5.03
9–10	5.30	4.89	5.35	4.95
11–12	5.23	4.81	5.25	4.84
13–14	5.07	4.64	5.12	4.69
15–16	5.03	4.59	5.07	4.64
18	4.95	4.50	5.05	4.62

C_1 and C_2 are the terms in percent fat equation to substitute in the Siri (1956) equation for the calculation of percent fat:

$$\% \, BF = [C_1/D_b - C_2] \cdot 100.$$

thus, the effects of physical activity on attainment of chemical maturity and the associated density of FFM remain unresolved.

In the adult athletic male population, two studies using the 4C model indicate the density of FFM is significantly different from the non-athletic population (Modlesky *et al.* 1996, Prior *et al.* 2001). In male weight trainers, a high water content (74.8%) and lower protein (19.9%) and mineral (5.3%) content was found compared to non-athletes (72.6% water, 21.5% protein, and 5.9% mineral). Thus, the density of FFM was 1.089 rather than 1.099 g·mL^{-1} (non-athletic sample). Use of the Siri equation in this adult athletic population results in a 4% overestimation of body fat. In other male and female athletic groups the work of Prior *et al.* (2001) shows a range of 1.087–1.114 g·mL^{-1} in the density of FFM, with female gymnasts having the highest FFM density and male and female swimmers having the lowest FFM density. Thus, different training programs and different male and female athletic groups vary considerably in their FFM composition. Further work in this area is summarized by Heyward and Wagner (2004).

As a systematic study of the density of FFM using the 4C model in prepubescent, pubescent, and post-pubescent athletes for both males and females has not been carried out, whenever possible, 3C and 4C models are recommended for body composition assessment in child and adolescent athletes, or 2C methods that have been validated against a multi-component model.

Densitometry

Body density, like the density of any material, is defined as the ratio of its mass to volume. While mass is easily estimated, estimation of body volume is more challenging. Indeed, most so-called densitometric techniques are methods devised to estimate body volume. Historically, hydrostatic weighing has been the most common method. With the recent development of the Bod Pod, it is possible to estimate body volume and density via air displacement plethysmography. In compliant subjects, both methods give acceptable estimates of body density. However, both are limited by the validity of assumptions underlying the models and equations used to convert body density to estimates of FM and FFM.

Body density is inversely related to body fatness and the simplest approaches take advantage of this relationship to derive equations for converting density to percent body fat (Fig. 30.1). For example, the often-used Siri equation, based on the 2C model, was derived by assuming the densities of body fat (d_f) and fat-free mass (d_{ffm}) were equal to 0.9 and 1.1 g·mL^{-1}, respectively. For over 30 years densitometry has been used as a criterion method for developing practical equations from anthropometry and bioelectrical impedance assuming the 2C model is effective in all populations. Chemical analyses support these estimates in healthy, young adults (Brozek *et al.* 1963) but recent work with multicomponent models (Evans *et al.* 2001; Prior *et al.* 2001) show considerable heterogeneity in the protein, water, and mineral fractions of FFM, and thus its density in growing children and adolescents. The accuracy of any densitometric approach is therefore limited.

Population-specific equations (gender- and age- or maturation-specific) can be derived when the

Basic equation for estimating percent BF from body density (D_b):

$$\% \ BF = \left[\frac{1}{D_b} \times \frac{D_{FFM} \times D_F}{D_{FFM} - D_F} - \frac{D_F}{D_{FFM} - D_F} \right] \times 100$$

D_{FFM}, density of the fat-free mass; D_F, density of the fat mass.

For a hypothetical child, using D_{FFM} = 1.082 g·mL^{-1} and D_F = 0.901 g·mL^{-1}

$$\% \ BF = \left[\frac{1}{D_b} \times \underset{0.181}{\frac{1.082 \times 0.901}{1.082 - 0.901}} - \frac{0.901}{1.082 - 0.901} \right] \times 100$$

$$\% \ BF = \left[\frac{5.37}{D_b} - 4.98 \right] \times 100$$

With a D_b = 1.05 g·mL^{-1}, the common Siri 2C equation estimates % BF = 21.4%, whereas the new equation gives % fat = 13.4%.

Following this approach, Lohman (1989) has derived population-specific equations for boys and girls, 1–18 years of age (Table 30.4).

Fig. 30. 1 Derivation of equations to estimate percent body fat (BF) using specific densities of the fat-free mass.

FFM composition for a particular group is known (Fig. 30.1). Lohman (1986, 1989) has described the typical developmental changes in protein, water, and mineral content, and their contributions to FFM composition and density. Using these constants, Lohman derived population-specific equations for children and adolescents that are more valid than equations based on adult models (Table 30.4). Population-specific 2C equations are recommended when multicomponent equations are not possible. Population-specific equations for children are more accurate than application of adult equations, because they are based on appropriate constants.

Underwater weighing

Underwater weighing has been the most common approach to measuring body volume and estimating body density. Based on Archimedes' principle, volume is estimated from the difference between body weight on land and weight under water (Going 2005). Ideally, weights are obtained following an 8–12 h fast and after emptying the bladder and bowels. Accurate determinations of body density require correction for gas in the lungs and the gastrointestinal tract. The latter is often assumed to equal 100 mL. Gas in the lungs must be measured, and this requirement presents the biggest challenge and potentially introduces the largest error into the estimate of body density. The best practices to determine pulmonary gas volume and the typical errors associated with measurement of weight, underwater weight, and residual lung volume have been described elsewhere (Going 1996, 2005). Under ideal conditions, body density can be measured to within ± 0.0017 g·mL^{-1} which is equivalent to an error of ≈1.0% body fat.

The estimation of body fat from body density has larger errors when inappropriate equations are used to convert body density to percent body fat. It is critical that a population-specific formula be used that is valid for the gender and maturation (or age, as a surrogate) group of interest. Numerous reports have been published of methods and equations developed against underwater weighing and the 2C model as the criterion method. When choosing a method, it is important to investigate whether an appropriate 2C model and population-specific equation was used to minimize model error, which is passed on to the method being validated.

Air displacement plethysmography

The recent development of the Bod Pod has made air displacement plethysmography (ADP) a reasonable alternative to underwater weighing for estimation of body density (Going 2005). Although the initial investment is somewhat more than underwater weighing, the Bod Pod is affordable, portable, and useful in individuals who cannot be submerged in water. To measure body volume with adequate accuracy, it is necessary to either eliminate or account for the effects of clothing, hair, skin surface area, and lung volume. The effects of clothing and hair are adequately dealt with by wearing minimal clothing (bathing suits) and compressing the hair with a swim cap. The isothermal effects related to skin surface area are minimized by adjusting the raw body volume for the surface area artefact. The raw body volume is also adjusted for the thoracic gas volume, which is measured during the test using a technique very similar to the plethysmographic measurement of thoracic gas volume used in pulmonary function testing (Ruppell 1994).

The reliability and validity of Bod Pod ADP has now been assessed in a number of studies (Demerath *et al.* 2002; Fields *et al.* 2002; Going 2005). Excellent precision and accuracy have been demonstrated for estimating the volume of an inanimate object. Across studies of adults, reliability of Bod Pod is good to excellent. Between-day test–retest correlation coefficients for body density and percent fat generally exceed r = 0.90; within-subject coefficients of variation (CV) for percent fat range from 1.7–4.5% within a day and from 2.0–2.3% between days. These CVs are within the range of CVs reported for underwater weighing (Going 2005) and dual energy X-ray absorptiometry (DEXA) (Lohman & Chen 2005).

Validation studies of estimates of body composition by the Bod Pod against underwater weighing and DEXA have generally shown acceptable average agreement between methods (Going 2005). Reliability and validation studies of Bod Pod in children have generally yielded results similar to those in adults, showing good-to-excellent reliability, good average agreement with other methods, and large individual variations in differences between methods. Thus, Bod Pod ADP is a viable alternative to underwater weighing for estimating body volume and body density. As with underwater weighing, ADP is susceptible to model error, unless age-appropriate formulae are used to convert body density to percent body fat.

Hydrometry

Total body water (TBW) can be estimated accurately via isotope dilution in children and adolescents. Deuterium, which is non-toxic, is used more frequently than tritium because of concerns about radiation exposure, although both can be used safely in small doses in boys and non-pregnant girls. Once TBW is known, it can be used in combination with body density in 3C or 4C models to estimate percent fat and then FFM, or TBW can be converted directly

to FFM (and the percent fat can be estimated) using the water fraction of FFM as the conversion constant. As shown in the example in Table 30.2, the Siri 3C model combining TBW and body density provides a significant improvement over the traditional 2C model in children and is a useful criterion method in this population. However, the water fractions of the FFM are well established for different ages and levels of maturation (Table 30.3), and FFM can be estimated from TBW as long as population-specific conversion constants are used. The main challenges are the isotope expense, the need to collect multiple specimens (blood, saliva, or urine) over 3–4 h, and the cost and technical expertise required for processing the samples and estimating isotope concentration. Protocols for both laboratory and field applications (Schoeller 2005) have been developed and, when feasible, hydrometry is the preferred 2C approach. Other 2C models include ADP or indirect methods such as skinfolds or whole body impedance.

Dual energy X-ray absorptiometry

DEXA is increasingly available and easily performed on children. Based on a 3C model (bone mineral, lean soft tissue, and fat), DEXA provides an ideal method to assess body composition in children and youth (Lohman 1986). Radiation exposure is low and, unlike other methods that are confounded by changes in FFM composition during growth and development (e.g., body density, body water, bioelectrical impedance analysis, and anthropometry), DEXA estimates of bone mineral, soft tissue, and fat are not greatly affected by the hydration level of FFM. Theoretical analyses in adults (Pietrobelli *et al.* 1996) and in children from infancy to 10 years of age (Testolin *et al.* 2000) have shown that the typical variation in FFM hydration affects DEXA estimates of percent fat by less than 1% during growth and development.

Ellis *et al.* (2000) have developed reference models for children and adolescents using DEXA in a population of black, white, and Hispanic children 5–19 years of age. In general, their results confirm older estimates of FFM and FM by Fomon *et al.*

(1982) and Haschke (1989) using indirect estimates of body composition from the literature. Sopher *et al.* (2004) recently compared DEXA with a 4C model, adjusting for mineral and water in a large sample of children and adolescents ($n = 411$) 6–18 years of age. Close average (~1%) agreement was found between methods, they were highly correlated ($R^2 = 0.85$), and prediction accuracy was good (standard error of estimate [SEE] = 3.7%). In this sample, DEXA overestimated percent fat in children above 30% fat by 3–5% and underestimated percent fat in children below 10% fat by 1–2%.

Bioelectrical impedance analysis

Bioelectrical impedance analysis (BIA) is based on the relationship between the volume of the conductor (the body) and the conductor's length (height) and its impedance, which reflects the resistance to the flow of an electric current. In the common tetrapolar arrangement, impedance measurements are made with an individual lying supine on a non-conducting surface with surface electrodes attached to specific sites on the hand and foot of the right side of the body. A low-dose (800 μA), single frequency (50 kHz) current is passed through the individual and the value for impedance is measured. Because the resistive component of impedance is so much larger than reactance, resistance is often substituted for impedance in prediction equations. Because impedance is inversely proportional to the cross-sectional area of the conductor, prediction equations that include resistance or impedance plus height^2 (cm^2) are used to estimate FFM. Fat mass and percent fat can then be derived from FFM and body weight. Alternatively, percent fat can be predicted directly if body weight is also included in the equation.

Many prediction equations have been validated against 2C models. The accuracy of prediction equations for children and adolescents is improved when population-specific equations validated and cross-validated against multicomponent criterion methods are used to estimate FFM and percent fat. The validity of BIA measurements can be substantially altered if electrode placement is incorrect,

if body temperature is elevated, if the subject is under- or overhydrated, or has eaten within 3–4 h of the measurement. Gender, body fatness, race/ ethnicity, and athletic status are other factors that influence prediction accuracy and these factors should be included in the prediction equation if population-specific equations are not used.

In recent years, new instruments and alternative electrode placements have been developed, allowing for standing measurements and alternative conduction pathways (e.g., arm-to-arm and leg-to-leg, rather than whole body). Although more convenient, overall measurement errors for these techniques are somewhat higher than the standard protocol and further cross-validation work is needed. With multiple electrodes it is possible to obtain impedance and resistance measures for body segments (arm, legs, trunk). The inclusion of segmental resistance in prediction equations has theoretical advantages, although in practice the improvement is small.

For the athletic adult population, several BIA equations have been developed. One of the most successful approaches was developed by Fornetti *et al.* (1999) from a large sample of athletic women aged 18–27 years. Additional BIA equations in the athletic population have been summarized by Heyward and Wagner (2004). Little systematic research has been carried out to cross-validate BIA equations in child and adolescent athletes, although Eckerson *et al.* (1992) reported that some previously published BIA equations gave acceptable errors in high school aged gymnasts, and Pichard *et al.* (1997) found acceptable errors in elite female runners. The equation from Van Loan *et al.* (1990) was particularly useful in teenage female gymnasts. Oppliger *et al.* (1991a) have also validated a potentially useful equation for high school aged wrestlers (males), although to our knowledge it has not been cross-validated. The BIA method is highly dependent on testing under controlled conditions; however, the physiology of athletes is often altered or in an "uncontrolled" state. For example, any condition that results in fluid shifts and altered electrolyte concentrations can alter impedance measurements. Given that it may be difficult for an athlete in training to comply with controlled conditions (e.g., 2-h post-consumption of a light meal; euhydration; no preceding exercise), the BIA method may not be the most suitable field method for testing athletes.

Multifrequency impedance analysis

Multifrequency BIA, or bioelectrical impedance spectroscopy (BIS) as it is sometimes called, differs from the more common single frequency BIA in its use of multiple measures of impedance or resistance over a range of frequencies to estimate body composition (Chumlea & Sun 2005). Single-frequency impedance analyzers are limited in their ability to distinguish the distribution of body water into its intracellular (IC) and extracellular (EC) compartments. The ability of multifrequency impedance to differentiate TBW into intracellular water (ICW) and extracellular water (ECW) is potentially an important advantage to describe fluid shifts and balance and to explore variations in levels of hydration that confound single frequency analyses. Theoretically, impedance values measured across a spectrum of frequencies, at several discrete frequencies or some combination of frequencies, can explain interindividual variations in body composition more precisely than impedance measurements at a single frequency. The most appropriate combination of frequencies and multivariate methods of using multifrequency impedance values in estimating body composition are still being investigated. Recently, Chumlea and Sun (2005) have reviewed advances in multifrequency BIA. New developments in multifrequency analysis come with the use of the Cole–Cole and Hanai models. With these new approaches, multifrequency BIA has expanded the use of impedance to quantify the distributions of TBW, ECW, and ICW in clinical and nutritional studies. However, in general, multifrequency impedance has not improved estimates of fat and FFM over the use of single-frequency impedance (Dittmar & Reber 2001; Simpson et al. 2001), but it has been able to provide accurate and precise estimates of TBW and ECW under conditions of varying levels of hydration, which limits single-frequency 50-kHz impedance This may be an advantage in the application of the 2C model based on TBW in athletes, but further research is needed to be certain.

Anthropometry

The use of weight, height, skinfolds, circumferences, and skeletal widths are the most common field measures of body composition in various populations of children and youth, including athletic youth. Of the several approaches to be summarized in the next sections, skinfold equations have emerged as the most valid approach for the athletic population.

Body mass index

The widespread use of body mass index (BMI) in nutrition and growth surveys over the last 30 years makes it an important candidate for a growth survey. Height and weight can be measured precisely and accurately in large samples with inexpensive equipment. Both are non-invasive and can be easily assessed in children. Height is essential to document linear growth with age and thus is an important part of any survey designed to obtain normative data. Weight gives additional information over and above height as an estimate of growth in mass and thus reflects the sum of muscle, bone, organs, and fat. While weight in relation to height (BMI) can be used as a measure of under- and overnutrition, it is especially valuable as a measure of undernutrition, because at low levels of BMI there is less variation in muscle, bone, and fat because all three compartments have been depleted to arrive at the low value.

In contrast, high levels of BMI can be reached as a result of varying amounts of muscle, bone, and fat, and thus one cannot discern the composition of the increased mass relative to height. Thus, while BMI is correlated with fatness, it has limited ability to detect excess adiposity because of its failure to detect obesity (lack of sensitivity) in 20–50% of children who are obese by more direct methods (Lazarus et al. 1996; Pietrobelli et al. 1998; Sardinha et al. 1999; Sarria et al. 2001; Mei et al. 2002; Bedogni et al. 2003; Zimmermann et al. 2004), depending on the BMI cutpoints used to define obesity. In support of this point, Siervogel et al. (2000) documented the change in FFM and FM in relation to height as a function of maturation and leg and trunk length in the longitudinal data collected in Fels Longitudinal Study. They clearly show that variation in FFM/height increases BMI with age independent of adiposity.

Racial and ethnic differences in the composition of weight per unit height also confound interpretation of the BMI. Several studies have shown significant racial and/or ethnic differences in body composition, especially in bone and muscle mass. For example, Cohn et al. (1977) showed that total body potassium and calcium were 5–10% higher in black women than white women, indicating greater muscle mass and bone mass in black people per unit of height. Similar findings have been reported in children and adolescents. For example, Novotny et al. (2005) recently reported differences in body composition between Asian girls and other groups that persisted after adjustment for differences in maturation, and Going et al. (2005) showed these differences translated into differences in the BMI–percent fat relationship.

Skinfolds

The use of skinfolds to estimate percent fat and, indirectly, FFM in children and adults is well established. Many studies have included skinfolds along with height and weight to better describe changes in body fat with growth and development. Skinfold sites, such as the triceps and subscapular, are leading candidates representing extremity and trunk subcutaneous fat depots.

Studies relating skinfolds to body fatness in children using 2C, 3C, and 4C models have shown a prediction error of 3–4% body fat (SEE) and many equations have been developed to assess body fat from skinfold measurements (Boileau et al. 1981; Rolland-Cachera et al. 1982; Lohman 1986; Slaughter et al. 1988; Deurenberg et al. 1990). Roemmich et al. (1997) emphasized the need for multicomponent models as criterion methods for the development of skinfolds equations and found that equations based on 3C or 4C models were more valid than those based on 2C models, which lead to a large systematic overestimation (≥5%) of body fat in children.

The relationship between skinfolds and body fat varies with age, maturation (Slaughter et al. 1988; Deurenberg et al. 1990) obesity, athletic group, and ethnicity (Heyward & Wagner 2004). Thus, it is important to select equations validated and cross-validated using the athletic population.

The most extensive work in the athletic population has been carried out in high school wrestlers (Housh et al. 1989; Thorland et al. 1991). In the former study, Housh et al. (1989), using a sample of 409 high school wrestlers in Nebraska, cross-validated 23 equations drawn from previous studies in youth and young male adults. The authors found four equations using skinfold thickness and two equations with skinfolds and circumferences to be cross-validated successfully. The authors recommend the quadratic equation using the sum of three skinfolds from the combined work of Sinning, Sloan, Lohman, and Boileau (Lohman 1981). In the second cross-validation study, Thorland et al. (1991) analyzed data collected from five universities ($n = 806$ high school wresters). The sample of high school wrestlers from Iowa, Nebraska, Illinois, Minnesota, and Ohio was measured by selected anthropometric dimensions and for body density. Thorland et al. (1991) found several effective equations (Katch & McArdle 1973; Lohman 1981; Thorland et al. 1984) and cross-validated these equations within three age groups and three weight groups.

Circumferences

Because intersubject variation in circumferences reflects variation in muscle, fat, and bone, they have limited utility when applied across a broad age range including different levels of maturation. Leg, and especially upper arm circumferences, when corrected for relevant subcutaneous fat via skinfold thicknesses, are useful for estimating muscle plus bone cross-sectional area. Because there is greater variation in muscle than bone, corrected upper arm area is a relatively good index of muscularity and has been often used as an index of nutritional status and growth. The approach has merit given the importance of describing changes in different components of body composition during growth and development. Muscle is the largest tissue component of FFM, and variation in muscle resulting from age, maturation, gender, race/ethnicity, nutrition, and activity certainly contributes to variation in BMI and confounds its interpretation as an index of fatness across different groups. Somatograms, developed from circumferences (Behnke & Wilmore 1974), provide a useful approach for describing muscle and fat distribution, and have been used to characterize athletic groups and establish norms for various sports (Behnke & Wilmore 1974).

The waist circumference may also be particularly useful, given the interest in abdominal fatness and its association with metabolic disorders and chronic disease risk (Seidell *et al.* 1987). The association is much better established in adults, although emerging evidence suggests abdominal fatness is also a risk factor in children and adolescents. Use of waist circumference as an index of fatness avoids some of the problems associated with interpretation of BMI, as variation in waist circumference is expected to reasonably track variation in fatness. Only limited normative data exist for children and adolescents (Heyward & Stolarczyk 1996; McCarthy *et al.* 2001), and certainly more work is needed to better define the relationship between waist circumference, intra-abdominal and subcutaneous fatness, and chronic disease risk factors in children and adolescents. In general, the athletic youth population has less abdominal fat in association with an overall low body fatness, and thus lower chronic disease risk factors.

Establishing body fat ranges for athletic youth

Optimal fatness ranges for good health and high level performance are difficult to establish, given the wide individual variation in fatness in healthy individuals and the many factors, in addition to body composition, that contribute to physical performance. All of the methods described above have been applied in young athletes, although typically in limited samples, and few studies have used the recommended multicomponent models that are needed for accurate estimates of fatness in developing boys and girls. Fatness ranges are better described for adult athletes (Going & Mullins 2000; Heyward & Wagner 2004), although ranges in young athletes (males, ~5–20%; females, ~9–28%, depending on athletic group) are similar to adults. Whether these

Table 30.5 Percent fat standard for athletic youth.

	Body fat level (%)		
	Low	Mid	Upper
Boys			
Prepubescent	10	13	18
Post-pubescent	7	10	14
Girls			
Prepubescent	16	20	25
Post-pubescent	14	17	20

ranges are truly optimal and should be recommended is difficult to conclude, as it is impossible to be certain that all of the study participants were healthy and performing at a high level. In our view, standards for youth must be set to provide protection against establishing low body fat levels during the time of peak growth and development of the musculoskeletal system. With this in mind, we propose that boys maintain 10% body fat and girls maintain at least 16% body fat (Table 30.5). Undoubtedly, more systematic research is needed to establish optimal fatness ranges for child and adolescent athletes.

Estimation of minimal weight in athletes

Behnke (1965) proposed that there is an essential amount of fat necessary for health. He defined lean body mass (LBM) as fat-free body mass plus essential fat (for males, 2–3% of LBM is essential fat). Thus, LBM represents the absolute lowest weight that an individual should attain. As a result of measurement error and the belief that male wrestlers should have some subcutaneous fat in addition to essential fat, 5% fat has become accepted as the minimal percent fat for college-aged athletes for optimal performance and health and to prevent the loss of lean body mass (American College of Sports Medicine 1985). Minimal weight for males is therefore calculated as fat-free body mass divided by 0.95. In males 16 years and younger (American College of Sports Medicine 1985), minimal fat has been defined as 7% fat, although we recommend a slightly higher value of 10% because of growth concerns (Table 30.5).

Several anthropometric approaches have been used to estimate the minimal weight for health and performance in athletes. In practice, skeletal dimensions and circumferences, and more recently skinfolds and body weight, have been used to develop generalized equations for high school wrestlers.

Early work with anthropometric dimensions focused on the association of skeletal dimensions and lean body mass. Sinning (1974), in a critical evaluation of the diameter approach as compared to skinfolds, used densitometry in 35 college wrestlers to predict minimal weight. He found that the Tcheng and Tipton (1973) equations using skeletal diameters predicted fat-free body mass with an SEE of 4.0 kg, a result remarkably similar to that found by Tcheng and Tipton (1973), who did not use densitometry. Similar results were found by Sinning (1974) using the Behnke approach (Behnke 1959) of eight skeletal diameters and constants derived from other samples.

Sinning (1974) also showed that fat-free body mass of wrestlers could be predicted with an SEE of 2.1–2.9 kg using skinfolds (subscapular and abdominal) along with skeletal diameters. This contrast of a 4.0–2.1 kg SEE between approaches is very significant, these findings suggest that a skinfold equation could be developed for high school wrestlers that would estimate FFM with an SEE of 2 kg (4 lb) or less, and that this approach could be used by coaches and students to achieve more realistic weight loss goals. However, Thorland et al. (1991) cautioned that, at best, the typical estimate of fat-free body mass and minimal weight has an error of 2.4 kg (5.3 lb). Further reduction of error is found within specific age groups and weight classes, with errors as low as 1.7 kg (3.7 lb) in the lightweight groups, using the better equations. However, part of this error is associated not with the error in estimating percent fat from body density in this population, but with individual variation in hydration status and bone mineral content.

Population-specific anthropometric equations for other athletic groups

There is a great need to develop population-specific equations for estimating body composition in young athletes of different ages, genders, ethnicity, and athletic groups. These equations could then be used to develop optimal as well as minimal weight predictions for a given sport. The equation developed from several samples (Lohman 1981) has been found to be valid for high school wrestlers (15–17 years). To apply the equation to the college wrestling population (18–22 years), we must change the intercept (Sinning 1974).

High school white male wrestling population (15–17 years):

$$D = 1.097 - 0.000815 \ (\Sigma \ 3sk) = 0.00000084 \ (\Sigma \ 3sk)^2$$

College white male wrestling population (18–21 years):

$$D = 1.1030 - 0.000815 \ (\Sigma \ 3sk) + 0.00000084 \ (\Sigma \ 3sk)^2$$

The three skinfolds are triceps + subscapular + abdomen (Lohman 1981). Once D (body density) is calculated, then percent fat can be derived from the Siri equation: percent fat = (495/D) − 450. Minimal weight (kg) we assume a lower limit of body fat at 10% as:

Minimal weight (kg) for 10% fat = [Body weight − percent fat/100 (body weight)]/0.90

Further modification of this high school wrestlers equation for Hispanic and black wrestlers at the high school and college level may be needed, because the variations in fat patterning across ethnic groups affects the skinfold–fat content relationship, resulting in a slightly different equation for skinfolds versus fatness (Roby et al. 1991). Additional skinfold equations for the athletic population have been recommended by Heyward and Wagner (2004).

The estimation of minimal weight in the female population has been investigated to a lesser extent, and the cross-validation of various skinfold equations in female athletes is needed. The work of Sinning and Wilson (1984) applies to the female population. They found that the equation of Jackson et al. (1980) using the sum of four skinfolds predicted very close to the mean density in the athletic population and had low SEE and a good standard deviation of prediction values. Thus, in the female athletic population (ages 15–21 years), the following skinfold equation is recommended:

$$D = 1.0961 - 0.000695 \text{ (sum of four skinfolds:}$$
$$\text{triceps, abdomen, suprailiac, thighs)}$$
$$+ 0.0000011 \, (\Sigma \, 4sk)^2 - 0.0000714 \text{ (age, years)}$$

Given that the FFM density is close to 1.100 g·mL^{-1} in college women, an estimate a minimal weight at 16% fat from the sum of four skinfolds can be made as follows:

$$\text{Minimal weight (kg) for 16\% fat} = [\text{body weight}$$
$$- \text{percent fat}/100 \text{ (body weight)}]/0.84$$

Further work along the line of Prior *et al.* (2001) is essential to establish the FFM density in pre-pubescent and post-pubescent athletic girls or to develop equations using DEXA and anthropometry where bone mineral, fat, and lean tissue mass are independently estimated.

Assessment of musculoskeletal size

Various methods have been proposed to estimate musculoskeletal size in both athletic and non-athletic populations. In general, greater musculoskeletal development is associated with better performance in sports such as wrestling, gymnastics, weight lifting, and swimming. The Health–Carter anthropometric somatotype has been widely used to estimate mesomorphy (greater musculoskeletal mass per unit of height) over the past 30 years (Carter 1982). Slaughter *et al.* (1988) proposed a method using the regression of FFM on height as another approach to estimate musculoskeletal size in the athletic population and using this approach described considerable variation among athletic groups.

More recently, the use of FFM (FFM/height^2) and FM (FM/height^2) indices, derived in a fashion analogous to BMI have been proposed as a more descriptive method of musculoskeletal development in all populations of youth when estimates of FFM or FM are available. Hattori *et al.* (1997) proposed these indices to adjust FM and FFM for size (height) as a better method for evaluation of growth in children (Hattori *et al.* 1997). Work by Wells (2001) and Maynard *et al.* (2001) further supports the validity of this approach. Siervogel *et al.* (2000)

have clearly shown that changes in FFM/height^2 confounded interpretation of BMI as a measure of adiposity in adolescence, especially around the time of peak height velocity.

Conclusions

The assessment of body composition in children and youth has been reviewed, emphasizing the young athlete. The more promising and common laboratory and field methods have been described and efforts to study the complex aspects of body composition during development have been explored. Practical field measures of estimating body fatness and minimal weight are also presented. While body composition is clearly an important contributor to performance, and certainly underlies good health, the relationships are complex and wide interindividual variability exists. The frequent use of less than optimal assessment methods (e.g., reliance on the 2C model and field methods validated against the 2C model) have confounded attempts to validate assessment methods in growing children and adolescents and inhibited efforts to describe optimal ranges for body fat. Often, emphasis is placed on describing percent fat, and while body fat is certainly an important compartment, the musculoskeletal compartment is at least equally important and deserves greater emphasis. While we describe typical ranges of percent fat, there is clearly a need for more systematic research in athletic males and females of all ages, ethnicities, and athletic groups to better define the optimal ranges of body fat and FFM associated with good health and high level performance. We cautiously propose body fat ranges. Past estimates have been derived from considerations of minimal weight, a concept reasonably well developed in wrestlers that is assumed to relate to other groups as well. There is a great need to apply multicomponent models in young athletes to better describe the relationships between body composition, growth, and performance, and to understand the minimal weight (fat) that is compatible with normal growth. Also, there continues to be a need to validate methods for assessing body fat and FFM against appropriate criterion methods in order to achieve the goal of understanding these relationships.

References

American College of Sports Medicine (1985) *Position Stand and Opinion Statements (1975–85)*, 3rd edn. Indianapolis, IN.

Bedogni, G., Iughetti, L., Ferrari, M., *et al.* (2003) Sensitivity and specificity of body mass index and skinfold thicknesses in detecting excess adiposity in children aged 8–12 years. *Annals of Human Biology* **30**, 132–139.

Behnke, A.R. (1959) The estimation of lean body weight from "skeletal" measurements. *Human Biology* **31**, 295–315.

Behnke, A.R. (1965) Discussion. In: *Radioactivity in Man* (Menecky, G.R. & Linde, S.M., eds.) C.C. Thomas, Springfield, IL.

Behnke, A.R. & Wilmore, J.H. (1974) *Evaluation and Regulation of Body Build and Composition*. Prentice Hall, Englewood Cliffs, NJ.

Boileau, R.A., Wilmore, J.H., Lohman, T.G., Slaughter, M.H. & Riner, W.F. (1981) Estimation of body density from skinfold thicknesses, body circumferences and skeletal widths in boys aged 8 to 11 years: comparison of two samples. *Human Biology* **53**, 575–592.

Brozek, J., Grande, F. & Anderson, J.T. (1963) Densitometric analysis of body composition: revision of some quantitative assumptions. *Annals of the New York Academy of Sciences* **110**, 113–140.

Carter, J.E.L. (1982) Physical structure of Olympic athletes. Part I. *Medicine and Sport*. Vol. 16. S. Karger, New York.

Chumlea, W.C. & Sun, S.S. (2005) Bioelectrical impedance analysis. In: *Human Body Composition*, 2nd edn. (Heymsfield, S.B. *et al.* eds.) Human Kinetics, Champaign, IL.

Cohn, S.H., Abesamis, C., Zanzi, I., Aloia, J.F., Yasumura, S. & Ellis, K.J. (1977) Body elemental composition: comparison between black and white adults. *American Journal of Physiology* **232**, E419–E422.

Demerath, E.W., Guo, S.S., Chumlea, W.C., Towne, B., Roche, A.F. & Siervogel, R.M. (2002) Comparison of percent body fat estimates using air displacement plethysmography and hydrodensitometry in adults and children. *International Journal of Obesity and Related Metabolic Disords* **26**, 389–397.

Deurenberg, P., Pieters, J.J. & Hautvast, J.G. (1990) The assessment of the body fat percentage by skinfold thickness measurements in childhood and young adolescence. *British Journal of Nutrition* **63**, 293–303.

Dittmar, M. & Reber, H. (2001) New equations for estimating body cell mass from bioimpedance parallel models in healthy older Germans. *American Journal of Physiology. Endocrinology and Metabolism* **281**, E1005–E1014.

Eckerson, J.M., Housh, T.J. & Johnson, G.O. (1992) Validity of bioelectrical impedance equations for estimating fat-free weight in lean males. *Medicine and Science in Sports and Exercise* **24**, 1298–1302.

Eliakim, A. & Beyth, Y. (2003) Exercise training, menstrual irregularities and bone development in children and adolescents. *Journal of Pediatric and Adolescent Gynecology* **16**, 201–206.

Ellis, K.J., Shypailo, R.J., Abrams, S.A. & Wong, W.W. (2000) The reference child and adolescent models of body composition. A contemporary comparison. *Annals of the New York Academy of Sciences* **904**, 374–382.

Evans, E.M., Prior, B.M., Arngrimsson, S.A., Modlesky, C.M. & Cureton, K.J. (2001) Relation of bone mineral density and content to mineral content and density of the fat-free mass. *Journal of Applied Physiology* **91**, 2166–2172.

Fields, D.A., Goran, M.I. & McCrory, M.A. (2002) Body-composition assessment via air-displacement plethysmography in adults and children: a review. *American Journal of Clinical Nutrition* **75**, 453–467.

Fomon, S.J., Haschke, F., Ziegler, E.E. & Nelson, S.E. (1982) Body composition of reference children from birth to age 10 years. *American Journal of Clinical Nutrition* **35**, 1169–1175.

Fornetti, W.C., Pivarnik, J.M., Foley, J.M. & Fiechtner, J.J. (1999) Reliability and validity of body composition measures in female athletes. *Journal of Applied Physiology* **87**, 1114–1122.

Going, S., Novotny, R., McCabe, G., *et al.* (2005) Relationship of body mass index to percent fat in Asian, Hispanic and non-Hispanic adolescent girls. In: *Experimental Biology*. Federation of American Societies for Experimental Biology, San Diego, CA: 108.

Going, S.B. (1996) Densitometry. In: *Human Body Composition* (Roche, A.F., Heymsfield, S.B. & Lohman, T.G., eds.) Human Kinetics Publishers, Champaign, IL: 3–23.

Going, S.B. (2005) Hydrodensitometry and air displacement plethysmography. In: *Human Body Composition*, 2nd edn. (Heymsfield, S.B., *et al.*, eds.) Human Kinetics, Champaign, IL: 17–33.

Going, S.B. & Mullins, V.A. (2000) Body composition of the endurance performer. In: *International Olympic Committee Encyclopedia*, Vol II. *Endurance in Sport* (Shepard, R. & Astrand, P.O., eds.) Blackwell Scientific, Oxford, UK.

Gordon-Larsen, P., Adair, L.S., Nelson, M.C. & Popkin, B.M. (2004) Five-year obesity incidence in the transition period between adolescence and adulthood: the National Longitudinal Study of Adolescent Health. *American Journal of Clinical Nutrition* **80**, 569–575.

Haschke, F. (1989) Body composition during adolescence. In: *98th Ross Conference on Pediatric Research. Body Composition Measurements in Infants and Children* (Klish, W.J. & Kretchmer, N., eds.) Ross Laboratories, Columbus, OH: 76–83.

Hattori, K., Tatsumi, N. & Tanaka, S. (1997) Assessment of body composition by using a new chart method. *American Journal of Human Biology* **9**, 573–578.

Heyward, V. & Stolarczyk, L. (1996) *Applied Body Composition Assessment*. Human Kinetics, Champaign, IL.

Heyward, V.H. & Wagner, D.R. (2004) *Applied Body Composition*, 2nd edn. Human Kinetics, Champaign, IL.

Housh, T.J., Johnson, G.O., Kenney, K.B., *et al.* (1989) Validity of anthropometric estimations of body composition in high school wrestlers. *Research Quarterly for Exercise and Sport* **60**, 239–245.

Jackson, A.S., Pollock, M.L. & Ward, A. (1980) Generalized equations for predicting body density of women. *Medicine and Science in Sports and Exercise* **12**, 175–181.

Katch, F.I. & McArdle, W.D. (1973) Prediction of body density from simple anthropometric measurements in college-age men and women. *Human Biology* **45**, 445–455.

Lazarus, R., Bauer, L., Webb, K. & Blyth, F. (1996) Body mass index in screening for adiposity in children and adolescents: systematic evaluation using receiver operating characteristic curves. *American Journal of Clinical Nutrition* **63**, 500–506.

Lohman, T.G. (1981) Skinfolds and body density and their relationship to body fatness: a review. *Human Biology* **53**, 181–255.

Lohman, T.G. (1986) Applicability of body composition techniques and constants for children and youths. In: *Exercise and Sports Science Reviews* (Holloszy, J.O., ed.) Williams & Wilkins, Baltimore: 325–357.

Lohman, T.G. (1989) Assessment of body composition in children. *Pediatric Exercise Science* 1, 19–30.

Lohman, T.G. (1992) Advances in body composition assessment. *Current Issues in Exercise Science Series*. Monograph No. 3, Human Kinetics, Champaign, IL.

Lohman, T.G. & Chen, Z. (2005) Dual-energy X-ray absorptiometry. In: *Human Body Composition*, 2nd edn. (Heymsfield, S.B., *et al.*, eds.) Human Kinetics, Champaign, IL.

Maynard, L.M., Wisemandle, W., Roche, A.F., Chumlea, W.C., Guo, S.S. & Siervogel, R.M. (2001) Childhood body composition in relation to body mass index. *Pediatrics* 107, 344–350.

McCarthy, H.D., Jarrett, K.V. & Crawley, H.F. (2001) The development of waist circumference percentiles in British children aged 5.0–16.9 y. *European Journal of Clinical Nutrition* 55, 902–907.

Medicine, A.C.O. (1997) Weight loss in wrestlers: Position stand. *Medicine and Science in Sports and Exercise* 29, ix–xii.

Mei, Z., Grummer-Strawn, L.M., Pietrobelli, A., Goulding, A., Goran, M.I. & Dietz, W.H. (2002) Validity of body mass index compared with other body-composition screening indexes for the assessment of body fatness in children and adolescents. *American Journal of Clinical Nutrition* 75, 978–985.

Modlesky, C.M., Cureton, K.J., Lewis, R.D., Prior, B.M., Sloniger, M.A. & Rowe, D.A. (1996) Density of the fat-free mass and estimates of body composition in male weight trainers. *Journal of Applied Physiology* 80, 2085–2096.

Novotny, R., Going, S., Teegarden, D., *et al.* (2005) Asian, Hispanic and White adolescent body size, composition and fat distribution. In: *Experimental Biology*. Federation of American Societies for Experimental Biology, San Diego, CA: 108.

Oppliger, R.A., Nielsen, D.H., Hoegh, J.E. & Vance, C.G. (1991a) Bioelectrical impedance prediction of fat-free mass for high school wrestlers validated. *Medicine and Science in Sports and Exercise* 23, S73 [abstract].

Oppliger, R.A., Nielsen, D.H. & Vance, C.G. (1991b) Wrestlers' minimal weight: Anthropometry, bioimpedance, and

hydrostatic weighing compared. *Medicine and Science in Sports and Exercise* 23, 247–253.

Pichard, C., Kyle, U.G., Gremion, G., Gerbase, M. & Slosman, D.O. (1997) Body composition by X-ray absorptiometry and bioelectrical impedance in female runners. *Medicine and Science in Sports and Exercise* 29, 1527–1534.

Pietrobelli, A., Faith, M.S., Allison, D.B., Gallagher, D., Chiumello, G. & Heymsfield, S.B. (1998) Body mass index as a measure of adiposity among children and adolescents: A validation study. *Journal of Pediatrics* 132, 204–210.

Pietrobelli, A., Formica, C., Wang, Z. & Heymsfield, S.B. (1996) Dual-energy X-ray absorptiometry body composition model: review of physical concepts. *American Journal of Physiology* 271, E941–E951.

Prior, B.M., Modlesky, C.M., Evans, E.M., *et al.* (2001) Muscularity and the density of the fat-free mass in athletes. *Journal of Applied Physiology* 90, 1523–1531.

Roby, F.B., Kempema, J.M., Lohman, T.G., Williams, D.P. & Tipton, C.M. (1991) Can the same equation be used to predict minimal wrestling weight in Hispanic and non-Hispanic wrestlers? *Medicine and Science in Sports and Exercise* 23, S29.

Roemmich, J.N., Clark, P.A., Weltman, A. & Rogol, A.D. (1997) Alterations in growth and body composition during puberty. Comparing multicompartment body composition models. *Journal of Applied Physiology* 83, 927–935.

Rolland-Cachera, M.F., Sempe, M., Guilloud-Bataille, M., Patois, E., Pequignot-Guggenbuhl, F. & Fautrad, V. (1982) Adiposity indices in children. *American Journal of Clinical Nutrition* 36, 178–184.

Ruppell, G. (1994) *Manual of Pulmonary Function Testing*. Mosby, St. Louis, MO.

Sardinha, L.B., Going, S.B., Teixeira, P.J. & Lohman, T.G. (1999) Receiver operating characteristic analysis of body mass index, triceps skinfold thickness, and arm girth for obesity screening in children and adolescents. *American Journal of Clinical Nutrition* 70, 1090–1095.

Sarria, A., Moreno, L.A., Garcia-Llop, L.A., Fleta, J., Morellon, M.P. & Bueno, M. (2001) Body mass index, triceps skinfold and waist circumference in screening for adiposity in male children and adolescents. *Acta Paediatrica* 90, 387–392.

Schoeller, D.A. (2005) Hydrometry. In: *Human Body Composition*, 2nd edn. (Heymsfield, S.B., *et al.*, eds.) Human Kinetics, Champaign, IL: 35–49.

Seidell, J.C., Oosterlee, A., Thijssen, M.A.O., *et al.* (1987) Assessment of intra-abdominal and subcutaneous abdominal fat: Relation between anthropometry and computed tomography. *American Journal of Clinical Nutrition* 45, 7–13.

Selinger, A. (1977) The body as a three component system. Doctoral dissertation, University of Illinois, Urbana.

Siervogel, R.M., Maynard, L.M., Wisemandle, *et al.* (2000) Annual changes in total body fat and fat-free mass in children from 8 to 18 years in relation to changes in body mass index. The Fels Longitudinal Study. *Annals of the New York Academy of Sciences* 904, 420–423.

Simpson, J.A., Lobo, D.N., Anderson, J.A., *et al.* (2001) Body water compartment measurements: a comparison of bioelectrical impedance analysis with tritium and sodium bromide dilution techniques. *Clinical Nutrition* 20, 339–343.

Sinning, W.E. (1974) Body composition assessment of college wrestlers. *Medicine and Science in Sports* 6, 139–145.

Sinning, W.E. & Wilson, J.R. (1984) Validation of "generalized" equations for body composition analysis in women athletes. *Research Quarterly for Exercise and Sport* 55, 153–160.

Siri, W.E. (1956) The gross composition of the body. In: *Advances in Biological and Medical Physics* (Tobias, C.A. & Lawrence, J.H., eds.) Academic Press, New York: 239–280.

Siri, W.E. (1961) Body composition from fluid spaces and density: Analysis of methods. In: *Techniques for Measuring Body Composition* (Brozek, J. & Henschel, A., eds.) National Academy of Sciences, Washington, DC: 223–244.

Slaughter, M.H., Lohman, T.G., Boileau, R.A., *et al.* (1988) Skinfold equations for estimation of body fatness in children and youth. *Human Biology* 60, 709–723.

Sopher, A.B., Thornton, J.C., Wang, J., Pierson, R.N. Jr., Heymsfield, S.B. & Horlick, M. (2004) Measurement of percentage of body fat in 411 children and adolescents: a comparison of dual-energy X-ray absorptiometry with a four-compartment model. *Pediatrics* 113, 1285–1290.

Srinivasan, S.R., Bao, W., Wattigney, W.A. & Berenson, G.S. (1996) Adolescent overweight is associated with adult overweight and related multiple cardiovascular risk factors: the Bogalusa Heart Study. *Metabolism* **45**, 235–240.

Stout, J.R., Housh, T.J., Johnson, G.O., Housh, D.J., Evans, S.A. & Eckerson, J.M. (1995) Validity of skinfold equations for estimating body density in youth wrestlers. *Medicine and Science in Sports and Exercise* **27**, 1321–1325.

Tcheng, T.K. & Tipton, C.M. (1973) Iowa wrestling study: anthropometric measurements and the prediction of a "minimal" body weight for high school wrestlers. *Medicine and Science in Sports* **5**, 1–10.

Testolin, C.G., Gore, R., Rivkin, T., *et al.* (2000) Dual-energy X-ray absorptiometry: analysis of pediatric fat estimate errors due to tissue hydration effects. *Journal of Applied Physiology* **89**, 2365–2372.

Thorland, W.G., Johnson, G.O., Tharp, G.D., Housh, T.J. & Cisar, C.J. (1984) Estimation of body density in adolescent athletes. *Human Biology* **56**, 439–448.

Thorland, W.G., Tipton, C.M., Lohman, T.G., *et al.* (1991) Midwest wrestling study: prediction of minimal weight for high school wrestlers. *Medicine and Science in Sports and Exercise* **23**, 1102–1110.

Tipton, C.M. & Oppliger, R.A. (1984) The Iowa wrestling study: lessons for physicians. *Iowa Medicine* **74**, 381–385.

Wang, Z.-M., Pierson, R.N. & Heymsfield, S.B. (1992) Extracellular fluid and solids. *American Journal of Clinical Nutrition* **56**, 19–28.

Wells, J.C. (2001) A critique of the expression of paediatric body composition data. *Archives of Disease in Childhood* **85**, 67–72.

Zimmermann, M.B., Gubeli, C., Puntener, C. & Molinari, L. (2004) Detection of overweight and obesity in a national sample of 6–12-y-old Swiss children: accuracy and validity of reference values for body mass index from the US Centers for Disease Control and Prevention and the International Obesity Task Force. *American Journal of Clinical Nutrition* **79**, 838–843.

Chapter 31

Growth and Maturation: Methods of Monitoring

ROBERT M. MALINA AND GASTON BEUNEN

Growth and maturation are related concepts. Growth refers to the increase in the size of the body as a whole or in the size-specific parts or segments of the body from conception to adulthood. Maturation, on the other hand, refers to the tempo and timing of progress towards the mature biologic state. Growth and maturation are target-seeking; the target is the adult or mature state. The processes underlying growth and maturation are quite plastic and respond to a variety of conditions in the environments in which children are reared.

This chapter presents an overview of procedures of monitoring the growth and maturation of children and youth. It is based largely on Malina *et al.* (2004), which contains all of the primary references. Focus is largely on height, weight, and skeletal, sexual, and somatic maturation. Other body dimensions are briefly considered.

Growth

Overall body size

The monitoring of growth of children and youth in the context of sport is most often limited to weight and stature. Body weight is a measure of body mass, which is a composite of independently varying tissues. Stature or standing height is a linear measurement of the distance from the floor or standing surface to the top (vertex) of the skull. It is a composite of linear dimensions contributed by the lower extremities, the trunk, the neck, and the head. Both stature and weight show diurnal variation, which refers to variation in the dimension during

the course of a day. This can be a problem in short-term longitudinal studies, in which apparent changes might simply reflect variation in the time of the day at which the measurement was taken.

Measurements of stature and weight indicate size attained or growth status at a given chronologic age (CA). Hence, it is imperative to have accurate birth dates. The size of a child or a group of children is ordinarily compared with corresponding data derived from a large sample of children free from overt disease. These data, commonly referred to as growth charts, are reference data (i.e., they are the reference of comparison in evaluating the growth status of a child or group of children). Reference data for statures and weights of a nationally representative sample of American children and youth are available at www.cdc.gov/growthcharts.htm (Kuczmarski *et al.* 2000).

Measuring the same child or children at regular intervals over time provides an estimate of growth rate or velocity (i.e., cm·year^{-1} or kg·year^{-1}). Rates of growth vary considerably among children and with season of the year. They are also influenced by the interval between observations.

National reference values for growth rates are not available. Annual velocities for the height and weight and associated percentiles for Swiss (Prader *et al.* 1989), Belgian (Hauspie & Wachholder 1986), Polish (Chrzastek-Spruch *et al.* 1989), Japanese (Suwa *et al.* 1992), and US black and white (Berkey *et al.* 1993) youth are available. Percentiles for 6-monthly increments in stature and weight of US children from the Fels Longitudinal Study are also available (Baumgartner *et al.* 1986).

The use of increments between adjacent ages must be used with care. The rather continuous growth process is overlooked by simply connecting adjacent points and two measurement errors are involved. Distributions of increments also tend to be skewed. In addition, successive increments are negatively related (Van 't Hof *et al.* 1976). Although the use of increments has limitations, when used carefully, they can provide useful information on growth rates.

The pattern of change in stature and weight is generally similar in all children. However, size attained at a given age, rates of growth, and the timing of the adolescent growth spurt vary considerably among children. The smoothed curves of height velocity for US youth include the 3rd, 50th, and 97th percentiles for girls having peak velocity at 9, 11, and 13 years and for boys having peak velocity at 11, 13, and 15 years (Berkey *et al.* 1993). Charts that include adjustments for individual differences in the timing and tempo of the adolescent spurt are called tempo-conditional. The timing of the adolescent spurt is considered in more detail with indicators of maturation.

It has been suggested that the overall pattern of growth in height during childhood is somewhat cyclical, with a mean peak interval of about 2 years in boys and girls (Butler *et al.* 1990). Cycles continue until interrupted by the onset of the adolescent spurt. More recently, variation in growth velocity over very short periods of time (days or weeks) in infants (Lampl *et al.* 1992) and an adolescent boy (Lampl & Johnson 1993) has been demonstrated. Growth in length or height apparently proceeds in a "saltatory" manner with series of stepwise increases or jumps separated by variable periods of no growth (stasis). The superimposition of "mini growth spurts" on a continuous growth pattern has also been suggested (Hermanussen *et al.* 1988).

Other body dimensions

Much of the variation in human morphology during growth and maturation relates to the development of skeletal, muscle, and adipose tissues, as well as the viscera. Thus, in addition to stature and weight, other dimensions taken in the monitoring of growth

often focus on bone, muscle, and fat. Skeletal breadths are taken across specific bone landmarks and therefore provide an indication of the robustness or sturdiness of the skeleton. Skeletal lengths are also taken between specific landmarks, but the most commonly used length measurement, leg length, is ordinarily estimated by subtracting sitting height from stature. Limb circumferences are indicators of relative muscularity. A circumference includes bone, surrounded by a mass of muscle tissue, which is ringed by a layer of subcutaneous fat. Thus, limb circumferences do not provide measures of muscle tissue per se; however, because muscle is the major tissue comprising the circumference, limb circumferences indicate relative muscular development. Skinfold thicknesses are indicators of subcutaneous fat and are measured as a double fold of skin and underlying subcutaneous tissue.

The purpose of a study (i.e., the specific question(s) under consideration) should dictate the dimensions to be measured. Thus, no single battery of measurements will meet the needs of every study. Procedures for taking a variety of measurements are described elsewhere (Lohman *et al.* 1988; Malina *et al.* 2004).

Most body dimensions, with the exception of subcutaneous fat and dimensions of the head and face, follow the same general pattern of growth in size attained and rate as do stature and weight. This general pattern is characteristic of a variety of trunk and extremity dimensions (e.g., lengths, widths, and circumferences) (Beunen *et al.* 1980; Malina & Roche 1983; Roche & Malina 1983; Beunen & Simons 1990). Longitudinal data indicate adolescent spurts in these dimensions (Beunen *et al.* 1988; Gasser *et al.* 1991, 1993) which vary in timing between the sexes and relative to the age at peak height velocity (PHV). Some dimensions also show a mid-growth spurt of lesser intensity (Gasser *et al.* 1991, 1993).

Measurement variability

Implicit in studies utilizing body measurements is the assumption that every effort is made to ensure reliability and accuracy of measurement and standardization of technique. It is assumed that measurements are made by trained observers and that equipment is regularly calibrated. Reliable and accurate data are particularly critical in serial studies, short term or long term, in which the definition of rather small changes is necessary and errors of measurement can mask the true changes. Therefore, quality control and careful monitoring of the measurement process are essential. Duplicate measurements taken independently on the same individual by either the same technician or by two different technicians can be used to estimate measurement error within and between observers. It is not sufficient to indicate that technicians were trained by criterion anthropometrists.

The *technical error of measurement* is a widely used measure of replicability. It is the square root of the sum of the squared differences of replicates divided by twice the number of pairs (i.e., the within-subject variance) (Malina *et al.* 1973):

$$\sigma_e = \sqrt{\Sigma d^2 / 2N}$$

where d is the difference between replicate measurements, and N is the number of pairs of replicates. The statistic assumes that the distribution of replicate differences is normal and that errors of all pairs can be pooled. It indicates that about two-thirds of the time, the measurement in question should fall within ± the technical error of measurement. Examples of within-technician (intraobserver) and between-technician (interobserver) technical errors of measurement are summarized in Malina (1995).

Ratios and proportions

In addition to providing specific information in their own right, measurements can be related to each other in the form of indices or ratios. Thus, ratios provide information on body shape and proportions. Two commonly used ratios are described, although any two measurements can be related to each other.

The relationship between weight and stature is commonly expressed in the form of the *body mass index (BMI)*: weight (kg)/stature (m)^2. Although the BMI grades reasonably well on total body fatness and finds wide use in studies of overweight and obesity, its utility with young athletes is limited and questionable.

The ratio of sitting height to stature, sitting height/height × 100, provides an estimate of relative trunk length, and conversely relative leg length. The ratio decreases from infancy to adolescence and increases slightly in late adolescence. It also shows variation in the proportional contribution of lower extremity length to stature among populations and perhaps among athletes participating in different sports and/or events and positions within a sport.

Maturation

Maturation varies according to the biologic system used, but the more commonly used maturity indicators in growth studies are reasonably well related. They include maturation of the skeleton, sexual maturation, timing of the adolescent growth spurt, and percentage of adult stature attained at a given age.

Skeletal maturation

The bones of the hand and wrist provide the primary basis for assessing skeletal maturation, which is based upon changes in the developing skeleton which can be easily viewed and evaluated on a standardized radiograph. Traditionally, the left hand and wrist is used. The hand is placed flat on the X-ray plate with the fingers slightly apart. Hence, when a film is viewed, the hand-wrist skeleton is observed from the dorsal (posterior) as opposed to the palmar (anterior) surface.

The changes that each bone goes through from initial ossification to adult morphology are fairly uniform and provide the basis for assessing skeletal maturation. These are referred to as *maturity indicators*, specific features of individual bones which can be noted on a hand-wrist X-ray and which occur regularly and in a definite, irreversible order (Greulich & Pyle 1959).

Three methods are available for assessing skeletal maturity of the hand and wrist, the Greulich–Pyle (Greulich & Pyle 1959), Tanner–Whitehouse (Tanner *et al.* 1975, 1983, 2001), and Fels (Roche *et al.* 1988) methods. The authors of each method defined and described specific maturity indicators used to make the assessments.

GREULICH–PYLE METHOD

The Greulich–Pyle (GP) method is based on the original work of Todd (1937) and is sometimes called the atlas or inspectional method. It entails the matching of a hand-wrist X-ray of a specific child as closely as possible with a series of standard X-ray plates, which correspond to successive levels of skeletal maturation at specific chronologic ages. Assessments should be performed bone by bone and the skeletal age (SA) should be based on the median of the SAs assigned to each individual bone of the hand-wrist (there are 29 bones). In practice, however, a GP SA is generally, but improperly, based on the SA of the standard plate to which the film of a child most closely matches, thus excluding variation among bones of the hand-wrist.

TANNER–WHITEHOUSE METHOD

The Tanner–Whitehouse (TW) method, sometimes called the bone-specific approach, entails matching features of 20 individual bones to a series of written criteria for stages through which each bone passes from initial appearance on a radiograph to the mature state. The 20 bones include 7 carpals (excluding the pisiform) and 13 long bones (radius, ulna, and metacarpals and phalanges of the first, third and fifth digits). Each stage has a specific point score. In the first version of the method (TW1), the scores are summed to give a skeletal maturity score, which can be converted to a SA (TW1 20 Bone SA). The TW2 method provides a Carpal SA based on the 7 carpals and a radius, ulna, short bone (RUS) SA, in addition to the 20 Bone SA. The TW3 version provides for separate assessments of the 13 long bones and 7 round bones, but does not provide for a 20 bone skeletal maturity score (sum of scores for 13 long and 7 round bones). Reference samples for TW3 also differ from TW1 and TW2 (see below).

FELS METHOD

The Fels method is based on the same 20 bones as the TW method plus the pisiform and adductor sesamoid. The authors defined their own maturity indicators and specific criteria for each. They are based on a variety of shape changes and ratios of linear width measurements of the diaphyses and epiphyses of the long bones. Grades are assigned to the indicators for each bone by matching the film being assessed to the described criteria. The method uses different bones to estimate SA depending on the age and sex of the child, and provides an SA with a standard error, which provides an estimate of the error inherent in an assessment. The latter is a unique feature which is not available with the other methods. The computation procedure for determining SA in the Fels method weights the contributions of specific indicators depending on age and sex of the child.

COMPARISON OF METHODS

Methods of skeletal maturity assessment are similar in principle. All entail matching a hand-wrist radiograph of a child to a set of criteria: pictorial, verbal, or both. However, the three methods vary in maturity indicators, criteria for making assessments, procedures used to construct a scale of skeletal maturity from which SAs are assigned, and reference samples upon which each method was based.

In the GP method, a child's hand-wrist film is matched to standard plates in the atlas, while in the TW and Fels methods, the child's film is matched to specific criteria for each bone. The Fels method also uses ratios between linear measurements of the long bones. The GP method uses all bones of the hand and wrist (Greulich & Pyle 1959). The TW and Fels methods use 20 bones; however, the Fels method also uses the pisiform and the adductor sesamoid of the first metacarpal.

The GP method assigns an SA based on either on the median of the SA assigned to each individual bone or the standard plate that the film of a child most closely matches. The TW method results in a maturity point score which is based on the sum of the point scores for each of the 20 bones, or for the 7 carpals, or for the 13 long bones. TW3 provides only for carpal and RUS SAs, and the age at attainment of skeletal maturity for the radius, ulna, and short bones was lowered to 15.0 years in girls and 16.5 years in boys (it was 16.0 and 18.2 years, respectively, in TW2). The Fels method provides an SA with a standard error; this is a unique feature which is not available with the GP and TW methods. The computation procedure for determining SA in the Fels method weights the contributions of specific indicators depending on age and sex of the child.

The reference samples upon which each method for the assessment of skeletal maturity is based also differ. The GP method was based on 31 white boys and 29 white girls from the Cleveland area of Ohio born between 1917 and 1942. The sample thus represents the grandparents and great-grandparents of present day children.

The TW method was based on a sample of British children, 1392 boys and 1317 girls from orphanages and public schools, most of whom were born between 1940 and 1955. As noted, the method has had two major revisions. The reference values of TW3 are based on samples of European (British, Belgian, Italian, Spanish), Argentine, Japanese, and well-off US youth from the Houston (Texas) area.

The Fels method is based on 13,823 serial posterior-anterior radiographs of the left hand-wrist of children in the Fels Longitudinal Study, middle class US children from south-central Ohio, studied between 1932 and 1972.

SKELETAL AGE

All of the methods for the estimation of skeletal maturity yield an SA, which corresponds to the level of skeletal maturity attained by a child relative to the reference sample. Given the differences in the methods as well as in the reference samples for each, the skeletal maturity status of a child rated by all three methods may be quite different. It is important that the method used to estimate SA be specified.

SA is expressed relative to a child's chronologic age (CA). It may simply be compared to CA (e.g., a child's CA is 10.5 years while his or her SA is 12.3 years). In this instance, the child has attained the skeletal maturity equivalent to that of a child of 12.3 years, and is advanced in skeletal maturity. Or, a child's CA may be 10.5 years but his or her SA is 9.0 years. The child is chronologically 10.5 years of age, while he or she has only attained the skeletal maturity of a 9-year-old child; this child is late in skeletal maturity. SA may also be expressed as the difference between SA and CA (i.e., SA – CA).

Thus, in the first example given above, $12.3 - 10.5 = +1.8$ years, while in the second example, $9.0 - 10.5 = -1.5$ years. Skeletal maturity is advanced in the former by 1.8 years and is late in the latter by 1.5 years relative to CA.

SA assessment is basically a method to estimate the level of maturity that a child has attained at a given point in time relative to reference data for healthy children. The three methods for assessing skeletal maturity have their strengths and limitations. SAs derived from the GP, TW, and Fels methods as well as from each version of the TW method are not equivalent. The methods differ in criteria and scoring, and the reference samples upon which they are based. There also is population variation in skeletal maturation (Malina *et al.* 2004). Changes in each bone from initial formation to epiphyseal union or adult morphology are the same; the rate at which the specific changes progress varies among populations.

Sexual maturation

The assessment of sexual maturation is based upon the development of the secondary sex characteristics (i.e., breast development and menarche in girls, penis and testes (genital) development in boys, and pubic hair in both sexes). The use of secondary sex characteristics as indicators is obviously limited to the pubertal or adolescent phase of growth and maturation.

BREAST, GENITAL, AND PUBIC HAIR DEVELOPMENT

The development of secondary sex characteristics is ordinarily summarized into scales of five stages or grades for each character. The most commonly used criteria for pubic hair, breast, and genital maturation are those described by Tanner (1962). Stage 1 indicates the prepubertal state (i.e., the absence of development of each characteristic). Male genitalia, for example, are approximately the same size as in early childhood. Stage 2 indicates the initial development of each characteristic (i.e., the initial elevation of the breasts in girls, the initial enlargement of the genitals in boys, and the initial appearance of pubic hair in both sexes). Stages 3 and 4 indicate continued maturation of each characteristic, and are somewhat more difficult to evaluate. Stage 5 indicates the adult or mature state of development for each characteristic. Stages of breast, genital, and pubic hair development are readily available in textbooks of physical growth (Tanner 1962; Malina *et al.* 2004). Excellent color illustrations of the stages are available in the national survey of Dutch children (Roede & Van Wieringen 1985). The photographs are accompanied by schematic illustrations and descriptive criteria in Malina *et al.* (2004).

Ratings of the stages of sexual maturation are ordinarily made by direct observation at clinical examination. As such, these ratings have limitations because the method requires invasion of the individual's privacy which is a matter of concern for many adolescents. At times, evaluations are made from standardized, nude photographs of high quality. As good as the photographs may be it is often quite difficult to detect the initial appearance of pubic hair. For example, commonly used reference data from the Harpenden Growth Study of British youth (Marshall & Tanner 1969, 1970) have somewhat later ages for stage 2 of pubic hair development. This high value reflects the difficulty in detecting first appearance of pubic hair on photographs. Clinical observation gives better estimates.

There is need for quality control in assessment of secondary sex characteristics. How concordant are assessments made by two different examiners or by the same examiner on two independent occasions? Such data are rarely reported.

In practice ratings are used as follows. A girl, for example, may be rated as in stage 2 of breast development (B2) and stage 1 for pubic hair (PH1). Thus, breast development has begun, while pubic hair has not yet appeared. This girl is just in the beginning of puberty, because the budding or initial elevation of the breasts (B2) is most often the first overt sign of sexual maturation in girls. Similarly in males, a boy may be rated in stage 2 of genital development (G2) and stage 1 for pubic hair (PH1). He is likewise just beginning puberty, because the initial enlargement of the testes (G2) is most often the first overt sign of sexual maturation in boys.

It should be noted that the development of secondary sex characteristics is a continuous process upon which the stages are superimposed. Thus, the five stages are somewhat arbitrary. For example, a boy just entering G3 of genital development is rated the same as a boy nearing the end of G3 (i.e., they are both rated as being in G3). The latter boy is really more advanced in maturation than the former, but given the limitations of the procedure, both are rated as being in G3.

It is common in the pediatric literature to refer to the assessment of secondary sex characteristics as "Tanner staging." This is erroneous. Secondary sex characteristics are assessed using the criteria of Tanner. Further, the stages of pubertal development are specific to breasts, genitals, and pubic hair. It is incorrect, for example, to take the average of breast and pubic hair stages to characterize the level of sexual maturation of a girl or group of girls. In a related issue, individuals should not be assessed as being in "puberty stage 2" or in "Tanner stage 3"; the specific secondary sex characteristic and its stage should be noted (e.g., genital stage 4 [G4] or pubic hair stage 3 [PH3]).

A more direct estimate of genital maturation in males is provided by measurements of testicular volume. It is estimated from the size of the testes using a series of models of known volume which have the shape of the testes (Prader orchidometer). Application of the models requires direct manipulation of the testes at clinical examination as the physician attempts to match the size of the testis with the ellipsoid model that most closely matches it. This procedure, although quite useful, has limited utility in surveys. It is most often used clinically to evaluate boys with extremely late maturation or disorders of growth and sexual maturation.

SELF-REPORTED ASSESSMENT OF SECONDARY SEX CHARACTERISTICS

Given the difficulty in direct assessment of sexual maturation status in non-medical settings, self-assessments by youth are often used. Youth are asked to rate their stage of sexual development relative to schematic illustrations and/or photographs of stages of breast, genital, and/or pubic hair development. The quality of schematic illustrations and photographs varies among studies.

There are limited data on the concordance of self-ratings of youth and those of experienced assessors. Correlations between self-ratings and physician ratings of breast and pubic hair were moderate, ranging from 0.52 to 0.74 (Brooks-Gunn *et al.* 1987; Matsudo & Matsudo 1994). Some data suggest a tendency for youngsters to overestimate early stages and underestimate later stages of pubertal development (Schlossberger *et al.* 1992). The reproducibility of clinical assessments by physicians or other experienced raters is not generally reported, when in fact it should be.

If self-assessments are used, good quality photographs of the stages with simplified descriptions should be used (for a combination of photos and schematic illustrations of each stage see Malina *et al.* 2004). Self-assessments should not be used in a group setting. Rather, they should be carried out individually in a quiet room after careful explanation of the purpose of the assessment.

MENARCHE

Menarche, the first menstrual period, is the most commonly reported indicator of female puberty. Significant value judgments are associated with the attainment of menarche in many cultures. There is no corresponding physiologic event in the sexual maturation process of boys, although the psychologic importance of puberty in boys cannot be overlooked.

Age at menarche can be estimated in three ways: longitudinally (prospective), status quo, and retrospectively. In longitudinal studies, the girl or her mother is interviewed on each occasion whether menarche has or has not occurred; if it occurred, the girl or her mother is asked when. Given that the interval between examinations in most longitudinal studies is relatively short, age at menarche so derived is quite reliable. The method provides an estimate for individual girls. However, sample sizes in longitudinal studies are not ordinarily large enough to derive population estimates and may not reflect the normal range of variation.

The status quo method provides an estimate and range of variation for a sample or population. A representative sample of girls 9–17 years of age is surveyed. Two pieces of information are required: first, the exact age of each girl, and second, whether or not she has attained menarche (i.e., yes or no). Probits or logits for the percentage of girls who have attained menarche in each age group are plotted and a straight line is fitted to the points. The point at which the line intersects 50% is the estimated median age at menarche for the sample; the method also provides confidence intervals.

The prospective and status quo methods are also used to estimate ages for the attainment of each stage of pubic hair, breast, and genital development. These estimates indicate the ages at which a child is in a particular stage and do not necessarily indicate when the stage began. Estimates of the duration of an age require longitudinal data.

In contrast to the status quo method for estimating the age at menarche, many studies use the retrospective method, which requires the girl to recall the age at which she attained menarche. If the interview is performed at close intervals as in longitudinal studies, the method is quite accurate. If it is performed some time after menarche, it is affected by error in recall. However, with careful interview procedures (e.g., attempting to place the event in the context of a season or event of the school year or holiday) reasonably accurate estimates of the age at menarche can be obtained from most adolescents and young adults. Data on ages at menarche in athletes are largely obtained with the retrospective method, and as such, have a margin of error. Prospective and status quo data for young athletes in a variety of sports are limited (Malina *et al.* 2004).

GONADOTROPIC AND GONADAL HORMONES

The use of circulating levels of gonadotropic (follicle-stimulating hormone and luteinizing hormone) and gonadal (estrogens in females and testosterone in males) hormones is occasionally suggested as a maturity indicator. Single serum samples have extremely limited utility in this regard because virtually all hormones are episodically secreted. Studies in which 24-h levels of hormones are monitored or in which actual pulses of the hormones are sampled every 20 min or so are needed to provide a more accurate indication of a child's hormonal status. Further, the simple presence of a hormone does not necessarily imply that it is physiologically active. Variation in the responsiveness of hormone receptors at the tissue level is an additional factor.

Somatic maturation

The use of stature as an indicator of maturity requires longitudinal data that span the adolescent years. This permits estimates of the timing and tempo of the adolescent growth spurt. If adult stature is available, the percentage of mature or adult size attained at different ages during growth can also be used as a maturity indicator.

PEAK HEIGHT VELOCITY

PHV refers to the maximum rate of growth in height during the adolescent spurt, and the age when PHV occurs is an indicator of somatic maturity. Longitudinal data are necessary to estimate age at PHV and related parameters of the adolescent growth. The spurt in stature refers to the acceleration in stature which in boys begins at about 10–11 years, peaks at about 14 years, and stops at about 18 years. In girls the spurt starts at about 9–10 years, peaks at about 12 years, and stops at about 16 years.

There is an earlier mid-growth spurt in height at 6.5–8.5 years in many children. This spurt is much smaller and some evidence suggests that it also occurs in other body dimensions. A sex difference in the timing of the maximum velocity of the mid-growth spurt is not apparent, but the spurt occurs more frequently in boys than in girls (Gasser et al. 1985; Tanner & Cameron 1980; Sheehy et al. 1999). Not all children show a mid-growth spurt, which may reflect normal biologic variability, the frequency of and interval between measurements, and/or methods of estimation.

Fitting growth curves to individual growth records is indicated for estimation of velocities and accelerations, and in turn, for calculation of the timing and magnitude of the spurt, although it is not the only approach to the analyses of longitudinal growth data (Goldstein 1979). Several models have been described and new models are being proposed to quantify individual growth. However, most models

have been developed for statural growth. In fitting mathematical models to growth curves for height a distinction has to be made between structural models and polynomials (Marubini 1978; Hauspie & Chrzastek-Spruch 1999). The former have a pre-selected form of the growth curve and the parameters or constants of the function have biologic meaning. Structural models include the Gompertz function; single, double, and triple logistic functions; the Preece–Baines family of growth functions; and a number of others. Although the use of polynomials has been severely criticized, several applications have been useful for describing growth over large age periods and characteristics with no uniform continuous increase. These applications include moving polynomials, cubic splines, and kernel estimations.

Regardless of the model used, curve fitting provides a convenient means of characterizing and comparing individual or group differences in adolescent growth in a biologically meaningful manner (Beunen & Malina 1988; Malina et al. 2004). The parameter of the fitted curve relevant to the estimation of maturity status is the age at PHV. Fitted curves also provide an estimate of peak velocity of growth at this time. Ages at PHV, peak velocity of growth, and other parameters of the growth spurt for samples of European and North American adolescents are summarized in Malina et al. (2004). Girls are advanced, on average, about 2 years in ages at onset of the spurt and at PHV. The magnitude of the spurt is generally smaller in girls than in boys, although the difference is not so large as the differences in mean ages at take-off and PHV. Standard deviations around the mean ages are about 1 year or a little more in most studies. This indicates considerable variation among individuals in the timing of the adolescent spurt and also in the magnitude. Within the range of normal variation, an early maturing girl can experience her PHV at the age of 9.5 years, whereas a late maturing girl can experience the same milestone at the age of 13.9 years (Malina et al. 2004).

Age at PHV is an indicator when maximum growth occurs during the adolescent spurt. It also serves as a landmark against which attained sizes and velocities of other body dimensions, physical performance, and the development of secondary sex characteristics can be expressed. Menarche, for example, occurs after PHV in girls, while peak strength development occurs after PHV in boys. The relationship of performance to age PHV is discussed in more detail in Beunen and Malina (see Chapter 1; Malina *et al.* 2004).

Some of the models that have been used to describe height growth have also been applied to other body dimensions. Ages at peak velocity in other body dimensions are most often related to the age at PHV to demonstrate the sequence of changes occurring during the adolescent spurt. The available evidence for external body dimensions can be summarized as follows. Maximum velocity in body weight (PWV) generally occurs after PHV, and standard deviations of age at PWV are about 1 year. Peak velocity for leg length occurs earlier than PHV, while peak velocity for trunk length or sitting height occurs after PHV. Rapid growth in lower extremities is characteristic of the early part of the adolescent growth spurt (Malina *et al.* 2004).

MATURITY OFFSET

A method for predicting time from PHV (maturity offset, years) has also been developed as a maturity indicator (Mirwald *et al.* 2002). The method requires age, height, sitting height, leg length (height minus sitting height), weight : height ratio, weight (girls only), and interaction terms. Maturity offset has been cross-validated in a sample of Belgian children (Mirwald *et al.* 2002). The method has been used in studies of physical activity (Thompson *et al.* 2003) and bone mineral accrual in female gymnasts (Nurmi-Lawton *et al.* 2004). The addition or subtraction of maturity offset to CA provides a predicted age at PHV. However, there is a need for cross-validation of predicted ages at PHV (i.e., difference between the predicted age at PHV and a criterion age at PHV based on individually fitted longitudinal records of height).

PERCENTAGE OF MATURE (ADULT) STATURE

Another indicator of somatic maturity is the percentage of mature stature attained at a given age.

Children who are closer to their mature stature compared to other children of the same chronologic age are advanced in maturity status. For example, two 7-year-old boys have attained the same stature, 122 cm. For one of the boys this stature accounts for 72% of his adult stature, while for the other, it accounts for only 66% of his adult stature. The former is closer to the mature state (i.e., maturationally advanced, compared to the latter). Percentage of mature stature is based on size attained, and is thus the result of variation in tempo of growth and is not an indicator of tempo per se as is age at PHV. In other words, a child who reaches PHV early is also closer to adult size, while a child who reaches PHV later is also farther from adult size.

Estimates of the percentage of mature stature attained at a given age during growth require longitudinal data. As such, this maturity indicator has limited utility. However, it may have some application if a child's stature at the time of examination is expressed as a percentage of his or her predicted mature stature. Such an approach may be useful in distinguishing youngsters who are tall at a given age because they are genetically tall or who are tall because they are maturationally advanced compared to their peers (i.e., they have attained a greater percentage of their predicted adult stature at a given chronologic age).

Three methods are commonly used to predict mature stature: the Bailey–Pinneau (BP; Bailey & Pinneau 1952; Bayer & Bayley 1959), Roche, Wainer and Thissen (RWT; Roche *et al.* 1975a,b), and Tanner–Whitehouse (TWSP; Tanner *et al.* 1983, 2001) methods. TWSP (Tanner–Whitehouse stature prediction) is used to distinguish it from the TW method for the assessment of skeletal maturity.

The BP method utilizes stature and GP SA, and provides an estimate of the percentage of adult stature. The RWT method uses CA, recumbent length (not stature), weight, mid-parent stature (stature of the mother and father divided by 2), and GP SA (based on median bone specific SAs) to predict stature at 18 years of age. The RWT method has been modified for use with SAs based on the Fels method (Khamis & Guo 1993) and also for use when SA is not available (Roche *et al.* 1983; Khamis & Roche 1994). Parental statures provide a target range for the mature height of their child, and mature stature can be predicted from current age, height and weight, and mid-parent height. A protocol for the prediction of mature height in adolescent boys 12.5–16.5 years of age that does not include SA has also been developed (Beunen *et al.* 1997). Mature height is predicted from age, height, sitting height, and the subscapular and triceps skinfolds. Prediction methods that do not require an estimate of SA have potential for application in youth sport (Malina *et al.* 2005).

The TWSP method utilizes RUS maturity scores (see above). In girls below 7.0 years and boys below 10.0 years, prediction of mature height is based on CA and current height. Thereafter, prediction of mature height is based on RUS maturity scores and current height. Different equations are used for pre- and post-menarcheal girls. Inclusion of the height increment for the previous year reduces the standard error of the prediction (Tanner *et al.* 2001).

All predictions have an associated error, usually within the range of 3–5 cm. The error may be larger and all prediction models occasionally have outlying predictions. Individual differences in the timing and tempo of the growth spurt and error associated with the assessment of SA contribute to the variation among methods. Systematic errors may occur in prediction of mature height when the three methods are applied to the same individual (Roemmich *et al.* 1997). Accuracy of estimates of mature height may be somewhat less for short children or for children with short parents (Maes *et al.* 1997; Luo *et al.* 1998) and for children with delayed growth and puberty (Bramswig *et al.* 1990). The issue of height prediction of short children is relevant to gymnasts of both sexes who have the characteristics of short, normal, late maturing children with short parents (see Chapter 1; Malina 1999).

Interrelationships among maturity indicators

Biologic maturation is often discussed in terms of status and timing. Status refers to the state of maturation of the individual at a given point in time; timing refers to when specific maturational events occur. Indicators of maturity status include skeletal age; stage of breast, pubic hair and/or genital development; prepubertal vs. pubertal; premenarcheal vs. menarcheal; and percentage of mature height attained at a given age. Indicators of maturational timing include age at menarche, age at attaining a specific stage of breast, pubic hair and/or genital development; age at PHV; and maturity offset. An additional concern is tempo of maturation (i.e., the pace at which biologic maturation proceeds). Estimates of tempo require longitudinal data.

Two questions are important when using different maturity indicators. The first deals with relationships among indicators (i.e., do they measure the same kind of biologic maturity?) The second relates to the consistency of maturity ratings over time (i.e., is a child who is maturationally late at, for example, 6 years of age, also late at 11 years of age?) The same question can be asked of those advanced and average in maturity status.

The issue of interrelationships is complex because only skeletal maturation spans childhood through adolescence, while indicators of sexual maturation and age at PHV are limited to the pubertal period. Further, evidence suggests that prepubertal growth and maturation may be somewhat independent of pubertal growth and maturation. For example, a cluster analysis of indicators of *sexual* (ages at attaining genital and pubic hair stages 2 and 4); *skeletal* (skeletal maturity at 11–15 years of age); and *somatic* (ages at peak velocity for stature, weight, leg length, and trunk length; age at initiation of the stature spurt; ages at attaining 80%, 90%, 95%, and 99% of adult stature) maturity among 111 Polish boys who were followed longitudinally from 8 to 18 years of age (Bielicki *et al.* 1984) indicated two clusters. The first was a general maturity factor during adolescence. Ages at peak velocities and at attainment of stages of sexual maturation, SAs at 14 and 15 years, ages at attaining 90%, 95%, and 99% of mature stature, and age at initiation of the stature spurt all clustered together. Such a general maturity factor suggests that the tempo of maturation during adolescence is under common control. The second cluster concerned late prepubertal growth and maturation and the transition into adolescence. It included SAs at 11, 12, and 13 years and age at attaining 80% of mature stature, and was independent of the other maturity indicators. Similar analyses of the patterns of relationships among maturity indicators in Polish girls and in other longitudinal studies have produced generally similar results (Nicolson & Hanley 1953; Bielicki 1975).

There is thus a general maturity factor that underlies growth and maturation during adolescence. This factor appears to discriminate among individuals who are early, average, or late in the timing of adolescent events. However, there is variation among maturity indicators, which suggests that no single system, sexual, skeletal, or somatic, provides a complete description of the tempo of growth and maturation of an individual boy or girl during adolescence. This is related to the observation that there is no consistent relationship between the age at which a specific stage of a secondary sex characteristic develops and the rate of progress from one stage to the next. Some boys may pass from genital stages G2 through G5 in about 2 years, while others may take about 5 years (Malina et al. 2004).

Part of the variation in such analyses is caused by the methods used to assess maturation. The five grade scales for rating secondary sex characteristics are somewhat arbitrary. Different intervals between observations among studies also contribute to the variable results. Methods of estimating ages at peak velocities and ages at attainment of specific stages of sexual and skeletal maturation also differ. Measurement variation is an additional contributing factor.

The independence of prepubertal growth from the events of adolescence raises the question of maturity indicators during childhood. Skeletal maturation is the primary indicator for the prepubertal years and, if longitudinal data are available, the percentage of adult stature may be useful. Relationships between skeletal maturity and the attained percentage of adult stature are moderately high and positive during the prepubertal years. Children advanced in SA are, on average, closer to adult stature at all ages during childhood and adolescence than those who are delayed in SA relative to CA. In late adolescence, catch-up of those later in skeletal maturation occurs. The child who is advanced in skeletal maturation attains adult stature earlier and thus stops growing earlier, while the child later in skeletal maturation attains adult stature later and grows over a longer period of time.

On average, both groups attain similar adult statures, but one attains it more rapidly than the other.

Although processes of maturation during prepuberty and puberty are somewhat independent, indicators of sexual and somatic maturity are positively related with each other during puberty (Malina et al. 2004). Correlations are moderate to high, which suggests that youngsters early or late in sexual maturation are, respectively, early or late in the timing of the adolescent growth spurt in stature. Similarly, if the youngster is early or late in the appearance of one indicator of sexual maturation, he or she is early or late, respectively, in the appearance of the others. The correlations, although reasonably consistent across studies, are not perfect, which suggests variation in timing of somatic and sexual maturation.

Skeletal maturity is also related to the development of secondary sex characteristics and PHV. Variation in SA is considerably reduced at menarche and PHV in girls and boys, respectively (Marshall 1974; Hauspie et al. 1991). However, that SA may vary as much as CA at the onset of sexual maturation in girls and the growth spurt in stature (take off) in boys, but as sexual maturation and the growth spurt proceed, skeletal maturity becomes more strongly related to these maturational events.

Challenges in future research

The following are suggested as areas that need further study and application:

• Refinement of non-invasive methods for the assessment of maturity status. Methods and the criteria need to be standardized.

• The use of predicted mature stature as an indicator of maturity status needs to be further explored, especially methods that do not require an estimate of SA.

• Cross-validation of predicted age at PHV from maturity offset with criterion estimates of age at PHV from individually fitted longitudinal height records.

• Evaluation of the influence of measurement variability (error) on various predictions. For example, estimated leg length is derived as height minus sitting height. Hence, two measurements and associated errors are involved.

- Routinely measure parental statures and incorporate these into the evaluation of growth and maturity status. Reported statures, although useful, have limitations.
- Regularly update reference values for both size-attained and growth rate (velocity), and implement them in both clinical and sport science research.

- Improve designs of longitudinal studies of sufficient duration to better understand the adolescent spurt and sexual maturation, and incorporate appropriate analytical strategies.
- Undertake further short-term longitudinal studies to better understand saltatory growth versus continuous mini-growth spurt.

References

Baumgartner, R.N., Roche, A.F. & Himes, J.H. (1986) Incremental growth tables: supplementary to previously published charts. *American Journal of Clinical Nutrition* **43**, 711–722.

Bayer, L.M. & Bayley, N. (1959) *Growth Diagnosis: Selected Methods for Interpreting and Predicting Development from One Year to Maturity.* University of Chicago Press, Chicago.

Bayley, N. & Pinneau, S.R. (1952) Tables for predicting adult height from skeletal age: revised for use with the Greulich–Pyle hand standards. *Journal of Pediatrics* **40**, 423–441.

Berkey, C.A., Dockery, D.W., Wang, X., Wypij, D. & Ferris, B. (1993) Longitudinal height velocity standards for US adolescents. *Statistics in Medicine* **12**, 403–414.

Beunen, G. & Malina, R.M. (1988) Growth and physical performance relative to the timing of the adolescent spurt. *Exercise and Sport Science Reviews* **16**, 503–540.

Beunen, G.P., Malina, R.M., Lefevre, J., Claessens, A.L., Renson, R. & Simons, J. (1997) Prediction of adult stature and noninvasive assessment of biological maturation. *Medicine and Science in Sports and Exercise* **29**, 225–230.

Beunen, G.P., Malina, R.M., Van't Hof, M.A. *et al.* (1988) *Adolescent Growth and Motor Performance. A longitudinal Study of Belgian Boys.* HKP Sport Science Monographs Series. Human Kinetics, Champaign, IL.

Beunen, G., Simons, J., Renson, R., Van Gerven, D. & Ostyn, M. (1980) Growth curves for anthropometric and motor components. In: *Somatic and Motor Development of Belgian Secondary Schoolboys. Norms and Standards* (Ostyn, M., Simons, J., Beunen, G., Renson, R. & Van Gerven, D., eds.) Leuven University Press, Leuven.

Beunen, G.P. & Simons, J. (1990) Physical growth, maturation and performance. In: *Growth and Fitness of Flemish Girls. The Leuven Growth Study.* HKP Sport Science Monographs Series. (Simons, J., Beunen, G.P., Renson, R., Claessens, A.L.M., Vanreusel, B. & Lefevre, J.A.V., eds.) Human Kinetics, Champaign, IL.

Bielicki, T. (1975) Interrelationships between various measures of maturation rate in girls during adolescence. *Studies in Physical Anthropology* **1**, 51–64.

Bielicki, T., Koniarek, J. & Malina, R.M. (1984) Interrelationships among certain measures of growth and maturation rate in boys during adolescence. *Annals of Human Biology* **11**, 201–210.

Bramswig, J.H., Fasse, M., Holthoff, M.-L., van Lengerke, H.J., van Petrykowski, W. & Schellong, G. (1990) Adult height in boys and girls with untreated short stature and constitutional delay of growth and puberty: Accuracy of five different methods of height prediction. *Journal of Pediatrics* **117**, 886–891.

Brooks-Gunn, J., Warren, M.P., Rosso, J. & Gargiulo, J. (1987) Validity of self-report measures of girls' pubertal status. *Child Development* **58**, 829–841.

Butler, G.E., McKie, M. & Ratcliffe, S.G. (1990) The cyclical nature of prepubertal growth. *Annals of Human Biology* **17**, 177–198.

Chrzastek-Spruch, H., Susanne, C., Hauspie, R. & Kozlowska, M.A. (1989) Individual growth patterns and standards for height and height velocity based on the Lublin (Poland) Longitudinal Growth Study. In: *Auxology '88: Perspectives in the Science of Growth and Development* (Tanner, J.M., ed.) Smith-Gordon, London: 161–166.

Gasser, T., Kneip, A., Ziegler, P., Largo, R., Molinari, L. & Prader, A. (1991) The dynamics of growth of width in distance, velocity and acceleration. *Annals of Human Biology* **18**, 449–461.

Gasser, T., Müller, H.G., Köhler, W., Prader, A., Largo, R. & Molinari, L. (1985) Analysis of the midgrowth and adolescent spurts in height based on acceleration. *Annals of Human Biology* **12**, 129–149.

Gasser, T., Ziegler, P., Kneip, A., Prader, A., Molinari, L. & Largo, R.H. (1993) The dynamics of growth of weight, circumferences and skinfolds in distance, velocity and acceleration. *Annals of Human Biology* **20**, 239–259.

Goldstein, H. (1979) *The Design and Analysis of Longitudinal Studies.* Academic Press, London.

Greulich, W.W. & Pyle, S.I. (1959) *Radiographic Atlas of Skeletal Development of the Hand and Wrist,* 2nd edn. Stanford University Press, Stanford, CA.

Hauspie, R., Bielicki, T. & Koniarek, J. (1991) Skeletal maturity at onset of the adolescent growth spurt and at peak velocity for growth in height: a threshold effect. *Annals of Human Biology* **18**, 23–29.

Hauspie, R. & Chrzastek-Spruch, H. (1999) Growth models: Possibilities and limitations. In: *Human Growth in Context* (Johnston, F.E., Eveleth, P.B. & Zemel, B., eds.) Smith-Gordon, London: 15–24.

Hauspie, R.C. & Wachholder, A. (1986) Clinical standards for growth velocity in height of Belgian boys and girls, aged 2 to 18 years. *International Journal of Anthropology* **1**, 339–348.

Hemanussen, M., Geiger-Benoit, K., Burmeister, J. & Sippel, W.G. (1988) Periodical changes of short term growth velocity ("mini growth spurts") in human growth. *Annals of Human Biology* **15**, 103–109.

Khamis, H.J. & Guo, S. (1993) Improvement in the Roche–Wainer–Thissen stature prediction model: A comparative study. *American Journal of Human Biology* **5**, 669–679.

Khamis, H.J. & Roche, A.F. (1994) Predicting adult stature without using skeletal age: The Khamis–Roche method. *Pediatrics* **94**, 504–507. [Errata in *Pediatrics* (1995) **95**, 457.]

Kuczmarski, R.J., Ogden, C.L., Grummer-Strawn, L.M., *et al.* (2000) *CDC growth charts: United States.*

Advance Data from Vital and Health Statistics, no. 314. National Center for Health Statistics, Hyattsville, MD (www.cdc.gov/growthcharts.htm).

Lampl, M. & Johnson, M.L. (1993) A case study of daily growth during adolescence: A single spurt or changes in the dynamics of saltatory growth? *Annals of Human Biology* **20**, 595–603.

Lampl, M., Veldhuis, J.D. & Johnson, M.L. (1992) Saltation and stasis: a model of human growth. *Science* **258**, 801–803.

Lohman, T.G., Roche, A.F., & Martorell, R., eds. (1988) *Anthropometric Standardization Reference Manual*. Human Kinetics, Champaign, IL.

Luo, Z.C., Albertaaon-Wikland, K. & Karlberg, J. (1998) Target height as predicted by parental heights in a population study. *Pediatric Research* **44**, 563–571.

Maes, M., Vandeweghe, M., Du Caju, M., Ernould, C., Bourguignon, J.-P. & Massa, G. (1997) A valuable improvement of adult height prediction methods in short normal children. *Hormone Research* **48**, 184–190.

Malina, R.M. (1995) Anthropometry. In: *Physiological Assessment of Human Fitness* (Maud, P.J. & Foster, C., eds.) Human Kinetics, Champaign, IL: 205–219.

Malina, R.M. (1999) Growth and maturation of elite female gymnasts: is training a factor? In: *Human Growth in Context* (Johnston, F.E., Zemel, B. & Eveleth, P.B. eds.). Smith-Gordon, London: 291–301.

Malina, R.M., Bouchard, C. & Bar-Or, O. (2004) *Growth, Maturation and Physical Activity*, 2nd edn. Human Kinetics, Champaign, IL.

Malina, R.M., Cumming, S.P., Morano, P.J., Barron, M. & Miller, S.J. (2005) Maturity status of youth football players: A noninvasive estimate. *Medicine and Science in Sports and Exercise* **37**, 1044–1052.

Malina, R.M., Hamill, P.V.V. & Lemeshow, S. (1973) Selected body measurements of children 6–11 years. *Vital and Health Statistics*, Series 11, No. 123.

Malina, R.M. & Roche, A.F. (1983) *Manual of Physical Status and Performance in Childhood*, Vol. 2. Plenum, New York.

Marshall, W.A. (1974) Interrelationships of skeletal maturation, sexual development and somatic growth in man. *Annals of Human Biology* **1**, 29–40.

Marshall, W.A. & Tanner, J.M. (1969) Variations in pattern of pubertal changes in girls. *Archives of Disease in Childhood* **44**, 291–303.

Marshall, W.A. & Tanner, J.M. (1970)

Variations in the pattern of pubertal changes in boys. *Archives of Disease in Childhood* **45**, 13–23.

Marubini, E. (1978) Mathematical handling of long-term longitudinal data. In: *Human Growth*. Vol. 1. *Principles and Prenatal Growth* (Falkner, F. & Tanner, J.M., eds.) Plenum Press, New York: 209–225.

Matsudo, S.M.M. & Matsudo, V.K.R. (1994) Self-assessment and physician assessment of sexual maturation in Brazilian boys and girls: Concordance and reproducibility. *American Journal of Human Biology* **6**, 451–455.

Mirwald, R.L., Baxter-Jones, A.D.G., Bailey, D.A. & Beunen, G.P. (2002) An assessment of maturity from anthropometric measurements. *Medicine and Science in Sports and Exercise* **34**, 689–694.

Nicolson, A.B. & Hanley, C. (1953) Indices of physiological maturity: derivation and interrelationships. *Child Development* **24**, 3–38.

Nurmi-Lawton, J.A., Baxter-Jones, A.D.G. & Mirwald, R.L. (2004) Evidence of sustained skeletal benefits from impact-loading exercise in young females: A 3 year longitudinal study. *Journal of Bone and Mineral Research* **19**, 314–322.

Prader, A., Largo, R.H., Molinari, L., & Issler, C. (1989) Physical growth of Swiss children from birth to 20 years of age. Helvetica Paediatrica Acta, suppl. 52.

Roche, A.F., Chumlea, W.C. & Thissen, D. (1988) *Assessing the Skeletal Maturity of the Hand-Wrist: Fels Method*. C.C. Thomas, Springfield, IL.

Roche, A.F. & Malina, R.M. (1983) *Manual of Physical Status and Performance in Childhood*, Vol. 1. Plenum, New York.

Roche, A.F., Tyleshevski, F. & Rogers, E. (1983) Non-invasive measurement of physical maturity in children. *Research Quarterly for Exercise and Sport* **54**, 364–371.

Roche, A.F., Wainer, H. & Thissen, D. (1975a) *Predicting Adult Stature for Individuals*. Monographs in Paediatrics 3. Karger, Basel.

Roche, A.F., Wainer, H. & Thissen, D. (1975b) The RWT method for the prediction of adult stature. *Pediatrics* **56**, 1026–1033.

Roede, M.U. & van Wieringen, J.C. (1985) Growth diagrams 1980: Netherlands Third Nationwide survey. *Tijdschrift voor Sociale Gezondheidszorg* **63** (Supplement 1), 1–34.

Roemmich, J.N., Blizzard, R.M., Peddada, S.D. *et al.* (1997) Longitudinal assessment of hormonal and physical alterations during normal puberty in boys. IV. Predictions of adult height by the Bayley-Pinneau, Roche-Wainer-Thissen and Tanner-Whitehouse methods compared. *American Journal of Human Biology* **9**, 371–380.

Schlossberger, N.M., Turner, R.A. & Irwin, C.E. (1992) Validity of self-report of pubertal maturation in early adolescents. *Journal of Adolescent Health* **13**, 109–113.

Sheehy, A., Gasser, T., Molinari, L. & Largo, R. (1999) An analysis of variance of the pubertal and midgrowth spurts for length and width. *Annals of Human Biology* **26**, 309–331.

Suwa, S., Tachibana, K., Maesaka, H., Tanaka, T. & Yokoya, S. (1992) Longitudinal standards for height and height velocity for Japanese children from birth to maturity. *Clinical Pediatrics and Endocrinology* **1**, 5–13.

Tanner, J.M. (1962) *Growth at Adolescence*, 2nd edition. Blackwell, Oxford.

Tanner, J.M. & Cameron, N. (1980) Investigation of the mid-growth spurt in height, weight and limb circumference in single-year velocity data from the London 1966–67 growth survey. *Annals of Human Biology* **8**, 495–517.

Tanner, J.M., Healy, M.J.R., Goldstein, H. & Cameron, N. (2001) *Assessment of Skeletal Maturity and Prediction of Adult Height (TW3 Method)*, 3rd edn. Saunders, London.

Tanner, J.M., Whitehouse, R.H., Cameron, N., Marshall, W.A., Healy, M.J.R. & Goldstein, H. (1983) *Assessment of Skeletal Maturity and Prediction of Adult Height*, 2nd edn. Academic Press, New York.

Tanner, J.M., Whitehouse, R.H., Marshall, W.A., Healy, M.J.R. & Goldstein, H. (1975) *Assessment of Skeletal Maturity and Prediction of Adult Height (TW 2 Method)*. Academic Press, New York.

Thompson, A.M., Baxter-Jones, A.D.G., Mirwald, R.L. & Bailey, D.A. (2003) Comparison of physical activity in male and female children: Does maturation matter? *Medicine and Science in Sports and Exercise* **35**, 1684–1690.

Todd, T.W. (1937) *Atlas of Skeletal Maturation*. Mosby, St. Louis, MO.

Van't Hof, M.A., Roede, M.J. & Kowalski, C.J. (1976) Estimation of growth velocities from individual longitudinal data. *Growth* **40**, 217–240.

Chapter 32

Testing for Aerobic Capacity

HELGE HEBESTREIT AND RALPH BENEKE

The term "aerobic capacity" denotes the maximal ability of an individual, a limb, or an organ to utilize oxygen. Commonly, "aerobic capacity" refers to the maximal whole body rate of oxygen consumption ($\dot{V}o_2$), which can be achieved during a defined number of seconds of an all-out exercise using a large fraction of the total muscle mass. In a wider perspective, aerobic capacity also includes other conceptual determinants of endurance performance (i.e., the maximal lactate steady state) and also the efficiency or economy of locomotion. Furthermore, the speed of $\dot{V}o_2$ adaptation to a change in metabolic demand may be viewed as an aspect of aerobic capacity. For the scope of this chapter, a broad definition of aerobic capacity will be adopted. However, because whole body peak oxygen uptake ($\dot{V}o_{2peak}$) is by far the most common measurement of aerobic capacity, emphasis will be given to this indicator of aerobic capacity. As it has become custom in exercise physiology, the term "$\dot{V}o_{2peak}$" is used in this chapter to describe the highest $\dot{V}o_2$ of an individual during an incremental exercise test because a plateau of $\dot{V}o_2$ despite an increase in exercise intensity is not routinely achieved when testing children (for details, see below).

This chapter provides practical information on how to measure aerobic capacity in children and how to interpret the findings. The reader is also referred to Chapters 4 and 5, which provide a more general discussion of the development of aerobic capacity and our understanding of factors affecting $\dot{V}o_{2peak}$.

Peak oxygen uptake

$\dot{V}o_{2peak}$ is determined by far more often than any other indicator of aerobic capacity in young athletes. It is usually measured as the highest $\dot{V}o_2$ over 15–30 s during a continuous incremental exercise task to volitional fatigue. Protocols with rest periods between exercise stages—so called discontinuous protocols—are rarely used.

The equipment necessary to measure gas exchange parameters during exercise in children is commercially available. Nowadays, the systems offer breath-by-breath analysis and provide detailed information on ventilation and respiration parameters. The use of the equipment in children requires—relative to the adult sizes—smaller facemasks and/or mouth pieces—the emphasis is on low dead space—in addition to minor modifications in the software set-up for testing small children.

Preparing for exercise testing

Before an exercise test is conducted, a short medical history should be obtained to identify possible contraindications such as an upper respiratory tract infection. The testing protocol and possible risks of the test are explained to the child and her or his guardian and consent should be obtained.

Experienced staff trained in emergency measures should conduct the exercise test. For tests of athletes with a health problem, a physician should be available and the laboratory must be equipped with well-maintained emergency equipment. In any case, it is recommended to provide a metered-dose inhaler of a short-acting β_2-agonist to treat a possible exercise-induced bronchoconstriction.

The children should not have eaten a large meal for at least 2 h prior to testing. Familiarization of the child with the testing equipment and procedures is highly recommended to obtain optimal test results.

The exercise test should be terminated if the child does not want to continue or if (severe) adverse effects of exercise occur.

Which ergometer?

Treadmill exercise and cycle ergometry are mostly used for exercise testing in children (Rowland 1993). Furthermore, to test the ability of an athlete to perform tasks relevant for his or her discipline, sports-specific ergometers such as rowing ergometers or swimming flumes are also used. If several types of ergometers are available and the child is training systematically to compete in a specific event, the system that resembles best the tasks during competition should be selected.

Both treadmill and cycle ergometer have advantages and disadvantages in children. While the treadmill can be used for exercise testing in children as young as 3 years of age, cycle ergometry is usually not possible in children younger than 5 years. Further advantages of the treadmill are that walking and running are much more important activities for most young athletes than cycling. Finally, a larger muscle mass is involved in walking and running than cycling, usually resulting in a higher stress on the cardiorespiratory system and a higher $\dot{V}o_{2peak}$. However, space and staff requirements of cycle ergometry are less than treadmill exercise. In addition, there is no risk of injury during cycle ergometry and therefore it is unlikely that the subject terminates the test prematurely because of fear. Furthermore, the cycle ergometer allows measurement of power directly, and, last but not least, it is easier to obtain valid readings of electrocardiogram (ECG), blood pressure, or oxygen saturation and to collect blood samples during cycle ergometry.

Most cycle ergometers need to be modified for use with smaller children. The seat should move in

horizontal and vertical position and the crank arm length should be adjustable between 9 and 17 cm (Hebestreit *et al.* 1997).

Which exercise protocol?

Numerous exercise protocols have been used in children to determine $\dot{V}o_{2peak}$. In a survey of 30 pediatric cardiac exercise-testing facilities, the treadmill (17 laboratories) was used more often than the cycle ergometer (13 laboratories) (Rowland 1993). Most laboratories used the Bruce treadmill protocol or modifications thereof. The Godfrey, James, and McMaster protocols were used for cycle ergometry.

The choice of the protocol depends on the age and body size of the child to be tested, the measurements planned, and the equipment available. In general, total exercise duration should be kept to 6–12 min in normal children to avoid premature muscle fatigue. In adolescent (endurance trained) athletes, longer test durations may be acceptable.

BRUCE PROTOCOL

The Bruce treadmill protocol can be used for individuals of all ages, although there may be problems with small children and very fit adults. Table 32.1 summarizes the changes in speed and grade during the Bruce treadmill protocol. Some laboratories use 2-min instead of 3-min stages. For the Bruce protocol, normal values for children aged 4–14 years have been established by Cumming *et al.* (1978).

Table 32.1 The Bruce treadmill protocol.

Stage	Speed (km·h^{-1})	Grade (%)	Stage duration (min)
1	2.7	10	3
2	4.0	12	3
3	5.5	14	3
4	6.8	16	3
5	8.0	18	3
6	8.8	20	3
7	9.7	22	3

BALKE PROTOCOL

In the Balke treadmill protocol, the speed of the belt is held constant while the slope is increased. Several variations of the Balke protocol have been used with children. For example, Riopel *et al.* (1979) used a modified Balke protocol with a walking speed of about 5 km·h^{-1} and an increase in slope of 2% every minute for their normative study. However, this protocol has been challenged for use in young athletes, because of the uncomfortably steep slopes at peak exercise and long test duration (Rowland 1993).

JAMES PROTOCOL

This cycle ergometer protocol is often used for cardiac exercise testing in children. Initial power is set to ≈33 W, power is than increased every 3 min by ≈16 W, if body surface area (BSA) is <1 m^2, by ≈33 W for BSA between 1 and 1.2 m^2, or by ≈50 W for BSA >1.2 m^2. After the third stage, power is increased by ≈16–33 W every minute. Normative data have been published by James *et al.* (1980) and Washingston *et al.* (1988).

GODFREY PROTOCOL

This protocol for cycle ergometry has been widely used for the exercise evaluation of patients with cystic fibrosis (Nixon *et al.* 1992). Stage duration is 1 min; work rate increases depend on the height of the person tested. Children who are smaller than 120 cm will start with a work rate of 10 W, which is increased minute-by-minute by 10 W until the child cannot maintain a cycling cadence of 60 rev·min^{-1}. Initial work rate and work rate increments in children 120–150 cm tall are 15 W. In children taller than 150 cm, the respective value is 20 W. Normal values for maximal power and $\dot{V}O_{2peak}$ can be estimated from equations reported by Godfrey *et al.* (1971) and Orenstein (1993), respectively.

Other progressive continuous cycling protocols, usually with 2-min stages, are also commonly employed. Often, the increments in work rate are based on body weight (i.e., 0.5 or 0.75 W·kg^{-1}). In the McMaster cycling protocol, on the other hand, initial work rate and work rate increments vary between 12.5 and 50 W, depending on body height and gender (Bar-Or & Rowland 2004).

Considerations when interpreting $\dot{V}O_{2peak}$ data

DEFINING A MAXIMAL EFFORT

It is obvious that if no maximal effort has been achieved during the exercise test, $\dot{V}O_{2peak}$ cannot be determined. However, defining that a test was maximal may sometimes be difficult. Traditionally, the main criterion for the achievement of an individual's maximal $\dot{V}O_2$ has been that a plateau of $\dot{V}O_2$ is observed during an incremental exercise task despite an increase in work rate. The plateau is usually defined as an increase in $\dot{V}O_2$ during the final completed stage of an incremental exercise test of less than 2 mL·kg^{-1}·min^{-1} for a 5–10% increase in exercise intensity or of less than 2 standard deviations of the average increase in $\dot{V}O_2$ during the preceding stages (Sheehan *et al.* 1987). However, in 14 pediatric studies summarized by Rowland (1996), a plateau was detected only in 56% of children. Furthermore, there is some evidence that children who demonstrate a plateau do not differ in their maximal $\dot{V}O_2$ or maximal heart rate from those who do not (Cunningham *et al.* 1977; Cooper *et al.* 1984; Rivera-Brown *et al.* 1992). Based on these observations, it is clear that the achievement of a plateau in $\dot{V}O_2$ cannot be the exclusive criterion to define a maximal effort. However, if it occurs, the achievement of the individual's maximal oxygen uptake for this exercise mode can be assumed. If not, the investigator has to rely on other criteria. One important criterion is the impression of the investigator conducting the test that a maximal effort has occurred. Further criteria suggested as indicators of a maximal test on the treadmill in healthy children and adolescents include a maximal heart rate of at least 200 min^{-1} or a maximal respiratory exchange ratio during exercise of at least 1.00 (Rowland 1996). The respective values for cycle ergometry are 195 min^{-1} and 1.03 (Rowland 1996). The use of (post-exercise) lactate levels to define a maximal effort in children has been discouraged (Armstrong & Welsman 1997).

INFLUENCE OF EXERCISE MODE AND TESTING PROTOCOL

The choice of the ergometer influences the $\dot{V}O_{2peak}$ measured. In most but not all subjects $\dot{V}O_{2peak}$ is about 6–10% higher if determined during treadmill running than with cycle ergometry (Boileau *et al.* 1977; Cumming & Langford 1985). Running protocols generate higher $\dot{V}O_{2peak}$ values than walking protocols. For example, Cumming and Langford (1985) could show that, using treadmill exercise, the Bruce (running) protocol elicited higher $\dot{V}O_{2peak}$ values than the Balke (walking) protocol (52.9 ± 7.7 vs. 48.2 ± 6.6 mL·kg^{-1}·min^{-1}) in 23 children aged 9–13 years. Supine cycling resulted in about 15–20% lower $\dot{V}O_{2peak}$ measurements than upright cycling in the same group of subjects (Cumming & Langford 1985). As demonstrated by Cumming and Langford (1985), $\dot{V}O_{2peak}$ measured during four upright cycle protocols was not dependent on the protocol used, therefore different upright cycling protocols may result in comparable $\dot{V}O_{2peak}$ measurements.

RELIABILITY

Test–retest reliability coefficients of $\dot{V}O_{2peak}$ reported in children range 0.81–0.95 for cycle ergometry and 0.57–0.99 for treadmill running (Freedson & Goodman 1993). The reliability employing a treadmill walking protocol appears to be lower (Paterson *et al.* 1981).

INTERPRETING $\dot{V}O_{2PEAK}$/NORMALS

$\dot{V}O_{2peak}$ increases, not only with increasing aerobic fitness, but also with body size and age. There are also gender differences. Thus, if the $\dot{V}O_{2peak}$ data of two individuals are to be compared or the $\dot{V}O_{2peak}$ of an individual is to be related to normative data, these factors need to be taken into account.

Traditionally, $\dot{V}O_{2peak}$ has been expressed per kilogram body weight in children. Using this approach, several meta-analyses of studies have shown that $\dot{V}O_{2peak}$ expressed in mL·kg^{-1}·min^{-1} is relatively independent of age in males during childhood and adolescence, while there is a decline in $\dot{V}O_{2peak}$ relative to body mass in females (Krahenbuhl *et al.* 1985; Armstrong & Welsman 1994). Krahenbuhl

et al. (1985) reported average values for treadmill running in males of around 52 mL·kg^{-1}·min^{-1} while $\dot{V}O_{2peak}$ decreased in females from 51 mL·kg^{-1}·min^{-1} at the age of 7 years to 40 mL·kg^{-1}·min^{-1} at the age of 16 years.

However, as pointed out by Welsman and Armstrong in Chapter 5, the use of the "per kilogram body weight" ratio standard has repeatedly been challenged. Allometric scaling techniques might be much more appropriate to compare $\dot{V}O_{2peak}$ among individuals or to follow changes over time (for details see Chapter 5). Unfortunately, there are only few reports on $\dot{V}O_{2peak}$ using allometric scaling which could be used to obtain normative $\dot{V}O_{2peak}$ data in children.

RELATIONSHIP BETWEEN $\dot{V}O_{2PEAK}$ AND ENDURANCE PERFORMANCE

Several studies have shown that $\dot{V}O_{2peak}$ expressed relative to body weight can predict running performance of children in endurance tasks (Nevill *et al.* 1992, 2004; Pettersen *et al.* 2001). However, Pettersen *et al.* (2001) showed that the use of allometric scaling of $\dot{V}O_{2peak}$ (i.e., expressed in mL·kg$^{-0.67}$·min^{-1} or mL·kg$^{-0.75}$·min^{-1}) correlated stronger with the total distance covered during a progressive treadmill test than $\dot{V}O_{2peak}$ expressed in mL·kg^{-1}·min^{-1} ($r = 0.72$ vs. 0.59) in 107 males and 88 females aged 8–17 years. In contrast, Nevill *et al.* (1992, 2004) found in two independent studies that an allometric approach had little advantage over the traditional ratio standard in the prediction of running speed in a 1-mile or 5-km run from $\dot{V}O_{2peak}$ in children.

Maximal lactate steady state, ventilatory threshold, lactate threshold

During prolonged exercise tasks, children and adults cannot maintain a work rate equivalent to $\dot{V}O_{2peak}$. The maximal constant work rate that can be performed for relatively long time periods presumably corresponds to the highest work rate where lactate production and lactate oxidation are still in equilibrium or, in other words, the highest work rate that can be fuelled by oxidative metabolism alone. This phenomenon is called the maximal lactate steady state (MLSS). To determine the MLSS, several

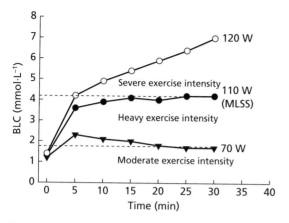

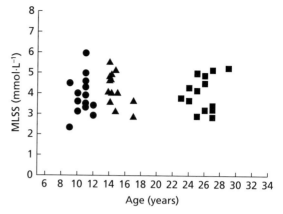

Fig. 32.1 Test to determine maximal lactate steady state (MLSS) in a 14-year-old boy. Three 30-min constant load exercise tests were performed and lactate concentrations were measured from capillary blood samples every 5 min. The exercise intensity of 110 W corresponds to the MLSS. A higher exercise intensity leads to an increase in lactate concentration.

Fig. 32.2 Lactate concentration at maximal lactate steady state (MLSS) in 15 boys (circles), 12 adolescents (triangles), and 17 young men (squares). There is no difference among groups. Data from Beneke *et al.* (1996a,b, unpublished).

20- to 30-min constant work rate exercise tasks are performed, and blood lactate levels are determined every 4–5 min (Fig. 32.1). An exercise shorter than 20 min would result in significantly lower power and $\dot{V}O_2$ at the determined MLSS (Beneke *et al.* 1996b; Beneke 2003). The test with the highest constant work rate with an increase in blood lactate less than 0.05 mmol·L^{-1}·min^{-1} between minutes 10 and 20 (or 30) provides the MLSS.

Only a few studies have assessed MLSS in children (Mocellin *et al.* 1991; Williams & Armstrong 1991; Beneke *et al.* 1996a,b). In these studies, MLSS corresponded to approximately 77 ± 7% of $\dot{V}O_{2peak}$ (Williams & Armstrong 1991) or 50–85% of peak power output (Beneke *et al.* 1996a), with no effect of gender or age. Using a 10-min constant load protocol, reported whole blood lactate concentrations at MLSS measured by electroenzymatic technique were 2.1 ± 0.5 mmol·L^{-1} in boys and 2.3 ± 0.6 mmol·L^{-1} in girls, respectively (Williams & Armstrong 1991). Given the slow lactate on-kinetics, these relative low levels of MLSS may partly reflect the exercise time of 10 min which is insufficient to reach a lactate steady state (Beneke *et al.* 1996b; Beneke 2003). Using 20- or 30-min constant load protocols and an enzymatic photometric method to measure blood lactate, values of 4.2 ± 0.7 mmol·L^{-1} (range 2.8–5.5 mmol·L^{-1}) have been reported in boys aged

11–20 years (Beneke *et al.* 1996a). No significant relationship between lactate concentration at MLSS and age was reported (Fig. 32.2).

Because the determination of the MLSS is time consuming and invasive, other methods such as the ventilatory threshold (VAT) or the lactate threshold (LT) are commonly used to identify the point at which lactate production exceeds lactate elimination. The VAT is determined from gas exchange data collected during an incremental exercise task. Two criteria to determine VAT are commonly used:

1 A sudden increase in the ventilatory equivalent for O_2 occurs without an increase in the ventilatory equivalent for CO_2; and

2 A sudden change occurs in the slope of the regression line between $\dot{V}O_2$ and $\dot{V}CO_2$ (V-slope method).

Some investigators also use changes in respiratory exchange ratio (RER) to detect VAT. In any case, it is recommended to use 10- to 15-s data averages instead of breath-by-breath data (Washington 1993) and to plot the gas exchange data over $\dot{V}O_2$ rather than over time (Hebestreit *et al.* 2000). Figure 32.3 shows a typical plot of gas exchange data during an incremental exercise test on the cycle ergometer, the respective VAT is highlighted. Although the detection of VAT seems to be rather simple, there are two problems that limit the practical use of VAT:

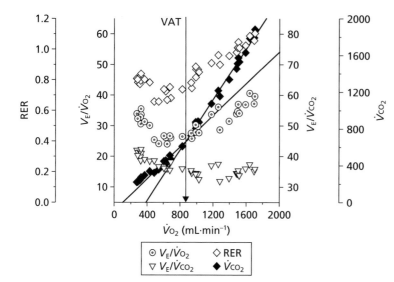

Fig. 32.3 Determining ventilatory anaerobic threshold from parameters of gas exchange plotted over $\dot{V}o_2$. The option to use several different criteria (V-slope method for $\dot{V}co_2$ over $\dot{V}o_2$, increase in $V_E/\dot{V}o_2$ without an increase in $V_E/\dot{V}co_2$, increase in respiratory exchange ratio [RER]) has good intra- and interobserver reliability (Hebestreit *et al.* 2000).

1 VAT cannot be determined from a single exercise test in about 10% (to 20%) of children; and

2 Two investigators may identify different VAT values from the same data set.

However, if more than one criterion is used to determine VAT (Fig. 34.3), intra- and interobserver reliability is high (Hebestreit *et al.* 2000).

Lactate threshold is determined from a series of blood lactate measurements during an incremental exercise task, often employing 3-min stages or a discontinuous protocol. Based on the fact that a definite lactate cut-off threshold of 4 mmol·L^{-1} overestimated

MLSS workload significantly if usual stage durations were used, a variety of different lactate threshold concepts have been developed. Many of them have been validated for specific incremental load test protocols and exercise modes in adults. There are no corresponding validations for children and adolescents. However, there is evidence that, on average, MLSS workload was best described by the workload corresponding to a blood lactate concentration of 3 mmol·l^{-1} measured during an incremental load test with increases in work rate every 2 min by 25 W in children, adolescents, and adults (Fig. 32.4).

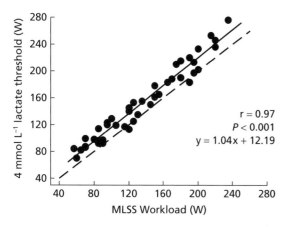

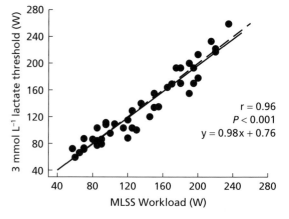

Fig. 32.4 Predicting work rate at maximal lactate steady state (MLSS) from lactate threshold determined during an incremental cycling task with 2-min stages in children and adults. The 3 mmol·L^{-1} threshold (right panel) has a better predictive value compared with a 4 mmol·L^{-1} threshold (left panel). Data from Beneke *et al.* (1996a,b, unpublished).

Considerations when assessing MLSS, VAT, or LT

MEASURING BLOOD LACTATE CONCENTRATION

Measuring lactate requires blood sampling. Given the small amount of blood needed (maximally 25 µL), arterial, venous, or capillary blood could be used. Theoretically, arterial sampling should be preferred because arterial lactate concentration best reflects femoral venous lactate concentration and thus lactate release from active muscle. However, because of the invasive nature of arterial punctures this option has been only occasionally employed in children and venous sampling is used although it may yield lower lactate concentrations (Armstrong & Welsman 1994). By far the most common method is to sample arterialized capillary blood, preferably from the hyperemic ear lobe. These samples well reflect arterial blood lactate concentration.

The lactate concentration in plasma is higher than in red blood cells. Consequently, the measured lactate decreases from plasma to hemolyzed blood to erythrocytes, and the blood lactate concentration depends on hematocrit (Foxdal *et al.* 1990). The latter needs to be carefully considered if different methods are used for the analysis.

Currently, three different methods are used to measure blood lactate concentrations:
1 UV-absorption photometry;
2 An enzymatic amperometric method; and
3 Reflection photometry (Beneke *et al.* 1994, Lormes *et al.* 1995).

All methods are sufficiently reliable and have been extensively validated. The equipment for the first two methods is expensive compared to the third method. However, this may be more than compensated by relatively low costs for consumables per sample if high sample numbers are processed.

RELIABILITY

The test–retest reliability of VAT in children is relatively high (Mahon & Marsh 1992). No data are available for the reliability of LT or MLSS.

VALIDITY

Only very few data are available in children comparing lactate levels and work rate among MLSS, VAT, and LT. Moccelin *et al.* (1991) found lower lactate concentrations and workloads at LT than at MLSS. Correlations between VAT, LT, and MLSS were poor. These results reflect pitfalls of MLSS predictions using selected LT concepts and MLSS definitions (Beneke *et al.* 1996b, Beneke 2003). Appropriate testing procedures seem to provide high correlations between LT and MLSS irrespective of age (Fig. 32.4).

Mechanical efficiency and economy of locomotion

During endurance type activities, performance does not only depend on $\dot{V}O_{2peak}$ and the MLSS (in percent of $\dot{V}O_{2peak}$) but also on an individual's oxygen requirements for a given work rate or speed. The term "mechanical efficiency" is commonly used for the quotient of external work divided by metabolic energy turnover. To calculate gross mechanical efficiency, total metabolic energy expenditure is used as denominator. Net mechanical efficiency refers to external work divided by total energy expenditure minus resting metabolic rate, and delta mechanical efficiency is calculated relative to a baseline low intensity exercise. The term "economy" or "energy cost of locomotion" describes the caloric requirements of a given exercise task (i.e., running at a certain speed).

Mechanical efficiency

Mechanical efficiency is usually assessed using cycle ergometry by measuring the $\dot{V}O_2$ and the RER at several steady state work rates below the lactate or ventilatory threshold. $\dot{V}O_2$ is then translated into calories, based on RER and assuming that no protein metabolism occurs. The caloric equivalent of 1 L oxygen varies between 19.586 kJ·L^{-1} (RER = 0.70) and 21.131 kJ·L^{-1} (RER = 1.00). Often, a caloric equivalent of oxygen of 20.306 kJ·L^{-1} is used irrespective of RER.

Net efficiency increases in prepubertal boys with increasing exercise intensity up to about 60% $\dot{V}O_{2peak}$

(Rowland *et al.* 1990). For exercise intensities above 60% $\dot{V}O_{2peak}$, typical values for net mechanical efficiency during cycling are around 17–20% in children, the respective values for delta efficiency are around 22–30% (for review see Rowland 1996). There seems to be no difference in delta efficiency between children and adults during cycling.

Economy or energy cost of locomotion

The terms "economy" or "energy cost of locomotion" are used to describe the energy requirements for activities such as running, in which external work cannot be determined precisely. As in the assessment of mechanical efficiency, the metabolic energy expenditure is determined during steady state conditions and usually expressed as $\dot{V}O_2$ (in mL·kg^{-1}·min^{-1}). This value is then divided by the running speed (in km·min^{-1}). However, as in any ratio, there are significant disadvantages of this procedure. In consequence, this measure of running economy can only be used—and needs to be reported—for one specific running speed. It may be better to assess the $\dot{V}O_2$ at various running speeds and plot $\dot{V}O_2$ over speed. Although this approach does not provide a single number to describe an individual's running economy, changes with increase in age can be monitored.

Oxygen requirements for a given walking or running speed (in mL·kg^{-1}·min^{-1}) decrease with growth during childhood. Females require less oxygen per kilogram body weight for a given speed than males (Ariens *et al.* 1997; Morgan *et al.* 1999). While the relationship between running economy and performance in distant runs is well established in adults, data in children are equivocal (for review see Rowland 1996). Possibly, allometric scaling techniques will simplify the use and interpretation of running economy in the future.

Oxygen uptake kinetics

Many athletic activities do not require a prolonged effort with a continuously high intensity. In contrast, these activities consist of short bursts of high intensity activities interspersed by intervals of low intensity activities or rest. The usual methodology of exercise testing for aerobic fitness does not assess the ability of an individual to adapt to these quick changes in metabolic demand.

Over the last 25 years, many studies have evaluated the responses of oxygen uptake to changes in exercise intensities in children and adults (Hebestreit *et al.* 1998; Fawkner *et al.* 2002). Usually, several tests with a sudden change in exercise intensity and stages of 3–6 min duration at each intensity are applied to determine $\dot{V}O_2$ on- or off-kinetics. $\dot{V}O_2$ is determined breath-by-breath and data are then superimposed to reduce noise.

Following an abrupt increase in work rate, the first rise in $\dot{V}O_2$ is a result of the rise in venous return (phase 1). After about 15–20 s, $\dot{V}O_2$ increases further. This $\dot{V}O_2$ response (phase 2) reflects the increase in oxygen uptake by the muscle. The phase 2 response can be described by a mono-exponential equation, which is characterized by a time delay, an amplitude, and a time constant (Fig. 32.5). For exercise intensities below the anaerobic threshold, $\dot{V}O_2$ reaches a plateau. For work rates above the anaerobic threshold, an additional increase in $\dot{V}O_2$ occurs after about 100–180 s, which is usually referred to as the "slow component." Mathematically, the slow component is usually also modeled by an exponential (Fig. 32.5b). Off-transients are usually modeled by a single exponential equation.

Studies suggest that the time constants of the phase 2 response are similar or faster in children than in active young adults (Hebestreit *et al.* 1998; Fawkner *et al.* 2002). For moderate intensity exercise, phase 2 time constants are similar in boys and girls (Fawkner *et al.* 2002), while for high intensity exercise they differ between genders with shorter time constants in boys (Fawkner & Armstrong 2004).

Quality of test and parameters

The number of test repetitions used to generate the data set influences the data-to-noise ratio and thus the fit of the exponential(s). Usually, four identical tasks with changes in work rate are performed. The algorithm chosen to treat outliers and to smooth data may also affect parameter estimates of the exponential function. Furthermore, the selection of the break point between phases 1 and 2 (and between phase 2 and the slow component for exercise intensities

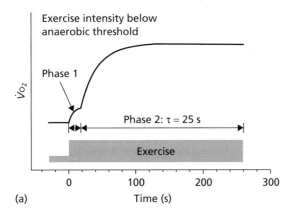

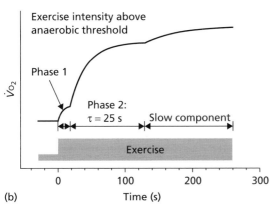

Fig. 32.5 Adjustment of oxygen uptake to an increase of exercise intensity: (a) below anaerobic threshold; and (b) above anaerobic threshold. τ, time constant.

beyond the anaerobic threshold) will influence the parameters. No studies have been performed to calculate the magnitude of the "error" imposed by different approaches to data reduction.

In children, test–retest reliability data for $\dot{V}O_2$ on- or off-transients have not been published.

The validity of time constants describing $\dot{V}O_2$ on-transients have been assessed by correlation analysis with $\dot{V}O_{2peak}$ in several studies (Fawkner *et al.* 2002; Hebestreit *et al.* unpublished data). In contrast to reports on adults, the relationship between time constants of $\dot{V}O_2$ on-transient and $\dot{V}O_{2peak}$ is weak in children.

Challenges for future research

The interpretation of $\dot{V}O_{2peak}$ measured in an individual is limited because normative data spanning a large age range and based on the principles of allometric scaling are missing. This information may be derived from a large cross-sectional or longitudinal study.

The relationships between the various threshold concepts—lactate threshold, ventilatory threshold, maximal lactate steady state—their validity and thus applicability are mostly unknown in children. More research is needed before sound recommendations can be issued regarding their use in active children and youth athletes.

Tests to measure aerobic fitness in children usually aim to assess endurance capacity. However, many disciplines, such as ball games, require fast changes in metabolic demand. Although some research has been carried out using oxygen uptake transients to describe the ability of an individual to adjust to such changes in energy requirements, studies on validity and reliability of this approach are still lacking.

References

Ariens, G.A., van Mechelen, W., Kemper, H.C. & Twisk, J.W. (1997) The longitudinal development of running economy in males and females aged between 13 and 27 years: the Amsterdam Growth and Health Study. *European Journal of Applied Physiology* **76**, 214–220.

Armstrong, N. & Welsman, J.R. (1994) Assessment and interpretation of aerobic fitness in children and adolescents. *Exercise and Sport Sciences Reviews* **22**, 435–476.

Armstrong, N. & Welsman, J. (1997) The assessment and interpretation of aerobic fitness in children and adolescents: an update. In: *Exercise and Fitness: Benefits and Risks. Children and Exercise*, Vol. XVIII (Froberg, K., Lammert, O., Hansen, H.S. & Blimkie, C.J.R., eds.) Odense University Press, Odense: 173–180.

Bar-Or, O. & Rowland, T.W. (2004) *Pediatric Exercise Medicine. From Physiologic Principles to Health Care Application.* Human Kinetics, Champaign, IL.

Beneke, R. (2003) Methodological aspects of maximal lactate steady state: implications for performance testing. *European Journal of Applied Physiology* **89**, 95–99.

Beneke, R., Boldt, F., Richter, T.H., Kress, A., Leithäuser, R. & Behn, C. (1994) Laktatmessung in der Sportmedizin: drei Geräte im Vergleich. *Deutsche Zeitschrift für Sportmedizin* **45**, 60–64, 69.

Beneke, R., Heck, H., Schwarz, V. & Leithäuser, R. (1996a) Maximal lactate steady state during the second decade of age. *Medicine and Science in Sports and Exercise* **28**, 1474–1478.

Beneke, R., Schwarz, V., Leithäuser, R., Hütler, M. & von Duvillard, S.P. (1996b) Maximal lactate steady state in children. *Pediatric Exercise Science* **8**, 328–336.

Boileau, R.A., Bonen, A., Heyward, V.H. & Massey, B.H. (1977) Maximal aerobic capacity on the treadmill and bicycle ergometer of boys 11–14 years of age. *Journal of Sports Medicine* **17**, 153–162.

Cooper, D.M., Weiler-Ravell, D., Whipp, B.J. & Wasserman, K. (1984) Aerobic parameters of exercise as a function of body size during growth in children. *Journal of Applied Physiology* **56**, 628–634.

Cumming, G.R., Everatt, D. & Hastman, L. (1978) Bruce treadmill test in children: normal values in a clinic population. *American Journal of Cardiology* **4**, 69–75.

Cumming, G.R. & Langford, S. (1985) Comparison of nine exercise tests used in pediatric cardiology. In: *Children and Exercise* Vol. XI (Binkhorst, R.A., Kemper, H.C.G. & Saris, W.H.M., eds.) Human Kinetics, Champaign, IL: 58–68.

Cunningham, D.A., Van Waterschoot, B., Paterson, D.H., Lefcoe, M. & Sangal, S.P. (1977) Reliability and reproducibility of maximal oxygen uptake measurements in children. *Medicine and Science in Sports* **9**, 104–108.

Fawkner, S.G. & Armstrong, N. (2004) Sex differences in the oxygen uptake kinetic response to heavy-intensity exercise in prepubertal children. *European Journal of Applied Physiology* **93**, 210–216.

Fawkner, S.G., Armstrong, N., Pooter, C.R. & Welsman, J.R. (2002) Oxygen uptake kinetics in children and adults after the onset of moderate-intensity exercise. *Journal of Sports Sciences* **20**, 319–326.

Foxdal, P., Sjödin, B., Rudstam, H., Östman, C., Östman, B. & Hedenstierna, G.C. (1990) Lactate concentration differences in plasma, whole blood, capillary finger blood erythrocytes during submaximal graded exercise. *European Journal of Applied Physiology* **61**, 218–222.

Freedson, P.S. & Goodman, T.L. (1993) Measurement of oxygen consumption. In: *Pediatric Laboratory Exercise Testing* (Rowland, T.W., ed.) Human Kinetics, Champaign, IL: 91–113.

Godfrey, S., Davies, C.T.M., Wozniak, E. & Barnes, C.A. (1971) Cardiorespiratory response to exercise in normal children. *Clinical Science* **40**, 419–431.

Hebestreit, H., Kriemler, S., Hughson, R.L. & Bar-Or, O. (1998) Kinetics of oxygen uptake at the onset of exercise

comparing boys and men. *Journal of Applied Physiology* **85**, 1833–1842.

Hebestreit, H., Lawrenz, W., Zelger, O., Kienast, W. & Jüngst, B.-K. (1997) Ergometrie im Kindes und Jugendalter. *Monatsschrift Kinderheilkunde* **145**, 1326–1336.

Hebestreit, H., Staschen, B. & Hebestreit, A. (2000) Ventilatory threshold: a useful method to determine aerobic fitness in children? *Medicine and Science in Sports and Exercise* **32**, 1964–1969.

James, F.W., Kaplan, S., Glueck, C.J., Tsay, J.Y., Knight, M.J.S. & Sarwar, C.J. (1980) Responses of normal children and young adults to controlled bicycle exercise. *Circulation* **61**, 902–912.

Krahenbuhl, G.S., Skinner, J.S. & Kohrt, W.M. (1985) Developmental aspects of maximal aerobic power in children. *Exercise and Sport Sciences Reviews* **13**, 503–538.

Lormes, W., Steinacker, J.M. & Stauch, M. (1995) Laktatbestimmung mittels ACCUSPORT und vollenzymatisch-photometrisch bei leistungsdiagnostischem Mehrstufentest und bei Langzeitbelastung. *Deutsche Zeitschrift für Sportmedizin* **46**, 3–11.

Mahon, A.D. & Marsh, M.L. (1992) Reliability of the rating of perceived exertion at ventilatory threshold in children. *International Journal of Sports Medicine* **13**, 567–571.

Mocellin, R., Heusgen, M. & Gildein, H.P. (1991) Anaerobic threshold and maximal steady-state blood lactate in prepubertal boys. *European Journal of Applied Physiology* **62**, 56–60.

Morgan, D.W., Tseh, W., Caputo, J.L., Craig, I.S., Keefer, D.J. & Martin, P.E. (1999) Sex differences in running economy of young children. *Pediatric Exercise Science* **11**, 122–128.

Nevill, A.M., Ramsbottom, R. & Williams, C. (1992) Scaling physiological measurements for individuals of different body size. *European Journal of Applied Physiology* **65**, 110–117.

Nevill, A.M., Rowland, T., Goff, D., Martel, L. & Ferrone, L. (2004) Scaling or normalising maximum oxygen uptake to predict 1-mile run time in boys. *European Journal of Applied Physiology* **92**, 285–288.

Nixon, P.A., Orenstein, D.M., Kelsey, S.F. & Doershuk, C.F. (1992) The prognostic value of exercise testing in patients with cystic fibrosis. *New England Journal of Medicine* **327**, 1785–1788.

Orenstein, D.M. (1993) Assessment of exercise pulmonary function. In: *Pediatric Laboratory Exercise Testing:*

Clinical Guidelines (Rowland, T.W., ed.) Human Kinetics, Champaign, IL: 141–163.

Paterson, D.H., Cunningham, D.A. & Donner, A.P. (1981) The effect of different treadmill speeds on the variability of $\dot{V}o_{2max}$ in children. *European Journal of Applied Physiology* **47**, 113–122.

Pettersen, S.A., Fredriksen, P.M. & Ingjer, F. (2001) The correlation between peak oxygen uptake ($\dot{V}o_{2peak}$) and running performance in children and adolescents. Aspects of different units. *Scandinavian Journal of Medicine and Science in Sports* **11**, 223–228.

Riopel, D.A., Taylor, A.B. & Hohn, A.R. (1979) Blood pressure, heart rate, pressure rate product and electrocardiographic changes in healthy children during treadmill exercise. *American Journal of Cardiology* **44**, 697–704.

Rivera-Brown, A.M., Rivera, M.A. & Frontera, W.R. (1992) Applicability of criteria for $\dot{V}o_{2max}$ in active adolescents. *Pediatric Exercise Science* **4**, 331–339.

Rowland, T.W. (1993) Aerobic exercise testing protocols. In: *Pediatric Laboratory Exercise Testing* (Rowland, T.W., ed.) Human Kinetics, Champaign, IL: 19–41.

Rowland, T.W. (1996) *Developmental Exercise Physiology*. Human Kinetics, Champaign, IL.

Rowland, T.W., Staab, J.S., Unnithan, V.B., Rambusch, J.M. & Siconolfi, S.F. (1990) Mechanical efficiency during cycling in prepubertal and adult males. *International Journal of Sports Medicine* **11**, 452–455.

Sheehan, J.M., Rowland, T.W. & Burke, E.J. (1987) A Comparison of four treadmill protocols for determination of maximal oxygen uptake in 10–12 year old boys. *International Journal of Sports Medicine* **8**, 31–34.

Washington, R.L. (1993) Anaerobic threshold. In: *Pediatric Laboratory Exercise Testing: Clinical Guidelines* (Rowland, T.W., ed.) Human Kinetics, Champaign, IL: 115–129.

Washington, R.L., van Gundy, J.C., Cohen, C., Sondheimer, H.M. & Wolffe, R.R. (1988) Normal aerobic and anaerobic exercise data for North American school-age children. *Journal of Pediatrics* **112**, 223–233.

Williams, J.R. & Armstrong, N. (1991) Relationship of maximal lactate steady state to performance at fixed blood lactate reference values in children. *Pediatric Exercise Science* **3**, 333–341.

Chapter 33

Testing Anaerobic Performance

EMMANUEL VAN PRAAGH

Compared to the study of aerobic performance, little attention has been given in the scientific pediatric literature to short-burst activities (sprinting, jumping, throwing) lasting only a few seconds. This is surprising, considering that in almost all team ball games, the young athlete is more involved in short-term high-intensity exercise than in long-term activities. Moreover, today, many young athletes are encouraged to train intensely for sporting competitions from an early age. While during a 100-m dash only one single supramaximal exercise is performed, the young athlete has to achieve several series of repeated (intermittent) short-term high-intensity exercises during the weekly training sessions. During the growth process, the relative power ($W \cdot kg^{-1}$) of a typical child is approximately only 30% of that observed in power athletes (Ferretti *et al.* 1994). Van Praagh and França (1998) compared performance times for short distance (100-m, 200-m, 400-m) runs by 10-year-old US champion girls and boys with the respective world records by adults (Fig. 33.1; Tables 33.1 and 33.2). A difference of about 25% was observed in these sprint event times for both males and females.

This chapter focuses on testing the capability of children and adolescents to perform high-intensity (single or repeated) activities, which can range in duration from some milliseconds to 1 min. Exercises performed for several minutes will not be discussed in this chapter, because the main energy production for these endeavours comes from aerobic metabolic pathways.

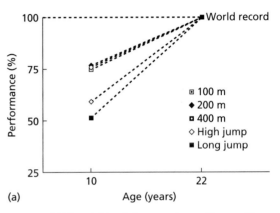

Fig. 33.1 (a) Elite child–adult comparisons: 10-year-old girls (US track and field champions) vs. 22-year-old women (world record holders 1989).

Table 33.1 Best performances of a 10-year-old US champion girl compared with a female world record holder. From Van Praagh & Franca (1998).

	10-year-old girl (1989)	22-year-old female world record holder (1989)	Performance difference (%)
100 m (s)	14.04	10.49	25
200 m (s)	28.17	21.34	24
400 m (s)	63.61	47.60	25
High jump (m)	1.40	2.09	33
Long jump (m)	4.13	7.52	45

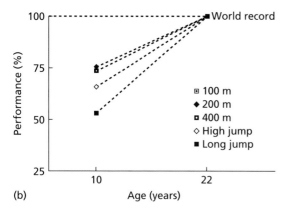

(b)

Fig. 33.1 (b) Elite child–adult comparisons: 10-year-old boys (US track and field champions) vs. 22-year-old men (world record holders 1989). From Van Praagh & França (1998) with permission.

Table 33.2 Best performances of a 10-year-old US champion boy compared with a male world record holder. From Van Praagh & Franca (1998).

	10-year-old boy (1989)	22-year-old male world record holder (1989)	Performance difference (%)
100 m (s)	13.39	9.92	26
200 m (s)	27.21	19.72	28
400 m (s)	59.15	43.29	27
High jump (m)	1.43	2.44	41
Long jump (m)	4.35	8.90	51

Definitions

In the literature, the terminology used to define muscle function and metabolism during short-term high-intensity exercise is very confusing (Van Praagh et al. 2000). Even in well-respected scientific journals, biochemical, physiologic, and mechanical concepts such as alactacid, lactacid, anaerobic power or capacity, anaerobic work capacity, instantaneous power output, peak or mean power output are sometimes indiscriminately used.

The term "power"—if used in conjunction with short-term exercise performance—refers to the ability of the body or a body segment to produce the greatest possible work in a given time period. However, Winter and Maclaren (2001) reported that power output is "only one measure of maximal intensity exercise, yet there is a tendency to assume it is the only measure of this type of performance." Adamson and Whitney (1971) suggested that, in explosive activities such as jumping, the use of power is meaningless and unjustified. Therefore, it is the impulse-generating capability, not the power-producing capability, that is determinant (e.g., during sprinting or jumping).

Power production is limited by the rate at which energy is supplied (adenosine triphosphate [ATP] production) for the muscle contraction (ATP utilization); in other words, the rate at which the myofilaments can convert chemical energy into mechanical work.

ATP production

ANAEROBIC POWER ($ATP \cdot s^{-1}$)

This is the maximal anaerobic ATP per second yield by the whole organism during a specific type of short duration, maximal exercise (Green 1994).

ANAEROBIC CAPACITY (ATP)

This is the maximal amount of ATP resynthesized via anaerobic (non-oxidative) metabolism (by the whole organism) during a specific type of short duration, maximal exercise (Green 1994).

Short-term anaerobic muscle metabolites can be investigated during exercise by the use of phosphorus magnetic resonance spectroscopy (^{31}P NMRS). In children, the use of this technique provides well-tolerated and non-invasive means of monitoring intracellular inorganic phosphate (Pi), phosphocreatine (PCr), and pH (Zanconato et al. 1993).

Power output (W)

Using work output to estimate or to reflect anaerobic capacity is less difficult than attempting to quantify the ATP yield using "direct methods" (e.g., needle biopsy, ^{31}P NMRS, or accumulated oxygen deficit techniques). However, interpreting the physiologic implications of work is certainly more awkward. This is especially true as the mechanical work estimates reflect not only anaerobic ATP supply, but also the contribution of oxidative sources of ATP, as well as the various factors involved in the transduction of chemical to mechanical energy (or work done). Thus, factors that influence work estimates of anaerobic capacity may not be completely anaerobic in nature (Van Praagh *et al.* 1991; Hebestreit *et al.* 1993). Anaerobic power is characterized by the generation of very high power outputs, from about 1.1 kW in untrained children aged 8–13 years (Ferretti *et al.* 1994) to about 6.0 kW in power athletes (Grassi *et al.* 1991).

The following terms are used in this chapter:

1 *Force* (mass × acceleration) is measured in newtons (N)

2 *Impulse* (force × time) is measured in newtons × s ($N \cdot s^{-1}$)

3 *Work* (force × distance) is measured in joules (J)

4 *Power* (work per unit of time, or force × velocity) is measured in watts (W)

5 *Fatigue* is defined as an inability to maintain the required or expected force or power (Edwards 1981). (For further details on exercise terminology see Winter & Maclaren 2001; Van Praagh & Doré 2002.)

Anaerobic testing in young people

Although quantitative measurements of non-oxidative (anaerobic) energy supply during short-term exercise can be made by invasive techniques in adults, this kind of investigation is ethically questionable in young athletes. Therefore, in this particular population, researchers have concentrated on measuring short-term power generated during standardized tests (Bar-Or 1996; Van Praagh & França 1998; Van Praagh & Doré 2002). In numerous sports the young athlete must activate and synchronize his or her motor units to throw a mass (e.g., shotput) or to displace his or her body mass against gravity (e.g., a basketball dunk). These activities need a burst of muscular contractions of very short duration (<1 s). This instantaneous power reflects the ability to transform ATP breakdown into external power (Ferretti *et al.* 1987). During a 400-m run race, high muscle power output may also be sustained over a longer time period. Moreover, young team games players need to be able to repeatedly produce brief maximal or near maximal sprints.

We may therefore consider:
• Single instantaneous anaerobic performance (<5 s duration);
• Single short-term anaerobic performance (>5–60 s);
• Repeated short-term anaerobic performance (repeated bouts of 5–10 s).

Fundamental considerations

Assessment of short-term power raises several methodologic problems (for review see Sargeant 1992; Van Praagh & Doré 2002).

First, because power is the product of force and velocity, the external load (e.g., body mass during jumping or load on the cycle ergometer) must closely match the capability of the active muscles so that they operate at their optimal velocity (Wilkie 1960). Clearly, this is a difficult condition to fulfil or to guarantee in freely accelerating or decelerating cycling or running sprint efforts. Several activities have been proposed for the measurement of short-term power output (STPO), including vertical jumping, running, or cycling. Of these activities, only cycle ergometry allows precise measurement of power independent of body mass as the imposed load.

Second, if 'true' maximal STPO is to be measured, the duration of the test must be as short as possible because power output decreases rapidly as a function of time (Fig. 33.2) (Wilkie 1960; Van Praagh *et al.* 1989, 1991). The measurement of "true" STPO requires measurements of instantaneous values of force and velocity. This condition is only satisfied in monoarticular force–velocity tests (Wilkie 1950), force platform tests (Davies & Rennie 1968; Ferretti *et al.* 1987), isokinetic cycle ergometry (Sargeant *et al.* 1981), cycling power tests including frictional force and flywheel inertia (Lakomy 1986; Doré *et al.* 1997), and inertial-load cycling ergometry (Martin *et al.* 1997). For instance, the well known 30-s Wingate cycling test does not provide instantaneous measures and is therefore unable to elicit "true" maximal STPO.

Third, anaerobic glycolysis and aerobic contribution are limited during instantaneous power tests. However, when using a 30-s Wingate cycling test in prepubescent and adolescent boys, Van Praagh *et al.* (1991) and Hebestreit *et al.* (1993) reported that the

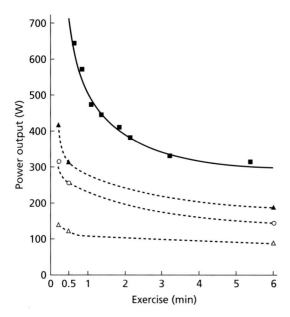

Fig. 33.2 Power–duration curves for one adult (Wilkie 1960) and children's data (Van Praagh *et al*. 1989, 1991). Solid square, adult; solid triangle, 12-year-old boys; open circle, 12-year-old girls; open triangle, 7-year-old boys.

aerobic fraction was high when compared to young men. Blood lactate production starts during the first seconds of a single supramaximal exercise (Saltin *et al*. 1971). This observation was confirmed by the study of Mercier *et al*. (1991) who reported a significant venous blood lactate increase during a single 6-s force–velocity cycling sprint in young trained male adolescents. According to Ferretti *et al*. (1987), only exercises lasting a few seconds can be considered as truly "alactacid." Direct measurements of "anaerobic capacity" or the maximum amount of ATP that can be supplied by the anaerobic energy pathways is still a matter for research, while the precise amount cannot actually be quantified in whole body short-term exercises.

Another problem is the reliability of short-term power tests. A reliable test allows confidence in the tracking of changes that occur during growth or training. To determine the reproducibility of a test, it has been shown that at least three trials need to be conducted (Hopkins 2000), and that the detection of a systematic bias (paired *t*-test or analysis of variance with repeated measures) and the use of

statistical methods based on correlation coefficients (Pearson's or intraclass correlation coefficient) are inadequate (Atkinson & Nevill 1998). Atkinson and Nevill suggested that the statistical techniques used to describe "absolute reliability," such as the standard error of measurement and coefficient of variation or limits of agreement (Bland & Altman 1986), are the most appropriate. Doré *et al*. (2003) recently reported the reproducibility of a short-term cycling power test (inertia included) in children and in young adults. The measurement of cycling peak power was found to be highly reliable (test–retest coefficient of variation of 2.8%). They therefore recommend:

1 Provision of a habituation session (motor learning);
2 Performance of three sprints by children and at least two sprints by young adults;
3 That high motivation in children is maintained to avoid performance alterations beyond two tests.

Finally, factors influencing STPO include the following:

1 Instantaneous or mean power is measured.
2 The legs act simultaneously (vertical jumping) or successively (cycling).
3 Total body mass or (active) muscle mass is taken into account (Van Praagh *et al*. 1990).
4 Peak power is measured in the beginning of exercise (stationary start) or after several seconds of a rolling start (Vandewalle *et al*. 1987). In all short-term power tests there are no objective criteria to confirm maximality and thus the scientist or trainer must rely on the willing cooperation of the individual to perform to his or her maximum.
5 STPO is assessed by field or laboratory testing. Field tests apparently cause maximal activation of the ATP-PCr energy system. These tests are generally referred to as power tests (i.e., work done per time unit: $J \cdot s^{-1} = W$). In the laboratory, these tests can be performed on several ergometric devices. Isokinetic devices can be used for monoarticular tests of peak torque and mean power. Force platforms are useful for the measurement of instantaneous leg power. Cycle ergometers (frictional or isokinetic) can be used for the measurement of instantaneous or average leg (arm) power. Finally, non-motorized treadmills can be used for short-term running power. All material must be carefully and regularly calibrated (Williams *et al*. 2003). Some commercial cycle

ergometers may show calibration errors of up to 40% (Van Praagh *et al.* 1992).

Short-term power output

In children and adolescents before publication of the Margaria staircase running protocol (Margaria *et al.* 1966), most, if not all, short-term tests measured work (e.g., vertical jump), time (e.g., 30–50-m dash), or distance (e.g., softball throw), but not mechanical power. Since then, many other tests have been developed. When considering a specific test one must keep in mind that:

• Anaerobic tests are highly specific to the muscle group being evaluated; and

• Anaerobic performance of a muscle group depends highly on the force and the velocity of its contraction. Therefore, force and speed of movement must be matched (Hill 1938). Maximal muscle power is thus obtained at optimal values of force and velocity. The relationship between force, velocity, and power can be more or less accurately assessed during growth with various protocols:

   1 *Staircase running tests* (Margaria *et al.* 1966);

   2 *Cycling tests* (Bar-Or 1987; Van Praagh *et al.* 1990; Doré *et al.* 2000);

   3 *Vertical jump tests* (Davies & Young 1984; Bosco 1992); and

   4 *Non-motorized treadmill running tests* (Fargeas *et al.* 1993a; Sutton *et al.* 2000).

One single maximal short-term exercise

Until recently, most of the pediatric scientific literature investigated a single short-burst exercise (e.g., only one cycling sprint; only one running sprint; only one vertical jump, etc.).

Running tests

LABORATORY TESTS

Sprinting upstairs

The first study that investigated STPO in children was reported by Margaria *et al.* (1966). They measured the vertical component of the "maximum" constant speed in boys and girls aged 10–15 years by having the individual sprint up a staircase. Body mass (kg) of the child represented the external force. To measure the power output time was recorded, with typical durations of about 400–500 ms. Absolute maximal anaerobic power (MAP) was higher in boys, although the difference disappeared when MAP was expressed relative to body mass. There is a fairly linear increase in absolute MAP up to the age of approximately 13 years in both genders. After that age the values for boys continue to increase, while those for girls level off (Davies *et al.* 1972). The authors concluded that psychomotor, biomechanical, and/or biochemical changes that occur at the age of approximately 13 years contribute to this development. Despite the statements made by the authors, running performances in this particular test may be influenced by several factors including body mass, step height, leg length, stride pattern, and the skill of climbing stairs at maximal velocity. In young children, because of risk of injury in taking two steps at a time, the test administrator might consider the 30-m dash with a standing start as an alternative. Because of the abovementioned limitations, few data using the Margaria stair-running test have been recently reported.

Acceleration in sprint running

The effects of three different training regimens: (i) "isometrics" who trained with isometric knee extensions; (ii) "jumpers" who trained using vertical jumps; and (iii) "runners" who trained by sprinting, on STPO and the possible transfer of training among the different complex motor functions have been examined by Nielsen *et al.* (1980). A total of 249 girls aged 7–19 years took part in the training experiments. The girls trained for only 5 weeks, three times per week. In each training session, the "runners" performed maximally about 100 steps in 10 starts, employing maximal force with each leg. Each girl made a standing start and ran 10 m as fast as possible. Running velocity was measured by means of three adjustable photocell systems placed at the hip height. Accelerations were calculated using the time recordings from the cells placed at 0.2 and 4 m from the starting line. In this study, the actual contraction times were very short (200–300 ms) in both vertical jumping and fast stepping during the sprint start. Results showed that in girls, but not in boys (Asmussen 1973), the acceleration in sprint running was independent of height. This is in contrast to what occurs with vertical jump performance, which increases with height. All three training programs had a positive transfer effect on isometric leg extension and the height of a vertical jump, but there was no significant effect on acceleration in sprint running. It is interesting to notice that the improvement was considerably more pronounced in the test tasks that were identical with the training program, again with the exception of the sprint training.

Non-motorized horizontal treadmill running

Performing on a cycle ergometer is ideal for cyclists, but it has less practical value for the investigation of running performances. Attempts have therefore been made to measure maximal velocity and power output during brief high-intensity exercise in adult populations on non-motorized treadmills (Lakomy 1987; Tong *et al.* 2001). In the author's laboratory the same methodology has been used to assess, for the first time, short-term running power output in untrained and trained children (Van Praagh *et al.* 1993). Fargeas *et al.* (1993b), studied the longitudinal running and cycling power of girls and boys aged 8–14 years. The child develops maximal velocity while connected to a belt at the waist. The belt, which is attached to a horizontal bar, is connected to a potentiometer (vertical displacement) and strain gauges (horizontal traction force). A constant torque motor installed in the rear wheel of the treadmill is not used to drive the treadmill, but to compensate for belt friction or to simulate different loads (Fig. 33.3).

Signals from the potentiometer, the transducers, and from the treadmill (belt speed) allows mechanical power (potential + kinetic power) to be calculated. Although this test seems promising with respect to its specificity (sprint running or team games), it has limitations such as the assessment of "true" kinetic power and the difficulty in keeping balance. In adults, the test was found reliable (Lakomy 1987). In children, three studies have reported high reliability coefficients (r > 0.90) for this test (Fargeas *et al.* 1993b; Falk *et al.* 1996; Sutton *et al.* 2000).

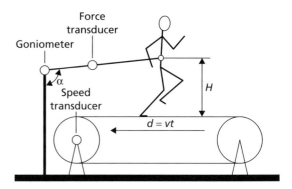

Fig. 33.3 Schematic representation of the non-motorized treadmill. *d*, distance; *H*, height; *t*, time; *v*, velocity. From Belli & Lacour 1989.

FIELD TESTS

30- to 50-m sprint running

Historically, in the USA, Europe, and in most other countries, physical educators and coaches have used a 30- to 50-m dash as a measure of running velocity. The test is easy to administer, can be performed indoors and outdoors, and large pediatric populations can be assessed in a short time. This simple test enables individuals to be categorized as: slow, medium-slow, and rapid. However, it cannot be considered as a "real" power test, according to Wilkie (1960), as the force component is not measured. Several studies have described increases of sprint performance during growth and development. The American Alliance for Health, Physical Education, Recreation and Dance (1980) reported that average 50-yard sprint velocity improved by about 50% in boys and 23% in girls between the of 7 and 17 years (Fig. 33.4). Analysing sprint performance correlates in children, Rowland (2005) suggested that improvement in short-burst activities relies more on developmental changes in neuromuscular coordination, balance, and motor skill than changes in anaerobic metabolic capacity. Reliability coefficients of 0.66–0.94 (only for boys) have been reported. Learning effects for this test do not seem to have been investigated.

30-s shuttle run

In this test, the child runs to and fro (20 m for each lap). The average velocity is calculated from the

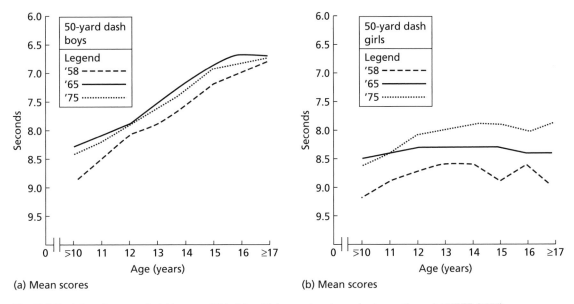

Fig. 33.4 Sprint performance in (a) boys and (b) girls with increasing chronologic age. From AAHPER (1975).

distance covered in 30 s. Non-significant differences in peak blood lactate were observed between a 30-s cycling Wingate test and the 30-s shuttle run test, suggesting that the field test was a rather strenuous effort for 12-year-old girls and boys (Van Praagh *et al.* 1990; Falgairette *et al.* 1994).

Cycling tests

In young people, external arm or leg power output (W) can be assessed on a cycle ergometer by measuring the velocity of cycling (*v*) for a given braking force (N).

ARM CYCLING

Few data are available concerning children. "Peak" power and local muscle endurance determined during arm cranking (Wingate protocol) appears to increase for boys, but not for girls during the adolescent period (Blimkie *et al.* 1988). More recently, Nindl *et al.* (1995) measured upper body anaerobic power in male and female adolescent athletes. Peak power normalized for body mass, fat-free mass, and cross-sectional area was significantly higher in boys than in girls.

LEG CYCLING

Several methods have been described for the assessment of STPO by cycle ergometry in the pediatric literature. Three main methods are discussed here. The popular Wingate anaerobic test (Cumming 1973; Inbar & Bar-Or 1986) measures "peak" power and mean power during 30-s intensive cycling. Short-term cycling power can also be measured by determining the relationship between force and velocity, the so-called "force–velocity test" (FVT). In children, the latter was successively performed without considering the flywheel inertia of the device for power calculations (Van Praagh *et al.* 1989; Bedu *et al.* 1991) and with consideration of inertia (Doré *et al.* 2000, 2001; Martin *et al.* 2003, 2004).

Regardless of the method chosen, the cycle ergometer must be adapted to the body dimensions of the child (crank length, frame, handlebars, and saddle height). The results of the tests also depend on the protocol. For instance, STPO is approximately 15% higher when the child can stand on the pedals, instead of sitting on the saddle. In children it is appropriate to express leg power corrected for active muscle (lean thigh volume or lean leg volume) instead of total body mass.

30-s wingate test

This supramaximal cycling test, which is derived from Cumming's test (1973) has been studied by many authors. The subject pedals on a cycle ergometer at a maximal velocity against a constant braking force for 30 s; the constant braking force has been pre-determined to produce mechanical power equivalent to two or three times the metabolic power obtained during a $\dot{V}o_{2max}$ test. According to the authors, peak power—the highest power achieved during a 3–5 s period during the test—reflects the ability of the leg muscles to produce short-term mechanical power, whereas mean power or total work performed during the entire 30 s of the test represents the local muscle endurance of the legs. The fixed external resistive force might not satisfy muscle force–velocity relationships and thus measured STPO values may be lower than in other tests. Furthermore, the 30-s cycling test needs strong motivation from the child, which is not always forthcoming. In our daily practice some tall and muscular adolescents experienced nausea and dizziness after the test. One way of decreasing these side effects is to cool down after the test by cycling against a low resistance for several minutes. However, it could be demonstrated that boys recovered faster than young men after performing a Wingate test. A resting period of 2 min was found sufficient for a full recovery after this test in healthy boys aged 9–12 years (Hebestreit *et al.* 1993).

The Wingate test has been examined more extensively than any other anaerobic performance test for several pediatric populations (abled, disabled, trained) and found to be highly valid and reliable. Test–retest reliability coefficients are in the range 0.89–0.97 (Tirosh *et al.* 1990). Representative values in children are available (Bar-Or 1996). For further information concerning the test protocol, the reader can consult recent reviews (Bar-Or 1996; Van Praagh & Doré 2002).

Force–velocity test without adjustment for flywheel inertia

With Wilkie's rationale in mind (maximal power = optimal force × optimal velocity), it does not appears

possible to measure STPO with a single braking force. In consequence, sprint cycling protocols that rely on variable loads have been proposed (Maréchal *et al.* 1979; Pirnay & Crielaard 1979). In these studies, individuals performed several all-out sprints (5–7 s) on a Monark cycle ergometer at incremental loads from 3 to 7 kp (approximately 30–70 N), followed by a 3-min recovery after each sprint. The highest value was assumed to correspond to peak power. Average peak power values of 7.6 and 10.1 W·kg^{-1} were observed in 11-year-old boys and 19-year-old young men, respectively. This test was the precursor of the load-optimization or force–velocity test (inertia not included). In adults, both Pérès *et al.* (1981) on a friction-loaded ergometer, and Sargeant *et al.* (1981) on a isokinetic-cycle ergometer, observed that cycling velocity decreased linearly as a function of increasing loads. In contrast to the *in vitro* studies, in which the relationship between force and velocity is exponential (Fenn & Marsh 1935) or hyperbolic (Hill 1938), a similar linear force–velocity and parabolic force–power relationship is generally observed in adults (Vandewalle *et al.* 1987) and children (Van Praagh *et al.* 1989) during cycling (Fig. 33.5).

The quasi-linear relationship allows the determination of internal test validation (Sargeant 1992). Moreover, single aberrant values within a series of experimental plots can be identified and analyzed. The coefficient of variation is around 12%. The procedure appears to satisfy muscle force–velocity relationships and produce theoretically sound STPO values. However, this procedure does not produce valid fatigue profiles. Furthermore, the 30-min total time required for completion (five sprints interspersed with 3-min recovery) is time consuming.

Inertial adjusted force–velocity test

Identification of an appropriate braking force is difficult during growth and maturation. Moreover, an ideal braking force at the beginning of a STPO exercise is not ideal at the end of a test. Fatigue decreases the pedaling rate and thus power output (Sargeant 1992). Few studies have investigated the optimal resistance required for children (Dotan & Bar-Or 1983; Van Praagh *et al.* 1990; Carlson & Naughton 1994). In addition, these studies have

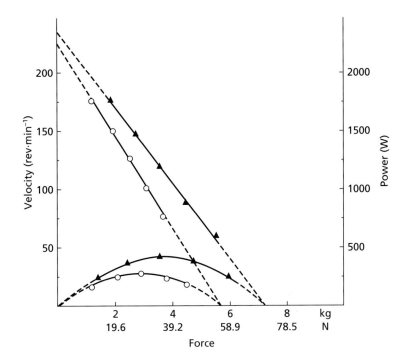

Fig. 33.5 Force–velocity (straight lines) and force–power (parabolas) relationships in 12-year-old girls (open circles) and boys (solid triangles). From Van Praagh *et al.* (1990).

not incorporated the force required to accelerate the flywheel of the cycle device (inertial force). Maximal power reported has been undoubtedly underestimated (Doré *et al.* 1997, 2000a,b). In contrast to previous protocols, the imposed total external force (braking force + inertial force) is not constant during the acceleration phase of sprint cycling. Therefore, recent concomitant measurements of forces, velocities and powers have been reported during the acceleration phase of sprint cycling (Fig. 33.6). This new test protocol allows the measurement of STPO and optimal velocity from only one sprint and does not require high resistances to be overcome. Doré *et al.* (2005) reported references for females ($n = 496$) and males ($n = 416$) aged 8–20 years. The present method is less affected by fatigue and motivational factors and is also less time consuming than current testing procedures.

Summary

If the aim is to measure STPO in untrained individuals, we recommend the less stressful FVT. Moreover, the FVT yields a higher peak power output because of

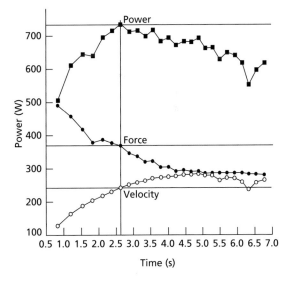

Fig. 33.6 Cycling power (W) as a function of time (s). Force (N) curve is decreasing, while the velocity (rev·min^{-1}) curve is increasing. In this particular case power is obtained in 26 s.

the shortness of the test. For instance, Doré *et al.* (2000) compared data reported by Inbar *et al.* (1996). It appears that in boys and girls aged 12–14 years the FVT (inertia included) showed 45% higher values than those obtained during the Wingate test (655 vs. 358 W, respectively). The Wingate protocol appears to be more useful in establishing fatigue profiles.

Jumping tests

FORCE PLATFORM (OR CONTACT MAT) TESTS

Vertical jump protocol

Since the early work of E.J. Marey (Marey & Demenÿ 1885), who recorded the simultaneous measurement of force (pneumatic force platform) and displacement during a vertical jump (Fig. 33.7), numerous authors have developed vertical jump protocols. Sophisticated instrumentation (force platform + computer analysis) allows the recording of the ground reaction forces and acceleration of the body's center of mass. STPO is calculated from the product of instantaneous force exerted by the individual on the force platform and the acceleration of the center of mass of the body. Davies and Young (1984) reported a high correlation ($r = 0.92$) between the height of a vertical jump and the data obtained on the force platform. They also reported fairly low intra-individual variation (7%). More recently, Ferretti *et al.* (1994) measured maximal leg power in children aged 8–13 years. They used the method described by Davies and Rennie (1968). However, the vertical jump started from a squatting position, to minimize counter-movements. The velocity was obtained by time integration of the instantaneous acceleration, which is equal to the ratio of force : individual mass. The test is considered as the "gold standard" in jump power testing and has been used for validation of other anaerobic power tests. However, the method requires an expensive force-plate technology, technical staff, and is time consuming.

Drop jump protocol

The individual (hands on hips throughout the entire jump) drops from heights of 0.2–0.8 m on

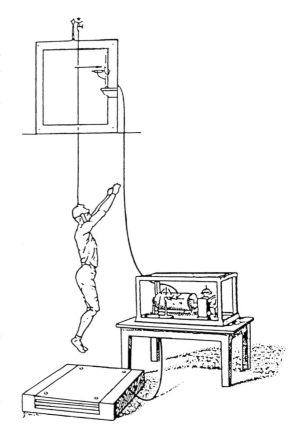

Fig. 33.7 The equipment used by E.J. Marey to record the simultaneous measurement of ground reaction force and displacement during a vertical jump. From Marey & Demenÿ (1885).

to the force platform with a subsequent upward jump. Each jump is recorded on magnetic tape and a vertical force–time curve produced by each jump is analyzed with computerized calculations (Komi & Bosco 1978). It is assumed that the "stretch–shortening cycle" which occurs during this type of jump, allows the stored elastic energy to be utilized during positive work and thus increases the vertical jump performance. The tolerance to progressive dropping height before injuries occur increases from childhood up to the age of 20–25 years (Bosco & Komi 1980). It is therefore recommended to protect the young untrained body against high stretch loads, especially when muscles and bones have not yet reached maturity and when ossification processes are not yet achieved.

Repeated rebound jumps

Bosco *et al.* (1983) proposed a 5- to 15-s vertical jump test to measure mechanical power output (W·kg⁻¹). In children aged 5–10 years, a 5-s test is recommended. In adolescents, the duration can be increased to 10–15 s. It was shown (Bosco 1992) that the repeated rebound test is highly relevant and sensitive to neuromuscular adaptations induced by training in relation to the individual characteristics and the specific sport activity practiced (specifically all jump activities). The purpose is to assess mean leg power or total work during a series of vertical jumps on a force platform or a contact mat. The performance is derived by plugging the total flight time and total number of vertical jump into a formula (Bosco *et al.* 1983). A high degree of logical validity was found in athletic populations (basketball or volleyball players), but it is lacking as a general power test. Even if the test is suitable for males from age 16 years, the reliability needs to be established for pediatric populations.

Hopping test

Power output measured during running or jumping events not only estimates the power of the chemo-mechanical conversion, but also gives information regarding the mechanical energy stored in the elastic elements of the muscles involved (Cavagna *et al.* 1965). Moritani *et al.* (1989) investigated neural and biomechanical variables during fast and maximal hopping tasks on a force platform in 9-year-old boys. Hopping represents a cyclical motor task, with repeated stretch–shortening cycles of the leg extensor muscles. Children were asked to hop on both legs, with either the fastest possible frequency or the maximal height in each jump recorded for 10–15 s. A rest interval of 1–2 min was allowed between trials. Mechanical power (normalized for body mass) was higher in adults than in boys during maximal hopping (26.0 vs. 15.4 W·kg⁻¹; $P < 0.01$). However, during fast hopping, boys generated significant higher power than adults (4.3 vs. 2.3 W·kg⁻¹; $P < 0.01$) (Fig. 33.8).

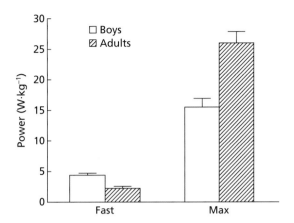

Fig. 33.8 Mechanical power (normalized to body mass) during fast and maximal hopping in boys and adults. From Moritani *et al.* (1989).

Counter-movement jump with added masses

Viitasalo *et al.* (1992) examined more than 300 male adolescent athletes aged 9–16 years and representing six different sports. After a warm-up, each individual performed 3–5 maximal counter-movement jumps with each of four different barbell loads; for the smallest children, the loads were 2, 50, 100, and 150 N, while the older children had to overcome loads of 2, 100, 200, and 400 N. Jumping height was calculated using the flight time (t) of the jump with the following formula:

$$hCG = (t^2 - g)/8$$

where hCG is the displacement of the center of gravity, t is the flight time, and $g = 9.81$ ms⁻².

The flight time was measured using a digital timer and a contact mat (Bosco *et al.* 1983). In a previous study (Viitasalo 1988), the coefficients of variation between determinations of the test decreased with age from 13% at 10 years of age to 6% at 16 years of age.

FIELD TESTS

Sargent test

Sargent (1921) developed the vertical jump test to measure maximal leg power in adults. Individuals are required to jump vertically as high as they can. At the peak of the jump, the administrator marks the measuring board with chalk. The individual's ability to exert leg power is derived from the height of the jump. The average value of three jumps is generally taken as the test score. Despite the fact that vertical velocity in jumping is determined by impulse (for discussion see Winter & Maclaren 2001), the vertical jump has been accepted as a valid measure of leg "power" and various vertical jump protocols have been derived from the Sargent test. Reliability coefficients of 0.91–0.93 suggest high intra-individual consistency (Glencross 1966). No test–retest reliability has been reported in pediatric populations. A major weakness is the lack of standardization in test administration. For instance, a counter-movement increases the vertical jump performance by about 10%. Moreover, a more rapid elevation of the arms also improves the height of a vertical jump (Bosco *et al.* 1983).

Standing long jump

Because of its easy execution and administration, this test is often used in pediatric populations, instead of the vertical jump test, as a measure of leg muscle "power." The problem with all field-based assessments, but also in laboratory-based measurements, is that the tests do not reflect a single factor (leg power, in this particular case), but also learning, coordination, and maturation in general. Thus, although the test appears to be objective as well as reliable, its validity is questionable. Correlation coefficients of 0.79 between standing long jump and vertical jump assume that either can be used as a criterion measure for the other. Docherty (1996) asserted that the specific issue of validity for either test has not been examined. The test is feasible for girls and boys from 6 years onwards (Council of Europe 1988). Normative data are available for both age and sex groups (AAHPER 1975).

Throwing test

Throwing power has traditionally been measured in field conditions with throwing tests such as ball throwing or medicine ball tests (Kirby 1991). In the latter "power" tests, it is assumed that the best distance attained reflects STPO of the arm. Viitasalo (1988) developed a new test to measure throwing velocity of balls with different masses. In this test, the young athlete throws balls of the same diameter but of different masses (0.3–4.0 kg) through a photocell gate to a 0.4×0.4 m contact mat hanging on the wall. The test was found to be reliable for 10- to 12-year-olds and had rather high correlations with their respective traditional field tests.

Repeated maximal short-term exercise

In almost all daily tasks, games in the playground, or "multiple sprint sports" (Williams 1987) such as football, rugby, basket-ball, field hockey, and other popular participation sports, the young athlete is repeatedly involved in short-term high-intensity exercises. One important question in this context is whether the young athlete is more fatiguible than a trained adult. Most of the studies related to this problem were recently carried out on repeated cycling (Hebestreit *et al.* 1993; Ratel *et al.* 2002a) and repeated running bouts (Ratel *et al.* 2006).

Intermittent cycling

During high intensity intermittent exercise (HIIE), the time course of peak power output is dependent on the time allowed for recovery. In adults, peak power strongly decreases during many repeated bouts of short-term HIIE with 30-s recovery intervals (Gaitanos *et al.* 1993). In contrast, when the recovery periods are longer (around 60 s), the decrease in peak power output is markedly lower and/or delayed (Wootton & Williams 1983). The decrease in peak power with short recovery intervals (30 s) was attributed to insufficient PCr resynthesis and/or muscle lactate accumulation. Ratel *et al.* (2002a) reported that prepubescent children could maintain their peak power output better than adults during several repeated bouts of high intensity intermittent cycling exercise separated by short recovery intervals. A group of prepubescent boys (Pre), pubescent boys (Pub) and men participated in the study. After a warm-up on the cycle ergometer followed by a 5-min rest, each individual then performed ten 10-s sprints separated by either 30-s (R30), 1-min (R1) or 5-min (R5) passive recovery intervals. These three

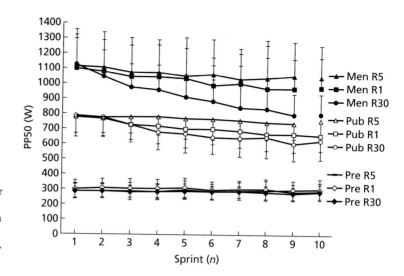

Fig. 33.9 Time course of peak power (PP50) during ten 10-s sprints separated by either 30-s (R30), 1-min (R1), or 5-min (R5) passive recovery intervals in prepubescent boys (Pre), pubescent boys (Pub) and men.

recovery durations were randomly assigned. Each sprint was performed against the friction load corresponding to 50% of the optimal braking force. Peak power (PP50) was calculated at each sprint (Doré *et al.* 2000). Results showed (Fig. 33.9) that in the prepubescent boys, whatever recovery intervals were used, cycling peak power remained unchanged during the ten 10-s sprints. In the pubescent boys, cycling peak power decreased by 18.5% with R30 and by 15.3% with R1 from the first to the tenth sprint but remained unchanged with R5. In adults, cycling peak power decreased respectively by 28.5% and 11.3% with R30 and R1 and slightly diminished with R5.

To conclude, prepubescent boys sustained their cycling peak power output during ten 10-s sprints with only 30-s recovery intervals. In contrast, pubescent boys and male adults needed 5-min recovery intervals. It is suggested that the faster recovery of peak power in the prepubescent group was because of their lower muscle gycolytic activity and their higher muscle oxidative capacity, allowing a faster resynthesis in PCr (Hebestreit *et al.* 1996; Taylor *et al.* 1997; Ratel *et al.* 2002b).

Intermittent running

Ratel *et al.* (2006) investigated the effects of age and recovery duration on performance during multiple treadmill sprints. Twelve boys (11.7 ± 0.5 years) and

13 men (22.1 ± 2.9 years) performed 10 consecutive 10-s sprints on a non-motorized treadmill separated by 15-s (R15) and 180-s (R180) passive recovery intervals. Mean power output (MPO), mean force output (MFO), running velocity, step length, and step rate were calculated for each sprint. Capillary blood samples were drawn from the fingertip at rest and 3 min after the tenth sprint to measure the lactate accumulation (Delta [La]). With R15, all mechanical parameters decreased significantly less in the boys than in the men over the 10 sprints (MPO: −28.9 vs. −47.0%, MFO: −13.1 vs. −25.6%, running velocity: −18.8 vs. −29.4%; all $P < 0.001$, respectively). With R180, all mechanical values remained unchanged in the boys. In the men, MPO and MFO significantly decreased over the 10 sprints (−7.8% and −4.6%; both $P < 0.05$, respectively). However, the running velocity did not decrease because the decrease in step rate ($P < 0.001$) was compensated by an increase in step length. For either recovery interval, Delta [La] values were higher in the men than the boys (R15: 12.7 vs. 7.7 mmol·L^{-1}, $P < 0.001$; R180: 10.7 vs. 7.7 mmol·L^{-1}, $P < 0.05$). To conclude, the boys more easily maintained their running performance than the men during repeated treadmill sprints with R15. Three-minute recovery periods were sufficient in the boys to repeat short running sprints without substantial fatigue. Despite the decrease in power and force outputs with R180, the young men were able to maintain their running velocity during the test.

Conclusions

In children, an universally accepted method that quantifies anaerobic energy supply is not yet available. Therefore, the measurement of STPO is a suitable alternative, although it is important to consider the limitations of each "power" test so that the results obtained can be properly interpreted. However, the final choice of a test must meet scientific (validity, reliability, objectivity) and practical (equipment, administration, age, category, suitability for research, norms) aspects.

Challenges for future research

Unlike the substantial body of results relating to the aerobic power in children or young athletes, there is a dearth of published results on anaerobic power and capacity as a result of methodologic and ethical constraints. Because of its fundamental importance in exercise and sports events, the following suggestions for short-term research are proposed:

• New technologies (e.g., nuclear magnetic resonance studies) may provide more insight into the underlying mechanism of anaerobic power output in a non-destructive way.

• Astonishingly few results in young untrained or trained girls are available. More research in this area will help to understand causes for gender differences.

• Most of the published reports are concerned with the assessment of anaerobic leg power. There is a lack of short-term arm crank ergometry.

• Today, many young athletes are being encouraged to train intensely for sporting competitions from an early age. More information about the effect of several series of repeated (intermittent) short-term high-intensity exercises on muscular fatigue is required.

References

Adamson, G.T. & Whitney, R.J. (1971) Critical appraisal of jumping as a measure of human power. In: *Medicine and Sport 6, Biomechanics* Vol. II. (Vredenbregt, J. & Wartenweiler, J., eds.) S. Karger, Basel, Switzerland: 208–211.

American Alliance for Health, Physical Education and Recreation (AAHPER) (1975) *Youth Fitness Test Manual.* AAHPER, Washington, DC.

American Alliance for Health, Physical Education and Recreation (AAHPER) (1980) *Youth Fitness Test Manual,* 2nd edn. AAHPERD, Washington, DC.

Asmussen, E. (1973) Growth in muscular strength and power. In: *Physical activity-human growth and development.* (Rarick, G.L., ed.) Academic Press, New York: 60–79.

Atkinson, G. & Nevill, A.M. (1998) Statistical methods for assessing measurement error (reliability) in variables relevant to sports medicine. *Sports Medicine* **26**, 217–238.

Bar-Or, O. (1996) Anaerobic performance. In: *Measurement in Pediatric Exercise Science* (Docherty, D., ed.) Human Kinetics, Champaign, IL: 161–182.

Bar-Or, O. (1987) The Wingate anaerobic test, an update on methodology, reliability and validity. *Sports Medicine* **4**, 381–394.

Bedu, M., Fellmann, N., Spielvogel, H.,

Falgairette, G., Van Praagh, E. & Coudert, J. (1991) Force–velocity and 30-s Wingate tests in boys at high and low altitudes. *Journal of Applied Physiology* **70**, 1031–1037.

Belli, A. & Lacour, J.R. (1989) Treadmill ergometer for power output measurements during sprint running. In: *Twelfth International Congress of Biomechanics.* University of California, Los Angeles: 391 (abstract).

Bland, J.M. & Altman, D.G. (1986) Statistical methods for assessing agreement between two methods of clinical measurement. *Lancet* **1**, 307–310.

Blimkie, C.J.R., Roache, P., Hay, J.T. & Bar-Or, O. (1988) Anaerobic power of arms in teenage boys and girls: relationship to lean tissue. *European Journal of Applied Physiology* **57**, 677–683.

Bosco, C. (1992) *Force Assessment by Means of the Bosco Test* [in French]. Società Stampa Sportiva, Rome.

Bosco, C. & Komi, P.V. (1980) Influence of aging on the mechanical behavior of leg extensor muscles. *European Journal of Applied Physiology* **45**, 209–219.

Bosco, C., Luhtanen, P. & Komi, P.V. (1983) A simple method for measurement of mechanical power in jumping. *European Journal of Applied Physiology* **50**, 272–282.

Carlson, J.S. & Naughton, G.A. (1994) Performance characteristics of children

using various braking resistances on the Wingate anaerobic test. *Journal of Sports Medicine and Physical Fitness* **34**, 362–369.

Cavagna, G.A., Saibene, P.F. & Margaria, R. (1965) Effect of negative work on the amount of positive work performed by an isolated muscle. *Journal of Applied Physiology* **20**, 157–158.

Council of Europe (1988) *European Test of Physical Fitness (Eurofit).* Edigrat Editionale Grafica, Rome.

Cumming, G.R. (1973) Correlation of athletic performance and aerobic power in 12–17-year-old children with bone age, calf muscles, total body potassium, heart volume and two indices of anaerobic power. In: *Pediatric Work Physiology* (Bar-Or, O., ed.) Wingate Institut, Natanya, Israel: 109–134.

Davies, C.T.M., Barnes, C. & Godfrey, S. (1972) Body composition and maximal exercise performance in children. *Human Biology* **44**, 195–214.

Davies, C.T.M. & Rennie, R. (1968) Human power output. *Nature* **217**, 770.

Davies, C.T.M. & Young, K. (1984) Effects of external loading on short-term power output in children and young male adults. *European Journal of Applied Physiology* **52**, 351–354.

Docherty, D. (1996) *Measurement in Pediatric Exercise Science.* Human Kinetics, Champaign, IL.

Doré, E., Bedu, M., Franca, N.M., Duché, P. & Van Praagh, E. (2000a) Testing peak cycling performance: effects of braking force during growth. *Medicine and Science in Sports and Exercise* **32**, 493–498.

Doré, E., Bedu, M., Franca, N.M., Duché, P. & Van Praagh, E. (2001) Anaerobic cycling performance characteristics in prepubescent, adolescent and young adult females. *European Journal of Applied Physiology* **84**, 476–481.

Doré, E., Diallo, O., Franca, N.M., Bedu, P. & Van Praagh, E. (2000b) Dimensional changes cannot account for all differences in short-term cycling power during growth. *International Journal of Sports Medicine* **21**, 360–365.

Doré, E., Duché, P., Rouffet, D., Ratel, S., Bedu, M. & Van Praagh, E. (2003) Measurement error in short-term power testing in young people. *Journal of Sports Science* **21**, 135–142.

Doré, E., França, N.M., Bedu, M. & Van Praagh, E. (1997) The effect of flywheel inertia on short-term cycling power output in children [Abstract]. *Medicine and Science in Sports and Exercise* **29**, S170.

Doré, E., Martin, R., Ratel, S., Duché, P., Bedu, M. & Van Praagh, E. (2005) Gender differences in peak muscle performance during growth. *International Journal of Sports Medicine* **26**, 274–280.

Dotan, R., & Bar-Or, O. (1983) Load optimization for the Wingate anaerobic test. *European Journal of Applied Physiology* **51**, 409–417.

Edwards, R.H.T. (1981) Human muscle function and fatigue. In: *Human Muscle Fatigue: Physiological Mechanisms* (Porter, R. & Whelan, J., eds.) Ciba Foundation Symposium, Pitman, London: 1–18.

Falgairette, G., Bedu, M., Fellman, N., Spielvogel, H., Van Praagh, E. & Coudert, J. (1994) Evaluation of physical fitness from field tests at high altitude in circumpubertal boys: comparison with laboratory data. *European Journal of Applied Physiology* **69**, 36–43.

Falk, B., Weinstein, Y., Dotan, R., Abramson, D.A., Mann-Segal, D. & Hoffman, J.R. (1996) A treadmill test of sprint running. *Scandinavian Journal of Medicine and Science in Sports* **6**, 259–264.

Fargeas, M.A., Lauron, B., Léger, L. & Van Praagh, E. (1993a) A computerized treadmill ergometer to measure short-term power output. *Proceedings of the Fourteenth International Congress of Biomechanics, Paris*: 394–395.

Fargeas, M.A., Van Praagh, E., Léger, L., Fellmann, N. & Coudert, J. (1993b) Comparison of cycling and running power output in trained children. *Pediatric Exercise Science* **5**, 415.

Fenn, W.O. & Marsh, B.S. (1935) Muscular force at different speeds of shortening. *Journal of Physiology (London)* **85**, 277–297.

Ferretti, G., Gussoni, M., di Prampero, P.E. & Cerretelli, P. (1987) Effects of exercise on maximal instantaneous muscle power of humans. *Journal of Applied Physiology* **62**, 2288–2294.

Ferreti, G., Narici, M.V., Binzoni, T., *et al.* (1994) Determinants of peak muscle power: effects of age and physical conditioning. *European Journal of Applied Physiology* **68**, 111–115.

Gaitanos, G., Williams, C., Boobis, L. & Brooks, S. (1993) Human muscle metabolism during intermittent maximal exercise. *Journal of Applied Physiology* **75**, 712–719.

Glencross, D.J. (1966) The nature of the vertical jump test and the standing broad jump. *Research Quarterly* **37**, 353–359.

Grassi, B., Cerretelli, P., Narici, M.V. & Marconi, C. (1991) Peak anaerobic power in master athletes. *European Journal of Applied Physiology* **62**, 394–399.

Green, S. (1994) A definition and systems view of anaerobic capacity. *European Journal of Applied Physiology and Occupational Physiology* **69**, 168–173.

Hebestreit, H., Meyer, F., Htay, H., Heigenhauser, G.J. & Bar-Or, O. (1996) Plasma metabolites, volume and electrolytes following 30-s high-intensity exercise in boys and men. *European Journal of Applied Physiology* **72**, 563–569.

Hebestreit, H., Mimura, K. & Bar-Or, O. (1993) Recovery of muscle power after high-intensity short-term exercise: comparing boys and men. *Journal of Applied Physiology* **74**, 2875–2880.

Hill, A.V. (1938) The heat of shortening and the dynamic constants of muscle. *Proceedings of the Royal Society* **126**, 136–195.

Hopkins, W.G. (2000) Measures of reliability in sports medicine and science. *Sports Medicine* **30**, 1–15.

Inbar, O. & Bar-Or, O. (1986) Anaerobic characteristics in male children and adolescents. *Medicine and Science in Sports and Exercise* **18**, 264–269.

Inbar, O., Bar-Or, O. & Skinner, S. (1996) *The Wingate Anaerobic Test*. Human Kinetics, Leeds, UK.

Kirby, R.F. (1991) *Kirby's Guide for Fitness and Motor Performance Tests*. Ben Oak, Cape Girardeau, MO.

Komi, P.V. & Bosco, C. (1978) Utilization of stored elastic energy in men and women. *Medicine and Science in Sport* **10**, 261–265.

Lakomy, H.K.A. (1986) Measurement of work and power output using friction-loaded cycle ergometers. *Ergonomics* **29**, 509–517.

Lakomy, H.K.A. (1987) The use of a non-motorized treadmill for analysing sprint performance. *Ergonomics* **30**, 627–638.

Maréchal, R., Pirnay, F., Crielaard, J.M. & Petit, J.M. (1979) *Influence of age on anaerobic power* [in French]. Economica, Paris.

Marey, E.J. & Demenÿ, G. (1885) Human locomotion: the jump mechanism [in French]. *Comptes Rendus des Séances de l'Academie des Sciences* 489–494.

Margaria, R., Aghemo, P. & Rovelli, E. (1966) Measurement of muscular power (anaerobic) in man. *Journal of Applied Physiology* **21**, 1662–1664.

Martin, J.C., Wagner, B.M. & Coyle, E.F. (1997) Inertial-load method determined maximal cycling power in a single exercise bout. *Medicine and Science in Sports and Exercise* **29**, 1505–1512.

Martin, R.J.F., Doré, E., Hautier, C.A., Van Praagh, E. & Bedu, M. (2003) Short-term peak power changes in adolescents of similar anthropometric characteristics. *Medicine and Science in Sports and Exercise* **35**, 1436–1440.

Martin, R.J.F., Doré, E., Twisk, J., Van Praagh, E., Hautier, C.A. & Bedu, M. (2004) Longitudinal changes of maximal short-term peak power in girls and boys during growth. *Medicine and Science in Sports and Exercise* **36**, 498–503.

Mercier, J., Mercier, B. & Préfaut, C. (1991) Blood lactate increase during the force–velocity exercise test. *International Journal of Sports Medicine* **12**, 17–20.

Moritani, T., Oddsson, L., Thorstensson, A. & Astrand, P.O. (1989) Neural and biomechanical differences between men and young boys during a variety of motor tasks. *Acta Physiolica Scandinavica* **137**, 147–155.

Nielsen, B., Nielsen, K., Behrendt Hansen, M. & Asmussen, E. (1980) Training of 'functional muscle strength' in girls 7–19 years old. In: *Children and Exercice*, Vol. IX (Berg. K. & Eriksson, B.O., eds.) University Park Press, Baltimore: 69–78.

Nindl, B.C., Mahar, M.T., Harman, E.A. & Patton, J.F. (1995) Lower and upper body anaerobic performance in male and female adolescent athletes. *Medicine and Science in Sports and Exercise* **27**, 235–241.

Pérès, G., Vandewalle, H. & Monod, H. (1981) Particular aspect of the load–velocity relationship during cycle ergometer pedalling [Abstract]. *Journal de Physiologie (Paris)* **77**, 10A.

Pirnay, F. & Crielaard, J.-M. (1979) Measurement of alacticid anaerobic power [in French]. *Médecine du Sport* **53**, 13–16.

Ratel, S., Bedu, M., Hennegrave, A., Doré, E. & Duché, P. (2002a) Effects of age and recovery duration on peak power output during repeated cycling sprints. *International Journal of Sports Medicine* **23**, 397–402.

Ratel, S., Duché, P., Hennegrave, A., Van Praagh, E. & Bedu, M. (2002b) Acid–base balance during repeated cycling sprints in boys and men. *Journal of Applied Physiology* **92**, 479–485.

Ratel, S., Williams, C.A., Oliver, J. & Armstrong, N. (2006) Effects of age and recovery duration on performance during multiple treadmill sprints. *International Journal of Sports Medicine* **27**, 1–8.

Rowland, T.W. (2005) *Children's Exercise Physiology*, 2nd edn. Human Kinetics, Champaign, IL.

Saltin, B., Gollnick, P.D., Eriksson, B.O. & Piehl, K. (1971) Metabolic and circulatory adjustments at onset of work. In: *Proceedings from Meeting on Pysiological Changes at Onset of Work* (Gilbert, A. & Guille, P., eds.) Toulouse, France: 46–58.

Sargeant, A.J. (1992) Problems in, and approaches to, the measurement of short term power output in children and adolescents. In: *Children & Exercise*. Vol. XVI. *Pediatric Work Physiology* (Coudert, J. & Van Praagh, E., eds.) Masson, Paris: 11–17.

Sargeant, A.J., Hoinville, E. & Young, A. (1981) Maximum leg force and power output during short-term dynamic exercise. *Journal of Applied Physiology* **53**, 1175–1182.

Sargent, D.A. (1921) The physical test of a man. *American Physical Education Reviews* **26**, 188–194.

Sutton, N.C., Childs, D.J., Bar-Or, O. & Armstrong, N. (2000) A nonmotorized treadmill test to assess children's short-term power output. *Pediatric Exercise Science* **12**, 91–100.

Taylor, D.J., Kemp, G.J., Thompson, C.H. & Radda, G.K. (1997) Ageing: effects on oxidative function of skeletal muscle *in vivo*. *Molecular and Cellular Biochemistry* **174**, 321–324.

Tirosh, E., Rosenbaum, P. & Bar-Or, O. (1990) A new muscle power test in neuromuscular disease: feasibility and reliability. *American Journal of Diseases of Childhood* **144**, 1083–1087.

Tong, R.J., Bell, W., Ball, G. & Winter, E.M. (2001) Reliability of power output measurements during repeated treadmill sprinting in rugby players. *Journal of Sports Science* **19**, 289–297.

Vandewalle, H., Pérès, G. & Monod, H. (1987) Standard anaerobic exercise tests. *Sports Medicine* **4**, 268–289.

Van Praagh, E. (2000) Development of anaerobic function during childhood and adolescence. *Pediatric Exercise Science* **12**, 150–173.

Van Praagh, E., Bedu, M., Falgairette, G., Fellmann, N. & Coudert, J. (1991) Oxygen uptake during a 30-s supramaximal exercise in 7 to 15 year-old boys. In: *Children and Exercise*. Vol. XV. *Pediatric Work Physiology* (Frenkl, R. & Szmodis, I., eds.) National Institute for Health Promotion, Budapest, Hungary: 281–287.

Van Praagh, E., Bedu, M., Roddier, P. & Coudert, J. (1992) A simple calibration method for mechanically braked cycle ergometers. *International Journal of Sports Medicine* **13**, 27–30.

Van Praagh, E. & Doré, E. (2002) Short-term muscle power during growth and maturation. *Sports Medicine* **32**, 701–728.

Van Praagh, E., Falgairette, G., Bedu, M., Fellmann, N. & Coudert, J. (1989) Laboratory and field tests in 7-year-old boys. In: *Children and Exercise*, Vol. XIII (Oseid, S. & Carlsen, K.-H., eds.) Human Kinetics, Champaign, IL: 11–17.

Van Praagh, E., Fargeas, M.A., Léger, L., Fellmann, N. & Coudert, J. (1993) Short-term power output in children measured on a computerised treadmill ergometer. *Pediatric Exercise Science* **5**, 482.

Van Praagh, E., Fellmann, N., Bedu, M., Falgairette, G. & Coudert, J. (1990) Gender difference in the relationship of anaerobic power output to body composition in children. *Pediatric Exercise Science* **2**, 336–348.

Van Praagh, E. & França, N.M. (1998) Measuring maximal short-term power output during growth. In: *Pediatric Anaerobic Performance* (Van Praagh, E., ed.) Human Kinetics, Champaign, IL: 155–189.

Viitasalo, J.T. (1988) Evaluation of explosive strength for young and adult athletes. *Research Quarterly for Exercise and Sport* **59**, 9–13.

Viitasalo, J.T., Rahkila, P., Österback, L. & Alén, M. (1992) Vertical jumping height and horizontal overhead throwing velocity in young male athletes. *Journal of Sports Science* **10**, 401–413.

Wilkie, D.R. (1950) The relation between force and velocity in human muscle. *Journal of Physiology (London)* **110**, 249–280.

Wilkie, D.R. (1960) Man as a source of mechanical power. *Ergonomics* **3**, 1–8.

Williams, C. (1987) Short-term activity. In: *Exercise: Benefits, Limits and Adaptations* (Macleod, D., *et al.*, eds.) Spon, London: 59–62.

Williams, C.A., Doré, E., James, A. & Van Praagh, E. (2003) Short term power output in 9 year old children: Typical error between ergometers and protocols. *Pediatric Exercise Science* **15**, 302–312.

Winter, E.M. & Maclaren, D.P. (2001) Assessment of maximal-intensity exercise. In: Eston, R.G. & Reilly, T., eds.) *Kinanthropometry and Exercise Physiology Laboratory Manual: Tests, Procedures and Data*. Vol. 2. *Exercise Physiology*, 2nd edn. Routledge, London: 263–288.

Wootton, S.A. & Williams, C. (1983) The influence of recovery duration on repeated maximal sprints. In: *Biochemistry of Exercise*. Vol. V. (Knuttgen, H.G., Vogel, J.A. & Poortmans J.J., eds.) Human Kinetics, Champaign, IL: 269–273.

Zanconato, S., Buchtal, S., Barstow, T.J. & Cooper, D.M. (1993) 31P-magnetic resonance spectroscopy of leg muscle metabolism during exercise in children and adults. *Journal of Applied Physiology* **74**, 2214–2218.

Chapter 34

Longitudinal Studies during Growth and Training: Importance and Principles

HAN C.G. KEMPER

Individual changes in growth, development, and fitness can only be studied if the same individuals are measured repeatedly over a period of time. This is called a longitudinal study. Two types of longitudinal research can be distinguished:

1 In non-interventive research, early characteristics are noted and changes over time analyzed on individual basis. Most of this prospective longitudinal research is descriptive and from such non-interventive research there can be no attempt made to establish causal relationships (Mednick & Baert 1981).

2 If one is interested in the effects of a training program on sporting youth, one has to take on longitudinal research with an interventive nature. This is called manipulative or experimental longitudinal research. Assuming that proper controls (e.g., no training) and research designs are used, certain causal statements can be made concerning the conclusions of such so-called randomized controlled trials (RCTs).

The great need for experimental longitudinal research in the child and adolescent athlete is because they are in a phase of continuous growth and development. Their morphologic, physiologic, and psychologic characteristics keep changing over the years and these changes are similar to training effects. For example, during growth and maturation children increase their muscle force, aerobic power, and motor coordination. Without control groups of children who do not train, the effects of sport cannot be evaluated.

Longitudinal research is also needed because non-interventive comparisons of children who train with those who do not train cannot discern the effects of sports training over a period of time. Self-selection is a serious problem in comparing sporting with non-sporting groups. It can be assumed that the sporting children are different from the non-sporting group because they are genetically better suited for sport performances than their non-sporting counterparts. Therefore, only RCTs in which the experimental and control group are randomly chosen and are compared over a period of time can give solid conclusions about the effects of participation in sport and training in growing youth.

In this chapter, the importance of longitudinal training studies is discussed, including the disadvantages of longitudinal designs such as testing and drop-out effects. A review is given of longitudinal studies in children and adolescents in which the effects of physical activity, sports participation, and training are evaluated. Because of the lack of studies in which girls have been tested using true experimental designs, this type of experiment needs further research with regard to gender.

Practical problems with longitudinal studies

The most common practical problems in longitudinal projects are as follow.

1 *Long-term financial commitment.* The period of repeated (e.g., annual) measurements must be preceded by an expensive training period for the staff. All the investigators must be hired before the start of the first measurements. Because there is no loss of subjects in the initial stage, there is a high cost of staff commitment.

2 *Long-term commitment of staff members and subjects.* The longer the duration of the study, the more chance there is that a large percentage of individuals will drop out, and if this dropout is selective, the population will no longer be representative. The same holds true when staff members leave and new investigators join the study. This may cause a test leader bias. The original purposes of the longitudinal research are sometimes modified by new ideas and interests.

3 *Techniques that become obsolete.* Although measures and techniques are thoroughly investigated at the start, they may become out of date several years later. Apparatus can fail over the years and new apparatus with other specifications can seriously disturb the individual curves. Likewise, new techniques that appear later cannot be included in the follow-up. It is also advisable to record the raw data rather than complex derivatives. Any new techniques of analysis and changes of interest during the project can be then be used on these raw data.

4 *Adherence of subjects.* To recruit subjects for repeated measurements over a longer period is a serious problem. During the first measurements all subjects are curious and eager to participate. Keeping their interest in the following years is a major challenge. Therefore, the subjects have to be informed and stimulated by special measures that are extrinsic to the research such as information sessions, general explanatory texts, personal reports with update of their own results, and, in the case of children, gifts (e.g., photographs, T-shirts).

5 *Final analysis and publication.* Only when the final measurements are completed can analysis begin and results published. The database will be large and the longitudinal analyses complicated, taking up considerable time and money. The importance of the final stage in a longitudinal study cannot be underestimated.

A longitudinal study therefore needs to be thoroughly planned. Starting a longitudinal study is not that difficult, but to finish it with repeated measurements in the same subjects over the foreseen follow-up period is the difficult task.

Individual changes

During youth, children and adolescents grow and develop to maturity at different paces. Children who grow fast and reach full maturity at an early chronologic age are called early maturers in contrast with late maturers, who reach full maturity at a later chronologic age. Both types of subjects are involved in longitudinal studies. Grouped data of children of the same chronologic age are composed of a mixture of subjects with different states of biologic maturation. The effects of a training or sport program may be different depending on the state of maturation (Vrijens 1978).

Changes that are related to biologic development can be measured. In growth studies, height and weight are measured at intervals of 2–6 months in order to calculate their velocities (change over time; e.g., height velocity in cm·year^{-1}). These velocities can be used as indicators for the biologic age of the growing child. During puberty, an increase in height occurs in both boys and girls and the peak height velocity (PHV) correlates well with other parameters of biologic maturation such as sexual maturation, menarche, and breast development in girls, and penis or testis development in boys. This is the case in both sexes with axillary and pubic hair development (Falkner & Tanner 1978).

Using longitudinal data, the changes in dependent variables such as aerobic power or muscle power can be related not only to chronologic age but also to other age scales that may be more relevant to the effects of physical activity on the human body. In the literature, age relative to PHV and skeletal age are used (Kemper 1985). Beunen and Malina (1988) also used different functional parameters such as peak muscle force velocity as age-related parameters (for details see Chapter 1).

In Fig. 34.1, 12-min endurance run performances are related both to skeletal age and chronologic age of a group of boys and girls. In Fig. 34.2, maximal arm pull muscle force is related to PHV age and to chronologic age in the same group of boys and girls as in Fig. 34.1.

Principles of longitudinal designs

In almost every study of growth, development and training confounding effects will occur, no matter which design has been used. Three classic designs have been most commonly used:

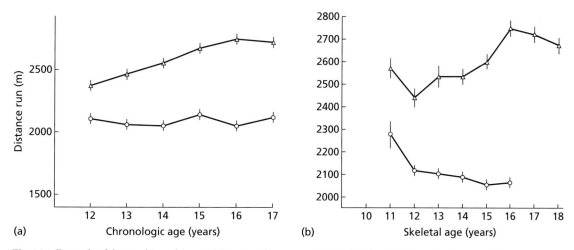

Fig. 34.1 Example of the aerobic endurance (12-min endurance run test) related to: (a) chronologic age; and (b) skeletal age. Open triangle, males; open circle, females. From Kemper (1985).

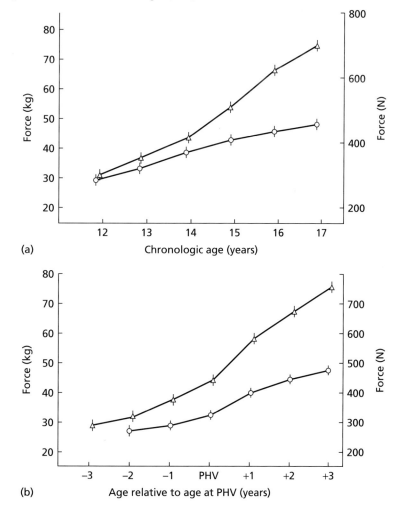

Fig. 34.2 Example of static arm strength (arm pull test) related to: (a) chronologic age; and (b) peak height velocity (PHV) age. Open triangle, males; open circle, females. From (Kemper) 1985.

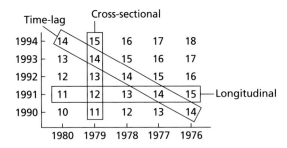

Fig. 34.3 Graphic representation of the three classic research designs: vertical bar, cross-sectional; diagonal bar, time-lag; and horizontal bar, longitudinal.

1 Cross-sectional design;
2 Time-lag design; and
3 Longitudinal design (Fig. 34.3).
Each measurement taken on a subject at a particular point of time is influenced by three factors:
1 Chronologic age of the subject, defined as the period that elapses between birth and time of measurement. Age effects produce the mean growth curve.
2 Birth cohort to which the subject belongs. This is defined as the group of individuals born in the same year. Cohort effects can be used to study secular trends.
3 Time of measurement (i.e., the moment at which the measurement is taken). Time of measurement effects are related to changes in environmental conditions that can occur over a period of time (such as changes in the methods of measuring in circumstances).

The three different designs are characterized in the following ways. In a cross-sectional study, the time of measurement is kept constant (cohort and age are varied), and different groups are measured at the same point of time (vertical bar in Fig. 34.3). Conversely, in a time-lag study, different groups of the same age are measured at different points of time, thus age is kept constant (cohort and time of measurement are varied; diagonal bar in Fig. 34.3). In a longitudinal study, information is gathered from one cohort at different points in time, thus at different ages. Because the cohort is kept constant (age and time of measurement are varied), the same group is measured repeatedly (horizontal bar in Fig. 34.3). None of these designs allows all three effects to be isolated (age, time of measurement, and cohort) (Schaie 1965).

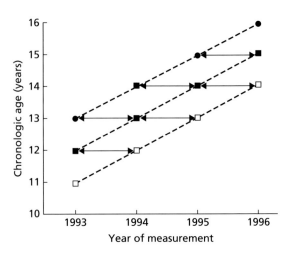

Fig. 34.4 Example of a multiple longitudinal design with three birth cohorts (1980, 1981, and 1982) which are measured in 4 consecutive years (1993, 1994, 1995, and 1996). Horizontal arrows indicate possible comparisons of different cohorts of the same age groups at different times of measurement.

Multiple longitudinal design

Descriptions can be found in the literature of several designs that try to overcome confounding effects (Tanner 1962; Rao & Rao 1966; Kowalski & Prahl-Andersen 1979). The "multiple longitudinal" design uses repeated measurements on more than one cohort (Kemper & Van 't Hof 1978), with overlapping ages during the study. This has the advantage of isolating the main effect (e.g. age effect) from interfering effects such as time of measurement and cohort.

In Fig. 34.4 an example is given of a multiple longitudinal design using three birth cohorts (1980, 1981, and 1982) which is measured over four consecutive years (1993–1996). Because there is an overlap in age, the cohorts can be compared with each other at different ages (horizontal comparisons in Fig. 34.4). A systematic difference between the cohorts at these ages is called a "cohort effect." At the same time, it is possible to distinguish another confounding factor in a longitudinal study; the time of measurement (Veling & Van 't Hof 1980). If there are no cohort effects, the time of measurement is blamed for a possible difference between the two groups. If it appears that there is no time

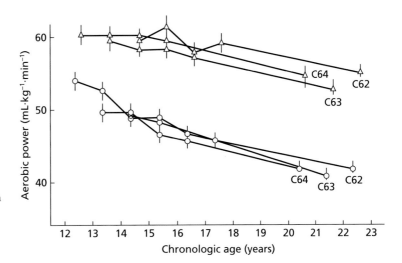

Fig. 34.5 Mean and standard error (SE) of maximal aerobic power, measured in the Amsterdam Growth and Health Study in males (open triangle) and females (open circle) from three birth cohorts (C62, C63, and C64).

of measurement effect and no cohort effect either, then the data of all cohorts at all points of time can be arranged in age groups and a real developmental pattern can be discerned (Bell 1954).

This pattern is illustrated in Fig. 34.5 with a data set from the Amsterdam Growth and Health Study. In this multiple longitudinal study, three birth cohorts (1962, 1963, and 1964) are used to measure $\dot{V}o_{2max}$ five times. Because of the overlap in age groups at the age of 13, 14, 15, and 16 years, the mean values of the cohorts can be combined (if there are no significant cohort effects) to construct the mean age curve. Another advantage of a multiple design is that in 4-yearly measurement periods a 5-year developmental pattern can be estimated (12–17 years in Fig. 34.5).

Testing or learning effects

Another problem with repeated measurements is a testing or learning effect. Many variables, physical as well as psychologic, require a certain motivation or habituation of the subject while being measured. This introduces differences between periods of measurement that are solely caused by the changes in attitude towards the measurement procedure itself. Such testing effects may be positive (i.e., when habituation or learning is important) or negative (i.e., when motivation decreases). Physical performance tests, where maximal motivation is needed, are

particularly threatened by these effects. Repeated measurements may therefore have a disturbing influence on the quantity measured and diminish the external validity of the results.

Systematic testing effects can be estimated if the design also includes a control group in which repeated measurements are not made. Cross-sectional data gathered from an identical population can be compared with those of the longitudinally measured population, except that they were not repeated measurements but derived from independent samples. In this design, when comparing data from both populations, systematic divergence of mean values in the course of the study is an indication of testing effect (Fig. 34.6).

Cohort effect, as well as time of measurement and testing effects, if established for a certain characteristic, will seriously hinder the interpretation of individual and mean growth curves. If neither cohort, time of measurement, nor testing effects can be found, the data of the different cohorts can simply be averaged and arranged in age groups to study the overall changes.

Longitudinal studies in growth, development, and physical fitness

In *A History of the Study of Human Growth*, Tanner (1981) reviewed the well-established growth studies since 1900. This section focuses on longitudinal

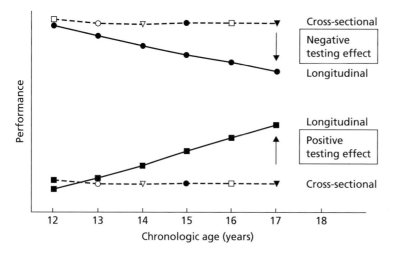

Cross-sectional

Negative
testing effect

Longitudinal

Longitudinal

Positive
testing effect

Cross-sectional

Fig. 34.6 Negative and/or positive testing effects can be studied by comparing cross-sectional data with longitudinal data. The same symbols represent mean values of same subjects; different symbols represent the mean values of different subjects.

studies in children and adolescents that include physical performance and fitness measurements over a period of more than 3 years.

Most of the major growth studies in the USA (e.g., the Harvard, Fels, and Denver studies) and in Europe (e.g., Harpenden study [Tanner *et al.* 1976] and several studies coordinated by the International Children's Centre [ICC]) are not reviewed because they did not include physical performance measurements and/or a physical activity component. In this chapter, the studies are divided into the five periods described below (for more details see also Kemper 1986, 1988).

First longitudinal approaches: USA 1920–1940

The first longitudinal approaches to growth studies were initiated in the USA by Baldwin (1921) who designed a mixed longitudinal study. This means that in the course of the study new subjects were recruited periodically and subsequently followed. He introduced a method of measuring standing height with a wall meter and initiated the measurement of height, weight, width, circumferences, vital capacity, and strength in Iowa children. After his death the work was continued by McCloy (1936) who introduced the first skinfold measurements, and Meredith (1935) who is well known for introducing accurate measurement procedures into anthropometrics.

The Berkeley growth study began in 1928 at the Institute of Child Welfare and was the first growth

study at the University of California. Bayley (1940) started with 31 boys and 30 girls recruited at birth from two Berkeley hospitals. Nearly 70% of them were followed successfully until maturity. This is a high percentage over a period of 18 years. Data were collected on physical and intellectual development. Photographs and radiographs of the hand and wrist were taken as a measure of a skeletal maturation.

The adolescent growth study at the University of California started in 1932 with 120 boys and girls, ended 7 years later with 60 subjects of each sex. This study is important for its orientation towards physiologic changes at puberty. Blood pressure, basal oxygen consumption, heart rate and strength, as well as skeletal maturation, were measured at 6-months intervals (Jones 1949). The results of motor performance tests on the same children were reported by Espenschade (1947). This growth study demonstrated for the first time that there was no pubertal period during which strength or motor performance declined.

Second period: Europe, 1940 to present

Before 1940 the important longitudinal studies came predominantly from North America. After 1940 European countries dominated in this field of growth research. Coordinated by the ICC, a group of representatives from different European research centers formulated a common baseline for measures, sampling procedures, and design in longitudinal studies on child growth (Falkner 1954).

The first two ICC growth studies were initiated by Moncrieff and Debré in Paris, who agreed that exactly the same somatic and psychologic methods should be used in the same cohorts of their London (Moore *et al.* 1954) and Paris growth studies (Falkner 1954). Other international child health centers showed an interest in coordinated longitudinal growth study research and soon the ICC studies were extended with growth studies in Stockholm/Gotheborg by Wallgren, in Zurich by Franconi, in Brussels by Graffar and Courbier (1966), and also some workers from outside Europe joined the group (from Dakar, Kampala, and Louisville). An overview of 25 years of internationally coordinated research was published containing a selection of the teams, their present status, and a bibliography (Falkner 1980).

In all ICC studies the investigations began with 3-monthly measurements in the first year after birth. During the second year there were 6-monthly measurements. The measurements were continued thereafter at yearly intervals until maturity. In the Zurich study, 6-month intervals were used during puberty (Largo *et al.* 1978). The baseline anthropometric measurements and radiographs of the hand and wrist were based on the Harpenden growth study techniques. Only the Paris and Stockholm/Gotheborg studies added activity histories and physical fitness measurements. Sample sizes differed quite considerably from one center to another, the smallest sample being the Stockholm/Gotheborg study with 90 girls and 122 boys (Karlberg *et al.* 1976) and the largest in the Paris study with 237 girls and 260 boys (Roy-Pernot *et al.* 1976). However, the selective dropout from the original samples was considerable, particularly in the Paris study: out of 497 babies, only 43 remained in the study until the age of 18 years.

Third period: North America and Europe

The initial objective for the Medford boys growth study was to investigate whether training practices pertaining to interschool competitive athletics among elementary schoolboys were harmful to the physical and emotional welfare of the participants.

In this North American mixed longitudinal growth study annual testing of strength and motor performances was conducted for 12 years from 1956 to 1968 (Clarke 1971), starting with children aged 7, 9, 12, and 15 years. The same boys were tested annually within 2 months of their birthdays until the age of 18 years.

The Prague growth study (Parizkova 1974; Sprynarova 1974) was initiated in 1961. A total of 143 boys with complete data were subdivided into two activity groups according to overall time spent on physical activity. Inspired by the World Health Organization, during the 1970s Lange Andersen, Seliger and Rutenfranz coordinated a longitudinal study of children in Norway and the former German Federal Republic. Two small rural communities were chosen (Lom and Fredeburg). The children were followed from the age of 8 to 16 years. Measurements included $\dot{V}o_{2max}$ (Lange Andersen *et al.* 1974c), heart rate and oxygen pulse during submaximal and maximal exercise (Lange Andersen *et al.* 1974a), respiratory response (Lange Andersen *et al.* 1974b) and influence of physical education (Lange Andersen *et al.* 1976).

In the former Czechoslovakia (Bratislava), Placheta (1980) performed a complex 3-year longitudinal examination of several groups of boys aged 12–15 years who were skilled at different motor activities including cyclists, rowers and ice-hockey players, plus a control group. To assess the influence of motor activity on development, the state of health, physique, physical fitness, blood chemistry, and lung functions were measured.

The Canadian stream

The Saskatchewan Growth and Development Study (Bailey 1968) began in 1964 with a group of 7-year-old boys. In 1965, 7-year-old girls were added, with the objective of following both groups for a period of 15 years. However, after 10 years of data collection for the boys, and 9 years for the girls, financial support was withdrawn. Although preliminary results in boys have been published (Carron & Bailey 1974; Mirwald 1980), a considerable amount of data remained unanalyzed. This study and the one in Prague were the first to produce longitudinal data on the maximal oxygen uptake of the same subjects over a considerable period of time.

Cunningham *et al.* (1977, 1981) completed a 5-year longitudinal study on 81 boys recruited from participants in organized ice-hockey (aged 10–15 years). This study included yearly testing of maximal oxygen uptake on a treadmill. Maturation level was determined by a hand-wrist X-ray at 10 and 14 years. The intent of the Canadian longitudinal study in the Trois Rivieres region (Jecquier *et al.* 1977) was not only to measure the physical and psychologic development of French Canadian schoolchildren, but also to study the effect of additional physical education upon their development between the ages of 5 and 12 years (the usual one lesson per week was changed to five). Over the 8 years of annual observation, almost 30% of the original sample was lost to the study. In the presence of many interfering factors such as experimental vs. control groups, urban vs. rural localities, it was not easy to evaluate the research hypotheses in this study (Shephard *et al.* 1980).

Benelux studies

The Leuven growth study of Belgian boys was designed to provide information on the physical fitness of normal boys from 12 to 20 years of age. In the Leuven study, children from entire classes of 59 schools were measured at yearly intervals at the same time of the year. Because of the design of the study it is understandable that from the original sample of 4278 boys observed for the first time in 1969 only 587 were followed throughout the 6-year period (Ostyn *et al.* 1980). In 1990 results were also published on the fitness of girls, but this was initially a cross-sectional design (Simons *et al.* 1990). Later on the girls were also followed (Simons *et al.* 1990).

A second Leuven study was initiated in 1969—the Leuven longitudinal experimental growth study (LEGS). This multidisciplinary study included children from 3 to 15 years of age (Hebbelinck *et al.* 1980). The Nijmegen growth study of the Netherlands was a large-scale interdisciplinary study, which has been limited to the 4–14 year age range. By stopping at 14 years of age, some valuable information was undoubtedly missed concerning the developmental

processes of boys and girls during puberty (Prahl-Andersen *et al.* 1979).

While the ICC studies and most of the North American studies used one single longitudinal cohort (except the Medford study), and the Harpenden, Leuven, and Trois Rivieres studies used mixed longitudinal designs, the Nijmegen study used a multiple longitudinal design. This design is a sophisticated compromise between the more traditional approaches to the study of development; namely, cross-sectional, longitudinal, and time-lag designs, as described above. The Amsterdam growth and health study is also a multiple longitudinal study. It started with three birth cohorts of boys and girls (from the first and second forms of a secondary school) in 1977 who were followed for 4 years (12–17 years) and measured again in 1985 (21 years) and 1991 (26–28 years), covering an age range of almost 15 years (Kemper 1995). In 1993, 1997, and 2000 the study was continued, following the subjects to age 35–37 years (Kemper 2004).

Most of the reviewed longitudinal studies are only descriptive and of a non-interventive type. A step further in the development of knowledge about training effects is to set up more experimental research; interventive longitudinal studies can be useful in revealing the influence of different types of training upon the health and performance of young people.

Overview of recent longitudinal studies on lifestyle and health from adolescence into adulthood

This overview is restricted to those with a follow-up of at least 8 years, covering measurements of lifestyle and biologic risk indicators of chronic diseases from adolescence into young adulthood (Koppes *et al.* 2004). Eleven studies that met the inclusion criteria were identified. Table 34.1 indicates for each study name, country, period and number of measurements, age range, gender, and number of participants, measured variables, and key publications.

The common feature of these studies is that they prospectively investigated the relationships between lifestyle behaviors and health characteristics over the important life transition from

Table 34.1 Overview of longitudinal studies on lifestyle and health from adolescence into adulthood.

Study	Country	Measurements		Participants				Measured variables										Key publications
		Period	No.	Age range	Gender	No. at Start	End	a	b	c	d	e	f	g	h	i	j	
Amsterdam Growth and Health Longitudinal Study	The Netherlands	1977–2000	9	13–36	M & F	600	375	X	X	X	X	X	X	X	X	X	X	Kemper (2004)
Cardiovascular Risk in Young Finns Study	Finland	1980–1992	5	3/18–15/30	M & F	3596	2370	X	X	X	X	X		X	X	X	X	Valimaki et al. (1994)
Children in the Community Study	USA	1983–1991	3	14–22	M & F	776	644			X	X	X			X	X		Cohen & Cohen (1996)
Danish Youth and Sports Study	Denmark	1983–1991	2	17–25	M & F	305	203	X		X	X	X	X	X				Andersen & Haraldsdottier (1993)
Dunedin Multidisciplinary Health and Development Study	New Zealand	1975–1998	10	3–26	M & F	1037	930	X	X	X	X	X	X	X		X	X	Silva & Stanton (1996)
Leuven Longitudinal Study on Lifestyle, Fitness and Health	Belgium	1969–1996	9	13–40	M	588	166	X	X	X	X	X	X	X	X	X	X	Lefevre et al. (2002)
Muscatine Study	USA	1971–1999	8	8–42	M & F	14,066	725	X		X	X	X	X	X	X	X	X	Lauer et al. (1988)
Northern Finland 1966 Birth Cohort	Finland	1980–1997	2	14–31	M & F	11,399	8767	X	X	X	X	X	X	X	X	X	X	Tammelin et al. (2003)
Northern Ireland Young Hearts Project	Northern Ireland	1989–1999	3	12–22	M & F	1015	508	X	X	X	X	X	X	X	X	X	X	Gallagher et al. (2002)
Québec Family Study	Canada	1980–1992	2	13–25	M & F	790	151	X		X	X	X	X	X	X	X		Katzmarzyk et al. (2001)
Swedish Activity and Fitness Study	Sweden	1974–1992	2	16–34	M & F	425	278	X		X	X	X	X	X		X	X	Barnekow-Bergkvist et al. (2001)

a, Physical activity; b, Dietary intake; c, Alcohol consumption; d, Tobacco smoking; e, Anthropometry; f, indicators of physical fitness; g, cardiovascular disease risk-factors (blood pressure, and/or cholesterol); h, indicators of bone health; i, other indicators of health status; j, psychologic/sociologic characteristics. From Koppes (2004).

adolescence into adulthood. Inevitably, these studies differ with respect to volume, quality, scope, accomplishments, and promise. In addition to the summary in Table 34.1, these studies are now discussed in alphabetic order.

The Amsterdam Growth and Health Longitudinal Study (AGAHLS), started as a 4-year mixed longitudinal study focusing on the growth, physical activity, and fitness of teenagers. None of the first- and second-year pupils from the two participating secondary schools refused to attend a first measurement at adolescence. About 35% dropped out over the following 23 years. The participants from one school were asked to attend all nine measurements, while those from the other school attended a maximum of one measurement at adolescence plus the two last measurements at the ages of 32 and 36 years. The measured variables a–g and j in Table 34.1 have been assessed at each measurement, and in addition to the listed variables, birth weight and arterial wall properties are important other measured variables in the AGAHLS (Kemper 1985, 1995, 2004).

The Cardiovascular Risk in Young Finns Study is a collaborative effort of all university departments of pediatrics and several other institutions in Finland to study the risk factors of coronary heart disease (CHD) and their determinants in children and adolescents (Valimaki *et al.* 1994). Boys and girls in the wide age range 3–18 years were included in the first measurement in 1980. The attrition rate was about 34% over the 12 years of follow-up. In addition to articles on the development with age and the interrelations of the assessed CHD risk factors, main articles are published on socioeconomic status, and clustering and tracking of CHD risk factors.

The focus of the Children in the Community Study was on the prevalence and risk factors for psychiatric symptoms in late childhood and adolescence (Cohen & Cohen 1996). The randomly sampled participants were sons and daughters of women who had been interviewed 11 years before the start of this study. Given the focus on psychiatric disorders, and demographic and other psychosocial variables, it is not surprising that physical activity, diet, and several aspects of health that are assessed in the other summarized studies were not assessed here.

The Danish Youth and Sports Study is a relatively small school-based study (Andersen & Haraldsdottier 1993). Only two-thirds of the initial population of 305 adolescent boys and girls attended the second measurement 8 years later. Published articles mainly focus on physical activity, fitness, and other CHD risk factors.

The Dunedin Multidisciplinary Health and Development Study consists of an unselected sample of boys and girls born between April 1972 and March 1973 in one hospital in New Zealand (Silva & Stanton 1996). The large number of publications on the birth cohort involve studies on birth weight, psychosocial aspects, problem behavior, dental health, and diverse other aspects of health.

The Leuven Longitudinal Study on Lifestyle, Fitness, and Health is the only included study that did not involve assessments in females (Lefevre *et al.* 2002). The 588 boys who were followed longitudinally were selected on pragmatic grounds from an original cross-sectional sample in 1969 of 4278 boys. Like the AGAHLS, it is a school-based study involving children from entire classes and was initially designed to provide information of the natural growth, physical activity, and fitness of teenagers. Other variables such as bone mineral density, stress, and coping have been added at adult age.

The Muscatine Study is a population-based investigation of cardiovascular disease risk factors (Lauer *et al.* 1988). It was originally designed as a cross-sectional school-based study. The initial follow-up measurements were performed only in the boys and girls who at that time were still at those schools. This resulted in the large attrition of participants. Although smoking and alcohol consumption have been assessed, practically all publications on lifestyle involve physical activity. Some other variables used in the Muscatine Study are fasting insulin and glucose, left ventricular mass, carotid intima media thickness, and coronary artery calcium.

Investigations in the Northern Finland 1966 Birth Cohort started with lifestyle, biologic, and sociologic measurements of the mothers of the cohort members in the sixth month of their pregnancy (Tammelin *et al.* 2003). The information obtained here was linked with perinatal and later outcomes obtained from measurements by the study group at ages of 14 and 31 years, and obtained from national registers. A large diversity of variables, such as social economic status, oral health habits, hormones, criminal behavior, mental disorders, and neurologic handicaps have formed the basis of publications. No data are available on adolescent dietary intakes, and the number of publications on adolescent physical activity and tobacco and alcohol use is small.

In order to search for causes of the high death rates from CHD in Northern Ireland, the Young Hearts Project was initiated (Gallagher *et al.* 2002). The original survey was completed in boys and girls from 16 randomly sampled representative schools of secondary education. About 50% of the original cohort participated in the last measurement so far at the age of 22 years. Not surprisingly, most publications on the project are about the socioeconomic, lifestyle, and biologic risk factors for CHD (including birth weight), whereas a few publications on adult age bone mineral status are available.

The Québec Family Study is designed to investigate genetic and environmental influences on several biochemical, physical, and physiologic characteristics (Katzmarzyk *et al.* 2001). Together with their parents, the participants were recruited using the local media. The participants were 8–18 years of age at the time of the first measurement. Only a few of the many publications on the Québec Family Study involved longitudinal data from adolescence into adulthood.

The participants in the Swedish Activity and Fitness Study were randomly selected pupils of randomly selected schools that were geographically and rural/urban representative, and of both practical and theoretical programs (Barnekow-Berkvist *et al.* 2001). Most publications on this study are about physical activity and/or fitness, while one publication is about neck, shoulder, and low back symptoms.

Longitudinal training studies in the child and adolescent

Longitudinal studies in children that aim to analyze the effects of training can be divided in two major types. In the first type, children are followed over a period of time. During that period some remain or become more physically active ("athletes") and the others remain or become inactive ("non-athletes"). At the end of the study, based on a retrospective determination, subgroups are made of children with differences in the observed or measured levels of physical activity. Children who showed a relatively high level of activity during the observation period are contrasted with children of the same sex, age, and other relevant characteristics who showed a relatively low level of activity during the same observation period. In four of the aforementioned studies (Saskatchewan Growth and Development Study, Prague Growth Study, Youth and Physical Activity Bratislava, and Amsterdam Growth and Health Longitudinal Study), the following tracking procedure was taken: subjects were divided into high activity (athletes) and low activity (non-athletes) groups on the base of their longitudinally collected data. In all these comparisons, active children demonstrated higher physiologic characteristics than the less active children. However, these results are not conclusive about the effects of physical activity; because the children made their own decisions about being active or not, self-selection may have influenced the results. Kemper (1986) showed that the aerobic power of adolescent boys and girls is significantly higher in active children, but the differences remain the same between 12- and 18-year-olds as should be expected as a result of higher training stimuli throughout the years. Therefore, the author concluded that the differences in $\dot{V}o_{2max}$ were not only caused by training, but also by heredity; active adolescents are more active because they have a higher aerobic power at their disposal.

The second type of training studies utilizes the school environment. A change is initiated in the school curriculum by adding physical education (PE) lessons as extra or as a replacement for other school subjects. Comparisons are made before and after the change with control classes that did not have curriculum modifications. Kemper *et al.* (1976) reviewed these and found in general no effects in physical fitness before puberty. The main reasons are as follow:

1 High training status of prepubertal children;
2 Low intensity of PE classes;
3 Small number of extra PE lessons;
4 Non-homogeneity of maturation between subjects; and

5 Low specificity of training stimulus: most of the PE lessons are devoted to motor coordination improvement and less to endurance and resistance training. This is reflected by the fact that in most of the studies motor coordination increased significantly in the experimental groups compared to control groups but not maximal aerobic power ($\dot{V}o_{2max}$) and maximal muscle force (F_{max}).

The only long-term intervention study (6 years) is the Trois Rivieres regional study in Canada (Shephard 1982). Children enrolled in the experimental program received five 40-min PE lessons per week integrated into the normal primary school curriculum. Control subjects received the usual one lesson of PE per week. This experiment followed boys and girls from 6 to 12 years of age.

$\dot{V}o_{2max}$ and other physical fitness characteristics increased significantly more in the experimental classes than in the control classes in the last 3 years, from age 8 to 11 years.

Aerobic training

Several critical reviews have been written about aerobic training effects in children. Sady (1986) reviewed more than 20 training studies. Only those studies were selected that made use of comparable control groups of children who were not trained. The increase in $\dot{V}o_{2max} \cdot$kg body weight^{-1} appears to vary considerably and there seem to be no differences in trainability between pubescent and postpubescent children. In Fig. 34.7 the percent increase of $\dot{V}o_{2max} \cdot$kg body weight^{-1} in the training group with respect to the increase in the control group is plotted for 27 studies against the duration of the aerobic training period: short term (<6 months) and long term (>6 months) were distinguished (Kemper & van de Kop 1994). The results show that in training studies with a duration of 4–15 weeks, effects vary between −2% (in two studies detraining was measured) and +20% of base-line $\dot{V}o_{2max} \cdot$kg body weight^{-1}. In training studies with a duration of 0.5–5 years, the effects vary from −10 to +10% of baseline $\dot{V}o_{2max} \cdot$kg body weight^{-1}.

Rowland (1985) stated that, when training programs in children are examined, those regimens failing to demonstrate a beneficial effect on aerobic fitness also do not comply with adult standards formulated by the American College of Sports Medicine (1990). Pate and Ward (1990) also concluded

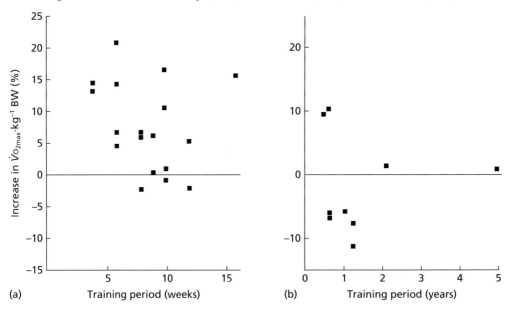

Fig. 34.7 Percentage increase of $\dot{V}o_{2max} \cdot$kg body weight^{-1} (BW) in training group with respect to control group of 27 training studies of different duration ranging from 4 weeks to 5 years. (a) Short-term training (<6 months); and (b) long-term training (>6 months). From Kemper and van de Kop (1994).

from 14 well-designed studies that both pre- and post-pubertal children are physiologically adaptive to endurance exercise training as demonstrated by statistically significant increases in $\dot{V}o_{2max}\cdot$kg body weight^{-1} in the training groups compared to the non-training groups. Although it is possible that a critical age exists before which the child is less trainable (before PHV age; Kobayashi *et al.* 1978; Mirwald & Bailey 1985), other authors (Weber *et al.* 1976; Cunningham *et al.* 1984; Froberg *et al.* 1991) cast considerable doubt on the hypothesis that greater training effects may be gained by exercise training during the period of PHV. Vaccaro and Mahon (1987) stated that the critical stage of maturity during which endurance training has its greatest influence on the cardiorespiratory system is still speculative. The degree of trainability seems to be dependent on: (a) motivation (prepubescents are less trainable); and (b) from pretraining levels (children can be very active even when not taking part in programmed sports training). Although in some studies no training effect or even a negative effect was shown in $\dot{V}o_{2max}\cdot$kg body weight^{-1} (Fig. 34.7), performance measures such as running time are always improved. Possible explanations for this apparent discrepancy are that training induces a higher mechanical efficiency and that the measurement of $\dot{V}o_{2max}$ in children does not reflect well the performance of children in endurance activities (Bar-Or 1989).

Strength training

Fewer studies have been performed on the effect of strength training than on aerobic training in children. While some authors have reported only a small degree of trainability before puberty (Vrijens 1978), more recent studies (Weltman 1984) demonstrated a significant strength-increase in boys aged 6–11 years following a period of strength training. The discrepancy can be explained by the way the strength effects were evaluated. Vrijens used non-specific testing by training with dynamic exercises and testing the effects isometrically; in contrast, Weltman trained and tested the effects isokinetically. The results of Weltman and of others (Pfeiffer & Francis 1986; Sewall & Micheli 1986) confirm that

increases in muscle strength are possible before puberty in boys and girls and are not related to maturity levels. Such increases are reached without the risk of musculoskeletal injuries. It has been recommended that strength training be used for prepubescent children only: (a) when it is indicated for well-defined athletic or rehabilitation purposes (Bar-Or 1989); (b) under the supervision of qualified instructors; and (c) using loads that can be repeated more than 7–10 times.

Anaerobic muscle performances, such as the Margaria stair-running test (Margaria *et al.* 1966) and the Wingate 30-s cycle test (Bar-Or 1987), can also be improved during childhood and adolescence regardless of maturation level.

Statistical methods for longitudinal data analyses

In longitudinal studies, the repeated observations of one individual are not independent of each other; they concern the same person. Therefore, statistical methods, which assume independent observations, such as linear and logistic regression analysis, cannot directly be used in longitudinal analyses (Twisk 2003; Twisk & Kemper 2004). For data analysis in longitudinal studies, special statistical methods have been developed, which take into account that the repeated observations of each individual (Zeger & Liang 1992). The most traditional methods for analysing longitudinal data are the paired *t*-test and (M)ANOVA for repeated measurements. With these methods it is possible to investigate changes in continuous outcome variables over time and to compare the development of a continuous outcome variable over time between different groups (Crowder & Hand 1990). In longitudinal research, however, there are many other questions to be answered (e.g., what is the relationship between the development of a continuous outcome variable and the development of several other variables?) and sometimes the longitudinal development of dichotomous (high or low risk for a disease) or categorical (stage of biologic maturation) outcome variables are of interest. In such more complicated situations, the paired *t*-test or (M)ANOVA for repeated measurements cannot be used.

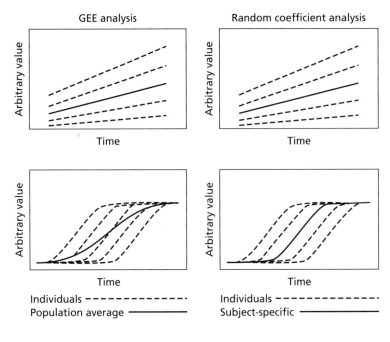

Fig. 34.8 Differences between generalized estimating equations (GEE) analysis (upper part) and random coefficient analysis (lower part) for a continuous and dichotomous outcome variable. From Twisk and Kemper (2004).

There are now other (more sophisticated) methods available that are suitable to answer these questions. Two of them frequently used are: generalized estimating equations (GEE) (Zeger & Liang 1986) and random coefficient analysis (Goldstein 1995). Both methods are suitable for the analysis of the longitudinal relationship between a continuous outcome variable and several time-dependent and time-independent covariates. Furthermore, these methods are suitable for the longitudinal analysis of a dichotomous (or categorial) outcome variable in relation to the development of other variables.

In Fig. 34.8 the difference between GEE analysis and random coefficient analysis is given for a continuous (upper part) and a dichotomous (lower part) outcome variable. For the analysis with a continuous outcome variable (i.e., linear regression analysis), both GEE and the random effect approach lead to the same results. For a dichotomous variable (i.e., logistic longitudinal regression analysis) both approaches lead to different results. From Fig. 34.8 it can be seen that the regression coefficients calculated with a logistic GEE analysis will always be lower than the coefficients calculated with a comparable random coefficient analysis.

The two sophisticated methods can also be used to analyze the stability (or tracking) of different variables over time, such as a physical activity pattern (Twisk *et al.* 1994). There is no widely accepted definition of tracking, but the following concepts are involved:

1 Relationship (correlation) between early measurements and measurements later in life, or the maintenance of a relative position within distribution of values in the observed population over time; and
2 Predictability of future values by early measurements.

The most traditional way of analyzing tracking of a continuous outcome variable is estimating the correlation coefficient between baseline and follow-up measurements. This is suitable for a longitudinal study with two measurements, but the more repeated measurements available, the more complicated it will be to use correlation coefficients to evaluate tracking over time. An alternative way is to use one of the sophisticated methods to analyze the relationship between the initial value of interest (e.g., a sport performance) and the total development of that variable using all the available data of that variable over time using GEE and estimating tracking coefficients, running from 0 (indicating no stability at all) to 1 (perfect stability).

Challenges for future research

Longitudinal research covering the whole period of puberty is relatively scarce. Therefore, in early or late maturing children it is not always possible to detect PHV, which is a yardstick of pubertal maturation. Comparison of the different longitudinal studies stresses the need for further standardization in sampling procedures, frequency of measurements, and measurement methods.

Most of the growth and training studies have used boys as subjects. Longitudinal growth and training studies have to be designed in which both sexes are included. Much knowledge is still lacking about the trainability of children.

To achieve a better understanding of trainability during growth and development the following research questions need to be resolved:

1 What are the best guidelines for adequate training stimuli in boys and girls?

2 What is the impact of biologic age on the training effects and is there a biologic age where trainability is minimal or maximal?

3 To what extent do aerobic power, anaerobic power, and strength track into adulthood?

4 Can adequate training started in early childhood lead to higher performance levels in adulthood?

5 Can intensive training during childhood and adolescence have detrimental effects on health in youth and/or in adulthood?

References

American College of Sports Medicine (1990) The recommended quantity and quality of exercise for developing and maintaining cardiorespiratory fitness and muscular fitness in healthy adults. *Medicine and Science in Sports and Exercise* **22**, 265–274.

Andersen, L.B. & Haraldsdottier, J. (1993) Tracking of cardiovascular disease risk factors including maximal oxygen uptake and physical activity from late teenage to adulthood: An 8-year follow-up study. *Journal of Internal Medicine* **234**, 309–315.

Bailey, D.A. (1968) *Saskatchewan Growth and Development Study*. Report of the College of Physical Education. University of Saskatchewan, Canada.

Baldwin, B.T. (1921) *The Physical Growth of Children from Birth to Maturity*. University of Iowa Studies in Child Welfare, Vol. 1. no. 1. University of Iowa, IO.

Barnekow-Bergkvist, M., Hedberg, G., Janlert, U. & Jansson, E. (2001) Adolescent determinants of cardiovascular risk factors in adult men and women. *Scandinavian Journal of Public Health* **29**, 208–217.

Bar-Or, O. (1987) The Wingate anaerobic test. An update on methodology, reliability an validity. *Sports Medicine* **4**, 381–394.

Bar-Or, O. (1989) Trainability of the prepubescent child. *Physician and Sports Medicine* **17**, 65–82.

Bayley, N. (1940) *Studies in the Development of Young Children*. University of California Press, Berkeley, CA.

Bell, R.Q. (1954) An experimental test of the accelerated longitudinal approach. *Child Development* **25**, 281–286.

Beunen, G. & Malina, B. (1988) Growth and physical performance relative to the timing of the adolescent growth sport. *Exercise and Sport Sciences Reviews* **16**, 503–541.

Carron, A.V. & Bailey, D.A. (1940) Strength development in boys from 10 through 16 years. *Monographs of the Society for Research in Child Development* **39** (Serial No. 157), 4.

Clarke, H.H. (1971) *Physical and Motor Tests in the Medford Boys' Growth Study*. Prentice Hall, Englewood Cliffs, NJ.

Cohen, P. & Cohen, J. (1996) The children in the community study. In: (Mahwah, N.J., ed.) *Life Values and Adolescent Mental Health*. Lawrence Erlbaum, New York: 203–210.

Crowder, M.J. & Hand, D.J. (1990) *Analysis of Repeated Measures*. Chapman & Hall, London.

Cunningham, D.A., Paterson, D.H. & Blimkie, C.J.R. (1984) The development of the cardiorespiratory system with growth and physical activity. In: *Advances in Pediatric Sport Sciences* (Boileau, R.A., ed.) Human Kinetics, Champaign, IL: 85–116.

Cunningham, D.A., Stapleton, J.J., MacDonald, I.C. & Paterson, D.H. (1981) Daily expenditure of young boys as related to maximal aerobic power. *Canadian Journal of Applied Sport Science* **6**, 207–211.

Cunningham, D.A., van Waterschoot, B.M., Paterson, D.H., Lefcoe, M. & Sangal S.P. (1977) Reliability and reproducibility of maximal oxygen uptake measurement in children. *Medicine and Science in Sports and Exercise* **9**, 104–108.

Espenschade, A. (1947) Development of motor coordination in boys and girls. *Research Quarterly* **18**, 13–40.

Falkner, F. (1954) Measurement of somatic growth and development in children. *Courrier* **4**, 169–181.

Falkner, F., ed. (1980) *Twenty-five Years of Internationally Coordinated Research: Longitudinal Studies in Growth and Development*. International Children's Centre, Courrier, Montreux, Switzerland.

Falkner, F. & Tanner, J.M., eds. (1978) *Human Growth*, Vol. 2. *Postnatal Growth*. Plenum Press, New York.

Froberg, K., Andersen, B. & Lammert, O. (1991) Maximal oxygen intake and respiratory functions during puberty in boy groups of different physical activity. In: *Children and Exercise, Pediatric Work Physiology*, Vol. XV (Frenkl, R. & Szmodis, L., eds.) NEVI, Budapest: 265–280.

Gallagher, A.M., Savage, J.M., Murray, L.J., *et al.* (2002) A longitudinal study through adolescence into adulthood: The Young Hearts Project, Northern Ireland. *Public Health* **11**, 332–340.

Goldstein, H. (1995) *Multilevel statistical models*, 2nd edn. Edward Arnold, London.

Graffar, M. & Courbier, J. (1966) Contribution a l'etude de l'influence des conditions socioeconomiques sur la croissance et le developpement [Contribution to the study of the effects of socioeconomic status on growth and development]. *Courrier* **16**, 1–25.

Hebbelinck, M., Blommaert, M., Borms, J., Duquet, W., Vajda, A. & van der Meer, J. (1980) A multidisciplinary longitudinal growth study: introduction of the project 'LLEGS'. In: *Kinanthropometry II. International Series of Sport Sciences*, Vol. 9 (Ostyn, M., Beunen, G. & Simons, J., eds.) University Park Press, Baltimore: 317–325.

Jequier, J., Lavallee, H., Rajic, M., Beaucage, C., Shephard, R.J. & Labarre, R. (1977) *The Longitudinal Examination of Growth and Development: History and Protocol of the Trois Rivieres Regional Study* in *Lavallee, Shephard, Frontiers of Activity and Child Health*. Pelican, Ottawa: 49–54.

Jones, H.E. (1949) *Motor Performance and Growth. A Developmental Study of Static Dynamometric Strength*. University of California Press, Berkeley, CA.

Karlberg, P., Taranger, J., Engstrom, L., *et al.* (1976) The somatic development of children in a Swedish urban community: a prospective longitudinal study. I. Physical growth from birth to 16 years and longitudinal outcome of the study during the same period. *Acta Paediatrica Scandinavica* **258** (Supplement), 7–76.

Katzmarzyk, P.T., Perusse, L., Malina, R.M., Bergeron, J. & Bouchard, C. (2001) Stability of indicators of the metabolic syndrome from childhood and adolescence to young adulthood. The Quebec Family Study. *Journal of Clinical Epidemiology* **54**, 190–195.

Kemper, H.C.G., ed. (1985) Growth, health and fitness of teenagers: longitudinal research in international perspective. *Medicine and Sport Science*, Vol. 20. Karger, Basel.

Kemper, H.C.G. (1986) Longitudinal studies on the development of health and fitness and the interaction with physical activity of teenagers. *Pediatrician* **13**, 52–59.

Kemper, H.C.G. (1988) Longitudinal studies in the development of physical fitness in teenagers. In: *Young Athletes, Biological, Psychological and Educational Perspectives* (Malina, R.M., ed.) Human Kinetics, Champaign, IL: 3–17.

Kemper, H.C.G., ed. (1995) The Amsterdam Growth Study, a longitudinal analysis of health, fitness, and lifestyle. *HK Sport Science Monograph Series*, Vol. 6. Human Kinetics, Champaign, IL.

Kemper, H.C.G., ed. (2004) Amsterdam Growth and Health Longitudinal Study, a 23-year follow-up from teenager to adult about lifestyle and health. *Medicine and Sport Science*, Vol. 47. Karger, Basel.

Kemper, H.C.G. & Van't Hoff, M.A. (1978) Design of a multiple longitudinal study of growth and health in teenagers. *European Journal of Pediatrics* **129**, 147–155.

Kemper, H.C.G., Verschuur, R., Ras, J.G.A., Snel, J., Splinter, P.G. & Tavecchio, L.W.C. (1976) Effect of 5 versus 3 lessons a week of physical education upon the physical development of 12 and 11 year old schoolboys. *Journal of Sports Medicine and Physical Fitness* **16**, 319–326.

Kobayashi, K., Kitamure, K., Miura, M., *et al.* (1978) Aerobic power as related to body growth and training in Japanese boys: a longitudinal study. *Journal of Applied Physiology* **44**, 666–672.

Koppes, L.L.J. (2004) Review of AGAHLS and other observational longitudinal studies on lifestyle and health from adolescence into adulthood. In: *Medicine and Sport Science*, Vol. 47 (Kemper, H.C.G., ed.) Basel, Karger: 21–29.

Kowalski, C.J. & Prahl-Andersen, B. (1979) General considerations in the design of studies of growth and development. In: *A Mixed Longitudinal Interdisciplinary Study of Growth and Development* (Kowalski, C.J., Prahl-Andersen, B. & Heyendael, P., eds.) Academic Press, New York: 3–13.

Lange Andersen, K., Seliger, V., Rutenfranz, J. & Berndt, L. (1974a) Physical perfonnance capacity of children in Norway: II. Heart rate and oxygen pulse in submaximal and maximal exercises. Population parameters in a rural community. *European Journal of Applied Physiology* **33**, 197–206.

Lange Andersen, K., Seliger, V., Rutenfranz, J. & Messel, S. (1974b) Physical performance capacity of children in Norway: III. Respiratory response to graded exercise loadings. Population parameters in a rural community. *European Journal of Applied Physiology* **33**, 265–276.

Lange Andersen, K., Seliger, V., Rutenfranz, J. & Mocellin, R. (1974c) Physical performance capacity of children in Norway: I. Population parameters in a rural inland community with regard to maximal aerobic power. *European Journal of Applied Physiology* **33**, 177–195.

Lange Andersen, K., Seliger, V., Rutenfranz, J. & Skrobak Kacyznski, J. (1976) Physical performance capacity of children in Norway: IV. The rate of growth in maximal aerobic power and the influence of improved physical education of children in a rural community. Population parameters in a rural community. *European Journal of Applied Physiology* **35**, 49–58.

Largo, R.H., Gasser, T., Prader, A., Stuetzle, W. & Humber, P.J. (1978) Analysis of the adolescent growth spurt, using smoothing spline functions. *Annals of Human Biology* 421–434.

Lauer, R.M., Lee, J. & Clarke, W.R. (1988) Factors affecting the relationship between childhood and adult cholesterol levels: The Muscatine Study. *American Journal of Epidemiology* **124**, 195–206.

Lefevre, J., Philippaerts, R., Delvaux, K., *et al.* (2002) Relation between cardiovascular risk factors at adult age, and physical activity during youth and and adulthood: The Leuven Longitudinal Study on Lifestyle, Fitness and Health. *International Journal of Sports Medicine* **23** (Supplement 1): S32–S38.

McCloy, C.H. (1936) *Appraising Physical Status. The Selection of Measurements.* University of Iowa Studies in Child Welfare, Vol. XII, No. 2. University of Iowa, IO.

Margaria, R., Aghemo, P. & Rovelli, E. (1966) Measurement of muscular power (anaerobic) in man. *Journal of Applied Physiology* **21**, 1662–1663.

Mednick, J.A. & Baert, A.E., eds. (1981) *Prospective Longitudinal Research: An Empirical Basis for the Primary Prevention of Psychosocial Disorders*. Oxford University Press, Oxford.

Meredith, H.V. (1935) *The Rhythm of Physical Growth*. University of Iowa Studies in Child Welfare, Vol. XI, No. 3. University of Iowa, IO.

Mirwald, R.L. (1980) Saskatchewan growth and development study. In: *Kinanthropometry II. International Series of Sports Science*, Vol. 9 (Ostyn, M., Beunen, G. & Simons, J., eds.) University Park Press, Baltimore: 289–305.

Mirwald, R.L. & Bailey, D.A. (1985) *Longitudinal Analyses of Maximal Aerobic Power in Boys and Girls by Chronological Age, Maturity and Physical Activity.* University of Saskatchewan, Saskatoon.

Moore, T., Hindley, G.B. & Falkner, F. (1954) A longitudinal research in child development and some of its problems. *British Medical Journal* **ii**, 1132–1137.

Ostyn, M., Simons, J., Beunen, G., Renson, R. & van Gerven, D. (1980) *Somatic and Motor Development of Belgian Secondary Schoolboys: Norms and Standards*. University Press, Leuven.

Parizkova, J. (1974) Particularities of lean body mass and fat development in growing boys as related to their motor activity. *Acta Paediatrica Belgica* **28** (Supplement), 233–243.

Pate, R.R. & Ward, O.S. (1990) Endurance exercise trainability in children and youth. In: *Advances in Sports Medicine and Fitness*, Vol. 3 (Grano, W.A., Lombardo, J.A., Sharkey, B.J. & Stone, J.A., eds.) Year Book Medical Publishers, Chicago: 37–55.

Pfeiffer, R. & Francis, R.S. (1986) Effects of strength training on muscle development in prepubescent, pubescent and postpubescent males. *Physician and Sports Medicine* **14**, 137–143.

Placheta, Z. (1980) *Youth and Physical Activity*. University of Purkyne, Bmo, CSSR.

Prahl-Andersen, B., Kowalski, C.J. & Heydendael, P. (1979) *A Mixed Longitudinal Interdisciplinary Study of Growth and Development*. Academic Press, New York.

Rao, M.N. & Rao, C.R. (1966) Linked cross-sectional study for determining norms and growth rates: a pilot survey of Indian school-going boys. *Saykgya* **68**, 237–258.

Rowland, T.W. (1985) Aerobic response to endurance training in prepubescent children: a critical analysis. *Medicine and Science in Sports and Exercise* **17**, 493–497.

Roy-Pernot, M.P., Sempé, M. & Filliozat, A.M. (1976) *Rapport d'Activité Terminal de l'Equipe Française. Compte Rendu de la 13 Reunion des Equipes Chargees des Etudes sur la Croissance et le Developpement de l'Enfant Normal* [Final report of the French group. Proceedings of the 13th conference of the groups involved with the growth and development of normal children.] Centre International de l'Enfance, Paris.

Sady, S.P. (1986) Cardiorespiratory exercise training in children. *Clinical and Sports Medicine* **5**, 493–514.

Schaie, K.W. (1965) A general model for the study of development problems. *Psychological Bulletin* **64**, 92–107.

Sewall, L. & Micheli, L.J. (1984) Strength training for children. *Journal of Pediatric Orthopedics* **6**, 143–146.

Shephard, K. (1982) *Physical Activity and Growth*. Medical Publishers, Chicago.

Shephard, R.J., Lavallee, H., Jequier, J., Rajic, M. & Labarre, R. (1980) Additional physical education in the primary school. A preliminary analysis of the Trois Rivieres regional experiment. In: *Kinanthropometry II International Series of Sports Science*, Vol. 9 (Ostyn, M., Beunen, G. & Simons, G., eds.) University Park Press, Baltimore: 306–316.

Silva, P.A. & Stanton, W.R. (1996) *The Dunedin Multidisciplinary Health and Development Study*. Oxford University Press, Auckland, New Zealand/London.

Simons, J., Beunen, G.P., Renson Claessen, A.L.M., van Reusel, B. & Lefevre, J.A.V. (1990) Growth and fitness of Flemish girls. The Leuven Growth Study HKP. In: *Sport Science Monograph Series*, Vol. 3. Human Kinetics, Champaign, IL.

Sprynarova, S. (1974) Longitudinal study of the influence of different activity on functional capacity or boys from 11–18 years. *Acta Paediatrica Belgica* **29** (Supplement), 204–213.

Tammelin, T., Nayha, S., Hills, A.P. & Jarvelin, M.R. (2003) Adolescent participation in sports and adult physical activity. *American Journal of Preventive Medicine* **24**, 22–28.

Tanner, J.M. (1962) *Growth at Adolescence*. Blackwell Scientific Publications, Oxford.

Tanner, J.M. (1981) *A History of the Study of Human Growth*. Cambridge University Press, London.

Tanner, J.M., Whitehouse, R.H., Marubini, E. & Rescle, L. (1976) The adolescent growth spurt of boys and girls of the Harpenden Growth Study. *Annals of Human Biology* **3**, 109–126.

Twisk, J.W.R. (2003) *Applied Longitudinal Data Analysis for Epidemiology: A Practical Guide*. Cambridge University Press, Cambridge.

Twisk, J.W.R. & Kemper, H.C.G. (2004) Longitudinal data analysis in the Amsterdam Growth and Health Longitudinal Study. *Medicine and Sport Science*, Vol. 47 (Kemper, H.C.G., ed.) Karger, Basel: 30–43.

Twisk, J.W.R., Kemper, H.C.G. & Mellenbergh, G.J. (1994) The mathematical and analytical aspects of tracking. *Epidemiological Reviews* **16**, 165–183.

Vaccaro, P. & Mahon, A. (1987) Cardiorespiratory response to endurance training in children. *Sports Medicine* **4**, 352–356.

Valimaki, M.J., Karkainen, M., Lamberg-Allardt, C., *et al.* (1994) Exercise, smoking, and calcium intake during adolescence and early adulthood as determinants of peak bone mass. Cardiovascular risk in young Finns study group. *British Medical Journal* **309**, 230–235.

Veling, S.H.S. & Van't Hof, M.A. (1980) Data quality control methods in longitudinal studies. In: *Kinanthropometry II. International Series of Sports Science*, Vol. 9 (Ostyn, M., Beunen, G. & Simons, J., eds.) University Park Press, Baltimore: 436–442.

Vrijens, J. (1978) Muscle strength development in the pre- and post pubescent ages. *Medicine and Sport* **11**, 152–158.

Weber, G., Kartodihardjo, W. & Klissouras, V. (1976) Growth and physical training with reference to heredity. *Journal of Applied Physiology* **40**, 211–215.

Weltman, A. (1984) Weight training in prepubertal children. Physiologic benefit and potential damage. In: *Advances in Pediatric Sports Sciences*, Vol. 3 (Bar-Or, O., ed.) Human Kinetics, Champaign, IL: 101–131.

Zeger, S.L. & Liang, K.-Y. (1986) Longitudinal data analysis for discrete and continuous outcomes. *Biometrics* **42**, 121–130.

Zeger, S.L. & Liang, K.-Y. (1992) An overview of methods, for the analysis of longitudinal data. *Statistics in Medicine* **11**, 1825–1839.

Index